Cold: limit edema, + bleeding

Tell me: is open ended invite pt ... on their concern

Paraphrasing = restates the content of pt message in similar words

Fundamentals **Success**

A Course Review Applying Critical Thinking to Test Taking

SECOND EDITION

Hypoxia = early sign ↑ heart rate

Chronic pain = may or may not have identifiable cause

Acute + chronic pain ⇓ immune system

Glucose 80 - 120 mg/dl

Older pt ↓ capacity to sense the pain + pressure

explain procedure help w/ anxiety

Ventrogluteal use the gluteus medius + minimus muscles in the hips

dorsogluteal site = use the gluteus maximus muscles in the buttock

Rectal supp inserted 4 inches + lubricated (Adult)

Etiology = is a term used to identify the factor/causes that is relate to

Healing 2a intention: = wet to damp allow epidermal cell to migrate more rapidly across the wound surface.

Anesthesia - reduced level consciousness. The pharyngeal laryngeal. gag reflexes. inability to cough or swallow can result in aspiration of oral secretion

Fundamentals Success

A Course Review Applying Critical Thinking to Test Taking

SECOND EDITION

Patricia M. Nugent, RN, MA, MS, EdD
Professor Emeritus
Nassau Community College
Garden City, New York
Private Practice – President of Nugent Books, Inc.

Barbara A. Vitale, RN, MA
Professor Emeritus
Adjunct Professor
Nassau Community College
Garden City, New York
Private Practice – Professional Resources for Nursing

F. A. DAVIS COMPANY • Philadelphia

F. A. Davis Company
1915 Arch Street
Philadelphia, PA 19103
www.fadavis.com

Printed in the United States of America

Last digit indicates print number: 10 9 8 7 6 5 4

Publisher, Nursing: Robert G. Martone
Director of Content Development: Darlene D. Pedersen
Project Editor: Padraic J. Maroney
Design and Illustrations Manager: Carolyn O'Brien

As new scientific information becomes available through basic and clinical research, recommended treatments and drug therapies undergo changes. The author(s) and publisher have done everything possible to make this book accurate, up to date, and in accord with accepted standards at the time of publication. The author(s), editors, and publisher are not responsible for errors or omissions or for consequences from application of the book, and make no warranty, expressed or implied, in regard to the contents of the book. Any practice described in this book should be applied by the reader in accordance with professional standards of care used in regard to the unique circumstances that may apply in each situation. The reader is advised always to check product information (package inserts) for changes and new information regarding dose and contraindications before administering any drug. Caution is especially urged when using new or infrequently ordered drugs.

ISBN 13: 978-0-8036-1921-0
ISBN 10: 0-8036-1921-9

Dedicated to

Joseph Vitale
and
Neil Nugent

For their love and support,
particularly during the production of this book

Acknowledgments

Many people at F. A. Davis were essential to the production of this book. We especially want to thank Bob Martone, Publisher for Nursing, whose skills of listening, focusing, and prodding were instrumental to the publication of this edition. He shared our enthusiasm for this project throughout the publishing process without losing his sense of humor, and we value his knowledge and friendship. We gratefully acknowledge Padraic Maroney, Project Editor, for his editorial expertise and keeping the project on task. Thanks also go to the entire F.A. Davis staff, especially to Louise Bierig, Developmental Editior; Lisa Thompson, Production Project Editor; and Bob Butler, Production Manager; all who competently transformed our manuscript into a book.

Special recognition goes to all the nursing students and faculty who participated in field-testing sessions and focus groups for their commitment to excellence and generosity in sharing their time, energy, and intellects. Finally, but most importantly, we would like to thank our husbands, Neil and Joseph, for their love, senses of humor, enthusiasm for life, and their attempts to keep our compulsive natures under control. Their support was essential to the completion of this book and they are loved and appreciated by us.

Reviewers

Gloria Coschigano, APRN-BC, MS
Assistant Professor
Westchester Community College
Valhalla, New York

Amy Elinskas, MS, RN
Nursing Instructor
St. Elizabeth College of Nursing
Utica, New York

Mindy Heutinick, MSN, RN, ANP-C
Instructor
William Jewell College
Liberty, Missouri

Barbara Maxwell, RN, MSN, MS
Associate Professor
State University of New York at Ulster
Stone Ridge, New York

A Message to Nursing Instructors

Following the popularity of the first edition of *Fundamentals Success: A Course Review Applying Critical Thinking to Test Taking*, we again conducted focus groups with nursing students and nursing faculty to determine if the book continued to meet their needs or if additional needs emerged.

- Nursing faculty still are concerned about assisting students with developing intellectual reasoning skills and supporting students' personal qualities that promote effective inquiry. Faculty continued to ask, "HOW CAN WE HELP OUR STUDENTS TO THINK CRITICALLY?"
- Although beginning nursing students alluded to the concerns identified by faculty, their greatest concern was the need for more fundamentals-of-nursing questions with which to practice test taking. Students still stated, "WE WANT MORE FUNDAMENTALS OF NURSING QUESTIONS!"
- Even though Alternate Item Formats have appeared on NCLEX examinations since the spring of 2003, both students and faculty continued to say, "WE WANT ADDITIONAL EXAMPLES OF ALTERNATE ITEM FORMATS!"
- In recent focus groups, students shared their concerns about preparing for and taking an examination at the end of a fundamentals of nursing course that addresses multiple fundamental concepts, principles, and theory. Students stated, "WE WANT TO PRACTICE TAKING A FUNDAMENTALS FINAL EXAMINATION!"
- With the advent of NCLEX examinations being administered on a computer, most students indicated that they now take their nursing examination on a computer. Students said, "WE WANT TO PRACTICE TEST TAKING USING A COMPUTER!"

This book addresses these felt needs.

"HOW CAN WE HELP STUDENTS TO THINK CRITICALLY?"

The entire premise of this book is based on the beliefs that:

- People use critical thinking all the time in their daily lives
- Nurses continue to use critical thinking in their professional lives
- People can enhance their critical-thinking skills
- Students can use critical-thinking skills when taking a nursing examination

Chapter 1, Fundamentals of Critical Thinking Related to Test Taking: The RACE Model, discusses the topic of critical thinking in relation to everyday living and introduces the Helix of Critical Thinking. **The Helix of Critical Thinking** schematically represents the cognitive and personal competencies involved in critical thinking. This model is then discussed relative to the cognitive processes used in nursing (the nursing process, problem solving, decision-making, diagnostic reasoning, and the scientific method). Maximizing your critical thinking abilities is presented in the context of personal competencies that foster critical thinking. Information related to being positive, reflective, inquisitive, and creative are explored, and strategies to overcome barriers to the development of these competencies are interwoven throughout the discussion. The application of critical thinking applied to test taking begins with a brief overview of educational domains, components of a multiple-choice test question, and the cognitive levels of nursing questions. Finally, the main component of this textbook is presented – The RACE Model. The **RACE Model** is a formula for using critical thinking when answering multiple-choice questions on a nursing examination. The theoretical framework of the RACE Model is explained and then applied to three sets of sample test items that span the cognitive domains of knowledge, comprehension, application, and analysis. This illustrates the increasing complexity of critical thinking required as the difficulty of questions increase in relation to the same nursing content.

"WE WANT MORE FUNDAMENTALS OF NURSING QUESTIONS!"

This book contains 1227 questions, which reflect a depth and breadth that comprehensively address the content commonly included in a fundamentals of nursing curriculum. They have been clustered by chapter into the related domains of: Chapter 2—Nursing Within the Context of Contemporary Health Care; Chapter 3—Psychosociocultural Nursing Care; Chapter 4—Essential Components of Nursing Care; and Chapter 5—Basic Human Needs and Related Nursing Care.

"WE WANT ADDITIONAL EXAMPLES OF ALTERNATE ITEM FORMATS!"

Chapter 6, Alternate Item Formats, presents information regarding the NCLEX item formats introduced in April 2003 by the National Council of State Boards of Nursing. Formats include: multiple-response items, fill-in-the-blank items, hot-spot items, chart/exhibit items, ordered-response (drag and drop) items, and standard multiple-choice questions that require the student to refer to a graphic image, picture, or chart/table to answer the question. In this edition, 78 additional Alternate Item Formats were added for a total of 103 items. In addition, numerous examples of the newly developed Chart/Exhibit Items by NCLEX have been included.

"WE WANT TO PRACTICE TAKING A FUNDAMENTALS FINAL EXAMINATION!"

To address this need, a 100-item Comprehensive Final Book Exam is presented in the text (Chapter 7). This provides students with an opportunity to integrate fundamental content learned in subunits of study into one examination.

"WE WANT TO PRACTICE TEST TAKING USING A COMPUTER!"

In this edition a CD-ROM, containing two, 75-item Comprehensive Course Exit Exams, has been included. This meets the need voiced by students to practice test taking on a computer as well as taking a comprehensive examination that integrates subunits of fundamentals of nursing content.

Questions for inclusion were selected considering content validity and the results of an elaborate field-testing process that included statistical item analyses and focus groups with student nurses and nursing faculty to ensure quality questions. Every question in the book has rationales for the correct and incorrect answers. These questions can be used to apply the **RACE Model** to answer the questions, practice test taking, and study or review nursing content. Each section of questions in Chapters 2 through 5 is preceded by a list of keywords commonly associated with the content included in that area. Knowing the definition of these words and understanding information, concepts, and principles associated with these words will build a theoretical base for answering the questions in the content area. In addition, a Glossary of more than 250 English words commonly encountered on nursing examinations is included in the back of the book for consideration by the reader. Familiarity with these words will refocus the challenge of a nursing examination away from the form of the test and back to the nursing content of the test.

SUMMARY

When we wrote the first edition, our goals were to produce more quality fundamentals of nursing questions and to design a model to assist nursing students to use critical-thinking strategies when taking a nursing test. Based on the feedback we received from students and faculty, we achieved these goals. In this edition, we addressed the emerging needs of students and faculty by including:

- 103 Alternate Item Formats (particularly Chart/Exhibit Format Items)
- A 100-item Comprehensive Final Book Exam
- A CD-ROM with two 75 Comprehensive Course Exit Exams

Patricia M. Nugent
Barbara A. Vitale

A Message to Nursing Students

Following the resounding success of the first edition of *Fundamentals Success: A Course Review Applying Critical Thinking to Test Taking*, we continue to hear the same comment from students, "MORE QUESTIONS, WE WANT MORE QUESTIONS!" We continue to hear from nursing faculty, "HOW CAN WE HELP OUR STUDENTS TO THINK CRITICALLY?" Even though Alternate Item Formats have appeared on NCLEX examinations since the spring of 2003, both students and faculty continue to say, "WE WANT ADDITIONAL EXAMPLES OF ALTERNATE ITEM FORMATS." In addition, emerging requests from students include, "WE WANT TO PRACTICE TAKING A FUNDAMENTALS FINAL EXAMINATION!" and "WE WANT TO PRACTICE TEST TAKING USING A COMPUTER!"

This book addresses these felt needs.

If you are similar to the average nursing student, you read assigned chapters in your textbook and articles in nursing journals, review your classroom notes, complete computer instruction programs related to nursing content, practice nursing skills in a simulated laboratory, and apply in the clinical area what you have learned. All of these activities are excellent ways for you to expand and strengthen your theoretical base and become a safe practitioner of nursing. However, they may not be enough for you to be successful when taking a nursing examination. You need to practice test taking as early as possible in your program of study and with questions appropriate for your level of nursing education. In addition, you must be aware of, strengthen, and expand your cognitive competencies (intellectual reasoning skills) and personal competencies (individual attitudes or qualities) reflected in **The Helix of Critical Thinking**, and then utilize these components of critical thinking when answering nursing questions.

In this book, we discuss personal competencies and present the **RACE Model** to provide you with a blueprint for applying critical thinking to answering multiple-choice questions in nursing. **The components of the RACE Model are:**

R — **R**ecognize what information is in the stem.
A — **A**sk, What is the question asking?
C — **C**ritically analyze the options in relation to the question asked in the stem.
E — **E**liminate as many options as possible.

The theoretical framework of the RACE Model is explained and then applied to three sets of sample test questions that span the cognitive domains of knowledge, comprehension, application, and analysis. This illustrates for you the increasing complexity of critical thinking required as the difficulty of questions increases in relation to the same nursing content. In addition, the book contains 1227 multiple-choice questions organized into 24 content areas commonly included in a fundamentals of nursing curriculum. When answering these questions you can use critical thinking by applying the RACE model and practice test taking. When examining the rationales for the correct and incorrect answers you can review fundamentals of nursing content and identify what you still need to study.

For your personal development, each of the fundamentals of nursing content areas is preceded by a list of keywords, nursing/medical terminology, concepts, principles, or information associated with the topics presented. In addition, a Glossary of 250 English words commonly found in nursing multiple-choice questions is included at the end of the textbook. Familiarity with these words will refocus the challenge of a nursing examination away from defining the words in a test question and back to the theoretical content being evaluated in the test question.

WHY YOU SHOULD READ THIS TEXTBOOK: FEATURES AND BENEFITS

FEATURE	BENEFITS
103 questions with formats other than multiple-choice.	These questions will: Expose you to the alternate types of question formats that appear on NCLEX examinations. Allow you to practice nursing questions that incorporate multiple-response items, fill-in-the-blank items, hot-spot items, chart/exhibit items, ordered-response (drag and drop) items, and questions that use graphic illustrations, tables/charts, or pictures. Reduce anxiety concerning alternate item formats you will be confronted with on NCLEX.
Key word lists at the beginning of each content chapter that include vocabulary, concepts, nursing/medical terminology, principles, and information.	These words encourage you to focus on the critical components of a topic of study. Understanding these critical components expands your theoretical base and provides a strong foundation for more advanced concepts.
Glossary that identifies and defines ordinary English words that appear frequently in nursing examinations.	Familiarity with these words reduces the challenge of a test question because you can center your attention on the theoretical content presented in the question.
A discussion of maximizing your critical-thinking abilities including the attitudes and qualities of successful critical thinkers and strategies to overcome barriers to critical thinking.	This discussion provides a basis for a self-assessment in relation to these qualities and introduces strategies that you can use to overcome barriers to your critical thinking. This discussion should motivate you to maintain a positive mental attitude and be reflective, inquisitive, and creative when thinking.
The RACE Model is introduced and applied to a variety of sample questions.	These concrete examples model the critical-thinking processes involved when answering increasingly complex multiple-choice questions in nursing. This facilitates the imitation of the critical-thinking activities used in the examples when you are confronted with answering a multiple-choice question in nursing. Ultimately, when you can critically analyze a question and answer it correctly, you will feel empowered and your test anxiety will decrease.
1227 quality fundamentals of nursing questions.	These questions allow you to practice test taking and apply the use of critical thinking via the use of the RACE model. This should increase your critical-thinking skills, promote your self-confidence, build your stamina when taking tests, and reduce test anxiety.
Rationales for the correct and incorrect answers for every question.	Reviewing the rationales for every question will: Reinforce what you know—This increases trust in your ability and promotes a sense of security. Teach you new information—This increases your knowledge and builds self-confidence. Identify what you still need to learn—This focuses and prioritizes your study activities so that the return on your effort is maximized.
100-item Comprehensive Course Exit Exam	This provides you with an opportunity to integrate fundamental content learned in subunits of study into one examination.
Two 75-item Comprehensive Course Exit Exams on a CD-ROM.	This provides you with an opportunity to practice test taking on a computer as well as taking a comprehensive examination that integrates subunits of fundamentals of nursing content.

To increase your knowledge of fundamentals of nursing theory and experience success on nursing examinations, it is important for you to use this book—***Fundamentals Success: A Course Review Applying Critical Thinking to Test Taking, Second Edition.*** Although this book is valuable for all nursing students regardless of their level of nursing education, it is essential for beginning nursing students. The related knowledge, attitudes, and skills that you develop early in your fundamental nursing courses influence your present and future educational performance. A house will stand and survive only when it is built on a strong foundation. The same concept can be applied to your nursing education. The components of a strong foundation in nursing are a comprehensive understanding of the fundamentals of nursing theory, well-developed critical-thinking abilities, and an inventory of strategies for successful test taking.

Another textbook that you may find helpful to maximize your success when preparing for and taking examinations in nursing is ***Test Success: Test-Taking Techniques for Beginning Nursing Students*** (Nugent & Vitale, F. A. Davis Company). This book focuses on empowerment, critical thinking, study techniques, the multiple-choice question, the nursing process, test-taking techniques, testing formats other than multiple-choice questions (including alternate item formats on NCLEX examinations), and computer applications in education and evaluation. It also contains 835 fundamentals of nursing questions with test-taking techniques and rationales for correct and incorrect answers for each question. It contains a 100-item Comprehensive Course Exit Exam and a CD-ROM that contains two 75-item Comprehensive Course Exit Exams.

We are firm believers in the old sayings, "You get out of it what you put into it!" and "Practice makes perfect!" The extent of your learning, the attitudes you develop, and the skills you acquire depend on the energy you are willing to expend. It is our belief that if you give this book your best effort you will strengthen and expand your theoretical foundation of fundamentals of nursing and your critical-thinking abilities in testing situations. We expect your efforts to be rewarded with success on your nursing examinations!

Table of Contents

1 Fundamentals of Critical Thinking Related to Test Taking: The RACE Model 1

INTRODUCTION 1

HYSTERICAL PERSPECTIVES 1

Definition of Critical Thinking 2

MAXIMIZE YOUR CRITICAL THINKING ABILITIES 5

Be Positive: You Can Do It! 5

Overcome Barriers to a Positive Mental Attitude 5

Be Reflective: You Need to Take One Step Backward Before Taking Two Steps Forward! 6

Overcome Barriers to Effective Reflection 8

Be Inquisitive: If You Don't Go There, You'll Never Get Anywhere! 8

Overcome Barriers to Being Inquisitive 10

Be Creative: You Must Think Outside the Box! 10

Overcome Barriers to Creativity 11

CRITICAL THINKING APPLIED TO TEST TAKING 12

Educational Domains 12

Components of a Multiple-Choice Question 12

Cognitive Levels of Nursing Questions 12

THE RACE MODEL: THE USE OF CRITICAL THINKING TO ANSWER MULTIPLE-CHOICE QUESTIONS 12

Knowledge Questions: Remember Information! 13

Cognitive Requirements 13

Use of the RACE Model to Answer Knowledge-Level Questions 14

Comprehension Questions: Understand Information! 15

Cognitive Requirements 15

Use of the RACE Model to Answer Comprehension-Level Questions 16

Application Questions: Use Information! 18

Cognitive Requirements 18

Use of the RACE Model to Answer Application-Level Questions 18

Analysis Questions: Scrutinize Information! 21

Cognitive Requirements 21

Use of the RACE Model to Answer Analysis-Level Questions 21

SUMMARY 24

2 Nursing Within the Context of Contemporary Health Care 25

THEORY-BASED NURSING CARE 25

KEYWORDS 25

QUESTIONS 25

ANSWERS AND RATIONALES 31

LEGAL ISSUES 40

KEYWORDS 40

QUESTIONS 41

ANSWERS AND RATIONALES 46

MANAGEMENT AND LEADERSHIP 52
KEYWORDS 52
QUESTIONS 53
ANSWERS AND RATIONALES 57
HEALTH-CARE DELIVERY 64
KEYWORDS 64
QUESTIONS 65
ANSWERS AND RATIONALES 70
COMMUNITY-BASED NURSING 79
KEYWORDS 79
QUESTIONS 79
ANSWERS AND RATIONALES 84

3 Psychosociocultural Nursing Care 93

NURSING CARE ACROSS THE LIFE SPAN 93
KEYWORDS 93
QUESTIONS 94
ANSWERS AND RATIONALES 99
COMMUNICATION 108
KEYWORDS 108
QUESTIONS 109
ANSWERS AND RATIONALES 114
PSYCHOLOGICAL SUPPORT 120
KEYWORDS 120
QUESTIONS 121
ANSWERS AND RATIONALES 126
TEACHING AND LEARNING 133
KEYWORDS 133
QUESTIONS 134
ANSWERS AND RATIONALES 139

4 Essential Components of Nursing Care 147

NURSING PROCESS 147
KEYWORDS 147
QUESTIONS 148
ANSWERS AND RATIONALES 152
PHYSICAL ASSESSMENT 158
KEYWORDS 158
QUESTIONS 160
ANSWERS AND RATIONALES 165
INFECTION CONTROL 172
KEYWORDS 172
QUESTIONS 173
ANSWERS AND RATIONALES 177
SAFETY 183
KEYWORDS 183
QUESTIONS 183
ANSWERS AND RATIONALES 188
MEDICATION ADMINISTRATION 194
KEYWORDS 194
QUESTIONS 195
ANSWERS AND RATIONALES 201
PHARMACOLOGY 207
KEYWORDS 207
QUESTIONS 208
ANSWERS AND RATIONALES 214

5 Basic Human Needs and Related Nursing Care 221
HYGIENE 221
KEYWORDS 221
QUESTIONS 222
ANSWERS AND RATIONALES 228
MOBILITY 235
KEYWORDS 235
QUESTIONS 236
ANSWERS AND RATIONALES 242
NUTRITION 248
KEYWORDS 248
QUESTIONS 249
ANSWERS AND RATIONALES 255
OXYGENATION 261
KEYWORDS 261
QUESTIONS 262
ANSWERS AND RATIONALES 268
URINARY ELIMINATION 275
KEYWORDS 275
QUESTIONS 276
ANSWERS AND RATIONALES 280
FLUIDS AND ELECTROLYTES 286
KEYWORDS 286
QUESTIONS 287
ANSWERS AND RATIONALES 292
GASTROINTESTINAL 298
KEYWORDS 298
QUESTIONS 299
ANSWERS AND RATIONALES 304
PAIN, COMFORT, REST, AND SLEEP 311
KEYWORDS 311
QUESTIONS 312
ANSWERS AND RATIONALES 318
PERIOPERATIVE NURSING 325
KEYWORDS 325
QUESTIONS 326
ANSWERS AND RATIONALES 332

6 Alternate Item Formats 341
ALTERNATE ITEM FORMATS 341
Multiple-Response Items 341
Hot-Spot Items 343
Fill-In-the-Blank Items 345
Items Using a Chart, Table, or Graphic Image 346
Drop and Drag/Ordered Response Items 349
Exhibit Items 350
ANSWERS AND RATIONALES 353

7 Comprehensive Final Book Exam 363
QUESTIONS 363
ANSWERS AND RATIONALES 376

Bibliography 393

Glossary of English Words Commonly Encountered on Nursing Examinations 395

Index 399

Fundamentals of Critical Thinking Related to Test Taking: The RACE Model

1

INTRODUCTION

The purpose of this book is to impress on you that you already use critical thinking in your everyday life. Since you already use critical thinking, you should be able to apply the same thinking to your professional life. This book will help you to:

- Enhance your critical thinking abilities when studying.
- Employ critical thinking skills when taking a nursing examination.

HYSTERICAL PERSPECTIVES

To prepare for writing this chapter I did what all writers should do. I performed a detailed search of the literature about critical thinking, I reviewed all the significant materials that related to test taking or nursing practice, and I wrote an outline for a comprehensive discussion of critical thinking in relation to nursing examinations. The introductory section of the chapter was to be titled "The Historical Perspective of Critical Thinking." When I typed the chapter heading and reread it, I had written "Hysterical" instead of "Historical." Having a relatively good sense of humor and the ability to laugh at myself, my response was peals of laughter. I realized that this was a Freudian slip! Loosely defined, a *Freudian slip* occurs when unconscious mental processes result in a verbal statement that reflects more accurately the true feelings of the speaker than does the originally intended statement. Being a true believer in the statement that *all behavior has meaning*, I could not continue until I explored why I wrote what I wrote.

When I looked up the word *hysterical* in the dictionary, its definition was *an uncontrollable outburst of emotion*, or *out of control* and *extremely comical* or *hilarious*. Associating the word hysterical to the concept of critical thinking raised 2 thoughts. Am I overwhelmed, frantic, and out of control when considering the relationship between critical thinking and nursing, or do I find this relationship funny, comical, and hilarious? If you feel overwhelmed, frenzied, or out of control when considering critical thinking, carefully read the section in this chapter titled *Be Positive: You Can Do It!* When I personalized the word to my own experiences, I recalled that when I believe that something is funny, my internal communication is "Isn't that hysterically funny?" So, now I was faced with the task of exploring why I thought reviewing the historical perspective of critical thinking was so funny or why it could be overwhelming. I actually spent several hours pursuing this goal. At the completion of this process, I arrived at three conclusions:

- The words *critical thinking* are just buzz words. Critical thinking is a skill that we all possess uniquely, and we use this skill routinely in all the activities of our daily living. It is funny to profess that critical thinking is something new and different.
- Who cares about the historical perspectives of critical thinking! Information about the abstract topic of critical thinking must be presented in a manner that the information learned today can be implemented tomorrow.
- Feelings of being overwhelmed can be conquered because critical-thinking abilities can be enhanced.

Definition of Critical Thinking

As I sat back and reflected on my morning's work in relation to Alfaro-LeFevre's (1995) definition of critical thinking, I recognized and appreciated the fact that I had been thoroughly involved with critical thinking. I had:

- Engaged in purposeful, goal-directed thinking.
- Aimed to make judgments based on evidence (fact) rather than conjecture (guesswork).
- Employed a process based on principles of science (e.g., problem solving, decision making).
- Used strategies (e.g., metacognition, reflection, Socratic questioning) that maximized my human potential and compensated for problems caused by human nature.

Critical thinking is a cognitive strategy by which you reflect on and analyze your thoughts, actions, and decisions. Critical thinking often is integrated into traditional linear processes. Linear processes usually follow a straight line, with a beginning and a product at the end. Some linear-like processes, such as the nursing process, are considered cyclical because they repeat themselves. Some formal reasoning processes include:

- **Problem Solving**—involves identifying a problem, exploring alternative interventions, implementing selected interventions, and arriving at the end product, which is a solution to the problem.
- **Decision Making**—involves carefully reviewing significant information, using methodical reasoning, and arriving at the end product, which is a decision.
- **Diagnostic Reasoning**—involves collecting information, correlating the collected information to standards, identifying the significance of the collected information, and arriving at the end product, which is a conclusion or nursing diagnosis.
- **The Scientific Method**—involves identifying a problem to be investigated, collecting data, formulating a hypothesis, testing the hypothesis through experimentation, evaluating the hypothesis, and arriving at the end product, which is acceptance or rejection of the hypothesis.
- **The Nursing Process**—involves collecting information (Assessment), determining significance of information and making a nursing diagnosis (Diagnosis), identifying goals, expected outcomes, and planning interventions (Planning), implementing nursing interventions (Intervention), and assessing the patient's response to interventions and comparing the actual to expected outcomes (Evaluation), ultimately arriving at the end product, which is meeting a person's needs.

Each of these methods of manipulating and processing information incorporates critical thinking. They all are influenced by intellectual standards, such as being focused, methodical, deliberate, logical, relevant, accurate, precise, clear, comprehensive, creative, and reflective. It is helpful to incorporate critical thinking into whatever framework or structure works for you.

The purpose of this discussion was to impress on you that you:

- Use critical thinking in your personal life.
- Will continue to use critical thinking in your professional life.
- Should enhance your critical-thinking abilities when studying.
- Can employ critical-thinking skills when taking a nursing examination.

In an attempt to make the abstract aspects of critical thinking more concrete, we have schematically represented our concept of critical thinking by the **Helix of Critical Thinking**. In Figure 1–1, the Helix of Critical Thinking has been unwound and enlarged so that the components of the cognitive competencies and personal competencies can be viewed easily. The cognitive competencies are the intellectual or reasoning processes employed when thinking. The personal competencies are the characteristics or attitudes of the individual thinker. These lists of competencies represent the cognitive abilities or personal qualities commonly associated with critical thinkers. No one possesses all of these competencies, and you may identify competencies that you possess that are not on these lists. The lists are not all-inclusive. Make lists of your own cognitive and personal competencies. Your lists represent your repertoire or inventory of thinking skills. As you gain knowledge and experience, your lists will expand. The more cognitive and personal competencies you possess, the greater your potential to think critically.

The Helix of Critical Thinking (Fig. 1–2) demonstrates the integration of cognitive competencies and personal competencies essential to thinking critically. Not all of these competencies are used in every thinking situation. You can pick or choose from them as

Cognitive Competencies	Personal Competencies
Dissect	Tolerant of ambiguity
Modify	Think independently
Analyze	Perseverance
Interpret	Self-confident
Examine	Open-minded
Correlate	Accountable
Synthesize	Courageous
Recall facts	Imaginative
Investigate	Disciplined
Categorize	Committed
Summarize	Inquisitive
Understand	Motivated
Demonstrate	Risk taker
Self-examine	Confident
Translate data	Reflective
Query evidence	Objective
Make inferences	Authentic
Manipulate facts	Assertive
Present arguments	Intuitive
Establish priorities	Rational
Make generalizations	Creative
Compare and contrast	Humble
Determine significance	Curious
Determine implications	Honest
Determine consequences	Moral

Figure 1–1. The Helix of Critical Thinking schematically elongated to demonstrate the components of cognitive competencies and personal competencies. The more cognitive competencies and personal competencies a person possesses, the greater the potential the person has to think critically.

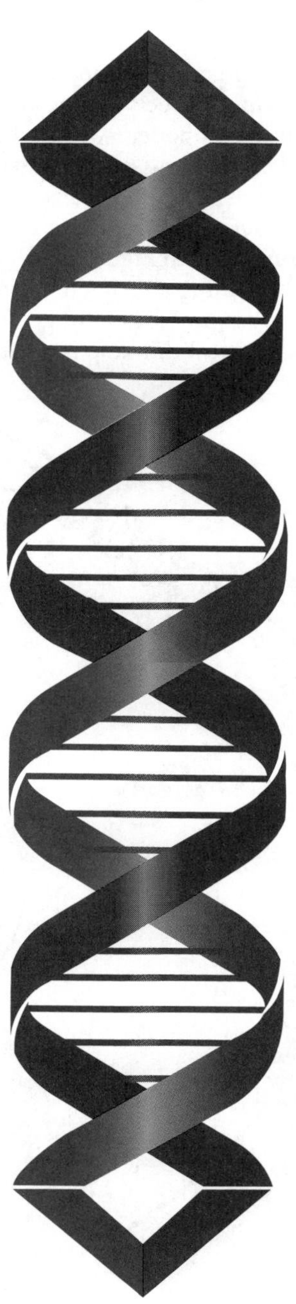

Figure 1–2. The Helix of Critical Thinking demonstrates the interwoven relationship between cognitive competencies and personal competencies essential to thinking critically. Throughout the thinking process there is constant interaction among cognitive competencies, among personal competencies, and between cognitive and personal competencies.

from a smorgasbord when you are confronted with situations that require critical thinking. Initially you may have to stop and consciously consider what cognitive competencies (i.e., intellectual skills) or personal competencies (i.e., abilities, attitudes) to use. As you gain knowledge and experience and move toward becoming an expert critical thinker, the use of these competencies will become second nature. The Helix will contract or expand depending on the competencies you utilize in a particular circumstance. In addition, there is constant interaction among cognitive competencies, among personal competencies, and between cognitive competencies and personal competencies.

The interactive nature of the Helix of Critical Thinking and the Nursing Process is demonstrated in Figure 1–3. The Nursing Process is a dynamic, cyclical process in which each phase interacts with and is influenced by the other phases of the process. The Nursing Process provides a precise framework in which purposeful thinking occurs. Critical thinking is an essential component within, between, and among the phases of the Nursing Process. Different combinations of cognitive and personal competencies may be used during the different phases of the Nursing Process.

The interactive nature of the Helix of Critical Thinking and the Problem-Solving Process is demonstrated in Figure 1–4. The Problem-Solving Process is a dynamic, linear process that has a beginning and an end, with a resolution of the identified problem. The Problem-Solving Process provides a progressive step-by-step method in which goal-directed thinking occurs. Critical thinking is an essential component within and between the steps of the

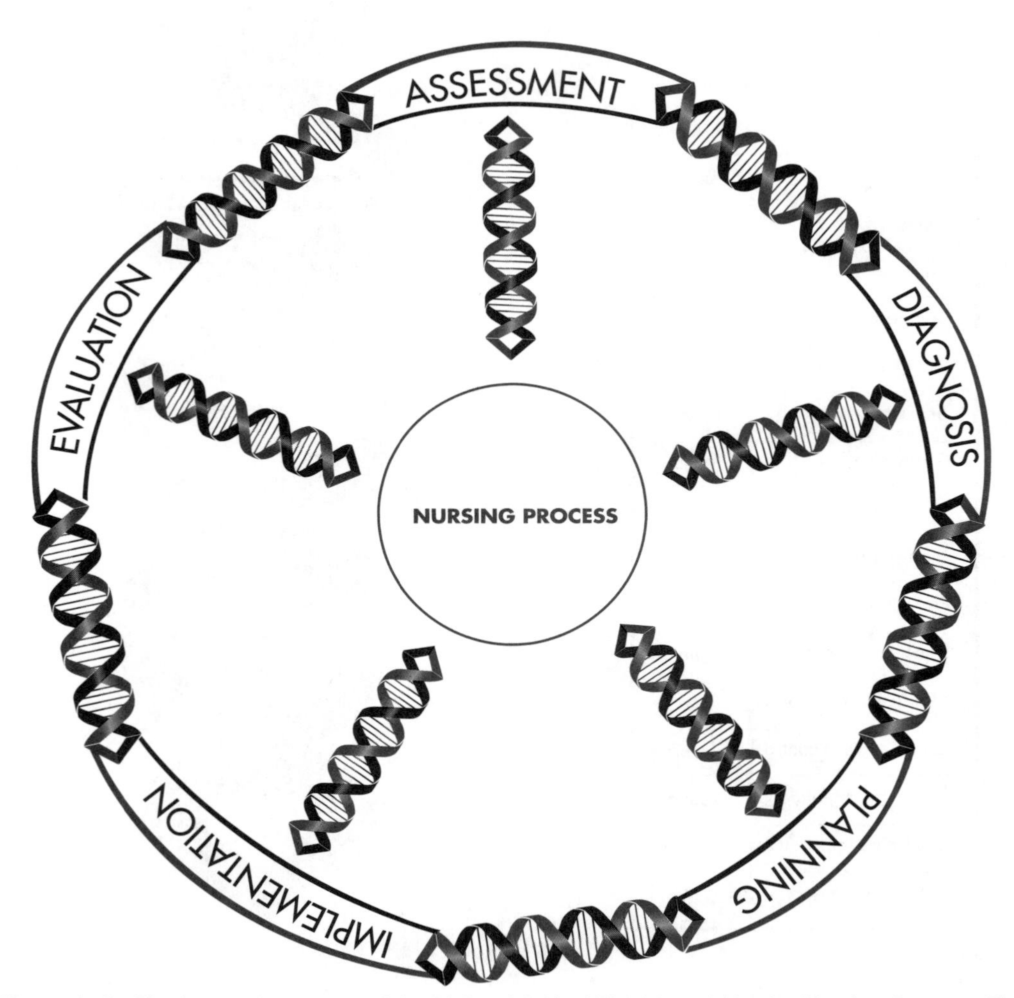

Figure 1–3. The interactive nature of the Helix of Critical Thinking within the Nursing Process. The Nursing Process is a dynamic, cyclical process in which each phase interacts with and is influenced by the other phases of the process. Critical thinking is an essential component within, between, and among phases of the Nursing Process. Different combinations of cognitive and personal competencies may be used during the different phases of the Nursing Process.

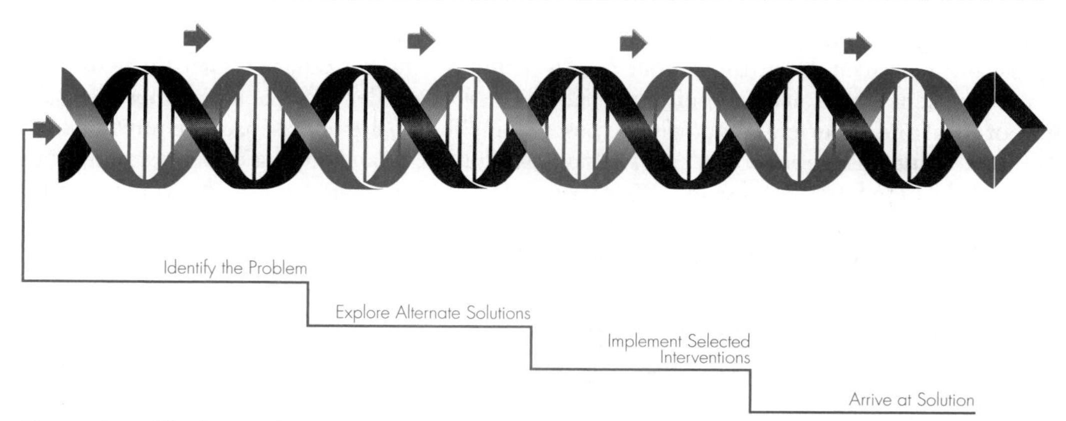

Figure 1–4. The interactive nature of the Helix of Critical Thinking within the Problem-Solving Process. The Problem-Solving Process is a dynamic, linear process that has a beginning and an end, with the resolution of the identified problem. Different combinations of cognitive and personal competencies may be used during the different steps of the Problem-Solving Process.

Problem-Solving Process. Different combinations of cognitive and personal competencies may be used during the different steps of the Problem-Solving Process.

MAXIMIZE YOUR CRITICAL THINKING ABILITIES

Be Positive: You Can Do It!

Assuming responsibility for the care one delivers to a patient and desiring a commendable grade on a nursing examination raise anxiety because a lot is at stake: to keep the patient safe; to achieve a passing grade; to become a nurse ultimately; and to support one's self-esteem. The most important skill that you can learn to help you achieve all of these goals is to be an accomplished critical thinker. We use critical thinking skills every day in our lives when we explore, "What will I have for breakfast?" "How can I get to school from my home?" and "Where is the best place to get gas for my car?" Once you recognize that you are *thinking critically* already, it is more manageable to *think* about *thinking critically*. If you feel threatened by the idea of critical thinking, then you must do something positive to confront the threat. You need to be disciplined and to work at increasing your sense of control, which contributes to confidence! YOU CAN DO IT!

OVERCOME BARRIERS TO A POSITIVE MENTAL ATTITUDE

Supporting a positive mental attitude requires developing discipline and confidence. **Discipline** is defined as self-command or self-direction. The disciplined person will work in a planned manner, explore all options in an organized and logical way, check for accuracy, and seek excellence. When you work in a planned and systematic manner with conscious effort, you are more organized, and therefore more disciplined. Disciplined people generally have more control over the variables associated with an intellectual task. Effective critical thinkers are disciplined, and discipline helps to develop confidence.

Confidence is defined as poise, self-reliance, or self-assurance. Confidence increases as one matures in the role of the student nurse. Understanding your strengths and limitations is the first step to increasing confidence. When you know your strengths you can draw on them, and when you know your limitations you know when it is time to seek out the instructor or another resource to help you in your critical thinking. Either way, you are in control! For example, ask the instructor for help when critically analyzing a case study, share with the instructor any concerns you have about a clinical assignment, and seek out the instructor in the clinical area when you feel the need for support. Failing to use your instructor is like putting your head in the sand. Learning needs must be addressed, not avoided. Although your instructor is responsible for your clinical practice and for stimulating your intellectual growth as a nursing student, you are the consumer of your nursing education. As the consumer, you must be an active participant in your own learning by ensuring that you get the assistance and experiences you need to build your abilities and confidence. When you increase your theoretical and experiential knowledge base, you will increase your sense of control, which ultimately increases your confidence. This applies not just to beginning nursing students but every level of practice because of the explosion in information and technology. When you are disciplined you are more in control, when you are more in control you are more confident, and when you are more confident you have a more positive mental attitude.

Be Reflective: You Need to Take One Step Backward Before Taking Two Steps Forward!

Reflection is the process of thinking back or recalling a situation or event to rediscover its meaning. It helps you to seek and understand the relationships among information, concepts, and principles and to apply them in future clinical or testing situations. Reflection can be conducted internally as quiet thoughtful consideration, in a one-on-one discussion with an instructor or another student, or in a group.

As a beginning nursing student, you are just starting to develop an experiential background from the perspective of a health-care provider. However, you have a wealth of experiences, personal and educational, that influence your development as a professional nurse. Your personal experiences include activities using verbal and written communication, such as delegating tasks to family members or coworkers, setting priorities for daily activities, using mathematics when shopping or balancing a checkbook, etc. A nursing program of study incorporates courses from a variety of other disciplines, such as anatomy and physiology, chemistry, physics, psychology, sociology, reading, writing, mathematics, and informatics, etc. Every single experience is a potential valuable resource for future learning. Recognize the value of "the you" you bring to your nursing education and incorporate it into your reflective processes.

Engaging in reflection is a highly individualized mental process. One form of reflection is writing a journal. A **journal** is an objective and subjective diary of your experiences. It is a chronicle that includes cognitive learning, feelings, and attitudes, and requires you to actively develop skills related to assessing, exploring the meaning of critical incidents, documenting, developing insights into thoughts and actions that comprise clinical practice, and evaluating. Journal writing is a rich resource that provides a written record of where you have been, where you are, and where you are going. It helps you to incorporate experiences into the development of your professional being. After an examination, explore your feelings and attitudes regarding the experience. Be honest with yourself. Did you prepare adequately for the test? Did you find the content harder or easier than content on another test? Were you anxious before, during, or after the test and, if so, was your anxiety low, medium, or high? What would a low score or high score on the test mean to you? When you were confronted with a question that you perceived as difficult, how did you feel, and how did you cope with the feeling? You do not necessarily have to ask yourself all of these questions. You should ask yourself those questions that have meaning for you.

Another form of reflection is making mental pictures. **Mental pictures** are visual images that can be recalled in the future. For example, when caring for a patient who has Parkinson's disease, compare the patient's adaptations to the classic adaptations associated with the disease. Then make a visual picture of this patient's classic adaptations in your mind. Visualize the pill-rolling tremors, mask-like face, drooling, muscle rigidity, etc., so that in the future you can recall the visual picture rather than having to remember a memorized list of symptoms.

Retrospective (after the event) reflection involves seeking an understanding of relationships between previously learned information and the application of this information in patient-care situations or testing experiences. This type of reflection helps you to judge your personal performance against standards of practice. A self-assessment requires the willingness to be open to identifying one's successful and unsuccessful interventions, strengths and weaknesses, and knowledge and lack of knowledge. The purpose of retrospective reflection is not to be judgmental or to second-guess decisions but rather to learn from the situation. The worth of the reflection depends on the abilities that result from it. When similar situations arise in subsequent clinical practice, previous actions that were reinforced or modified can be accessed to have a present successful outcome.

A *clinical postconference* is an example of retrospective reflection. Students often meet in a group (formally or informally) after a clinical experience to review the day's events. During the discussion, students have an opportunity to explore feelings and attitudes, consider interventions and alternative interventions, assess decision-making and problem-solving skills, identify how they and other students think through a situation, etc. You can also review your own thinking when reviewing a patient experience by speaking aloud what you were thinking. For example,

> "When I went into the room to take my postoperative patient's vital signs I realized that the patient had an IV in the right arm. I knew that if I took a blood pressure in the arm with an IV it could interfere with the IV so I knew I had to take the blood pressure in the left arm. When I looked at my patient, he looked very pale and sweaty. I got a little nervous but I continued to get the other vital signs. I put the thermometer in the patient's mouth and started to take his pulse. It was very fast and I knew that this was abnormal so I paid special attention to its rhythm and volume. It was very thready but it was regular. The temperature and respirations were within the high side of the expected range." A beginning nursing student may immediately respond by saying, "I don't know what is going on here so I better take this information to my instructor." A more advanced student might say, "What could be happening? Maybe the patient is bleeding or has an infection. I think I should inform my instructor but I'll inspect the incision first."

When you review an experience like this example, you can identify your thinking skills. Taking the blood pressure in the left arm and assessing the rate, rhythm, and volume of the pulse were habits because you did not have to figure out a new method when responding to the situation. Remembering the expected range for the various vital signs used the thinking skill of total recall because you memorized and internalized these values. Determining further assessments after obtaining the vital signs required inquiry. You collected and analyzed information and did not take the vital sign results at just face value. You recognized abnormalities and gaps in information, collected additional data, considered alternative conclusions, and identified alternative interventions.

Another example of retrospective reflection is reviewing an examination. When reviewing each question, determine why you got a question wrong. For example, several statements you might make are:

- I did not understand what the question was asking because of the English or medical vocabulary used in the question.
- I did not know or understand the content being tested.
- I knew the content being tested but I did not apply it correctly in the question.

When a limited English or medical vocabulary prevents you from answering a question correctly, you must spend time expanding this foundation. A list of English words that appear repeatedly in nursing examinations is included in a glossary at the end of this textbook. In addition, nursing/medical keyword lists have been included in each content area in this textbook. You can use these word lists to review key terminology used in nursing-related topics. To expand your vocabulary, keep English and medical dictionaries at your side when studying and look up new words, write flash cards for words you need to learn, and explore unfamiliar words that confront you on tests.

When you answered a question incorrectly because you did not understand the content, make a list so that you can design a study session devoted to reviewing this information. This study session should begin with a brief review of what you do know about the topic (5 minutes or less). The majority of your efforts should be devoted to studying what you identified as what you need to know. You should do this after reviewing every test. This exercise is based on the axiom *strike while the iron is hot*. The test is over, so your anxiety level is reduced and how nursing-related content is used in a test question is fresh in your mind. Study sessions that are goal directed tend to be more focused and productive.

When you know the content being tested but have applied the information incorrectly, it is an extremely frustrating experience. However, do not become deflated. It is motivating to recognize that you actually know the content! Your next task is to explore how to tap into your knowledge successfully. Sometimes restating or summarizing what the question is asking places it into your own perspective, which helps to clarify the content in relation to the test question. Also, you can view the question in relation to specific past experiences or review the information in two different textbooks to obtain different views on the same content. Another strategy to reinforce your learning is to use the left page of your notebook for taking class notes and leave the facing page blank. After an examination, use the blank page to make comments to yourself about how the content was addressed in test questions or add information from your textbook to clarify class notes. How to review thinking strategies in relation to cognitive levels of nursing questions is explored later in this chapter.

Examine your test-taking behaviors. For example, if you consistently changed your initial answers on a test, it is wise to explore what factors influenced you to change your answers. In addition, determine how many questions were converted to either right or wrong answers. The information you collect from this assessment should influence your future behaviors. If you consistently changed correct answers to incorrect answers, you need to examine the factors that caused you to change your answers. If you changed incorrect answers to correct answers, you should identify what mental processes were used to arrive at your second choice so that you can use them the first time you look at a question.

Reflection is an essential component of all learning. How can you know where you are going without knowing where you have been? Therefore, to enhance your critical thinking abilities you must TAKE ONE STEP BACKWARD BEFORE TAKING TWO STEPS FORWARD!

OVERCOME BARRIERS TO EFFECTIVE REFLECTION

Reflecting on your knowledge, strengths, and successes is easy, but reflecting on your lack of knowledge, weakness, and mistakes takes courage and humility. **Courage** is the attitude of confronting anything recognized as dangerous or difficult without avoiding or withdrawing from the situation. Courage is necessary because when people look at their shortcomings, they tend to be judgmental and are their own worst critics. This type of negativity must be avoided because it promotes defensive thinking, interferes with the reception of new information, and limits self-confidence.

Humility is having a modest opinion of one's own abilities. Humility is necessary because it is important to admit your limitations. Only when you identify what you do and do not know can you make a plan to acquire the knowledge necessary to be successful on nursing examinations and practice safe nursing care. Arrogance or a "know-it-all" attitude can interfere with maximizing your potential. For example, when reviewing examinations with students, the students that benefit the most are the ones who are willing to listen to their peers or instructor as to why the correct answer is correct. The students who benefit the least are the ones who consistently and vehemently defend their wrong answers. A healthy amount of inquiry, thoughtful questioning, and not accepting statements at their face value are important critical-thinking competencies; however, a self-righteous or obstructionist attitude more often than not impedes, rather than promotes, learning.

Be Inquisitive: If You Don't Go There, You'll Never Get Anywhere!

Inquiry means to question or investigate. The favorite words of inquisitive people are: *what*, *where*, *when*, and most importantly *how* and *why*; *if . . . then*; and *it depends*. When studying, ask yourself these words to delve further into a topic under consideration. Below are examples as illustrations.

- You raise the head of the bed when a patient is short of breath. You recognize that this intervention will facilitate respirations. Ask yourself the question, "*How* does this intervention facilitate respirations?" The answer could be, "Raising the head of the bed allows the abdominal organs to drop by gravity, which reduces pressure against the diaphragm, which in turn permits maximal thoracic expansion."

- You insert an indwelling urinary catheter and are confronted with the decision as to where to place the drainage bag. Ask yourself *what* questions. "*What* will happen if I place the drainage bag on the bed frame?" The answer could be, "Urine will flow into the drainage bag by gravity." "*What* will happen if I place the drainage bag on an IV pole?" The answer could be, "Urine will remain in the bladder because the IV pole is above the level of the bladder and fluid does not flow uphill, and if there is urine in the bag, it will flow back into the bladder."
- When palpating a pulse you should use gentle compression. Ask yourself the question, "*Why* should I use gentle compression?" The answer could be, "Gentle compression allows you to feel the pulsation of the artery and prevents excessive pressure on the artery that will cut off circulation and thus obliterate the pulse."
- The textbook says that in emergencies nurses should always assess the airway first. Immediately ask, "*Why* should I assess the airway first?" There may be a variety of answers. "In an emergency, follow the ABCs of assessment which always begins with airway. Maslow's Hierarchy of Needs identifies that physiologic needs should be met first. Because an airway is essential for the passage of life-sustaining gases in and out of the lungs, this is the priority." Although all of these responses answer the question *why*, only the last answer really provides an in-depth answer to the *why* question. If your response to the original *why* question still raises a *why* question, you need to delve deeper. "*Why* do the ABCs of assessment begin with airway?" "*Why* should physiologic needs be met first?"
- When talking with a patient about an emotionally charged topic, the patient begins to cry. You are confronted with a variety of potential responses. Use the method of *if . . . then* statements. *If . . . then* thinking links an action to a consequence. For example, *if* I remain silent, *then* the patient may refocus on what was said. *If* I say, "You seem very sad," *then* the patient may discuss the feelings being felt at the time. *If* I respond with an open-ended statement, *then* the patient may pursue the topic in relation to individualized concerns. After you explore a variety of courses of action with the *if . . . then* method, you should be in a better position to choose the most appropriate intervention for the situation.
- You will recognize that you have arrived at a more advanced level of critical thinking when determining that your next course of action is based on the concept of *It depends*. For example, a patient suddenly becomes extremely short of breath and you decide to administer oxygen during this emergency. When considering the amount and route of delivery of the oxygen, you recognize that *it depends*. You need to collect more data. You need to ask more questions such as, "Is the patient already receiving oxygen? Does the patient have a chronic obstructive pulmonary disease? Is the patient a mouth breather? What other adaptations is the patient exhibiting?" The answers to these questions will influence your choice of interventions.

When exploring the *how*, *what*, *where*, *when*, *why*, *if . . . then*, and *it depends* methods of inquiry, you are more likely to arrive at appropriate inferences, assumptions, and conclusions that will ensure safe, effective nursing care.

These same techniques of inquiry can be used when practicing test taking. Reviewing textbooks that have questions with rationales is an excellent way to explore the reasons for correct and incorrect answers. When answering a question, state why you think your choice is the correct answer and why you think each of the other options is an incorrect answer. This encourages you to focus on the reasons why you responded in a certain way in a particular situation. It prevents you from making quick judgments before exploring the rationales for your actions. After you have done this, compare your rationales to the rationales for the correct and incorrect answers in the textbook. Are your rationales focused, methodical, deliberate, logical, relevant, accurate, precise, clear, comprehensive, creative, and reflective? This method of studying not only reviews nursing content but it fosters critical thinking and applies critical thinking to test taking.

During or after the review of an examination, these techniques of inquiry also can be employed, particularly with those questions you got wrong. Although you can conduct this review independently, it is more valuable to review test questions in a group. Your peers and the instructor are valuable resources that you should use to facilitate your learning. Different perspectives, experiential backgrounds, and levels of expertise can enhance your inquiry. Be inquisitive. IF YOU DON'T GO THERE, YOU'LL NEVER GET ANYWHERE.

OVERCOME BARRIERS TO BEING INQUISITIVE

Effective inquiry requires more than just a simplistic, cursory review of a topic. Therefore, critical thinkers must have curiosity, perseverance, and motivation. **Curiosity** is the desire to learn or know and is a requirement to delve deeper into a topic. If you are uninterested in or apathetic about a topic, you are not going to go that extra mile. Sometimes you may have to "psych yourself up" to study a particular topic. Students frequently say they are overwhelmed by topics such as fluid and electrolytes, blood gases, or chest tubes. As a result, they develop a minimal understanding of these topics and are willing to learn by trial and error in the clinical area or surrender several questions on an examination. Never be willing to let a lack of knowledge be the norm because this results in incompetence, and never give away credits on an examination! Overcome this attitude by maximizing your perseverance.

Perseverance means willingness to continue in some effort or course of action despite difficulty or opposition. Critical thinkers never give up until they obtain the information that satisfies their curiosity. To perform a comprehensive inquiry when studying requires time. Make a schedule for studying at the beginning of the week and adhere to it. This prevents procrastination later in the week when you will prefer to rationalize doing something else and postpone studying. In addition, studying an hour a day is more effective than studying 7 hours in one day. Breaks between study periods allow for the processing of information, and they provide time to rest and regain focus and concentration. The greatest barrier to perseverance is a deadline. When working under a time limit, you may not have enough time to process and understand information. The length of time to study for a test depends on the amount and type of content to be tested and how much previous studying has been done. If you study 2 hours every day for 2 weeks during a unit of instruction, a 1-hour review may be adequate for an examination addressing this content. If you are preparing for a comprehensive examination for a course at the end of the semester, you may decide to study 3 hours a night for 1 to 2 weeks. If you are studying for the NCLEX-RN, you may decide to study 2 hours a day for 3 months. Only you can determine how much time you need to study or prepare for a test. Perseverance can be enhanced by the use of motivation strategies.

Motivation strategies inspire, prompt, encourage, instigate, or enthuse you to act. For example, divide the information to be learned into segments and set multiple short-term goals for studying. After you reach a goal, cross it off the list. Also, this is the time to use incentives. Reward yourself after an hour of studying. Think about how proud you will be when you earn an excellent grade on the examination. Visualize yourself walking down the aisle at graduation or working as a nurse during your career. Incentives can be more tangible (e.g., having a beverage, reading a book for 10 minutes, playing with your children, or doing anything that strikes your fancy). You need to identify the best pattern of studying that satisfies your needs; use motivation techniques to increase your enthusiasm, and then draw on your determination to explore in depth the *how*, *what*, *where*, *when*, and *whys*, *if . . . then*, and *it depends* of nursing practice.

Be Creative: You Must Think Outside the Box!

A **creative** person is imaginative, inventive, innovative, resourceful, original, and visionary. To find solutions beyond common, predictable, and standardized procedures or practices you must be creative. Creativity is what allows you to be yourself and individualize the nursing care you provide to each patient. With the explosion of information and technology, the importance of thinking creatively will increase in the future because the "old" ways of doing things will be inadequate. Nor are any two situations or people ever alike. Therefore, YOU MUST THINK OUTSIDE THE BOX!

OVERCOME BARRIERS TO CREATIVITY

To be creative you must be open-minded, have independence of thought, and be a risk-taker. It is difficult to think outside the box when you are not willing to color outside the lines! Being **open-minded** requires you to consider a wide range of ideas, concepts, and opinions before framing an opinion or making judgments. You need to identify your opinions, beliefs, biases, stereotypes, and prejudices. We all have them to one extent or another, so do not deny them. However, they must be recognized, compartmentalized, and placed on a "back burner." Unless these attitudes are placed in perspective, they will interfere with critical thinking. In every situation you need to remain open to all perspectives, not just your own. When you think that your opinion is the only right opinion, you are engaging in egocentric thinking. *Egocentric thinking* is based on the belief that the world exists or can be known only in relation to the individual's mind. This rigid thinking creates a barrier around your brain that obstructs the inflow of information, imaginative thinking, and the outflow of innovative ideas. An example of an instance in which you have been open-minded is one in which you have changed your mind after having had a discussion with someone else. The new information convinced you to think outside of your original thoughts and opinions.

Independence of thought means the ability to consider all the possibilities and then arrive at an autonomous conclusion. To do this you need to feel comfortable with ambiguity. *Ambiguous* means having two or more meanings and is therefore being uncertain, unclear, indefinite, and vague. For example, a nursing student may be taught by an instructor to establish a sterile field for a sterile dressing change by using the inside of the package of the sterile gloves. When following a sterile dressing change procedure in a clinical skills book, the directions may state to use a separate sterile cloth for the sterile field. When practicing this procedure with another student, the other student may open several 4×4 gauze packages and leave them open as their sterile fields. As a beginning nursing student, this is difficult to understand because of a limited relevant knowledge base and experiential background. Frequently, thinking is concrete and follows rules and procedures, is black and white, or is correct or incorrect. It takes knowledge and experience to recognize that you have many options and may still follow the principles of sterile technique. One nursing faculty member loves to say, "There is more than one road to Philadelphia!"

To travel a different path requires taking risks. Risk in the dictionary means the chance of injury, damage, or loss. However, **risk-taking** in relation to nursing refers to considering all the options, eliminating potential danger to a patient, and acting in a reasoned, logical, and safe manner when implementing unique interventions. Being creative requires intellectual stamina and a willingness to go where no one has been before. Risk-takers tend to be leaders, not followers. The greatest personal risk of creativity is the blow to the ego when confronted with failure. However, you must recognize that throughout your nursing career you will be faced with outcomes that are successful as well as those that are unsuccessful. How you manage your feelings with regard to each, particularly those that are unsuccessful, will influence your willingness to take future creative risks. Successful outcomes build confidence. If appropriately examined unsuccessful outcomes should not be defeating or prevent future creativity. The whole purpose of evaluation in the nursing process is to compare and contrast patient outcomes with expected outcomes. If expected outcomes are not attained, the entire process must be re-examined and than re-performed. You must recognize that:

- Unsuccessful outcomes do occur.
- Unsuccessful outcomes are not a reflection of your competence.
- The number of successful outcomes far outnumber the unsuccessful outcomes.

When you accept these facts, then you may feel confident to take risks with your creativity.

CRITICAL THINKING APPLIED TO TEST TAKING

Educational Domains

Nursing as a discipline includes three domains of learning—affective, psychomotor, and cognitive. The **affective domain** is concerned with attitudes, values, and the development of appreciations. An example of nursing care in the affective domain is the nurse quietly accepting a patient's statement that there is no God without the nurse imposing personal beliefs on the patient. The **psychomotor domain** is concerned with manipulative or motor skills related to procedures or physical interventions. An example of nursing care in the psychomotor domain is the nurse administering an intramuscular injection to a patient. The **cognitive domain** is concerned with recall, recognition of knowledge, comprehension, and the development and application of intellectual skills and abilities. An example of nursing care in the cognitive domain is the nurse clustering collected information and determining its significance. When discussing the application of critical thinking to test taking, the focus will be on the cognitive domain.

Components of a Multiple-Choice Question

A multiple-choice question is called an **item**. Each item has two parts. The **stem** is the part that contains the information that identifies the topic and its parameters and then asks a question. The second part consists of one or more possible responses, which are called **options**. One of the options is the correct answer and the others are wrong answers (also called **distractors**).

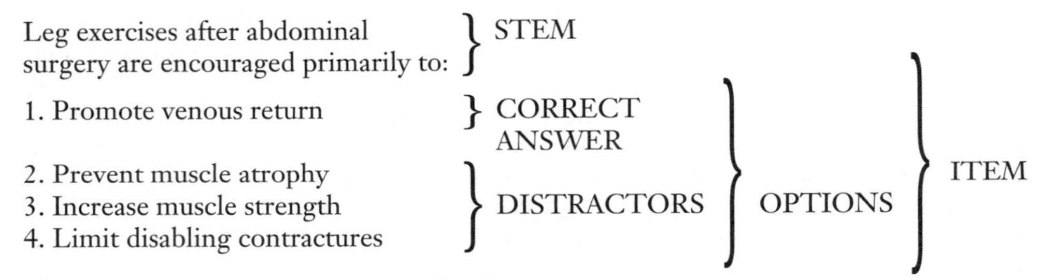

Cognitive Levels of Nursing Questions

Questions on nursing examinations reflect a variety of thinking processes that nurses use when caring for patients. These thinking processes are part of the cognitive domain and they progress from the simple to the complex, from the concrete to the abstract, and from the tangible to the intangible. There are four types of thinking processes represented by nursing questions.

- **Knowledge Questions**—the emphasis is on recalling remembered information.
- **Comprehension Questions**—the emphasis is on understanding the meaning and intent of remembered information.
- **Application Questions**—the emphasis is on remembering understood information and utilizing the information in new situations.
- **Analysis Questions**—the emphasis is on comparing and contrasting a variety of elements of information.

THE RACE MODEL: THE USE OF CRITICAL THINKING TO ANSWER MULTIPLE-CHOICE QUESTIONS

Answering a test question is like participating in a race. Of course, you want to come in first and be the winner. However, the thing to remember about a race is that success is not just based on speed but also on strategy and tactics. The same is true about success on nursing examinations. Although speed may be a variable that must be considered when taking a timed test so that the amount of time spent on each question is factored into the test strategy, the emphasis on **RACE** is the use of critical-thinking techniques to answer multiple-choice questions. The **RACE Model** presented below is a critical-thinking strategy to use when answering nursing multiple-choice questions. If you follow the **RACE Model** every time you examine a test question, its use will become second nature. This methodical approach will improve your abilities to critically analyze a test question and improve your chances of selecting the correct answer.

The **RACE Model** has four steps to answering a test question. The best way to remember the four steps is to refer to the acronym **RACE**.

R **R**ecognize what information is in the stem.
- **R**ecognize the key words in the stem
- **R**ecognize who the client is in the stem
- **R**ecognize what the topic is about

A **A**sk what is the question asking?
- **A**sk what are the key words in the stem that indicate the need for a response
- **A**sk what the question is asking me to do

C **C**ritically analyze the options in relation to the question asked in the stem.
- **C**ritically scrutinize each option in relation to the information in the stem
- **C**ritically identify a rationale for each option
- **C**ritically compare and contrast the options in relation to the information in the stem and their relationships to one another

E **E**liminate as many options as possible.
- **E**liminate one option at a time

The following discussion explores the **RACE Model** in relation to the thinking processes represented in multiple-choice nursing questions. Thoughtfully read the *Cognitive Requirements* under each type of question (e.g., Knowledge, Comprehension, Application, and Analysis). It is important to understand this content in order to apply the critical-thinking strategies inherent in each cognitive-level question as you apply the **RACE Model**. In addition, 3 sets of sample test questions are presented to demonstrate the increasing complexity of thinking reflected in the various levels focusing on specific fundamentals of nursing content.

Knowledge Questions: Remember Information!

COGNITIVE REQUIREMENTS

Knowledge is information that is filed or stored in the brain. It represents the elements essential to the core of a discipline. In nursing, this information consists of elements such as terminology and specific facts including steps of procedures, phenomena, expected laboratory values, classifications, and the expected ranges of vital signs. This type of information requires no alteration from one use or application to another because it is concrete. The information is recalled or recognized in the form in which it was originally learned. This information is the foundation of critical thinking. You must have adequate, accurate, relevant, and important information on which to base your more theoretical, abstract thinking in the future.

Beginning nursing students find knowledge-level questions the easiest because they require the recall or regurgitation of information. Information may be memorized, which involves repeatedly reviewing information to place it and keep it in the brain. Information also can be committed to memory through repeated experiences with the information. Repetition is necessary because information is forgotten quickly unless reinforced. When answering knowledge-level questions you either know the information or you don't. The challenge of answering knowledge questions is defining what the question is asking and tapping your knowledge. See the textbook *TEST SUCCESS: Test-Taking Techniques for Beginning Nursing Students*, F.A. Davis Company, for specific study techniques related to knowledge-level questions.

USE OF THE RACE MODEL TO ANSWER KNOWLEDGE-LEVEL QUESTIONS

1. What is the classification of the medication docusate sodium (Colace)?
   1. Diuretic
   2. Laxative
   3. Bronchodilator
   4. Antihypertensive

RACE:

Recognize key words. **R**ecognize who the client is. **R**ecognize what the topic is about.	What is the **classification** of the drug **docusate sodium (Colace)?** There is no client in this question. The drug docusate sodium (Colace).
Ask what the question is asking.	**What is the classification of docusate sodium (Colace)?**
Critically analyze options in relation to the question.	This question does not require complex understanding, comparative analysis or application skills, it only requires recall of information about docusate sodium (Colace). **Rationales:** 1. Diuretics are medications that increase urine secretion. Docusate sodium (Colace) is not a diuretic. **2. Laxatives are medications that promote the elimination of fecal material. Docusate sodium (Colace) is a laxative.** 3. Bronchodilators are medications that dilate the bronchi of the lungs. Docusate sodium (Colace) is not a bronchodilator. 4. Antihypertensives are medications that reduce the blood pressure. Docusate sodium (Colace) is not an antihypertensive.
Eliminate incorrect options.	Because 1, 3, and 4 are not the name of the classification of docusate sodium (Colace), they can be eliminated.

2. What is the description of the interviewing technique of paraphrasing?
   1. Asking the patient to repeat what was just said
   2. Condensing a discussion into an organized review
   3. Restating what the patient has said using similar words
   4. Asking goal-directed questions concentrating on key concerns

RACE:

Recognize key words. **R**ecognize who the client is. **R**ecognize what the topic is about.	What is the **description** of the interviewing technique of **paraphrasing?** There is no client in this question. The interviewing technique of paraphrasing.
Ask what the question is asking.	**What is the description of paraphrasing?**

Critically analyze options in relation to the question.	To answer this question you must know the definition or characteristic of paraphrasing. It is information that you must recall from your memory. You do not have to know other interviewing skills or their descriptions and characteristics to answer this question. **Rationales:** 1. Asking a patient to repeat what was just asked is known as clarifying, not paraphrasing. 2. Reviewing a discussion is known as summarizing, not paraphrasing. **3. Paraphrasing or restating is an interviewing skill where the nurse listens for a patient's basic message and then repeats the contents of the message in similar words. This validates information from the patient without changing the meaning of the statement and provides an opportunity for the patient to hear what was said.** 4. Asking goal-directed questions that concentrate on key concerns is known as focusing, not paraphrasing.
Eliminate incorrect options.	Options 1, 2, and 4 are not examples of paraphrasing and can be eliminated.

3. What is another name for a decubitus ulcer?
   1. Skin tear
   2. Pressure ulcer
   3. Surface abrasion
   4. Penetrating wound

RACE:

Recognize key words. **R**ecognize who the client is. **R**ecognize what the topic is about.	What is **another name** for **decubitus ulcer**? There is no client in this question. The names for decubitus ulcers.
Ask what the question is asking.	**What is another name for decubitus ulcer?**
Critically analyze options in relation to the question.	To answer this question you must know the alternate name for a decubitus ulcer. It is information you must recollect from your memory. You do not have to know the description or characteristics of other types of wounds to answer this question. **Rationales:** 1. A skin tear is a break in the continuity of thin, fragile skin caused by friction or shearing force. **2. A pressure ulcer is impaired skin (reddened area, sore, or lesion characterized by sloughing of tissue) over a bony prominence caused by pressure that interferes with the delivery of oxygen to body cells.** 3. An abrasion is the scraping or rubbing away of the superficial layers of the skin. 4. A penetrating wound occurs when a sharp object pierces the skin and injures underlying tissues.
Eliminate incorrect options.	Options 1, 3, and 4 are not other names for a decubitus ulcer and can be eliminated.

Comprehension Questions: Understand Information!

Cognitive Requirements

Comprehension is the ability to understand that which is known. To be safe practitioners, nurses must understand information such as reasons for nursing interventions, physiology and pathophysiology, consequences of actions, and responses to medications. To reach an understanding of information in nursing you must be able to translate information into your own words to personalize its meaning. Once information is rearranged in your own mind, you must interpret the essential components for their intent, corollaries, significance, implications, consequences, and conclusions in accordance with the conditions described in the original communication. The information is manipulated within its own context without being used in a different or new situation.

Beginning nursing students generally consider comprehension-level questions slightly more difficult than knowledge-level questions, but less complicated than application- and analysis-level questions. Students often try to deal with comprehension-level information by memorizing the content. For example, when studying local adaptations to an infection, students may memorize the following list: heat, erythema, pain, edema, and exudate. Although this can be done, it is far better to understand why these adaptations occur. Erythema and heat occur because of increased circulation to the area. Edema occurs because of increased permeability of the capillaries. Pain occurs because the accumulating fluid in the tissue presses on nerve endings. Exudate occurs because of the accumulation of fluid, cells, and other substances at the site of infection. The mind is a wonderful machine, but unless you have a photographic memory, lists of information without understanding often become overwhelming and confusing. The challenge of answering comprehension questions is understanding the information. See the textbook *TEST SUCCESS: Test-Taking Techniques for Beginning Nursing Students*, F.A. Davis Company, for specific study techniques related to comprehension-level questions.

USE OF THE RACE MODEL TO ANSWER COMPREHENSION-LEVEL QUESTIONS

1. The medication docusate sodium (Colace) facilitates defecation by:
   1. Softening stool
   2. Forming a bulk residue
   3. Irritating the intestinal wall
   4. Dilating the intestinal lumen

RACE:

Recognize key words. **R**ecognize who the client is. **R**ecognize what the topic is about.	The medication **docusate sodium (Colace) facilitates defecation by**: There is no client. The drug docusate sodium (Colace) and how it works.
Ask what the question is asking.	**How and why does docusate sodium (Colace) facilitate defecation?**
Critically analyze options in relation to the question.	The word in the stem that indicates this is a comprehension-level question is **facilitates**. What is the consequence of taking ducosate sodium (Colace)? You need to scrutinize each option to identify whether the description in the option correctly **explains how or why docusate sodium (Colace) works to facilitate defecation.** **Rationales:** **1. Docusate sodium (Colace) softens and delays the drying of feces by lowering the surface tension of water permitting water and fat to penetrate the feces.** 2. Bulk-forming laxatives, such as psyllium hydrophilic mucilloid (Metamucil) increase the fluid, gaseous, or solid bulk in the intestines. 3. Irritants or stimulants, such as bisacodyl (Dulcolax), irritate the intestinal mucosa or stimulate intestinal wall nerve endings, which precipitates peristalsis. 4. Large volume enemas, not medications, enlarge the lumen of the intestine, which precipitates peristalsis.

Eliminate incorrect options.	Options 2, 3, and 4 do not accurately describe the therapeutic action of docusate sodium (Colace) and can be eliminated.

2. The interviewing technique of paraphrasing promotes communication because it:
1. Requires patients to defend their points of view
2. Limits patients from continuing a rambling conversation
3. Allows patients to take their conversations in any desired direction
4. Offers patients an opportunity to develop a clearer idea of what they said

RACE:

Recognize key words. **R**ecognize who the client is. **R**ecognize what the topic is about.	The interviewing technique of **paraphrasing promotes communication because it**: There is no client. The interviewing technique of paraphrasing and how it works.
Ask what the question is asking.	**How and why does paraphrasing promote communication?**
Critically analyze options in relation to the question.	The word in the stem that indicates that this is a comprehension-level question is **promotes**. What is the consequence of paraphasing? You need to scrutinize each option to identify whether the description in the option correctly **explains how or why paraphrasing works to promote communication.** **Rationales:** 1. This describes the results of challenging statements that usually are barriers to communication. 2. This describes one purpose of the interviewing skill of focusing, which is the use of questions or statements to center on one concern mentioned within a wordy, confusing conversation. 3. This is the purpose of open-ended questions or statements. **4. Paraphrasing involves actively listening for patient concerns that are then restated by the nurse in similar words. This intervention conveys that the nurse has heard and understood the message and gives the patient an opportunity to review what was said.**
Eliminate incorrect options.	Options 1, 2, and 3 do not accurately describe how paraphrasing works to promote communication and can be eliminated.

3. Turning patients every 2 hours prevents pressure ulcers because:
1. Relieving weight on the capillaries allows oxygen to reach body cells
2. Moving promotes muscle contractions that increase the basal metabolic rate
3. Keeping the extremities dependent allows blood to flow to distal cells by gravity
4. Dropping of the abdominal organs by gravity relieves pressure against the diaphragm

RACE:

Recognize key words. **R**ecognize who the client is. **R**ecognize what the topic is about.	**Turning** patients every 2 hours **prevents pressure ulcers because**: The patient is the client. How turning a patient every 2 hours prevents pressure ulcers.
Ask what the question is asking.	**How and why does turning a patient prevent a pressure ulcer?**

continued

continued

Critically analyze options in relation to the question.	The word in the stem that indicates that this is a comprehension-level question is **prevents.** What is the consequence of turning patients every 2 hours? You need to scrutinize each option to identify whether the description in the option correctly **explains how or why turning a patient relieves pressure and prevents a pressure ulcer.** **Rationales:** **1. Capillary beds are compressed and blood flow is obliterated with excessive external pressure (12 to 32 mmHg). Changing position removes the weight of the body off dependent areas permitting blood to flow through the capillaries supporting gaseous exchange at the cellular level.** 2. Muscle contraction expends energy that raises the basal metabolic rate; however, this is unrelated to the development of pressure ulcers. 3. Blood flow to the extremities will increase when they are kept below the level of the heart; however, this is unrelated to the development of pressure ulcers. 4. Relieving pressure against the diaphragm by abdominal organs allows for greater thoracic expansion; however, this is unrelated to the development of pressure ulcers.
Eliminate incorrect options.	Options 2, 3, and 4 do not accurately explain how turning relieves pressure thereby preventing a pressure ulcer and can be eliminated.

Application Questions: Use Information!

COGNITIVE REQUIREMENTS

Application is the ability to use known and understood information in new situations. It requires more than just understanding information because you must demonstrate, solve, change, modify, or manipulate information in other than its originally learned form or context. With application questions you are confronted with a new situation that requires you to recall information and manipulate the information from within a familiar context to arrive at abstractions, generalizations, or consequences regarding the information that can be used in the new situation to answer the question. Application questions require you to make rational, logical judgments that result in a course of action.

Beginning nursing students frequently find these questions challenging because they require a restructuring of understood information into abstractions, commonalities, and generalizations, which are then applied to new situations. You do this all the time. Although there are parts of your day that are routine, every day you are exposed to new, challenging experiences. The same concept holds true for application questions. With application questions you will be confronted by situations that you learned about in a book, experienced personally, relived through other students' experiences, or never heard about or experienced before. This will happen throughout your entire nursing career. The challenge of answering application questions is going beyond rules and regulations and using information in a unique, creative way. See the textbook *TEST SUCCESS: Test-Taking Techniques for Beginning Nursing Students*, F.A. Davis Company, for specific study techniques related to application-level questions.

USE OF THE RACE MODEL TO ANSWER APPLICATION-LEVEL QUESTIONS

1. A patient complains about not having had a bowel movement in three days. Which classification of drugs is most helpful in relieving this problem?
   1. Diuretics
   2. Laxatives

3. Bronchodilators
4. Antihypertensives

RACE:

Recognize key words. **R**ecognize who the client is. **R**ecognize what the topic is about.	A patient complains about **not having a bowel movement in three days.** Which **classification** of **drug** is **most helpful** in **relieving** this problem? The patient is the client. A patient who has not had a bowel movement in three days and needs a drug from a classification of drugs that will be the most helpful in facilitating defecation.
Ask what the question is asking.	**Which classification of drugs is most helpful in facilitating defecation?**
Critically analyze options in relation to the question.	The words in the stem that indicate that this is an application question are **most helpful in relieving.** To choose which classification of drugs will be most helpful in relieving this patient's problem, you must know that a patient who has not had a bowel movement in three days may be constipated, the therapeutic action and outcome of various classifications of drugs, and which classification of drugs would be helpful in relieving constipation. **Rationales:** 1. Diuretics are medications that increase urine output. They are prescribed for people who retain excessive fluid. **2. Laxatives are medications that promote the elimination of fecal material. They are prescribed to prevent or treat constipation.** 3. Bronchodilators are medications that dilate the bronchi of the lungs. They are prescribed for patients who have difficulty breathing. 4. Antihypertensives are medications that reduce the blood pressure. They are prescribed for people who have high blood pressure (hypertension).
Eliminate incorrect options.	Because options 1, 3, and 4 are not the name of the classification of docusate sodium (Colace) they can be eliminated.

2. A patient scheduled for major surgery, who is perspiring and nervously picking at the bed linen, says, "I don't know if I can go through with this surgery." The nurse responds, "You'd rather not have surgery now?" Which interviewing technique was used by the nurse?
   1. Focusing
   2. Reflection
   3. Paraphrasing
   4. Clarification

RACE:

Recognize key words. **R**ecognize who the client is. **R**ecognize what the topic is about.	A patient scheduled for major surgery, who is perspiring and nervously picking at the bed linen, says, **"I don't know if I can go through with this surgery."** The nurse responds, **"You'd rather not have surgery now?" Which interviewing technique was used** by the nurse? The patient is the client. The name of a specific interviewing technique that repeats basically what the patient is saying.

continued

continued

Ask what the question is asking.	**What interviewing technique is being used by the nurse when the nurse says in response to the patient, "You'd rather not have surgery now?"**
Critically analyze options in relation to the question.	The words in the stem that indicate that this is an application question are **was used.** To identify which technique was used by the nurse you have to understand the elements of a paraphrasing statement and you need to be able to recognize a paraphrasing statement when it is used. Although it is helpful to understand the elements of the other interviewing techniques because it will help you eliminate incorrect options, it is not necessary to understand this information to answer the question. **Rationales:** 1. The example in the stem is not using focusing because the patient's statement was short and contained one message that was reiterated by the nurse. Focusing is used to explore one concern among many statements made by the patient. 2. The example in the stem is not using reflection because the nurse's statement is concerned with the content, not the underlying feeling, of the patient's statement. An example of reflection used by the nurse is, "You seem anxious about having major surgery." **3. The nurse used paraphrasing because the patient's and nurse's statements contain the same message but they are expressed with different words.** 4. The example in the stem is not using clarification. When clarification is used, the nurse is asking the patient to further explain what is meant by the patient's statement. An example of clarification used by the nurse is, "I am not quite sure that I know what you mean when you say you would rather not have surgery now."
Eliminate incorrect options.	Options 1, 2, and 4 can be eliminated because these techniques are different from the technique portrayed in the nurse's response in the stem.

3. The nurse identifies that a patient on prolonged bed rest may be developing a pressure ulcer when the skin over a bony prominence appears:
1. Red
2. Blue
3. Black
4. Yellow

RACE:

Recognize key words. **R**ecognize who the client is. **R**ecognize what the topic is about.	The nurse identifies that a patient may be developing a **pressure ulcer** when the **skin** over a bony prominence reveals: The patient is the client. Early signs and symptoms of a pressure ulcer.
Ask what the question is asking.	**Which early adaptation indicates a pressure ulcer caused by immobility?**

Critically analyze options in relation to the question.	The words in the stem that indicate this is an application question are **identifies** and **developing pressure ulcer.** To answer this question you have to understand how and why pressure can cause a pressure ulcer and know the common early adaptations that indicate the formation of a pressure ulcer. Although it would be helpful to know what is happening when the skin reflects each of the colors indicated so that you can eliminate incorrect answers, it is not necessary to comprehend this information to answer the question. **Rationales:** **1. Erythema is a red discoloration generally caused by local vasodilation in an attempt to bring more oxygen to the area.** 2. Cyanosis is a bluish color caused by an increased amount of deoxygenated hemoglobin associated with hypoxia not pressure. 3. Eschar generally appears black and is the scab or dry crust that results from the death of tissue. 4. Jaundice is a yellow-orange color caused by increased deposits of bilirubin in tissue, not a response to pressure.
Eliminate incorrect options.	Options 2, 3, and 4 are not early signs of a pressure ulcer and are incorrect answers. They can be eliminated.

Analysis Questions: Scrutinize Information!

COGNITIVE REQUIREMENTS

Analysis is the separation of an entity into its constituent parts and examination of their essential features in relation to each other. Analysis questions assume that you know, understand, and can apply information. They ask you to engage in higher-level critical-thinking strategies. To answer analysis-level questions, you first must examine each element of information as a separate entity. Secondly, you need to investigate the differences among the various elements of information. In other words, you must compare and contrast information. Thirdly, you must analyze the structure and organization of the compared and contrasted information to arrive at a conclusion or answer. Analysis questions often ask you to set priorities and in the stem use words such as *first*, *initially*, *best*, *priority*, and *most important*.

Beginning nursing students find analysis-level questions the most difficult to answer. Analysis questions demand scrutiny of individual elements of information as well as require identification of differences among elements of information. Sometimes students cannot identify the structural or organizational relationship of elements of information. The challenge of answering analysis questions is performing a complete analysis of all the various elements of information and their interrelationships without overanalyzing or "reading into" the question. See the textbook *TEST SUCCESS: Test-Taking Techniques for Beginning Nursing Students*, F.A. Davis Company, for specific study techniques related to analysis-level questions.

USE OF THE RACE MODEL TO ANSWER ANALYSIS-LEVEL QUESTIONS

1. A frail, malnourished older adult has been experiencing constipation. The nurse anticipates that the physician will most likely order:
   1. Bisacodyl (Dulcolax)
   2. Docusate sodium (Colace)
   3. Mineral oil (Haley's M-O)
   4. Magnesium hydroxide (milk of magnesia [MOM])

RACE:

Recognize key words. **R**ecognize who the client is. **R**ecognize what the topic is about.	A **frail**, **malnourished older adult** has been experiencing **constipation**. The nurse anticipates that **the physician will most likely order:** The patient is the client. Medications for constipation for a debilitated older adult.
Ask what the question is asking.	**Which cathartic or laxative is the least likely to cause problems in a debilitated older adult?**
Critically analyze options in relation to the question.	Analysis questions often ask you to set priorities as indicated by the words **most likely order** in the stem of this question. This question requires you to: understand that frail, malnourished older adults have minimal compensatory reserve in various body systems to manage responses to cathartics and laxatives; know the physiologic action, outcome, side effects, and toxic effects of all four medications presented in the stem; contrast and compare the drugs and the risks they pose in the older adult to arrive at which drug would be the least risky drug. The least risky drug is the one the physician is most likely to order. **Rationales:** 1. Dulcolax irritates the intestinal mucosa, stimulates nerve endings in the wall of the intestines, and causes rapid propulsion of waste from the body. Dulcolax is not the best choice of a laxative for an older adult because it can cause intestinal cramps, fluid and electrolyte imbalances, and irritation of the intestinal mucosa. **2. Colace permits fat and water to penetrate feces which soften stool. Of all the options, Colace has the fewest side effects in older adults.** 3. Mineral oil lubricates feces in the colon; however, it can inhibit the absorption of fat-soluble vitamins and is not the best laxative for an older adult. 4. Milk of magnesia (MOM) draws water into the intestine by osmosis, which stimulates peristalsis. It is contraindicated for an older adult because it can cause fluid and electrolyte imbalances and inhibit absorption of fat-soluble vitamins.
Eliminate incorrect options.	Options 1, 3, and 4 are more potent than the correct answer and therefore are least likely to be ordered to relieve constipation in a debilitated older adult.

2. The mother of a terminally ill child says, "I never thought that I would have such a sick child." The best initial response by the nurse is:
   1. "How do you feel right now?"
   2. "What do you mean by sick child?"
   3. "Life is not fair to do this to a child."
   4. "It's hard to believe that your child is so sick."

RACE:

Recognize key words. **R**ecognize who the client is. **R**ecognize what the topic is about.	The mother of a terminally ill child says, **"I never thought that I would have such a sick child."** The **best initial response by the nurse is:** The mother is the client. Interviewing skills the nurse can use when initially responding to a statement by the mother of a sick child.

Ask what the question is asking.	**Which is an example of the best interviewing skill to use when initially responding to a statement made by the mother of a sick child?**
Critically analyze options in relation to the question.	Analysis questions often ask you to set priorities as indicated by the words **best initial** response in the stem of this question. To answer this question you need to: identify which interviewing techniques are portrayed in the statements in each option; understand how and why each interviewing skill works; compare and contrast the pros and cons of each technique if used in this situation; identify which technique is the most supportive, appropriate, and best initial response by the nurse. **Rationales:** 1. Direct questions cut off communication and should be avoided. 2. This response focuses on the seriousness of the child's illness, which is not the issue raised in the mother's statement. 3. This statement reflects the beliefs and values of the nurse, which should be avoided. **4. This is a declarative statement that paraphrases the mother's beliefs and feelings. It communicates to the mother that the nurse is attentively listening and invites the mother to expand on her thoughts if she feels ready.**
Eliminate incorrect options.	Options 1, 2, and 3 can be eliminated because they are not the best initial response by the nurse of the options offered.

3. The patient with the greatest risk for developing a pressure ulcer is:
   1. An older adult on bed rest
   2. A toddler learning to walk
   3. A thin young woman in a coma
   4. An emotionally unstable middle-aged man

RACE:

Recognize key words. **R**ecognize who the client is. **R**ecognize what the topic is about.	The patient with the **greatest risk** for **developing** a **pressure ulcer** is: The patient is the client. Identifying risk factors for pressure ulcers and who would be at most risk.
Ask what the question is asking.	**Which patient in the various age groups is at the greatest risk for a pressure ulcer?**
Critically analyze options in relation to the question.	Analysis questions often ask you to set priorities as indicated by the words **greatest risk** in the stem of this question. To answer this question you need to: know what are the major risk factors that contribute to the development of a pressure ulcer; identify the risk factors for pressure ulcer development in all four of the specific categories of the life span represented in the options; and assign a level of risk to each of the individuals identified in the options in comparison with each of the other individuals. Once you complete this intellectual analysis, you will identify the individual at greatest risk.

continued

continued

	Rationales: 1. Although the skin of older adults is vulnerable to the development of pressure ulcers because of decreased subcutaneous fat, reduced thickness and vascularity of the dermis, and decreased sebaceous gland activity, older adults are still capable of changing position and moving around in bed, which relieves pressure on integumentary tissue. 2. A toddler learning to walk is not immobile. In addition, the skin of toddlers usually has adequate circulation, subcutaneous tissue, and hydration and is supple. A toddler may fall and develop bruises (contusions) or scrapes (abrasions), not pressure ulcers. **3. Of the options offered, this person is the most vulnerable for developing a pressure ulcer. A thin person has little protective subcutaneous fat over bony prominences, and a person in a coma is immobile and unable to move or turn purposefully. Immobility results in prolonged pressure, which interferes with the oxygen supply to body cells.** 4. Middle-aged men usually do not exhibit the effects of aging on the integumentary system. In addition, emotionally unstable people are able to move and change positions, which permits circulation to the cells of the skin.
Eliminate incorrect options.	Individuals presented in options 1, 2, and 4 are at less of a risk than a thin person who is immobile for the development of pressure ulcers.

SUMMARY

Thinking about thinking is more strenuous than physical labor. A physical task is always easier if you use the right tool. This concept is true also for mental labor. The **RACE Model** is a tool that provides a methodical format to apply critical thinking to answering multiple-choice questions in nursing. As with any tool, it takes practice and experience to perfect its use. Therefore, you are encouraged to use the **RACE Model** when practicing test taking or reviewing examinations.

Nursing Within the Context of Contemporary Health Care

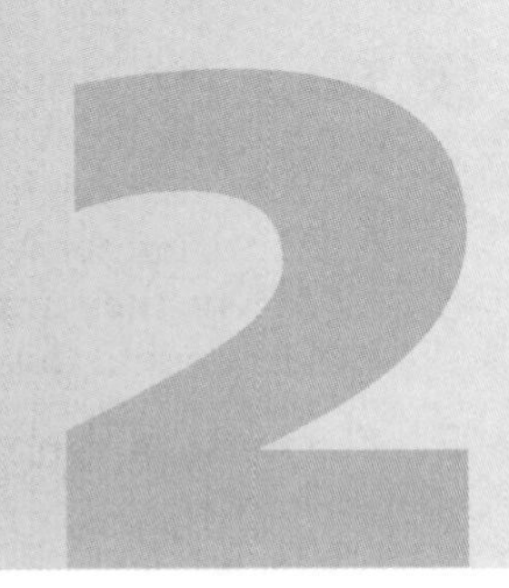

Theory-Based Nursing Care

KEYWORDS

The following words include English vocabulary, nursing/medical terminology, concepts, principles, or information relevant to content specifically addressed in the chapter or associated with topics presented in it. English dictionaries, nursing textbooks, and medical dictionaries such as *Taber's Cyclopedic Medical Dictionary*, are resources that can be used to expand your knowledge and understanding of these words and related information.

Actualization
Adaptation
Adaptive capacity
Beliefs
Compensatory reserve
Conceptual framework
Critical time
Defense mechanism
Developmental task
Ego differentiation
Erikson, Erik – Personality Development
Fixation
Free association
Freud, Sigmund – Psychoanalytic Theory
Gordon, Marjorie – Functional Health Patterns
Health
Health belief
Health-illness continuum
Holistic health
Homeostasis
Human behavior
Instinctual drive
Jung, Carl – Personality Theory
Kübler-Ross, Elisabeth – Stages of Grieving
Libido
Maslow, Abraham – Hierarchy of Basic Human Needs
Model
Moral development
Multiplicity of stressors
Philosophy of nursing
Piaget, Jean – Theory of Cognitive Development
Stress
Stressor (primary, secondary)
Theory
Values
Wellness

QUESTIONS

1. The nurse is assessing a patient who is experiencing prolonged stress. For which most serious complication should the nurse monitor the patient?
   1. Altered sleeping
   2. Impaired immunity
   3. Increased muscle tension
   4. Decreased intestinal peristalsis

2. The nurse is caring for a patient recently diagnosed with advanced cancer. Which patient statement reflects Kübler-Ross' stage of denial in the grief process?
   1. "Why did this have to happen to me now?"
   2. "My daughter will live with my sister after I am gone."
   3. "Maybe they mixed up my records with someone else's."
   4. "How could this happen when I quit smoking cigarettes?"

3. The nurse understands that the word that best describes the concept of adaptive capacity is:
   1. Change
   2. Etiology
   3. Remission
   4. Compliance

4. Maslow's Hierarchy of Needs theory helps the nurse to identify the patient's:
   1. Problem that has top priority
   2. Developmental level
   3. Coping patterns
   4. Health beliefs

5. The nurse is assessing the emotional needs of a variety of patients. In relation to the emotional needs of patients, the nurse understands that a concept reflective of the work of Sigmund Freud is:
   1. Human nature is essentially irrational
   2. Instinctual drives are the underlying stimuli for human behavior
   3. Universal moral principles are internalized as standards of behavior
   4. Moral development is based on concepts of caring and responsibility

6. The nurse is teaching a course about death and dying to a community group. The nurse should include that when preparing a child for the death of a grandparent it is most important for the parents to:
   1. Wait until the child asks a question about the situation
   2. Encourage the child to participate in mourning rituals
   3. Begin at the child's level of understanding
   4. Praise the child for being strong

7. A basic principle associated with Sigmund Freud and his work is that:
   1. Emotional or psychological events are not understandable
   2. Defense mechanisms are used to protect one's self-esteem
   3. The Id is the part of the psyche that imposes a conscience
   4. The conscious mind is unrelated to human behavior

8. When assessing patients, it is essential that the nurse understands that the most common human response to an emotional stressor is:
   1. Anger
   2. Denial
   3. Anxiety
   4. Depression

9. Which statement best reflects the relationship between stress and adaptation?
   1. Stressors usually cause maladaptive responses
   2. Addressing an adaptation will in turn limit the stressor
   3. Stress and adaptation are intertwined in a cyclic relationship
   4. Adaptations to stress are solely dependent on the nature of the stressor

10. The Health Belief Model attempts to explain and predict health behaviors and focuses on:
    1. One's ability to fulfill one's assigned roles
    2. Constructs associated with perceived threat and net benefit
    3. Locus of control being important in one making choices about health behaviors
    4. People moving along a continuum from health on one end to illness on the other end

11. Which psychodynamic theorist believed that an infant seeking pleasure through oral gratification is important to psychosocial growth?
    1. Sigmund Freud
    2. Erik Erikson
    3. Jean Piaget
    4. Carl Jung

12. According to Maslow's Hierarchy of Needs theory, a person who is no longer aware of a need has:
    1. Experienced emotional and physical health
    2. Had the need met to one's level of satisfaction
    3. Achieved one's role performance expectations
    4. Moved toward the healthy end of the health-illness continuum

13. The nurse is assessing patients in the postanesthesia care unit. For which physiological adaptation to stress should the nurse monitor this patient?
    1. Slow, bounding pulse
    2. Delayed response time
    3. Inability to concentrate
    4. Rapid, shallow breathing

14. The nurse is caring for numerous patients. It is important that the nurse understand that the person who may have the hardest time coping is the patient who is:
    1. Scheduled for a biopsy
    2. Unable to control the course of illness
    3. Experiencing a multiplicity of stressors
    4. Having to relocate to an assisted-living facility

15. A nurse inadvertently commits a medication error without the knowledge of other nursing team members. According to Freud, what part of the personality guides the nurse to initiate an incident report?
    1. Id
    2. Ego
    3. Libido
    4. Superego

16. When considering concepts related to the General Adaptation Syndrome, the nurse understands that adaptations:
    1. Depend on the nature of the stressor
    2. Can be conscious or unconscious
    3. Become secondary stressors
    4. Are maladaptive responses

17. A patient with terminal cancer is willing to try new therapies. The nurse identifies that the patient is in what stage of Kübler-Ross' Stages of Grieving?
    1. Denial
    2. Bargaining
    3. Depression
    4. Acceptance

18. The nurse gives a resident in a nursing home a choice about which color shirt to wear. What level need, according to Maslow's Hierarchy of Needs, has the nurse just met?
    1. Physiologic
    2. Self-esteem
    3. Safety and Security
    4. Love and Belonging

19. Which nursing intervention best supports a problem in the Role-Relationship Pattern category of Gordon's Functional Health Patterns?
1. Assessing a family member's readiness to provide care in the home
2. Referring a patient to a self-help group to learn colostomy care
3. Teaching the patient self-care in preparation for going home
4. Seeking the assistance of a spiritual advisor

20. When differentiating between primary and secondary stressors, the nurse identifies that an example of a secondary stressor is:
1. Pain
2. Cold weather
3. Death of a spouse
4. Ingested microorganisms

21. According to Maslow's Hierarchy of Needs theory, the nurse identifies that the level of need that should be met just before self-esteem needs can be met is:
1. Safety
2. Belonging
3. Physiologic
4. Self-actualization

22. Which statement best reflects a principle common to all theories of health, wellness, and illness?
1. Health is synonymous with a sense of well-being
2. People are able to control factors that affect health
3. Many variables influence a person's perception of health
4. Being able to meet the demands of one's role is necessary for health

23. The Public Health Nurse is considering the needs of members of a community. The nurse identifies which social stressor possesses the greatest risk for precipitating illness?
1. Change in marital status
2. Teenage motherhood
3. Single parent family
4. Living on the street

24. Which is an example of an adaptation to a physiologic stressor?
1. A sunburn after being outside all day
2. Diarrhea after eating contaminated food
3. Shortness of breath when walking up a hill
4. A rapid heart rate during a final examination

25. According to Maslow, which behavior least describes a person who is self-actualized? A person who:
1. Is autonomous
2. Is able to see the good in others
3. Has the ability to problem-solve
4. Has an external locus of control

26. The nurse understands that a concept basic to the health-illness continuum is that:
1. People can be both healthy and ill at the same time on the continuum
2. There is no distinct boundary between health and illness along the continuum
3. When variables are in balance, a person is in the exact center of the continuum
4. Actualization must be achieved to be placed on the healthy end of the continuum

27. A nurse completes a difficult day at work and feels satisfaction in performing well and helping others. According to Freud, this feeling of satisfaction is associated with what part of the personality?
 1. Ego
 2. Libido
 3. Fixation
 4. Superego

28. Which person is considered healthy when referring to the Role Performance Model of Health?
 1. Coach who continues to coach after becoming a paraplegic
 2. Coal miner who retires after having acquired black lung disease
 3. Brick layer who takes a leave of absence while recovering from hernia surgery
 4. Policeman who begins selling alarm systems after leaving the police force because of being shot while on duty

29. Freedom from which situation demonstrates a safety and security need in Maslow's Hierarchy of Basic Human Needs?
 1. Pain
 2. Hunger
 3. Ridicule
 4. Loneliness

30. The nurse identifies that the stressful life event that has the greatest potential to contribute to stress-related illness is:
 1. Retirement
 2. Pregnancy
 3. Adoption
 4. Divorce

31. When considering the principles of stress and adaptation, the nurse understands that the word that best describes the concept of adaptive capacity is:
 1. Safety
 2. Health
 3. Restore
 4. Imbalance

32. The nurse is facilitating a support group for people who are coping with the death of a significant other. The nurse identifies that the patient behavior that most reflects complicated grieving is:
 1. Remarrying within six months after the death of a wife
 2. Being continuously angry three months after the death of a parent
 3. Keeping a child's room unchanged for years after the death of the child
 4. Displaying clinical symptoms of depression nine months after the death of a husband

33. The nurse identifies that love and belonging needs associated with Maslow's Hierarchy of Needs are related to which of Gordon's Functional Health Patterns?
 1. Values-belief pattern
 2. Role-relationship pattern
 3. Cognitive-perceptual pattern
 4. Sexuality-reproductive pattern

34. The nurse understands that the word that best describes the concept of adaptive capacity is:
 1. Role
 2. Cope
 3. Stimuli
 4. Energy

35. The nurse understands that a basic principle associated with Sigmund Freud and his work is that:
1. The reality principle reflects man's need for immediate gratification
2. Defense mechanisms are a common means of conscious coping
3. No human behavior is accidental
4. The Id controls the personality

36. A concept that nurses need to appreciate about health is that:
1. Perceptions of health vary among cultures
2. To be considered healthy a person needs to be productive
3. There must be an absence of illness for a person to be considered healthy
4. Underlying consensus exists among theorists about the definition of health

37. When assessing a patient's behavioral responses to stress from the Freudian perspective, the nurse understands that conflicts that arise from inner impulses are dealt with through:
1. Free association
2. Ego differentiation
3. Developmental tasks
4. Defense mechanisms

38. An immobilized patient develops a pressure ulcer. The nurse identifies that the type of stressor that precipitated the ulcer is:
1. Microbiological
2. Physiological
3. Chemical
4. Physical

39. Which are examples of a health belief? Check all that apply.
1. _____ Eating foods that are low in fat
2. _____ Accepting positive results of diagnostic tests
3. _____ Concluding that illness is the result of being bad
4. _____ Recognizing that smoking can cause lung cancer
5. _____ Respecting a patient's decision regarding therapeutic treatment

40. Kübler-Ross' theory on grieving is a process that progresses through stages to final acceptance. List these patient statements in order according to Kübler-Ross' theory on grieving.
1. "I am going to get a second opinion."
2. "I find it so hard to think about the fact that I don't have long to live."
3. "I've never smoked in my life. I shouldn't be the one with lung cancer."
4. "I'll have the chemotherapy because I want to see my children grow up."
5. "I don't want a big funeral because I want people to remember me and be happy."
Answer: _______________

ANSWERS AND RATIONALES

1. 1. Difficulty sleeping is a common adaptation to stress, but it is not life threatening. Although it can contribute to fatigue, it is not as serious a concern as one of the other options offered.
   2. **Impaired immunity is a serious threat caused by prolonged periods of stress. Stressors elevate blood cortisone levels, which decrease anti-inflammatory responses, deplete energy stores, lead to a state of exhaustion, and decrease resistance to disease.**
   3. This is a physiologic indicator of stress. However, it is not as serious a concern as one of the other options offered.
   4. When stressed, the patient's parasympathetic nervous system precipitates a decrease in intestinal peristalsis. Constipation is a concern, but it is not as serious as one of the other options offered.

2. 1. This statement characterizes the anger, not denial, stage in the grieving process. During the anger stage the person may vent hostile feelings or displace these feelings on others through acting out behaviors.
   2. This statement characterizes the bargaining, not denial, stage of the grieving process. During bargaining the person may put personal affairs in order, visit friends and relatives, and make final living arrangements for surviving family members.
   3. **This statement characterizes the denial stage of the grieving process. During denial the person is not ready to believe that the loss is happening. In denial, the person may isolate one's self from reality or repress the discussion about the loss.**
   4. This statement characterizes the anger, not denial, stage of the grieving process. During the anger stage the person may question, "Why me when I did everything right?"

3. 1. **Adaptive capacity refers to the quality and quantity of resources one can draw on to regain balance after one is threatened. This process requires an individual to change consciously or unconsciously in the physical, emotional, mental, or spiritual dimension in an effort to achieve balance or homeostasis.**
   2. Etiology refers to the stressor or threat to homeostasis that stimulates a person to draw upon personal resources within the physical, emotional, mental, or spiritual dimension.
   3. Remission refers to the abatement or lessened intensity of the symptoms of a disease or illness, not adaptive capacity.
   4. Compliance refers to adherence to an established therapeutic action plan, not adaptive capacity.

4. 1. **Patient problems/needs can be ranked in order of ascending importance according to how important they are for survival using Maslow's Hierarchy of Needs as a framework. Maslow identifies five levels of human needs. A person must meet lower-level needs before addressing higher-level needs. Physiologic needs are first-level needs: air, food, water, sleep, shelter etc.; safety and security needs are second; love and belonging needs are third; self-esteem needs are fourth; and self-actualization is the fifth-level need.**
   2. Erikson's Developmental Theory is designed to identify a patient's developmental level, not Maslow's Hierarchy of Needs.
   3. Maslow's Hierarchy of Needs is not designed to identify a person's coping patterns in response to illness.
   4. Rosenstock's and Becker's Health Belief Models identify the relationship between health beliefs and the use of preventive actions to promote health, not Maslow's Hierarchy of Needs.

5. 1. Freud's Psychoanaytical Theory of Personality Development does not include the thought that human nature is essentially irrational. Piaget believed that humans are rational, not irrational, and that a person's goal is to master the environment.
   2. **Freud believed that libidinal or instinctual drives are the underlying stimulus for human behavior in an attempt to gain pleasure or satisfaction through the mouth, anus, or genitals.**
   3. Freud's Psychoanaytical Theory of Personality Development does not include the concept of universal moral principles internalized as standards of behavior. He believed that the Superego is the center of the conscience that monitors and influences the behavior of the Ego.
   4. Carol Gilligan, not Sigmund Freud, described the importance of not overlooking the concepts of caring and responsibility in moral development.

6. 1. This is not a healthy way to deal with childhood grieving. Children are perceptive and capable of recognizing that something is wrong, but may not know what questions to ask. By avoiding discussing the loss with the child, the child may feel afraid, lonely, or even abandoned.
2. The child's age, level of understanding, feelings, and fears will determine how much the child should engage in mourning rituals. Children should not be forced to attend mourning rituals nor should they be pushed aside in an attempt to protect them from pain because this can lead to feelings of abandonment, fear, or loneliness.
3. Beginning at the child's level of understanding is essential when preparing a child for the death of a grandparent. Because there is such a difference regarding how children of different ages view the concept of death, it is important to first assess the child's level of understanding.
4. No one should be told how to feel or behave when it comes to reacting to loss. Expression of diverse feelings is essential if a child is to cope with the loss of the grandparent or develop positive coping strategies to deal with loss later as an adult.

7. 1. Freud believed that the underlying stimulus for all behavior was sexuality; therefore, all behavior can be explained and understood.
2. Defense mechanisms are unconscious coping patterns that deny, distort, or reduce awareness of a stressful event in an attempt to protect the Ego from anxiety. People tend to act in ways that support their self-esteem or how they feel about themselves. Anxiety, being a threat to self-esteem, stimulates the use of defense mechanisms to protect the Ego.
3. The Superego, not the Id, is the part of the psyche that imposes a conscience. The Id is the source of instinctive and unconscious urges seeking gratification.
4. Freud believed that all behavior has meaning and that behavior is directly related to unconscious as well as conscious motivation.

8. 1. Although anger may be identified as an adaptation to stress, it is not the most common response to stress. Anger is more commonly and classically seen in Kübler-Ross' second stage of dying/grieving.
2. Denial is more commonly seen in Kübler-Ross' first stage of dying/grieving, not as the most common response to stress.
3. Anxiety is the most common response to all new experiences that serve as an emotional threat.
4. Depression is an extreme response to prolonged stress and is not the most common human response to stress.

9. 1. Stress can cause a change in a person's balanced state, which can cause positive or negative responses. When an adaptation is maladaptive it reflects ineffective coping, which leads to illness. However, adaptations that result in a balanced state or promote personal growth are considered positive responses.
2. Adaptations do not limit stressors, but are responses to stressors. Internal or external stimuli (stressors) precipitate a positive or negative response (adaptation) that attempts to restore balance. If balance is not achieved, the stress continues resulting in disease/illness.
3. Adaptation occurs as a response to a stressor. It is an ongoing process that is constant and dynamic and is essential to physical, psychosocial, spiritual and emotional well-being.
4. The nature of a stressor is only one factor that influences a person's ability to adapt. Adaptations are an attempt to seek balance and are based on many variables which include a person's available physiological, psychosocial, spiritual, and emotional resources as well as interactive factors, not just the nature of the stressor.

10. 1. This is the focus of the Role Performance Model of health and wellness. This model states that health is defined in terms of a person's ability to fulfill societal roles; if roles are met, people perceive themselves as healthy even if they have an illness.
2. This theory focuses on perceived threats, severity, benefits, barriers, cues to action, and self-efficacy, which all influence a person's "readiness to act" in response to a health threat; Rosenstock first proposed this model during the 1950s.
3. This is the focus of the Health Locus of Control Model. If the nurse knows that a patient is motivated by either internal or external forces, then the nurse can plan internal or external reinforcement training to motivate a patient toward better health.
4. This is the focus of the Health-Illness Continuum model of health and wellness. This model focuses on health being on one end of the continuum and illness being on the

other end. People move back and forth along the continuum based on their own perceptions with no distinct boundary between health and illness.

11. 1. Sigmund Freud stressed the importance of instinctual human urges driving human behavior. Sucking, swallowing, chewing, and biting all give an infant pleasure, comfort, and a feeling of safety. If these needs are not met, the personality can become fixated at the oral stage. The adult may have difficulty trusting others and engage in dysfunctional behaviors, such as drug abuse, smoking, overeating, alcoholism, and overdependent behavior.

2. Erik Erikson does not focus on oral gratification but rather on the infant's need to resolve the conflict of trust versus mistrust. Erikson expands on Freud's theory and emphasizes the importance of environment on personality development.
3. Jean Piaget's Cognitive Theory does not focus on oral gratification as being important to psychosocial growth. Piaget believed that humans are rational and that a person's goal is to master the environment. Mastery depends on a person's ability to assimilate, accommodate and adapt as one responds to new situations and knowledge.
4. Carl Jung created a model called Analytical Psychology that focused on introverted and extroverted personalities. Also, he developed the concept of *Persona*, how a person appears to others in contrast to whom he or she actually is.

12. 1. Because a particular need is met it does not mean that the person is physically or emotionally healthy. A person who is ill and in pain can be medicated for the pain. The person will no longer be aware of the pain because the need for comfort is met; however, the person will still be ill.

2. Maslow's Hierarchy of Needs ranks human needs in order of ascending importance, with the basic needs first, according to how important the needs are for survival. When a need is met to one's level of satisfaction, the person is no longer aware of the need and can move on to the next level.

3. In spite of unmet needs, many people are able to achieve the expectations they and others set regarding their role performance.
4. Maslow's Hierarchy of Needs Model does not address where on a health-illness continuum a person is placed before or after a need is met. A person can have a need met and still be either healthy or ill somewhere along the continuum.

13. 1. While a bounding pulse is a physiological response to stress, a rapid pulse, not a slow pulse, is a physiological response to the body's neurohormonal reaction to stress. During the alarm phase of the General Adaptation Syndrome the autonomic nervous system initiates the fight-or-flight response and releases large amounts of epinephrine and cortisone into the body which contribute to a rapid pulse.

2. Level of alertness is considered a psychosocial, not physiological, response to stress. In addition, there is an increase, not a decrease, in response time as a result of an increase in alertness and energy associated with the alarm phase of the General Adaptation Syndrome.
3. Concentration is considered a psychosocial, not physiological, response to stress. Concentration and level of alertness are enhanced, not reduced, during the fight-or-flight response of the autonomic nervous system when large amounts of epinephrine and cortisone are released into the body.
4. **Rapid, shallow breathing is a physiological adaptation associated with the fight-or-flight response of the autonomic nervous system when large amounts of cortisone and epinephrine are released into the body as a person perceives a threat.**

14. 1. Although waiting for the results of a biopsy is stressful, it is not as stressful as one of the other options offered.

2. Although being unable to control the course of illness is stressful, it is not as stressful as one of the other options offered.
3. **As the multiplicity of stressors increases, the harder it is for a person to cope. As each stress is added, the accumulated impact is greater than just the sum of each individual stressor.**
4. Relocation is stressful whether it is voluntary or involuntary. However, it is not as stressful as one of the other options offered.

15. 1. The Id will not guide a nurse to initiate an incident report because the Id is the source of instinctive and unconscious urges, not the center of the conscience.

2. The Ego seeks compromise between the Id and Superego and represents the psychologic aspect of the personality, not the center of the conscience.
3. Libido refers to the psychic energy derived from basic biological urges, not the center of the conscience.

4. **The Superego monitors the Ego. The Superego is concerned with social standards, ethics, self-criticism, moral standards, and conscience. If the nurse initiates an incident report, it is the Superego that directs the achievement of ego-ideal behavior. If the nurse does not initiate an incident report it is the Superego that criticizes, punishes, and causes a sense of guilt.**

16. 1. The General and Local Adaptation Syndromes involve automatic nonspecific responses that are not dependent on specific stressors. The body automatically responds in the same way physiologically regardless of the nature of the stressor.
2. **Adaptations to stress are both conscious and unconscious. In the General and Local Adaptation Syndromes automatic physiologic responses are not under conscious control. Adaptations, such as behavioral responses, are often under conscious control.**
3. Although an adaptation may become a secondary stressor, many do not.
4. Adaptations can be maladaptive and fail to help a person achieve balance or they can be positive and help a person achieve balance.

17. 1. A patient in the denial stage of grieving refuses to believe that the event is happening and is unable to deal with practical problems such as trying new therapies.
2. **A patient in the bargaining stage of grieving seeks to avoid the loss and will try new therapies to gain more time.**
3. A patient in the depression stage of grieving usually will acknowledge the reality and inevitability of the impending loss, grieve the loss of present relationships and future experiences, and may stop all but palliative therapy.
4. The patient in the acceptance stage of grieving comes to terms with the loss. The patient begins to detach from surroundings and supportive people and generally no longer has the emotional or physical energy to try new therapies.

18. 1. This does not meet needs on the physiologic level of Maslow's Hierarchy of Needs. Physiologic needs are related to having adequate air, food, water, rest, shelter, and the ability to eliminate and regulate body temperature.
2. **Choosing which color shirt to wear provides a person with the opportunity to make a choice and supports feelings of independence, competence, and self-respect, which all contribute to a positive self-esteem.**
3. This does not meet needs on the safety and security level of Maslow's Hierarchy of Needs. Safety and security needs are related to being and feeling protected in the physiologic and interpersonal realms.
4. This does not meet needs on the love and belonging level of Maslow's Hierarchy of Needs. Love and belonging needs are related to giving and receiving affection, attempting to avoid loneliness and isolation, and wanting to feel as though one belongs.

19. 1. **This action supports achievement of a goal in the Role-Relationship category.**
2. This action supports the achievement of a goal in the Health Perception/Health Management category, not the Role-Relationship category.
3. This action supports achievement of a goal in the Cognitive-Perceptual category, not the Role-Relationship category.
4. This action supports the achievement of a goal in the Value-Belief category, not the Role-Relationship category.

20. 1. **Pain initially is an adaptation to some previous primary stressor, threat, or stimuli. However, when pain stimulates additional responses in an effort to manage the pain, the pain becomes a secondary stressor.**
2. Cold weather is a primary physical stressor, not an adaptation to some previous stressor.
3. Death of a spouse is a primary psychosocial stressor, not an adaptation to some previous stressor.
4. Ingested microorganisms is a primary microbiological stressor, not an adaptation to some previous stressor.

21. 1. Safety and security needs are not just before self-esteem needs on Maslow's Hierarchy of Needs. Safety and security needs are second-level needs and self-esteem needs are fourth-level needs.
2. **Belonging and love needs are directly below self-esteem needs on Maslow's Hierarchy of Needs. Belonging and love are third-level needs and self-esteem needs are fourth-level needs.**
3. Physiologic needs are not just before self-esteem needs on Maslow's Hierarchy of Needs. Physiologic needs are first-level needs and self-esteem needs are fourth-level needs.

4. Self-actualization needs are after, not before, self-esteem needs on Maslow's Hierarchy of Needs Model. Self-actualization is a higher-level need then self-esteem needs, therefore, self-esteem needs should be met before self-actualization needs.

22. 1. Not all models of health agree with this view of health. For example, the Clinical Model has a narrow interpretation which views health as the absence of signs and symptoms of disease or injury. Well-being is a subjective perception of energy and vigor. A person able to carry out daily tasks, interact successfully with others, manage stress and emotions, strive for continued growth and who has meaning or purpose in life has a sense of well-being, regardless of the severity of disease or infirmity.
2. Not all definitions of health identify that a person is able to control factors that affect health. The Adaptive Model is one of the few that addresses a person's ability to use purposeful adaptive responses and processes in response to internal and external stimuli to achieve health.
3. **There is little consensus about any one definition of health, wellness, and illness. However, all definitions of health, wellness, and illness address the fact that there are a number of factors that influence health.**
4. Not all definitions of health define health in terms of an individual's ability to fulfill societal roles. For example, the Clinical Model views people from the perspective of a physiologic system with related functions with health being the absence of disease or injury.

23. 1. A person with a changed marital status may experience several stressors but probably not be at as great a risk for developing an illness as a person in one of the other options.
2. A teenage mother may experience several stressors but probably not be at as great a risk to develop an illness as a person in one of the other options.
3. A single-parent family may experience several stressors but probably not be at as great a risk to develop an illness as a person in one of the other options.
4. **People living on the street most likely have a multiplicity of stressors in many different categories that places them at the greatest risk for developing an illness. For example, physiologic (poor nutrition and sleep patterns), physical (exposure to heat and cold), psychologic (fear of being a target for assault, robbery and abuse, lack of family support, and possible history of mental or emotional illness), economic (inadequate or no income), developmental (inability to complete developmental tasks), chemical (dependence on drugs, alcohol, and cigarettes), and microbiologic (exposure to pathogens from living on the street and not having access to adequate bathing and toileting environments).**

24. 1. A sunburn is an adaptation to the ultraviolet rays of the sun which is a physical, not a physiologic, stressor. Once the person has a sunburn, the sunburn is a physiologic stressor.
2. Diarrhea after eating contaminated food is an adaptation to a microbiologic, not a physiologic, stressor.
3. **Shortness of breath is an adaptation to the physiologic stress of walking up a hill. The body is reacting via physiological mechanisms to take in more oxygen to meet the oxygen demand of cells when walking.**
4. The threat or stressor is the final examination, a psychologic, not a physiologic, stressor. The rapid heart rate during a final examination is a physiological adaptation to a psychological stressor.

25. 1. Self-actualized people are autonomous, independent, self-directed, and governed from within.
2. Self-actualized people are friendly and loving. They respect themselves and others and seek out the good in others.
3. Self-actualized people are accurate in predicting future events, highly creative, open to new ideas and have superior perception. All these qualities contribute to problem-solving abilities.
4. **An external locus of control least describes self-actualized people. People with an external locus of control respond to rewards or recognition that come from outside the self. People who are self-actualized strive to develop their maximum potential based on motivation from within.**

26. 1. Where people place themselves on the health-illness continuum is a self-perception of their status in relation to health and illness. From their perspectives they cannot be healthy and ill at the same time.
2. **Health and illness are on opposite ends of the health-illness continuum and there is no distinct boundary between health and illness. Only a person can place her/himself somewhere along the health-illness continuum based on one's own**

perceptions about what constitutes health and illness.

3. Variables, such as genetic makeup, race, gender, age, lifestyle, risk factors, culture, environment, standard of living, support system, spiritual beliefs, and emotional factors, may be in balance and individuals view themselves at the extremes of the continuum or they may be out of balance and view themselves in the center of the continuum.
4. Only the Eudaemonistic Model of Health incorporates the concept of actualization or realization of a person's potential as the major component of a definition of health.

27. 1. The Ego is associated with mediating instinctual drives, social prohibitions, and reality and is not concerned with self-satisfaction.
2. **The Libido refers to the psychic energy derived from basic biologic urges. Desire for sex, life, pleasure, and satisfaction are attributed to the Libido.**
3. Fixation is the inability of the personality to develop to the next stage as a result of unresolved anxiety and is not the source of the pleasure principle.
4. The Superego monitors the Ego. The Superego is concerned with social standards, ethics, self-criticism, moral standards, and conscience, not achievement of self-satisfaction.

28. 1. **According to the Role-Performance Model of Health, as long as a person can perform work associated with societal roles, even if a person is limited physically, the person is considered healthy. A coach who continues coaching, even though ill or disabled, is considered healthy in light of the Role-Performance Model of Health.**
2. If a person retires because of illness, the person has not met society's expectation in terms of role performance and, therefore, is considered unhealthy in light of the Role-Performance Model of Health.
3. According to the Role-Performance Model of Health, a person who cannot fulfill responsibilities associated with one's job is considered sick. Therefore, a person who takes a leave of absence from work to recover is someone who is considered unhealthy in this model.
4. A strict interpretation of the Role-Performance Model of Health will most likely describe a policeman who changes jobs because of a physical or emotional inability to continue as unhealthy. Even though the former policeman is still a wage earner, it is not in the same job.

29. 1. **According to Maslow's Hierarchy of Needs, freedom from pain is considered a safety and security need. Confusion sometimes occurs because other theorists, such as R.A. Kalish, believe that pain should be categorized along with adequate air, food, water, rest/sleep, shelter, elimination, and temperature regulation as a first-level physiologic need.**
2. According to Maslow's Hierarchy of Needs, freedom from hunger is considered a first-level physiologic need, not a safety and security need.
3. According to Maslow's Hierarchy of Needs, freedom from ridicule is associated with self-esteem needs, not safety and security needs.
4. According to Maslow's Hierarchy of Needs, freedom from loneliness is associated with the need to feel loved and to belong, not to feel safe and secure.

30. 1. According to the Social Readjustment Rating Scale by Holmes and Rahe, retirement is ranked 10th on the list of life events likely to cause stress-related illness with a life-change-unit score of 45 out of 100. Retirement is considered less stressful than one of the other options offered.
2. According to the Social Readjustment Rating Scale by Holmes and Rahe, pregnancy is ranked 12th on the list of life events likely to cause stress-related illness with a life-change-unit score of 40 out of 100. Pregnancy is considered less stressful than two other options offered.
3. According to the Social Readjustment Rating Scale by Holmes and Rahe, the gaining of a new family member is ranked 14th on the list of life events likely to cause stress-related illness with a life-change-unit score of 39 out of 100. All of the other options are considered more stressful than gaining a new family member.
4. **According to the Social Readjustment Rating Scale by Holmes and Rahe, divorce is ranked 2nd on the list of life events likely to cause stress-related illness with a life-change-unit score of 73 out of 100. Only death of a spouse, ranked 1st on the scale with a score of 100, is considered more stressful than divorce.**

31. 1. Safety refers to a basic human need, not adaptive capacity.

2. Health refers to a relative state of a person at a particular moment in time in the physical, emotional, spiritual, and mental dimensions, not adaptive capacity.
3. **Adaptive capacity refers to the physical, emotional, mental, and spiritual resources one can draw on to reestablish or restore one's previous state or original condition.**
4. Imbalance occurs when a person is threatened by a stressor. Adaptive capacity refers to the physical, emotional, mental, and spiritual resources one can draw on to seek to correct the imbalance and return to a state of homeostasis.

32. 1. Moving on with one's life is a sign of successful grieving. Mourning periods may be abbreviated if the loss is replaced immediately by another equally respected person or if the person experienced anticipatory grieving, which is grieving experienced before the death.
2. Being continuously angry three months after the death of a parent is within the realm of expected grieving behavior and is not complicated grieving. If a person is continuously angry after one year, it is considered complicated grieving.
3. **Keeping a deceased child's room unchanged for years is outside the usual limits of grieving. Often a person can get stuck in a stage of grieving and is unable to progress to the next stage. Keeping a room unchanged for years reflects an inability to face the reality of the loss or to deal with the feelings associated with the loss.**
4. Depression of this length is not uncommon, particularly if the relationship was meaningful, intense, or no one was able to fill the role of the deceased. If depression does not resolve within a year after the death, it is considered complicated grieving.

33. 1. Love and belonging needs identified in Maslow's Hierarchy of Needs are not associated with Gordon's Value-Belief Pattern category. Gordon's Value-Belief Pattern category addresses topics such as spiritual distress and well-being, not love and belonging needs.
2. **Love and belonging needs identified in Maslow's Hierarchy of Needs are associated with Gordon's Role-Relationship Pattern category. Gordon's Role-Relationship Pattern category addresses topics such as social issues, loneliness, and relationships among family members and others.**
3. Love and belonging needs identified in Maslow's Hierarchy of Needs are not associated with Gordon's Cognitive-Perceptual Pattern category. Gordon's Cognitive-Perceptual Pattern category addresses topics such as comfort, confusion, conflict, knowledge deficit, disturbed thought processes and sensory perception, not love and belonging needs.
4. Love and belonging needs identified in Maslow's Hierarchy of Needs are not associated with Gordon's Sexuality-Reproduction Pattern category. Gordon's Sexuality-Reproduction Pattern category addresses topics such as altered sexuality patterns and dysfunction, not love and belonging needs.

34. 1. Role refers to a characteristic behavior in response to expectations of others or oneself, not adaptive capacity.
2. **Cope refers to an attempt to contend with or overcome some threat or stress, which directly depends on a person's potential or lack of potential to respond to a stress or threat. A person's potential or lack of potential to respond to a stress or threat is referred to as a person's adaptive capacity.**
3. The word stimuli refers to the stressor portion of the stress and adaptation relationship, not the adaptation portion of the relationship. Adaptive capacity refers to the adaptation portion of the stress and adaptation relationship.
4. Although all body activities require energy, including one's ability to adapt, one of the other three options is more clearly and directly related to the concept of adaptive capacity than is the word energy.

35. 1. The reality principle is a learned Ego function whereby a person is able to delay the need for pleasure rather than seek immediate gratification.
2. Defense mechanisms are unconscious, not conscious, coping patterns that deny, distort, or reduce awareness of a stressful event in an attempt to protect the personality from anxiety.
3. **Freud believed that all behavior has meaning and called this theory *psychic determinism*. He believed that every psychic event is determined by prior events. Behavior, mental phenomena, and even dreams are not accidental, but rather an expression of thoughts, feelings, or**

needs that have a relationship to the rest of a person's life.

4. The Ego, not the Id, controls the personality. The Ego mediates the urges of the Id and the conscience of the Superego and is therefore the part of the psyche that controls the personality.

36. 1. **Every individual is influenced by family, ethnic, and cultural beliefs and values. These beliefs and values influence a person's lifestyle through how one perceives, experiences, and copes with health, illness, and disability. The nurse needs to assess the impact of these influences on the patient's health and health practices.**
2. Only in the Role-Performance Model of Health is productivity or performance of one's role a necessary component to be considered healthy. While important to understand, it is a narrow definition of health and fails to include the multitude of other factors that impact on a definition of health.
3. Absence of disease or injury is the foundation of the Clinical Model of Health and fails to include the multitude of other factors that impact on a definition of health.
4. Health cannot be easily measured or defined in common terms. There is no consensus on a definition of health, because health is unique to each individual and is based on personal expectations and values.

37. 1. Free association, the free expression of thoughts or feelings just as they come to mind, is not a protective mechanism that is used in everyday life. It is a psychoanalytical technique used during therapy to lower a patient's defenses.
2. R. Peck proposed three developmental tasks during old age. Ego Differentiation versus Work-Role Preoccupation is the developmental task associated with adjusting to retirement from meaningful work. Individuals need to replace work roles with new roles that are a source of self-esteem.
3. Developmental Task Theory is attributed to R. J. Havighurst and is unrelated to Freud's Psychoanalytical Theory of Personality Development. According to Havighurst, developmental tasks associated with each age group are the source of conflict, not adaptations in an attempt to reduce anxiety.
4. **Defense mechanisms are unconscious coping techniques that deny, distort, or reduce awareness of a stressful event in an attempt to protect the Ego from anxiety.**

38. 1. Pressure is not a microbiological stressor. Microbiological stressors precipitate infection.
2. Pressure is not a physiological stressor. Physiological stressors are disturbances in structure or function of any tissue, organ, system, or body part.
3. Pressure is not a chemical stressor. Chemical stressors are drugs, poisons, and toxins.
4. **The force of pressure is a physical stressor. Pressure is the continuous force of a body part on a surface as a result of gravity; compression of tissue occurs between a bony prominence and the surface on which the body part is resting. This force is external to the body. The pressure ulcer which is the adaptation becomes a secondary stressor which is then physiologic in nature.**

39. 1. Eating foods low in fat is a health practice, not a health belief. A health behavior, such as eating a low-fat diet, reflects the belief that preventive measures will minimize risk factors that contribute to disease/illness.
2. Accepting positive results of diagnostic tests reflects a behavior in response to good news, rather than a behavior reflecting a health belief.
3. **This is an example of a health belief. A health belief is a conviction or opinion that influences health-care practices or decisions. If a person believes that illness is the result of being bad, the patient may feel the need to suffer in silence as a form of penance.**
4. **This is an example of a health belief. If a person believes that smoking cigarettes can cause lung cancer, then the person may refrain from smoking.**
5. Respecting a patient's decision is not an example of a health belief. It reflects the nurse's acceptance of a patient as a unique individual and recognizes the patient's right to make personal choices about one's own health care.

40. **Answer: 1, 3, 4, 2, 5**
1. **This statement reflects "doctor shopping," which is a form of denial, the first stage of Kübler-Ross' theory on grieving. The patient is experiencing shock and disbelief.**

3. **This statement reflects the anger stage, the second stage of Kübler-Ross' theory on grieving. The patient is aware of the reality of the situation and is resentful and angry.**
4. **This statement characterizes the bargaining stage, the third stage of Kübler-Ross' theory on grieving. The patient is negotiating for more time.**
2. **This statement reflects depression, the fourth stage of Kübler-Ross' theory on grieving. The patient is grieving over what is happening and what will never be.**
5. **This statement characterizes acceptance, the fifth stage of Kübler-Ross' theory on grieving. The patient has accepted the inevitable and is looking toward the future.**

Legal Issues

KEYWORDS

The following words include English vocabulary, nursing/medical terminology, concepts, principles, or information relevant to content specifically addressed in the chapter or associated with topics presented in it. English dictionaries, nursing textbooks, and medical dictionaries such as *Taber's Cyclopedic Medical Dictionary*, are resources that can be used to expand your knowledge and understanding of these words and related information.

Accountability
Accreditation
Act of commission/omission
Advanced directives
Do Not Resuscitate
Health-Care Proxy
Power of Attorney
American Nurses Association Standards of Nursing Practice
Americans With Disabilities Act
Assault
Autonomy
Autopsy
Battery
Beneficence
Breach of Duty
Certification
Civil law
Code of Ethics
Collective bargaining
Common law
Confidentiality
Constitution of United States
Contract
Contractual relationship
Controlled Substance Acts
Controlled substances
Crime
Criterion, Criteria
Death certificate
Defamation
Defendant
Defense
Disciplinary action
Document
Duty
Ethics
Euthanasia
False imprisonment
Federal legislation
Fidelity
Fraud
Functions of the nurse
Dependent
Independent
Interdependent
Futility
Good Samaritan Law
Health-Care Quality Improvement Act
Incident Report
Incompetent
Informed Consent
Invasion of privacy
Joint Commission on Accreditation of Healthcare Organizations (JCAHO)
Justice
Liability
Libel
Licensure
Litigation
Living Will
Malpractice
National Council Licensing Examinations (NCLEX)
National League for Nursing
National League for Nursing Accrediting Commission
Negligence
Nonmaleficence
North American Nursing Diagnosis Association (NANDA)
Nurse Practice Act
Occupational Safety and Health Acts
Organ donation
Patient's Bill of Rights
Plaintiff
Professional liability insurance
Professional misconduct
Public law
Quality of life
Reciprocity
Registration
Res ipsa loquitur
Respondeat superior

Risk management program
Sigma Theta Tau
Slander
Standards of care
State Board of Nursing
State legislation
Statutory law
Sue
Supreme Court
Testify
Tort
Veracity
Voluntary
Will
Witness

QUESTIONS

1. Licensure of Registered Professional Nurses is required primarily to protect:
1. Nurses
2. Patients
3. Common law
4. Health-care agencies

2. Which factor is unique to malpractice when comparing negligence and malpractice?
1. The action did not meet standards of care
2. The inappropriate care is an act of commission
3. There is harm to the patient as a result of the care
4. There is a contractual relationship between the nurse and patient

3. A patient falls while getting out of bed unassisted. When completing an Incident Report, the nurse understands that its main purpose is to:
1. Ensure that all parties have an opportunity to document what happened
2. Help establish who is responsible for the incident
3. Make data available for quality control analysis
4. Document the incident on the patient's chart

4. When the nurse administers a drug that has PRN after the order, the nurse functions:
1. Collegially
2. Dependently
3. Independently
4. Interdependently

5. A main purpose of the American Nurses Association is to:
1. Establish standards of nursing practice
2. Recognize academic achievement in nursing
3. Monitor educational institutions granting degrees in nursing
4. Prepare nurses to become members of the nursing profession

6. The nurse says, "If you do not let me do this dressing change, I will not let you eat dinner with the other residents in the dining room." This is an example of:
1. Assault
2. Battery
3. Negligence
4. Malpractice

7. State legislatures are responsible for:
1. Standardized care plans
2. Enactment of Nurse Practice Acts
3. Accreditation of educational nursing programs
4. Certification in specialty areas of nursing practice

8. The nurse should be aware of legal principles associated with nursing practice. Therefore, the nurse should understand that related to the doctrine of *respondeat superior*:
1. Nurses must respond to the Supreme Court when they commit acts of malpractice
2. Health-care facilities are responsible for the negligent actions of the nurses whom they employ
3. Nurses are responsible for their actions when they have contractual relationships with patients
4. The laws absolve nurses from being sued for negligence if they provide inappropriate care at the scene of an accident

9. When attempting to administer a 10:00 PM sleeping medication, the nurse assesses that the patient appears to be asleep. What should the nurse do?
1. Withhold the drug
2. Notify the physician
3. Awaken the patient to administer the drug
4. Administer it later if the patient awakens during the night

10. It is important for the nurse to be aware that the role of the American Nurses Association Standards of Nursing Practice is to:
1. Establish criteria for quality practice
2. Define the philosophy of nursing practice
3. Identify the legal definition of nursing practice
4. Determine educational standards for nursing practice

11. The physician asks the nurse to witness an informed consent. The nurse understands that a patient who is unable to give an informed consent for surgery is a:
1. 16-year-old boy who is married
2. 35-year-old woman who is depressed
3. 50-year-old woman who does not speak English
4. 65-year-old man who has received a narcotic for pain

12. When the nurse is administering a medication to a confused patient, the patient says, "This pill looks different from the one I had before." What should the nurse do?
1. Ask what the other pill looked like
2. Check the original medication order
3. Explain the purpose of the medication
4. Encourage the patient to take the medication

13. The nurse administers an incorrect dose of a medication to a patient. The nurse understands that the primary purpose of documenting this event in an Incident Report is to:
1. Record the event for future litigation
2. Provide a basis for designing new policies
3. Prevent similar situations from happening again
4. Ensure accountability for the cause of the accident

14. The physician writes an order for a medication that is larger than the standard dose. What should the nurse do?
1. Inform the supervisor
2. Give the drug as ordered
3. Discuss the order with the physician
4. Give the average dose of the medication

15. When the nurse attempts to administer a medication to a patient, the patient refuses to take the medication because it causes diarrhea. The nurse provides teaching about the medication, but the patient continues to adamantly refuse the medication. What should the nurse do first?
1. Document the patient's refusal to take the medication
2. Notify the practitioner of the patient's refusal to take the medication
3. Discuss with a family member the need for the patient to take the medication
4. Explain again to the patient the consequences of refusing to take the medication

16. A patient expresses the desire to commit suicide and asks the nurse for assistance. Based on the position of the American Nurses Association in relation to assisted suicide, the nurse should:
1. Not participate in active euthanasia
2. Participate based on personal values and beliefs
3. Participate when the patient is experiencing severe pain
4. Not participate unless two physicians are consulted and the patient has had counseling

17. Which is responsible for ensuring that Registered Nurses are minimally qualified to practice nursing?
1. Sigma Theta Tau
2. State Boards of Nursing
3. American Nurses Association
4. Constituent Leagues of the National League for Nursing

18. A nurse expert is called to testify in a lawsuit regarding professional nursing malpractice primarily to testify:
1. About standards of nursing care as they apply to the facts in the case
2. With regard to laws governing the practice of nursing
3. For the prosecution
4. For the defense

19. The nurse initiates a visit from a member of the clergy for a patient. When the nurse makes this call, the nurse is functioning:
1. Interdependently
2. Independently
3. Dependently
4. Collegially

20. A patient is asked to participate in a medical research study. The nurse describes to the patient and family members how the patient is protected by the:
1. Code of Ethics
2. Informed Consent
3. Nurse Practice Act
4. Constitution of the United States

21. The nurse is implementing an ordered bowel preparation for a patient who is scheduled for a colonoscopy. The nurse understands that the most serious consequence associated with an ineffective bowel preparation is:
1. Discomfort
2. Misdiagnosis
3. Wasted expense
4. Psychological stress

22. The physician orders OOB for a patient. When the nurse moves this patient out of bed to a chair, the nurse is working:
1. Dependently
2. Independently
3. Collaboratively
4. Interdependently

23. A Registered Nurse witnesses an accident and assists the victim who has a life-threatening injury. To meet the most important standard of acting as a Good Samaritan at the scene of an accident, the nurse should:
1. Stay at the scene until another qualified person takes over
2. Seek consent from the injured party before rendering assistance
3. Implement every possible critical-care intervention necessary to sustain life
4. Insist on helping because a nurse is the best qualified person to provide care

24. The graduate of an accredited Registered Nurse program understands that licensure to practice as an RN is:
1. Granted upon graduation from a nursing program
2. A standard of the American Nurses Association
3. Approved by the National League for Nursing
4. Required by state law

25. When considering legal issues the term "contract" is to "liable" as "standard" is to:
1. Rights
2. Negligence
3. Malpractice
4. Accountability

26. An anxious patient repeatedly uses the call bell to get the nurse to come to the room. Finally the nurse says to the patient, "If you keep ringing, there will come a time I won't answer your bell." This is an example of:
1. Slander
2. Assault
3. Battery
4. Libel

27. The nurse is informed that a credentialing team has arrived and is in the process of assessing quality of care delivered at the hospital. The nurse understands that the organization associated with the credentialing of the hospital is:
1. NCLEX
2. JCAHO
3. ANA
4. NLN

28. A patient asks the nurse, "What is a Living Will?" The nurse should respond that it is a document that:
1. Instructs a physician to withhold/withdraw life-sustaining procedures if death is near
2. Enables a person to request medication to end life in a humane and dignified manner
3. Gives consent to perform life-sustaining medical intervention during an emergency
4. Wills one's organs to help others who need a transplant to sustain life

29. A student nurse is about to graduate from an accredited nursing program. The student nurse understands that an action unrelated to a State Nurse Practice Act is:
1. Setting guidelines for nurses' salaries in the state
2. Establishing reciprocity for licensure between states
3. Determining minimum requirements for nursing education
4. Maintaining a list of nurses who can legally practice in the state

30. The nurse changes a patient's dry sterile dressing. When the nurse performs this task, the nurse is working:
1. Interdependently
2. Collaboratively
3. Independently
4. Dependently

31. The nurse must administer a medication. What should the nurse do first?
1. Determine the appropriateness of the medication
2. Ensure the medication is in the medication cart
3. Check the patient's identification armband
4. Verify the physician's order for accuracy

32. When choosing a nursing school in the United States that awards an associate degree, a future student nurse should consider schools that have met the standards of nursing education established by which organization?
1. National League for Nursing Accrediting Commission
2. North American Nursing Diagnosis Association
3. American Nurses Association
4. Sigma Theta Tau

33. The patient's diet order is "clear liquids to regular as tolerated." When the nurse progresses the diet to full liquid, the nurse is working:
1. Dependently
2. Independently
3. Collaboratively
4. Interdependently

34. A patient is scheduled to have surgery and informed consent is to be obtained. Place these steps in the order in which they should performed.
1. The patient is willing to sign the consent voluntarily
2. The patient signs the consent in the presence of the nurse
3. The physician informs the patient of the risks and benefits of the procedure
4. The nurse determines that the patient is alert and competent to give consent

Answer: ______

35. Identify the actions that are examples of slander. Check all that apply.
1. _____ Volunteer telling another volunteer a patient's age
2. _____ Nurse explaining to a patient that another nurse is incompetent
3. _____ Personal care assistant sharing information about a patient with another patient
4. _____ Unit Manager documenting a nurse's medication error in a performance appraisal
5. _____ Housekeeper who is angry at a nurse erroneously telling another staff member that the nurse uses cocaine

ANSWERS AND RATIONALES

1\. 1. Licensure does not protect the nurse. Licensure grants an individual the legal right to practice as a Registered Nurse.
   2. **Licensure indicates that a person has met minimal standards of competency, thus protecting the public's safety.**
   3. Licensure does not protect common law. Common law comprises standards and rules based on the principles established in prior judicial decisions.
   4. Licensure does not protect health-care agencies. The Joint Commission on Accreditation of Healthcare Organizations (JCAHO) determines if agencies meet minimal standards of health-care delivery, thus protecting the public.

2\. 1. There is a violation of standards of care with both negligence and malpractice.
   2. Negligence and malpractice both involve acts of either commission or omission.
   3. The patient must have sustained injury, damage, or harm with both negligence and malpractice.
   4. **Only malpractice is misconduct performed in professional practice, where there is a contractual relationship between the patient and nurse, which results in harm to the patient.**

3\. 1. The nurse who identifies or creates the potential or actual harm completes the Incident Report. The report identifies the people involved in the incident, describes the incident, and records the date, time, location, actions taken, and other relevant information.
   2. Documentation should be as factual as possible and avoid accusations. Questions of liability are the responsibility of the courts.
   3. **Incident reports help to identify patterns of risk so that corrective action plans can take place.**
   4. The report is not part of the patient's medical record, and reference to the report should not be made in the patient's medical record.

4\. 1. Collegial or collaborative interventions are actions the nurse carries out in conjunction with other health-care team members.
   2. Dependent interventions are those activities carried out under a practitioner's direction and supervision.
   3. Independent interventions are those activities the nurse is licensed to initiate based on knowledge and expertise.
   4. **An interdependent intervention requires a practitioner's order associated with a set parameter. The parameter, *whenever necessary*, requires that the nurse use judgment in implementing the order.**

5\. 1. **The American Nurses Association has established Standards of Care and Standards of Professional Performance. These standards reflect the values of the nursing profession, provide expectations for nursing practice, facilitate the evaluation of nursing practice, and define the profession's accountability to the public.**
   2. Sigma Theta Tau, the international honor society of nursing, recognizes academic achievement.
   3. The National League for Nursing Accrediting Commission, the Commission on Collegiate Nursing Education, and State Education Departments monitor educational institutions granting degrees in nursing.
   4. Schools of nursing (diploma, associate degree, and baccalaureate) educate individuals for entry into the practice of nursing.

6\. 1. **This statement is an unjust threat. Assault is the threat to harm another person without cause.**
   2. This is not an example of battery. Battery is the actual willful touching of another person that may or may not cause harm.
   3. This is not an example of negligence. Negligence occurs when harm or injury is caused by an act of either commission or omission.
   4. This is not an example of malpractice. Malpractice is negligence by a professional person as compared with the actions of another professional person in a similar circumstance when a contract exists between the patient and nurse.

7\. 1. Nursing team members or an interdisciplinary team of health-care providers write standardized care plans.
   2. **Every state has its own Nurse Practice Act that describes and defines the legal boundaries of nursing practice within the state.**

3. The National League for Nursing Accrediting Commission, the Commission on Collegiate Nursing Education and State Education Departments are the major organizations accrediting nursing education programs in the United States.
4. The American Nurses Association and other specialty organizations offer certification in specialty areas in nursing practice.

8. 1. This is unrelated to *respondeat superior.* Negligence and malpractice, which are unintentional torts, are litigated in local courts by civil actions between individuals.
2. The ancient legal doctrine *respondeat superior* means *let the master answer*. By virtue of the employer-employee relationship, the employer is responsible for the conduct of its employees.
3. Individual responsibility is unrelated to *respondeat superior.* A nurse can have an independent contractual relationship with a patient. When a nurse works for an agency, the contract between the nurse and patient is implied. In both instances, the nurse is responsible for the care provided.
4. This is unrelated to *respondeat superior*. Good Samaritan laws do not provide absolute immunity.

9. 1. This is a violation of the practitioner's order. Drug administration is a dependent nursing function.
2. This is unnecessary.
3. Administering a medication is a dependent function of the nurse, and the order should be followed as written if the order is reasonable and prudent. This medication was not a PRN medication but rather a standing order.
4. The drug should be administered as ordered, not at a later time.

10. 1. The ANA Standards of Clinical Nursing Practice describe the nature and scope of nursing practice and the responsibilities for which nurses are accountable.
2. A philosophy incorporates the values and beliefs about the phenomena of concern to a discipline. The ANA Standards of Clinical Nursing Practice reflect, not define, a philosophy of nursing. Each nurse and nursing organization should define its own philosophy of nursing.
3. The laws of each state define the practice of nursing within the state.
4. Educational standards are established by accrediting bodies, such as the National League for Nursing Accrediting Commission, the Commission on Collegiate Nursing Education, and State Education Departments.

11. 1. Legally, individuals younger than 18 years old can provide informed consent if they are married, pregnant, parents, members of the military, or emancipated.
2. A depressed person is capable of making health-care decisions until proven to be mentally incompetent.
3. This person can provide informed consent after interventions ensure that the person understands the facts and risks concerning the treatment.
4. Narcotics depress the central nervous system including decision-making abilities. This person is considered functionally incompetent.

12. 1. This action by itself is unsafe because the patient is confused and the information obtained may be inaccurate.
2. This is the safest intervention because it goes to the original source of the order.
3. This intervention ignores the patient's concern. Although this ultimately may be done, it is not the priority action.
4. This action ignores the patient's statement and is unsafe without first obtaining additional information.

13. 1. Although documentation of an incident may be used in a court of law, it is not the primary reason for an Incident Report.
2. This is not the primary reason for Incident Reports. New policies may or may not have to be written and implemented.
3. Risk-management committees use statistical data about accidents and incidents to identify patterns of risk and prevent future accidents and incidents.
4. Although nurses are always accountable for their actions, accountability for the cause of an incidence is the role of the courts.

14. 1. It is unnecessary to call the supervisor in this situation.
2. This is unsafe for the patient and may result in malpractice.
3. Nurses have a professional responsibility to know or investigate the standard dose for medications being administered. In addition, nurses are responsible for their own actions regardless of whether there is a written order. The nurse has a responsibility to question and/or refuse

to administer an order that appears unreasonable.
4. Changing a medication prescription is not within the scope of nursing practice.

15. 1. **Withholding the medication and documenting the patient's refusal and why are the appropriate interventions. Patient's have a right to refuse care.**
2. Notifying the practitioner eventually should be done, but it is not the priority at this time.
3. Discussing the situation with a family member without the patient's consent is a violation of confidentiality.
4. The patient has been taught about the medication and adamantly refuses the medication. Further teaching at this time may be viewed by the patient as badgering.

16. 1. **Nursing actions must comply with the law, and the law states that euthanasia is legally wrong. Euthanasia can lead to criminal charges of homicide or civil lawsuits for providing an unacceptable standard of care.**
2. A nurse's beliefs, values, or moral convictions should not be imposed on patients.
3. Compassion and good intentions are not an acceptable basis for actions beyond the scope of nursing practice.
4. These factors do not permit a nurse to be involved with euthanasia.

17. 1. Sigma Theta Tau, the international honor society of nursing, recognizes academic achievement and leadership qualities, encourages high professional standards, fosters creative endeavors, and supports excellence in the profession of nursing.
2. **The National Council of State Boards of Nursing is responsible for the NCLEX examinations; however, the licensing authority in the jurisdiction in which the graduate takes the examination verifies the acceptable score on the examination.**
3. The American Nurses Association (ANA) is the national professional organization for nursing in the United States. It fosters high standards of nursing practice; it does not grant licensure.
4. The National League for Nursing is committed to promoting and improving nursing service and nursing education.

18. 1. **The American Nurses Association Standards of Nursing Practice are authoritative statements by which the national organization for nursing describes the responsibilities for which its practitioners are accountable. An expert nurse is capable of explaining these standards as they apply to the situation under litigation. These professional standards are one criterion that helps a judge or jury determine if a nurse committed malpractice or negligence.**
2. An expert nurse is not an expert in the law. The expert nurse's role is not to make judgments about the laws as they apply to the practice of nursing.
3. A nurse expert can testify for either the prosecution or the defense.
4. A nurse expert can testify for either the defense or prosecution.

19. 1. The nurse does not need a physician's order to make a referral to a member of the clergy. An interdependent intervention requires a practitioner's order associated with a parameter.
2. **The nurse is initiating the referral to the member of the clergy and is therefore working independently. Nurses are legally permitted to diagnose and treat human responses to actual or potential health problems.**
3. This action is within the scope of nursing practice. The nurse does not need a physician's order to make a referral to a member of the clergy.
4. The nurse can make a referral to a member of the clergy without collaborating with another professional health-care team member.

20. 1. A code of ethics is the official statement of a group's ideals and values. It includes broad statements that provide a basis for professional actions.
2. **Informed consent is an agreement by a client to accept a course of treatment or a procedure after receiving complete information necessary to make a knowledgeable decision.**
3. Nurse Practice Acts define the scope of nursing practice; they are unrelated to informed consent.
4. The Constitution of the United States addresses broad individual rights and responsibilities. The rights related to nursing practice and patients include the rights of privacy, freedom of speech, and due process.

21. 1. Although this may occur, it is not the most serious outcome of an inappropriate preparation for a colonoscopy.
2. **Fecal material in the intestines can interfere with the visualization, collection,**

and analysis of data obtained through a colonoscopy, resulting in diagnostic errors.

3. A test may have to be cancelled or performed a second time if the patient has an ineffective bowel preparation. Although this is a serious consequence, it is not life threatening.
4. Although this is a serious consequence, it is not life threatening.

22. **1. Determining the extent of activity desirable for a patient is within the physician's, not nurse's, scope of practice. Following activity orders is a dependent function of the nurse.**

2. The responsibility to determine a patient's activity level is not within the legal scope of nursing practice.
3. A physician works independently when determining a patient's desired activity level.
4. The nurse is following the physician's order to get the patient OOB. There are no restrictions or parameters in relation to the order. However, the nurse must use judgment before, during, and after a transfer if a patient's condition changes.

23. **1. When a nurse renders emergency care, the nurse has an ethical responsibility not to abandon the injured person. The nurse should not leave the scene until the injured person leaves or another qualified person assumes responsibility.**

2. Depending on the injured person's physical and emotional status, the person may or may not be able to consent to care.
3. When a nurse helps in an emergency, the nurse is required to render care that is consistent with care that any reasonably prudent nurse would provide under similar circumstances. The nurse should not attempt interventions that are beyond the scope of nursing practice.
4. A nurse should offer assistance, not insist on assisting, at the scene of an emergency.

24. 1. When a person graduates from a school of nursing, the individual receives a diploma that indicates completion of a course of study; the diploma is not a license to practice nursing.

2. The ANA Standards of Professional Performance do not address licensure. They only indicate that a nurse should maintain current knowledge and competency.
3. The National League for Nursing promotes nursing service and nursing education, it is not involved with licensure.
4. **The Nurse Practice Act in a state stipulates the requirements for licensure within the state.**

25. 1. Although patients have a right to receive care that meets appropriate standards, the word *right* does not have the same relationship to the word *standard* as the relationship between the words *contract* and *liable*.

2. The words *standards* and *negligence* do not have the same relationship as *contract* and *liable*. Negligence involves an act (of commission or omission) that a reasonably prudent person would not do.
3. The words *standards* and *malpractice* do not have the same relationship as *contract* and *liable*. Malpractice is negligence by a professional person.
4. ***Liable* means a person is responsible (accountable) for fulfilling a contract that is enforceable by law. *Accountable* means a person is responsible (liable) for meeting standards, which are expectations established for making judgments or comparisons.**

26. 1. This is not an example of slander, which is a false spoken statement resulting in damage to a person's character or reputation.

2. **This is an example of assault. Assault is a verbal attack or unlawful threat causing a fear of harm. No actual contact is necessary for a threat to be an assault.**
3. This is not an example of battery, which is the unlawful touching of a person's body without consent.
4. This is not an example of libel, which is a false printed statement resulting in damage to a person's character or reputation.

27. 1. In the United States, graduates of educational programs that prepare students to become Licensed Practical Nurses or Registered Professional Nurses must successfully complete the National Council Licensure Examination-PN (NCLEX-PN) and the National Council Licensure Examination-RN (NCLEX-RN) respectively as part of the criteria for licensure.

2. **The Joint Commission of Accreditation of Healthcare Organizations (JCAHO) evaluates health-care organizations' compliance with JCAHO standards. Accreditation indicates that the organization has the capabilities to provide quality care. In addition, federal and state regulatory agencies and insurance companies require JCAHO accreditation.**

3. The American Nurses Association (ANA) is the national professional organization for nursing in the United States. Its purposes are to promote high standards of nursing practice and to support the educational and professional advancement of nurses.
4. The National League for Nursing (NLN) fosters the development and improvement of nursing education and nursing service.

28. 1. **A living will provides specific instructions about the care the person does or does not want to receive, including withholding or withdrawing life-sustaining procedures.**
2. Euthanasia, the act of painlessly putting to death a person who is suffering, is against the law in most states.
3. When an individual cannot provide written or oral consent (express consent) during an emergency, care is provided under the concept of *implied consent*.
4. Under the Uniform Anatomical Gift Act and the National Organ Transplant Act in the United States, individuals 18 years or older may donate all or part of their bodies for education, research, advancement of science, therapy, or transplantation. Consent for organ donation usually is made via a signed organ donation card.

29. 1. **State Nurse Practice Acts define and regulate the practice of nursing within the state. The salary of nurses is determined through negotiations between nurses or their representatives, such as a union or a professional nursing organization, and the representatives of the agency for which they work.**
2. A state's Nurse Practice Act determines the criteria for reciprocity for licensure.
3. A state's Nurse Practice Act stipulates minimum requirements for nursing education.
4. A state's Nurse Practice Act defines the criteria for licensure within the state. The actual functions may be delegated to another official body such as a State Board of Nursing or State Education Department.

30. 1. The changing of a dry sterile dressing is an interdependent action by the nurse when the physician's order for wound care states: *Dry Sterile Dressing PRN*.
2. In this situation, the nurse is not working with other health-care professionals to implement a physician's order.
3. This intervention is not within the scope of nursing practice without a physician's order.
4. **A nurse is not permitted legally to prescribe wound care. The nurse needs a practitioner's order to provide wound care.**

31. 1. A nurse is legally responsible for the safe administration of medications; therefore, the nurse should assess if a medication order is reasonable. However, this is not the first step when preparing to administer a medication to a patient.
2. Although this may be done as a time-management practice, it is not the first step when preparing to administer a medication to a patient.
3. Although this action is essential for the safe administration of a medication to a patient, it is not the first step of this procedure.
4. **The administration of medications is a dependent function of the nurse. The physician's order should be verified for accuracy. The order must include the name of the patient, the name of the drug, the size of the dose, the route of administration, and the number of times per day to be administered.**

32. 1. **The National League for Nursing Accrediting Commission (NLNAC) is an organization that appraises and grants accreditation status to nursing programs that meet predetermined structure, process, and outcome criteria.**
2. The North American Nursing Diagnosis Association (NANDA) developed a constantly evolving taxonomy of nursing diagnoses to provide a standardized language that focuses on the patient and related nursing care.
3. The American Nurses Association (ANA) is the national professional organization for nursing in the United States. It does not accredit schools of nursing.
4. Sigma Theta Tau, the international honor society of nursing, recognizes academic achievement. It does not accredit schools of nursing.

33. 1. This dietary order has parameters that exceed a simple dependent function of the nurse.
2. Prescribing a dietary order for a patient is outside the scope of nursing practice.
3. Collaborative or collegial interventions are actions the nurse carries out in conjunction with other health-care team members.
4. **The physician's order implies a progression in the diet as tolerated. The nurse uses judgment to determine the**

time of this progression, which is an interdependent action.

34. Answer: 3, 4, 1, 2
   3. **It is the responsibility of the practitioner to provide all the information necessary to make a knowledgeable decision. Patients have a legal right to have adequate and accurate information to make informed decisions.**
   4. **Patients must be competent to sign a consent form. The patient must be alert, competent, and in touch with reality. Confused, sedated, unconscious, or minor patients may not give consent.**
   1. **Patients must give their consent voluntarily and without coercion.**
   2. **The health-care provider witnessing the signing of the consent must ensure to the genuineness of the signature.**

35. 1. This is a violation of the patient's right to confidentiality, not slander.
   2. **This is an example of slander. Slander is a false spoken statement resulting in damage to a person's character or reputation.**
   3. This is a violation of the patient's right to confidentiality, not slander.
   4. This is not slander because it is a written, not spoken, statement and it documents true, not false, information.
   5. **This is an example of slander. It is a malacious, false statement that may damage the nurse's reputation.**

Management and Leadership

KEYWORDS

The following words include English vocabulary, nursing/medical terminology, concepts, principles, or information relevant to content specifically addressed in the chapter or associated with topics presented in it. English dictionaries, nursing textbooks, and medical dictionaries, such as *Taber's Cyclopedic Medical Dictionary*, are resources that can be used to expand your knowledge and understanding of these words and related information.

- Accountability
- Accountable
- Alternatives
- Assignment
- Bureaucratic
- Case management
- Change theory
- Controlling
- Consensus
- Cooperation
- Creative
- Cyclical process
- Decision
- Delegate
- Directing
- Documentation
- Efficiency
- Empower
- Feedback
- Five Rights of Delegation
  - Right Task
  - Right Person
  - Right Communication
  - Right Time
  - Right Supervision
- Flexible
- Human resource management
- Incentives
- Job description
- Leadership
- Leadership styles – classic
  - Autocratic – directive
  - Democratic – participative, consultative
  - Laissez-faire – nondirective, permissive
- Leadership styles – contemporary
  - Charismatic leadership
  - Connective leadership
  - Transactional leadership
  - Transformational leadership
  - Shared leadership
- Linear process
- Managers – types
  - First-line managers
  - Unit managers
  - Middle managers
  - Nurse executives
- Motivation
- Network
- Organization
- Performance evaluation
- Power – types of
  - Expert
  - Influence
  - Legitimate
  - Referent
  - Reward
- Preceptor
- Primary nursing
- Problem solving
- Productivity
- Resistance
- Resource
- Resource management
- Role model
- Solution
- Subordinate
- Systems theory
- Table of Organization
- Time management
- Trial and error

QUESTIONS

1. A nurse manager is informed that a large number of patients will be admitted in response to a terrorist attack. Which type of leadership style is most appropriate in this situation?
   1. Collaborative
   2. Authoritarian
   3. Laissez-faire
   4. Democratic
2. The nurse manager is experiencing staff resistance when implementing change. To overcome resistance to change, the most important action by the nurse manager is to:
   1. Identify the reason for the resistance
   2. Restate the purpose of the change concisely
   3. Modify the objectives to appeal to more key people
   4. Emphasize the positive consequences of the change
3. Leadership's major focus is on:
   1. Inspiring people
   2. Creating change
   3. Controlling others
   4. Producing a product
4. The primary difference between effective leaders and managers is that managers have:
   1. Vision
   2. Charisma
   3. Confidence
   4. Responsibility
5. Which situation is most reflective of the saying, *A stitch in time saves nine*?
   1. Obtaining the vital signs for the patients on the unit at the same time
   2. Collecting equipment for a procedure before entering the room
   3. Delegating some interventions to the Licensed Practical Nurse
   4. Documenting the nursing care given every two hours
6. The Registered Nurse delegates a procedure to a Licensed Practical Nurse. This act of delegation is used primarily to:
   1. Create change
   2. Establish a network
   3. Improve productivity
   4. Transfer accountability
7. The nurse manager plans to provide feedback to a subordinate who needs a change in behavior. The best intervention by nurse manager should be to:
   1. Be assertive
   2. Explore alternatives
   3. Identify the unacceptable behavior
   4. Document the content of the counseling session
8. The main reason the nurse manager achieves a consensus when making a decision within a group is to:
   1. Explore possible alternative solutions
   2. Demonstrate that staff members are flexible
   3. Facilitate cooperative effort toward goal achievement
   4. Ensure the use of effective autocratic decision making
9. The nurse manager evaluates the performance of a subordinate. Which management function is being implemented by the nurse manager?
   1. Planning
   2. Directing
   3. Organizing
   4. Controlling

10. Which is most related to systems theory?
   1. End result
   2. Linear format
   3. Trial and error
   4. Cyclical process
11. An accurate assessment drives the rest of the steps of the nursing process. The nurse in charge understands that the management function that drives effective management is:
   1. Planning
   2. Directing
   3. Organizing
   4. Controlling
12. The nurse works independently when:
   1. Limiting fluids when a patient has an order for 1000 mL fluid restriction
   2. Assigning another nurse to administer medications
   3. Irrigating a patient's wound with normal saline
   4. Applying a warm soak on an infiltrated IV site
13. Which is most basic for a nurse new to a management position?
   1. Strong interpersonal communication skills
   2. Awareness of when to be confrontational
   3. Knowledge of the role of a change agent
   4. Recognition by peers as a leader
14. A unit manager mentors a new unit manager as part of orientation to the position. Which type of power is being used by the unit manager mentor?
   1. Influence
   2. Coercive
   3. Referent
   3. Expert
15. A nurse manager understands that there are "Five Rights of Delegation," right task, right person, right communication, right time, and right:
   1. Supervision
   2. Feedback
   3. Route
   4. Place
16. When attempting to create change, the nurse manager meets resistance. To overcome resistance to change, the nurse manager must first:
   1. Ensure that the planned change is within the current beliefs and values of the group
   2. Provide incentives to encourage commitment to the change
   3. Implement change in small steps rather than large steps
   4. Use informational power to ensure that goals are met
17. A nurse manager who values the importance of positive role modeling will:
   1. Counsel subordinates who fail to meet expectations
   2. Hold team meetings to review rules of the agency
   3. Review job descriptions with employees
   4. Follow the policies of the agency
18. When considering leadership styles, an "autocratic" leader is to "authoritarian" as a "democratic" leader is to:
   1. Directive
   2. Permissive
   3. Oppressive
   4. Consultative
19. A nursing-care delivery model based on case management is:
   1. Primary nursing
   2. Critical pathways
   3. Diagnostic Related Groups
   4. Patient classification system

20. Which statement is most significant in relation to the concept of change theory in the health-care environment?
    1. Weigh the risks and benefits
    2. The stages of change are predictable
    3. Change in activity results in positive outcomes
    4. A large change is easier to adapt to than multiple smaller changes

21. Several nurses complain to the nurse manager that one of the patient care aides constantly takes extensive lunch breaks. The nurse manager should:
    1. Convene a group meeting of all the patient care aides to review their responsibilities related to time management
    2. Talk with the patient care aide to explore the reasons for the behavior and review expectations
    3. Arrange a meeting with the nurses so that they can confront the patient care aide as a group
    4. Document the patient care aide's behavior and place it in the aide's personnel file

22. To ensure efficiency when managing the daily workload, the Registered Nurse should:
    1. Give care to a patient in isolation first
    2. Plan activities to promote nursing convenience
    3. Organize care around legally required activities
    4. Perform routine bed baths between breakfast and lunch

23. A supervisor communicates expectations about a task to be completed and then delegates the task. Which management function is being implemented by the supervisor?
    1. Planning
    2. Directing
    3. Organizing
    4. Controlling

24. A student nurse in the clinical area is given an appropriate patient assignment by the instructor. The student nurse should:
    1. Accept the role of leader of the patient's health team
    2. Complete the care indicated on the patient's plan of care
    3. Assume accountability for the tasks that are assigned by the instructor
    4. Help other students to complete their assigned tasks whenever necessary

25. Between 80% and 90% of a manager's day is spent:
    1. Planning
    2. Assessing
    3. Evaluating
    4. Communicating

26. Which statement is most significant in relation to the concept of change theory in the health-care environment?
    1. Barriers to change can be overcome by embracing new ideas uncritically
    2. Change generates anxiety by moving away from the comfortable
    3. Behaviors are easy to change when change is supported
    4. Change is most effective when spontaneous

27. A patient is to be discharged from the hospital. A discharge task the nurse can delegate to a nursing assistant is:
    1. Teaching the patient how to measure weight using a standing scale
    2. Obtaining the patient's temperature, pulse, and respiratory rate
    3. Determining if the patient knows how to measure fluid intake
    4. Demonstrating to the patient how to use a walker

28. Management's major focus is on:
1. Accomplishing an objective
2. Empowering others
3. Problem solving
4. Planning

29. A staff nurse must solve a complex problem. The nurse's most effective resource is the:
1. Organizational Chart of the institution
2. Nursing Procedure Manual
3. Unit's Nurse Manager
4. Nursing Supervisor

30. When delegating a specific procedure to a patient care aide, the aide refuses to perform the procedure. The nurse should first:
1. Assign the procedure to another patient care aide
2. Explain that it is part of the patient care aide's job description
3. Explore why the patient care aide refused to perform the procedure
4. Send the patient care aide to the procedure manual to review the procedure

31. When planning to apply for a new position within an agency, what is the first thing the nurse should do?
1. Review the job description
2. Provide at least 3 positive references
3. Identify if power is associated with the position
4. Locate the position on the agency's Table of Organization

32. The most important reason why a nurse aide must fully understand how to implement a delegated procedure is because the nurse aide must be able to:
1. Teach the procedure to another nurse aide
2. Explain the procedure to the patient
3. Complete the procedure safely
4. Perform the procedure quickly

33. The nursing team leader delegates a wound irrigation to a Licensed Practical Nurse (LPN). It has been a long time since the LPN performed this procedure. To ensure patient safety the nursing team leader should:
1. Verbally describe to the LPN how to perform the procedure
2. Have the LPN demonstrate how to perform the procedure
3. Assign another LPN to assist with the procedure
4. Delegate the procedure to another LPN

34. Which tasks should be delegated to a Registered Nurse? Check all that apply.
1. _____ Obtaining vital signs
2. _____ Providing discharge teaching
3. _____ Evaluating a patient's response to morphine
4. _____ Administering a cleansing enema to a patient
5. _____ Transporting a patient to the operating room for surgery

35. Lewin's planned change theory progresses through phases. Order these statements by the nurse manager as change moves through the process.
1. "Let's implement a pilot project next week."
2. "This is a new venture that should be exciting."
3. "I know it may be difficult but you are doing a great job."

Answer: _______________

ANSWERS AND RATIONALES

1. 1. Collaborative is not a classic leadership style. Collaborative refers to the democratic leadership style. Democratic leaders encourage discussion and decision making within the group, which requires collaboration, coordination, and communication among group members.
   2. **This is the most appropriate leadership style in a crisis when urgent decisions are necessary. In a crisis, one person needs to assume the responsibility for decisions. Autocratic leaders give orders and directions and make decisions for the group.**
   3. This leadership style is not appropriate in a crisis when urgent decisions are necessary. Laissez-faire leaders are nondirective and permissive, which allows for self-regulation, creativity, and autonomy but limits fast-acting efficiency.
   4. This leadership style is not appropriate in a crisis when urgent decisions are necessary. Democratic leaders encourage discussion and decision making within the group, which takes time.

2. 1. **This is essential to overcome resistance to change. There are many different reasons people resist change. Each person will respond to different strategies. There are four different types of interventions to overcome resistance: providing information; disproving currently held beliefs; maintaining psychological safety; and by administrating an order or command.**
   2. Although it is important to state the purpose of the change clearly and concisely, another option is a more important action that can be implemented by the nurse manager to overcome resistance to change.
   3. Modifying a goal compromises the integrity of the planned change. All ramifications associated with the change should be explored before beginning and all contingencies planned for so that modifying a goal will be unnecessary.
   4. Although emphasizing the positive consequences of the change might be done, another option is a more important action that can be implemented by the nurse manager to overcome resistance to change.

3. 1. **Leaders can inspire others with their vision and gain cooperation through their persuasion and communication skills (influence power), the respect others have for their knowledge and abilities (expert power), and their charisma and prior success (referent power).**
   2. Creating change is the major function of a change agent, not a leader. Change agents are often managers rather than leaders because managers have responsibility for ensuring that the work of the organization is done.
   3. Controlling others is a function of a manager, not a leader.
   4. Producing a product is a function of a manager, not a leader. The manager is responsible for ensuring that the work of the organization is done, and this often requires the development of such things as a policy or procedure, management reports, and work schedules.

4. 1. Effective leaders and managers both should have vision.
   2. Effective leaders and managers both should have charisma.
   3. Effective leaders and managers both should have confidence.
   4. **Managers, not leaders, have responsibility. Leaders can be formal or informal. Informal leaders are not assigned to direct others. They are viewed as leaders by the members of the group because of their experience, vision, charisma, confidence, expertise, or age.**

5. 1. Taking the vital signs of all the patients on the unit at the same time is called functional nursing and is unrelated to the adage in the question.
   2. **This action is an appropriate example of the adage, "A stitch in time saves nine." It means that if you sew a tear when it is small, you need less stitches and time to repair it than when it is large. The same adage can be applied to the collection of equipment before a procedure. If the nurse has all the equipment that is needed before beginning a procedure, less time is used than when forgotten equipment is obtained later. Every time the nurse leaves the room for forgotten equipment, the patient is inconvenienced and time is wasted.**

3. Delegation is related to the efficient use of staff and is unrelated to the adage in the question.
4. This example is unrelated to the adage in the question.

6. 1. Delegation is unrelated to creating change. Delegation is the transfer of responsibility for the performance of a task to another while remaining accountable for the actions of the person to whom the task was delegated. Creating change is associated with responding to a stressor that is either planned or unplanned, which results in change that is positive or negative.
2. Delegation is unrelated to networking. Networking occurs when a person makes connections with others for sharing ideas, knowledge, information, and professional support.
3. Delegation allows the Registered Nurse to assign tasks to various individuals on the nursing team who are best qualified to complete the task. In today's health-care environment, nursing team members have different levels of educational preparation. The Registered Nurse must take into account the qualifications and scope of practice of each professional and nonprofessional nursing team member and assign tasks accordingly. When this is done, each person's skills and abilities are used most appropriately and productivity increases.
4. The person who is assigned a task is responsible for the outcome of the assigned task. However, the Registered Nurse delegating the task is not relieved of accountability but is responsible for the actions of the person to whom the task was delegated as well as the outcome of the intervention.

7. 1. The nurse manager can provide negative feedback in a manner that is firm without being assertive. Not yielding under pressure (firm) is less confrontational than being confident in a persistent way (assertive).
2. When providing negative feedback, the exploration of alternative solutions is performed later in the counseling session.
3. Feedback is essential to identify the problem. Problem recognition is the first step in the problem-solving process. Once the unacceptable behavior is identified and acknowledged, then the reasons for the problem can be explored, solutions suggested, and expectations reinforced.
4. Although this should be done, it is not feedback. Feedback is necessary for the nurse to recognize one's offending behavior. In addition, documentation is the last, not the first, step in the counseling process.

8. 1. Exploring possible alternative solutions occurs before achieving a consensus. A consensus is achieved when all, or most, agree or have the same opinion.
2. Consensus, not flexibility, is the goal. However, some members of the group may be flexible and change their opinion to ensure the achievement of a consensus.
3. Cooperation and teamwork is essential for the achievement of any goal. If a consensus is achieved about the value of the expected outcome, people are more likely to work together constructively.
4. Autocratic decision making does not seek a consensus when making a decision within a group. Autocratic leaders give orders and directions and make decisions for the group. There is little freedom within the group.

9. 1. Evaluating the performance of a subordinate does not fall under the planning function of management. Planning activities include assessment, problem identification, establishment of goals, planning interventions based on the priority identified, and how outcomes will be evaluated.
2. Evaluating the performance of a subordinate does not fall under the directing function of management. Directing activities involve getting the work accomplished and includes activities, such as assigning and communicating tasks and expectations, guiding and teaching, and decision making.
3. Evaluating the performance of a subordinate does not fall under the organizing function of management. Organizing activities include sharing expectations, identifying the chain of command, and determining responsibilities. In addition, since the manager is responsible for delegating tasks to subordinates, the manager is responsible for ensuring that policies and procedures clearly describe standards of care and expected outcomes.
4. The controlling function of management includes the evaluation of staff members. This is in addition to ensuring that plans are carried out and the outcomes evaluated.

10. 1. There is no end to a system. Individual parts of a system are interrelated and the whole system responds in an integrated way to changes within a part.
2. Systems do not function in a linear (straight-line) format. Systems are complex.
3. Trial and error is unrelated to Systems Theory. Trial and error is a problem-solving method whereby a number of solutions are tried until one is found that solves the problem.
4. Systems Theory is a cyclical process in which a whole is broken down into parts and the parts are studied individually as well as how they work together within the system. Every system consists of matter, energy, and communication. Because each part of a system is interconnected, the whole system reacts to changes in one of its parts. The concept of treating a patient holistically is based on an understanding of Systems Theory.

11. **1. Effective management depends on careful planning. Planning activities include deciding what is to be done, when to do it, where and how to do it, and who will do it and with what level of assistance. Planning is multifaceted and involves assessment, problem identification, establishment of goals, identifying interventions based on priorities, and how outcomes will be evaluated.**
2. Getting the work accomplished (directing) is associated with only one step in the management process.
3. Sharing expectations, identifying the chain of command, and determining responsibilities (organizing) are associated with only one step in the management process.
4. Ensuring that plans are carried out and the outcomes evaluated (controlling) is associated with only one step in the management process.

12. 1. Providing fluids based on a physician's order is a dependent, not independent, function of the nurse.
2. Delegating tasks within the scope of nursing practice is an independent function of the nurse and does not require a physician's order.
3. Wound care is a dependent function of the nurse and requires a physician's order.
4. Applying heat requires a physician's order and is a dependent function of the nurse.

13. **1. Strong communication skills are an essential competency of a nurse manager. Research demonstrates that 80% to 90% of a manager's day is spent communicating verbally and in writing. Managers need to express their thoughts clearly, concisely, and accurately.**
2. Although confrontation may be used occasionally, it can be learned as one socializes into the role of nurse manager and is not as important as a competency identified in another option.
3. Although knowledge of the role of change agent is important, it can be learned as one socializes into the role of nurse manager and is not as important as a competency identified in another option.
4. Recognition by peers as a leader is not as important as a competency identified in another option. A person generally is promoted to a management position because upper management recognizes leadership qualities. As a nurse manager grows into the role, peers will recognize the leadership ability of the nurse manager.

14. 1. This is not an example of influence power. Influence power is the use of persuasion and communication skills to exercise power informally without using the power associated with formal authority.
2. This is not an example of coercive power. The leader bases coercive power on the fear of the punitive withholding of rewards or retribution.
3. This is not an example of referent power. Referent power is associated with respect for the leader because of the leader's charisma and prior successes.
4. This is an example of expert power. Expert power is the respect one receives based on one's ability, skills, knowledge, and experience.

15. **1. The one who delegates a task is responsible for ensuring that the task is performed safely and according to standards of practice.**
2. Feedback is part of communication, which is one of the Five Rights of Delegation already cited in the stem of the question.
3. The right route refers to the Five Rights of Medication Administration, not the Five Rights of Delegation.
4. The right place is not one of the Five Rights of Delegation.

16. **1. Change that is consistent with current values and beliefs is easier to implement**

than change that is inconsistent with current values and beliefs. Values and beliefs are difficult to change.

2. This is not the priority intervention. Although incentives might motivate some individuals, it does not motivate all because some people have an internal rather than an external locus of control.
3. Although small steps are more effective than large steps because they are easier to achieve and once achieved are motivating, it is not the first thing the nurse should do to overcome resistance to change.
4. Although one person sharing explanations with another (informational power) is helpful when trying to change behavior, it is not the most effective type of power to use when trying to effect change. Another option identifies an action that the nurse should do first.

17. 1. Counseling subordinates who fail to meet expectations is not the best example of role modeling from the options offered.
2. Holding team meetings to review rules of the agency is not the best example of role modeling from the options offered.
3. Reviewing job descriptions with employees is not the best example of role modeling from the options offered.
4. **When the nurse manager follows policies and procedures, the manager is demonstrating the behavior that is expected. Role modeling is more effective than telling as a teaching strategy.**

18. 1. The word *directive* refers to the autocratic, not democratic, leadership style.
2. The word *permissive* refers to the laissez-faire, not democratic, leadership style.
3. *Oppressive* is the way some people refer to the autocratic, not democratic, leadership style. There is little freedom and a large degree of control by the autocratic leader, which frustrates motivated and professionally mature staff members.
4. **The word *consultative* is most closely related to the democratic leadership style. Democratic leaders encourage discussion and decision making within the group. The leader facilitates the work of the group by making suggestions, offering constructive criticism, and providing information.**

19. 1. **Primary nursing is a case management approach where one nurse is responsible for a number of patients 24 hours a day, 7 days a week. It is a way of providing comprehensive, individualized, and consistent nursing care.**
2. Critical pathways are not a nursing-care delivery model based on case management. Critical pathways are tools used in managed care that are sets of concurrent and sequential actions by nurses as well as other health-care professionals to achieve a specific outcome. They represent specific practice patterns in relation to specific medical populations.
3. Diagnostic Related Groups (DRGs) is not a nursing-care delivery model based on case management. Diagnostic Related Groups is a prospective reimbursement plan where patients are grouped based on medical diagnoses for the purposes of reimbursing the cost of hospitalization.
4. Patient classification systems are not a nursing-care delivery model based on case management. Patient classification systems are designed to assign an acuity level to patients based on their needs for the purpose of determining the number of nursing care hours required to provide care.

20. 1. **Risks and benefits must be carefully analyzed before initiating change. Some change is not worth the risk, because the consequences of failure are greater than the benefits.**
2. The stages of change are not always predictable. Although effective change moves through three zones—comfort, discomfort, and new comfort,—what happens in each stage is not always predictable and change is not always successfully achieved. Change is dynamic and the stages are not rigid.
3. Outcomes of change can be positive or negative. Sometimes well-planned change meets with resistance and the change effort can terminate in a loss of credibility, lack of achieving the goal, and confusion.
4. Smaller goals are much easer to achieve than a large goal. Smaller goals generally are designed to ensure achievement, which is motivating.

21. 1. It is the patient care aide who is late and takes extensive lunch breaks who needs to review the responsibilities related to time, not the patient care aides who follow the rules.
2. **Recognition of a problem is the first step in the problem-solving process. Once the unacceptable behavior is identified and acknowledged, then the reasons for the problem can be explored,**

solutions suggested, and expectations reinforced.

3. It is not the responsibility of others to confront the employee who is late for work and takes extensive lunch breaks. The employee reports to the nurse manager who is superior in the chain of command of the organization. The nurse manager should meet with the employee. In addition, counseling sessions with employees should be confidential and conducted in private.
4. This is premature. The nurse manager first needs to implement an action identified in another option.

22. 1. This may not be possible depending upon the needs of patients.
2. Patient needs are the priority, not the convenience of the nurse.
3. **Legally required activities must be accomplished because they are dependent functions that support the medical regimen of care. Although legally required activities should be accomplished first, many independent actions by the nurse also must be implemented to maintain a basic standard of care and patient safety. Some nursing interventions, which are not essential, can be implemented after the required activities.**
4. This may not be possible depending upon the needs of patients.

23. 1. This is not an example of the planning function of management. Planning involves assessment, problem identification, establishment of goals, designing interventions based on the priority identified, and how outcomes will be evaluated.
2. **This is an example of the directing function of management. Directing involves getting the work accomplished and includes activities, such as assigning and communicating tasks and expectations, guiding and teaching, and decision making.**
3. This is not an example of the organizing function of management. Organizing activities include sharing expectations, identifying the chain of command, and determining responsibilities. In addition, since the manager is responsible for delegating tasks to subordinates, the manager is responsible for ensuring that policies and procedures clearly describe standards of care and expected outcomes.
4. This is not an example of the controlling function of management. Controlling activities ensure that plans are carried out and the outcomes and staff are evaluated.

24. 1. Students are assigned to care for patients for a specific time period and generally are included as members, not leaders, of the nursing team.
2. Although students are expected to complete all planned care, the patient's condition can change or some unforeseen event may interfere with the plan. The student must keep the instructor or preceptor informed about the patient's condition, and use the instructor or preceptor as a resource person when the unexpected occurs or guidance is needed.
3. **Students are accountable for the tasks assigned by the instructor or preceptor. As part of accountability, students are obligated to keep the instructor or preceptor informed about the status of the patient, how the assignment is progressing, and whether all interventions are implemented as planned.**
4. Students should not help other students unless specifically assigned to do so by the instructor or preceptor. An exception occurs when assistance is needed to ensure patient safety in an emergency.

25. 1. Planning does not consume 80% to 90% of a manager's day.
2. Assessing does not consume 80% to 90% of a manager's day.
3. Evaluating does not consume 80% to 90% of a manager's day.
4. **Research demonstrates that this is true. Strong communication skills are an essential competency of a nurse manager. They communicate verbally and in writing and need to express their thoughts clearly, concisely, and accurately.**

26. 1. Before initiating change, barriers need to be anticipated and addressed. All aspects of the new idea are best accomplished when critically analyzed.
2. **Change causes one to move from the comfortable to the uncomfortable and is known as *unfreezing* in Lewin's Change Model. It involves moving away from that which is known to the unknown, from the routine to the new, and from the expected to the unexpected. The unknown, new, and unexpected can be threatening, which can increase anxiety.**
3. Behavior is not easy to change even when supported. Most people do not like to function in an unfamiliar environment. In addition,

change challenges one's comfort zone in each level of Maslow's Hierarchy of Needs.

4. Planned, not spontaneous, change is most effective because it is organized, systematic, and purposeful.

27. 1. Teaching requires the knowledge and judgment of a Registered Nurse. Teaching requires a complex level of interaction with the patient, problem solving, and innovation in the form of an individually designed teaching plan of care that addresses the specific learning needs of the patient. In addition, the outcome is unpredictable and it has the potential to cause harm if the skill is taught incorrectly.
2. **Obtaining vital signs can be delegated to a nursing assistant because it is not a complex task. It requires simple problem-solving skills and a simple level of interaction with the patient. Although this task has the potential to cause harm if the critical elements of the skill are not implemented appropriately, it is within the scope of practice of an unlicensed nursing assistant. It does not require the more advanced competencies of a Registered Nurse.**
3. Assessing a patient's level of understanding is a complex task that requires knowledge and judgment and is within the scope of practice of a Registered Nurse. This task requires a complex level of interaction with the patient, problem solving, and innovation in the form of an individually designed teaching plan of care that addresses the specific learning needs of the patient.
4. Teaching requires the knowledge and judgment of a Registered Nurse. Teaching requires a complex level of interaction with the patient, problem solving, and innovation in the form of an individually designed teaching plan of care that addresses the specific learning needs of the patient. In addition, the outcome is unpredictable and it has the potential to cause harm if the skill is taught incorrectly.

28. 1. **Although planning, problem solving, and empowering others are tasks of a manager, the bottom line is for the manager to accomplish the work of the organization.**
2. Although empowering others is one of the tasks of a manager, the major objective is identified in another option.
3. Although problem solving is one of the tasks of a manager, the major objective is identified in another option.
4. Although planning is one of the tasks of a manager, the major objective is identified in another option.

29. 1. The Organizational Chart schematically plots the reporting relationship of every position within the organization. It does not help a staff nurse identify a solution to a complex problem.
2. The Nursing Procedure Manual is not designed to help a staff nurse identify a solution to a complex problem. The Nursing Procedure Manual contains details of policies relative to nursing practice and nursing procedures along with the purpose and all the steps that one must follow to implement the procedure safely.
3. **Generally, in the chain of command of an organization the staff nurse works under the direction of and reports to the unit's nurse manager. The nurse manager generally is an experienced nurse and is the primary resource person for the staff nurse. The staff nurse should seek guidance from the nurse manager when assistance is needed to solve a complex problem.**
4. The nursing supervisor is higher up the chain of command in a Table of Organization than another employee who is the best person for the staff nurse to seek assistance from when needing help to solve a complex problem.

30. 1. Assigning the procedure to another staff member is premature. Another option has priority.
2. The employee may be fully aware of the requirements of the job description and not need to have them described. Even though a task is within one's job description, a person can refuse to perform a procedure because of a reason that is considered acceptable.
3. **This is the issue that the nurse manager needs to explore. The employee may have an acceptable reason for refusing to comply. When the reason is identified, then the nurse manager can take an informed action.**
4. The reason for refusal may have nothing to do with the lack of understanding of the procedure.

31. 1. **This is one of the most important actions by the nurse seeking a new position. The job description provides an overview of the requirements and responsibilities of the role. Job descriptions include factors, such as educational and experiential**

requirements, job responsibilities, subordinates to be supervised, and whom one reports to in the chain of command.

2. Requesting references protects the hiring agency, not the nurse. This is not the most important thing the nurse should do when applying for a new position within an agency.
3. Although understanding the power of the position may help a person meet the responsibilities associated with the job description, it is not the priority when applying for a new position.
4. Although it is important to recognize where the new position fits into the organization's Table of Organization, it is not the priority when applying for a new position. A Table of Organization schematically plots the reporting relationship of every position within the organization.

32. 1. Nurse aides are trained and supervised by the nurse, not other nurse aides.
2. Although this is important, it is not the priority.
3. **Safety of the patient is the priority. The nurse aide must perform only the skills that are within the legal role of the nurse aide, are understood, have been practiced, and have been performed correctly on a return demonstration.**
4. Although this may be desirable, it is not the priority.

33. 1. Providing just a verbal description is unsafe. This does not ensure that cognitive information can be converted to a psychomotor skill.
2. **Demonstration is the safest way to assess whether a person has the knowledge and skill to safely perform a procedure. A superior delegating care is responsible for ensuring that the person implementing the care is legally qualified and competent.**
3. A peer should not be held responsible for the care assigned to another team member. The Registered Nurse who delegates a procedure to a subordinate is directly responsible for ensuring that the care is safely delivered to patients.
4. This intervention does not address the original LPN's need to know how to perform the procedure safely. This procedure is within the legal scope of practice of a Licensed Practical Nurse.

34. 1. Taking routine vital signs is not complex, has little potential for harm, requires only simple problem-solving skills, involves a simple level of interaction with the patient, and is within the scope of practice of an unlicensed nursing assistant. It requires the more advanced competencies of a Registered Nurse only when previous vital signs have been outside the expected range.
2. **Discharge teaching requires the knowledge and judgment of a Registered Nurse. It requires synthesizing and summarizing information as well as coordinating a variety of community health-care services to meet patient needs.**
3. **Evaluation requires the knowledge and judgment of a Registered Nurse. The skill of evaluation requires reassessing, synthesizing and analyzing data, determining significance of data, and diagnosing and responding to the data. In addition, it involves an unpredictable outcome and requires problem solving that may call for innovation in the form of an individually designed plan of care to address the patient's need for pain relief if pain is still being experienced.**
4. Administering an enema is not a complex task. It requires simple problem-solving skills, involves a predictable outcome, and employs a simple level of interaction with the patient. Although this task has the potential to cause harm if the critical elements of the skill are not implemented, it is within the scope of practice of an unlicensed nursing assistant. It does not require the more advanced competencies of a Registered Nurse.
5. Transporting a patient is not a complex task. It requires simple problem-solving skills, involves a predictable outcome, and a simple level of interaction with the patient. Although this task has the potential to cause harm if the critical elements of the skill are not implemented, it is within the scope of practice of an unlicensed nursing assistant. It does not require the more advanced competencies of a Registered Nurse.

35. Answer: 2, 1, 3
2. **The first phase is called "unfreezing" and is concerned with identifying the need for change, exploring alternative solutions, and stimulating enthusiasm.**
1. **The second phase is called "moving/changing" and is concerned with creating actual visible change.**
3. **The third phase is called "refreezing" and is concerned with providing feedback, encouragement, and constructive criticism to reinforce new behavior.**

Health-Care Delivery

KEYWORDS

The following words include English vocabulary, nursing/medical terminology, concepts, principles, or information relevant to content specifically addressed in the chapter or associated with topics presented in it. English dictionaries, nursing textbooks, and medical dictionaries, such as *Taber's Cyclopedic Medical Dictionary*, are resources that can be used to expand your knowledge and understanding of these words and related information.

Access to health care
Acuity
Advocate
Baby boomers
Beliefs
Burnout
Career ladder
Case management, case manager
Comprehensive care
Continuity of care
Cost containment
Counselor
Critical pathways
Demographics
Diagnostic Related Groups (DRGs)
Functional nursing
Health-care professionals
- Activity Therapist
- Certified Social Worker
- Clinical Nurse Specialist
- Licensed Practical Nurse
- Nurse Anesthetist
- Nurse Assistant
- Nurse Midwife
- Nurse Practitioner
- Occupational Therapist
- Pastoral care provider
- Patient
- Patient's family members
- Physical Therapist
- Physician
- Physician's Assistant
- Registered Dietitian
- Registered Nurse
- Speech Therapist

Health-care settings
- Acute care – hospitals
- Adult day care
- Ambulatory care centers
- Assisted-living residence
- Clinics
- Extended care
- Home health services
- Hospice (inpatient, residential, in the home)
- Industrial or occupation settings
- Life-care community
- Long-term care – nursing homes
- Neighborhood community health center
- Physician's offices
- Psychiatric facilities
- Rehabilitation centers
- School settings
- Urgent visit centers

Health Maintenance Organization
Hospice
Indigent
Length of stay
Levels of health care
- Primary health care
- Secondary health care
- Tertiary health care

Levels of prevention
- Primary prevention
- Health promotion
- Health protection
- Preventive health services
- Secondary prevention
- Tertiary prevention

Managed care
Medicaid
Medicare
Metropolitan
Multidisciplinary
Patient classification system
Population
Poverty
Preauthorization
Preferred Provider Organization
Primary nursing
Prospective payment system
Provider
Reengineering
Reimbursement
Resource Utilization Groups (RUGs)

Rural
Sandwich generation
Socialized health care
Suburban
Surrogate
Third-party payers
Types of agencies
  Official – governmental
  Proprietary – for profit
  Voluntary – not for profit
Underserved population
Undocumented immigrants (aliens)
Urban

QUESTIONS

1. The nurse identifies and meets the health needs of a patient. Which word best describes this role of the nurse?
1. Teacher
2. Advocate
3. Surrogate
4. Counselor

2. The nurse is examining research results regarding receipt of health-care benefits in the United States. Which group of people is the most underserved?
1. Children
2. Older adults
3. Pregnant women
4. Middle-aged men

3. A patient with an infection receives medical intervention and nursing care in a hospital setting. Which level health-care service has been provided in this situation?
1. Emergency
2. Secondary
3. Tertiary
4. Primary

4. The nurse identifies that the cornerstone of *Nursing's Agenda For Health Care Reform* is:
1. A standardized package of health-care services must be provided by the federal government
2. Advanced practice nurses should play a prominent role in the provision of primary care
3. Services need to be provided in environments that are accessible, familiar, and friendly
4. Nursing must provide for the central focus for the health-care delivery system

5. A home health-care nurse is functioning as a Case Manager for a patient recently discharged from the hospital. What is the primary role of the nurse when functioning as a Case Manager?
1. Coordinator
2. Counselor
3. Provider
4. Teacher

6. Which is the best example of an inpatient care setting where nursing care is delivered?
1. Ambulatory care center
2. Extended-care facility
3. Day-care center
4. Hospice

7. Which change identified by the nurse will most affect health-care delivery in the United States in the future?
1. Less emphasis will be placed on prolonging life
2. The proportion of older adults in society will increase
3. More people will seek health care in an acute care setting
4. Genetic counseling will dramatically decrease the number of ill infants born

8. It is important for the nurse to understand that Diagnostic Related Groups mainly were instituted by the federal government to reduce the:
   1. Number of professionals working in hospitals
   2. Focus on illness and place it on prevention
   3. Fragmentation of care
   4. Cost of health care

9. What characteristic is unique to the nurse–patient relationship?
   1. Patient's needs are satisfied
   2. There is a social component
   3. The nurse is the leader of the team
   4. Both are working toward a common goal

10. A recently licensed Registered Nurse is working the night shift on an active medical unit in the hospital. What is the best thing this nurse can do to prevent professional burnout?
    1. Challenge the how and why of one's role
    2. Get adequate sleep and exercise each day
    3. Clarify expectations, strengths, and limitations
    4. Seek a balance among seriousness, humor, and aloofness

11. In the emerging health-care delivery system in the United States, a professional who can provide independent health care with third-party reimbursement is a:
    1. Licensed Registered Nurse
    2. Clinical Nurse Specialist
    3. Physician's Assistant
    4. Nurse Practitioner

12. The nurse understands that critical pathways in health care refer to:
    1. Educational career ladders for health-care professionals
    2. Multidisciplinary plans with predetermined patient outcomes
    3. Times during life when certain health problems are more likely to occur
    4. Organizations that provide services that progress from acute care to long-term care

13. The nurse understands that the setting that is the organizational center of the United States health-care system is the:
    1. Clinic setting
    2. Acute care setting
    3. Community setting
    4. Long-term care setting

14. The nurse is functioning as a direct caregiver for a patient with multiple health problems. Which word is most associated with the caregiver role of the nurse?
    1. Facilitate
    2. Evaluate
    3. Counsel
    4. Teach

15. When reviewing articles in health-care journals, the nurse identifies that a major trend in health care is that:
    1. Individuals and the family have primary responsibility for making health-care decisions
    2. Health-care providers control the direction and development of health-care services
    3. Striving for longevity will take on greater concern than quality-of-life issues
    4. Social issues are taking a back seat as a result of the advances in technology

16. The nurse is explaining mammography screening to a patient who is reluctant to have the diagnostic test. The nurse understands that this diagnostic test reflects which Level of Prevention?
    1. Secondary
    2. Tertiary
    3. Primary
    4. Acute

17. The nurse should begin rehabilitative care after the patient is:
    1. Conscious
    2. Diagnosed
    3. Discharged
    4. Ambulatory

18. Nurses should be role models for healthy living because nurses:
    1. Need to be as healthy as possible to fight invasion of pathogens
    2. Know that the immune system can be affected by an unhealthy lifestyle
    3. Recognize that patients often look at what nurses do rather than what they say
    4. Must be able to deal with the physiological demands of the profession of nursing

19. The nurse Case Manager is counseling an older adult patient about the resources available to assist with the cost of health care. The nurse should inform the patient that the majority of the health-care costs for people over 65 years of age is provided by:
    1. Medicare
    2. Medicaid
    3. Blue Cross
    4. Blue Shield

20. Which result of reengineering in hospital settings has raised the greatest concerns for patient safety?
    1. Decreased hospital occupancy rates
    2. Increased acuity of hospitalized patients
    3. Hospitals merging with larger institutions
    4. Substitution of less skilled workers for nurses

21. A patient is discharged from the hospital three days after abdominal surgery because of the influence of Diagnostic Related Groups (DRGs). The nurse performing the discharge teaching should be most concerned about:
    1. Providing for continuity of care
    2. Ordering equipment to be used in the home
    3. Accepting discharge by the patient and family
    4. Ensuring hospital reimbursement for services rendered

22. Together the nurse and patient are setting a goal during health-care planning. Which factor generates the most anxiety with this process?
    1. Change
    2. Beliefs
    3. Values
    4. Role

23. Three hospitals agree to work collectively to provide a full range of health-care services in their neighborhoods. What type of relationship has been entered?
    1. Integrated health-care service network
    2. Third-party reimbursement system
    3. Health Maintenance Organization
    4. Diagnostic Related Groups

24. The nurse is planning actions that address a patient's health-care needs. Which statement is most important for the nurse to consider?
    1. Health and illness clearly are separated at the middle of the Health-Illness Continuum
    2. Demographics of the population of the United States are changing drastically
    3. External factors mainly are the cause of most illnesses
    4. Most people view health as the absence of disease

25. The home care nurse is coordinating the delivery of health-care services to an older adult in the home. The nurse understands that the factor that most affects health-care delivery to the older-adult population is that older adults:
    1. Need the services of long-term care institutions
    2. Tend to fall, requiring expensive hospital services
    3. Suffer from significant cognitive deficits as they age
    4. Live below the economic poverty level, requiring financial assistance

26. Which nursing activity reflects care on the Primary Level of Health-Care Delivery?
    1. Arranging for hospice services
    2. Delivering care in a Coronary Care Unit
    3. Providing emergency care at a local hospital
    4. Encouraging attendance at a Smoke Enders' meeting

27. Which action is common to the majority of Registered Nurse positions in different settings in which nurses work?
    1. Serving in an administrative capacity
    2. Developing patient plans of care
    3. Providing direct physical care
    4. Assisting the physician

28. The nurse is planning a community outreach program about the variety of health-care professionals and the services they provide. The nurse should include that the largest group of health-care professionals in the United States is:
    1. Social workers
    2. Nurse aides
    3. Physicians
    4. Nurses

29. Nurses should understand that the major factor that prevents an overhaul of the health-care delivery system of the United States is the:
    1. Need for elected officials to respond to the pressure of political constituencies
    2. Explosion of technical advances within the profession of medicine
    3. Complexity of the problems associated with health-care reform
    4. Resistance of physicians to reform

30. Which is emphasized in the traditional health-care delivery system in the United States?
    1. Health promotion
    2. Illness prevention
    3. Diagnosis and treatment
    4. Rehabilitation and long-term care

31. At the end of a shift the nurse in charge must evaluate each patient in relation to the hospital's classification system. The nurse understands that a patient classification system is designed to:
    1. Document resource needs for the purpose of establishing reimbursement
    2. Provide data about patient acuity to help assign nursing staff
    3. Establish that quality standards have been met
    4. Identify standardized expected outcomes

32. The nurse identifies the major responsibilities of various health-care professionals and identifies that the person best prepared to track a patient's progress through the health-care system is the:
    1. Home Care Nurse
    2. Primary Nurse
    3. Case Manager
    4. Manager Nurse

33. The nurse is reviewing a variety of surveys regarding the delivery of health care within the United States. Which statement reflects a significant change in the thinking of the general public about concepts related to health-care delivery?
   1. "Institutional-based care will have to be increased as baby boomers age."
   2. "More services need to address the secondary health-care needs of the community."
   3. "Individuals can influence their own health through behavior and lifestyle changes."
   4. "Health-care providers should be charged with the primary responsibility to provide appropriate health-care services."

34. Nurses identify that the size of which group is the greatest challenge to the financing of health care in the United States?
   1. Undocumented immigrants
   2. Medically uninsured
   3. Preterm infants
   4. Older adults

35. A patient asks the nurse, "What is the difference between Medicare and Medicaid?" Which statement best describes the Medicaid program?
   1. A federally funded health insurance program for individuals with low incomes
   2. A United States' federal health insurance program for individuals aged 65 years or older
   3. A state program requiring physicians to be providers of care to people living below the designated poverty level
   4. A retrospective health-care reimbursement program that pays for the costs incurred by health-care agencies for the care of the indigent

36. The nurse is functioning as a patient advocate. What word best describes this nursing role?
   1. Provider
   2. Nurturer
   3. Protector
   4. Evaluator

37. A patient is told that preauthorization is required before surgery can be performed. The patient asks the nurse, "What does preauthorization mean?" The nurse's best response is, "It means:
   1. Third-party payers have approved the surgery and the facility will be reimbursed for costs."
   2. The preoperative checklist has been completed and verified by a nurse."
   3. Required preoperative diagnostic tests have been performed."
   4. You have signed the legal consent form for the surgery."

38. A patient is to return from the operating room to a semiprivate room. Before the transfer, the nurse should ensure that the patient's roommate is:
   1. Emotionally stable
   2. Able to communicate
   3. In the bed by the window
   4. Physiologically compatible

39. A patient receiving a special diet is given a meal tray that does not contain a food requested by the patient. What should the nurse do? Place these interventions in order of priority.
   1. Check the diet manual
   2. Verify the practitioner's diet order
   3. Schedule a conference with the dietitian
   4. Explore with the physician the possibility of including this food preference in the diet

   Answer: ______________

40. Which are examples of an official agency? Check all that apply.
   1. _____ Department of Health
   2. _____ American Heart Association
   3. _____ National League for Nursing
   4. _____ Nonprofit community hospital
   5. _____ Veterans Administration Hospital

ANSWERS AND RATIONALES

1. 1. The role of teacher is only one area of nursing practice; a word in another option has a stronger relationship with the role of the nurse when identifying and meeting the needs of the patient. Teaching is related only to helping patients learn about their health and health-care practices.
   2. **The role of advocate is the most important role of the nurse because in this role the nurse protects and supports patients' rights. Advocacy combines the roles of teacher, counselor, and leader so that the best interests of patients are protected, particularly when patients are most vulnerable.**
   3. The surrogate role is not a professional role of the nurse. A surrogate role is assigned to a nurse when a patient believes that the nurse reminds them of another person and projects that role and the feelings for the other person onto the nurse.
   4. The role of counselor is only one area of nursing practice and a word in another option has a stronger relationship with the role of the nurse when identifying and meeting the needs of the patient. Counseling is related only to helping a patient recognize and cope with emotional stressors, improve relationships, and promote personal growth.

2. 1. **In the United States, the current health-care system neglects the overall needs of children. One in 5 children lives in poverty and only half of these children receive Medicaid. One in 5 children does not have health insurance. More than 35% of preschool children are not immunized. In addition, children are vulnerable because they cannot be their own advocates.**
   2. Although older adults are a vulnerable population, they are not as underserved as a group in another option because of the availability of Medicare.
   3. Although pregnant women are a vulnerable population, they are not as underserved as a group in another option.
   4. Middle-aged men are the least underserved population of the options offered.

3. 1. Emergency care is not a level of care in the health-care system. Emergency care is a description of one type of service provided on the Secondary Health-Care level in the health-care system.
   2. **This is an example of the Secondary Health-Care level of the health-care system. Secondary Health Care is associated with intense and elaborate diagnosis and treatment of disease or trauma and includes critical care and emergency treatment. The Levels of Health Care should not be confused with Levels of Prevention. The health-care system has three Levels of Health Care that describe the scope of services and settings where health care is provided and includes Primary, Secondary, and Tertiary. The Levels of Prevention identify three levels of prevention that focus on health-care activities, such as Primary Prevention (avoiding disease through health promotion and disease prevention), Secondary Prevention (early detection and treatment), and Tertiary Prevention (reducing complications, rehabilitation, restoration, and maintenance of optimal function).**
   3. This is not an example of the Tertiary Health-Care level of the health-care system. Tertiary Health Care is associated with the provision of specialized services.
   4. This is not an example of the Primary Health-Care level of the health-care system. Primary Health Care is associated with early detection and routine care.

4. 1. Although this is a component of *Nursing's Agenda for Health Care Reform*, it is not the cornerstone of the document.
   2. Although this is a component of *Nursing's Agenda for Health Care Reform*, it is not the cornerstone of the document.
   3. **This is the cornerstone of *Nursing's Agenda For Health Care Reform*. All people have a right to receive health care, but this right is useless unless the care is easily reached and used.**
   4. Although this is a component of *Nursing's Agenda for Health Care Reform*, it is not the cornerstone of the document.

5. 1. **The primary role of a Case Manager is to coordinate the activities of all the other members of the health-care team and ensure that the patient is receiving care in the most appropriate setting.**
   2. Counseling is not the primary role of a Case Manager. When counseling, the nurse helps

a patient recognize and cope with emotional stressors, improve relationships, and/or promote personal growth.

3. Providing care is not the primary role of the Case Manager. When providing care, the nurse is in the direct caregiver role. Caregiving involves identifying and meeting the patient's needs by helping the patient regain health through the caring process.
4. Teaching is not the primary role of the Case Manager. When teaching, the nurse helps the patient learn about health and health-care practices.

6. 1. Ambulatory care centers are not an inpatient care setting. Although some may be located in a hospital, they are more often in convenient locations, such as a shopping mall or storefront. They provide services such as emergency walk-in care, ambulatory surgery, and health prevention and health promotion interventions.
2. **An extended-care facility is an inpatient setting where a client lives while receiving subacute medical, nursing, or custodial care. It includes facilities, such as intermediate care and skilled nursing facilities (nursing homes), assisted living centers, rehabilitation centers, and residential facilities for the mentally or developmentally disabled.**
3. Day-care centers are not examples of inpatient care settings. Day-care centers provide care for people who arrive in the morning and go home at the end of the day. They provide care for healthy children or older adults so that significant others can work or they provide specialized services to specific populations, such as individuals with cerebral palsy or mental health problems.
4. Although hospice services may be provided in a hospital, a nursing home, or residential hospice setting, the majority of hospice services are provided in the home. Hospice agencies provide multiple specialized services to support the dignity and quality of life of individuals who are dying and their family members.

7. 1. Although this remains to be seen, the explosion in knowledge and technology usually results in treatments that prolong life.
2. **The percentage of older adults in the United States is expected to increase to 22% by the year 2030. Fourteen percent of the 22% will be people over the age of 85. Because chronic illness is more prevalent among older adults, additional health-care services will be needed in the future, raising costs.**
3. More people will seek health care in the home and community, not the acute care setting. In 1992 the National League for Nursing predicted that home care will become the center of health care and that community nursing centers and community health programs will focus on illness prevention and health promotion.
4. This may or may not occur because of a multiplicity of factors, such as religious beliefs, unplanned pregnancies, and a lack of seeking genetic counseling.

8. 1. This is not the reason why DRGs were instituted. In addition, the DRGs have increased the acuity of hospitalized patients requiring a lower ratio of nurses to patients. However, many hospitals have not increased the numbers of nurses because of reengineering and the lack of available qualified nurses.
2. This is not the reason why DRGs were instituted. Although there is a current trend in the United States with more people focusing on health promotion and illness prevention, it is unrelated to DRGs.
3. DRGs were not instituted to solve fragmentation of care. Fragmentation of care generally is caused by overspecialization and caregivers failing to address patients' needs holistically and comprehensively.
4. **The DRGs, pretreatment diagnoses reimbursement categories, were designed to decrease the average length of a hospital stay, reducing costs.**

9. 1. Because of circumstances, a nurse's intervention may not always be able to meet a patient's perceived needs.
2. The nurse–patient relationship is a therapeutic, not social, relationship.
3. The patient, not the nurse, is the leader of the health team.
4. **When planning patient care, the nurse and patient work together to identify appropriate goals and interventions to facilitate goal achievement.**

10. 1. How one practices nursing and why one is a nurse are based on enduring values and beliefs. Although it is important to be aware of how one practices nursing and why one is a nurse, confronting, taking exception to, and calling into question one's enduring values is not where the problem of burnout lies. Burnout generally occurs because nurses are

unable to practice nursing as they were taught based on principles and standards of practice. Nurses experience stress because of such factors as understaffing, increased patient care assignments, shift work, excessive mandatory overtime, inadequate support, and caring for more patients who are critically ill and dying.

2. Although it is important to reduce the effects of stress, these approaches do not reduce the contributing factors that cause stress.
3. **When faced with any stressful situation that can lead to feelings of burnout, the nurse must begin with self-awareness and identify personal expectations, strengths, and limitations associated with the job. After the assessment is complete and problems are identified, the nurse can explore options to reduce factors contributing to job-related stress. The nurse needs to employ strategies to manage stress to prevent the physical and emotional exhaustion associated with burnout and not wait until these responses occur.**
4. Although humor may temporarily defuse a stressful situation, it is not an effective strategy to cope with the major issues that contribute to burnout. The nurse should not be distant from the patient.

11. 1. Licensed Registered Nurses do not receive third-party reimbursement for their services.
2. Clinical Nurse Specialists are not health-care professionals who receive third-party reimbursement. Clinical Nurse Specialists have been involved in health-care delivery since the 1960s. They are master's-prepared nurses with a specialty in areas, such as medical–surgical nursing, pediatrics, psychiatry, etc., or they may have advanced education and experience in caring for individuals with special needs, such as wound care, enterostomal care, or care of the patient with diabetes.
3. Physician Assistants are not health-care professionals who receive third-party reimbursement directly. They work under the supervision of a physician in many different settings and are paid by the physician in private practice or by the organization that hired them. They assist physicians by carrying out common, routine medical treatments and they have prescriptive authority.
4. **This is a relatively new trend in health-care delivery. Nurse Practitioners generally are master's-prepared individuals who work independently or collaboratively with physicians to provide primary health-care services. Nurse Practitioners work independently under their own license, are accountable for their own practice, have prescriptive authority, and receive third-party reimbursement, depending on the state in which they work. In the states that do not permit this level of health-care delivery, Nurse Practitioners work under the license of a physician who supervises their practice.**

12. 1. Critical pathways are not an educational career ladder for health-care professionals. A career ladder is the organization of educational experiences so that professional growth progresses in a planned manner.
2. **Critical pathways are a case management system that identifies specific protocols and timetables for care and treatment by various disciplines designed to achieve expected patient outcomes within a specific time frame.**
3. This is a definition of critical time, not critical pathways.
4. This is unrelated to critical pathways.

13. 1. The clinic setting is not the organizational center of the United States health-care system.
2. **The acute care setting is the organizational center of the United States health-care system today. Specialized services (tertiary level of care) and emergency, critical care, and intense diagnosis and treatment (secondary level of care) of illness and disease are provided for in hospitals (acute care setting). In 1991, the American Nurses Association published *Nursing's Agenda for Health Care Reform*, which made recommendations for health-care reform in many areas. The major trend identified as a result of implementation of the recommendations is a shift of the focus of health care from illness and cure to one of wellness and care. If this occurs, the health-care system of the United States will shift from the acute care setting to the home and community.**
3. The community setting is not the organizational center of the United States health-care system.
4. The long-term care setting is not the organizational center of the United States health-care system.

14. 1. **The caregiver role is associated with *facilitating* the achievement of goals identified in the patient's plan of care.**

2. Of the options offered, the word *evaluate* is not the word most associated with the nurse functioning as a caregiver. Although, evaluation is important in relation to the nursing process and caregiving, it is only one aspect of caregiving.
3. Of the options offered, the word *counsel* is not the word most associated with the nurse functioning as a caregiver. When counseling, the nurse helps a patient recognize and cope with emotional stressors, improve relationships, and/or promote personal growth and it is only one aspect of care giving.
4. Of the options offered, the word *teach* is not the word most associated with the nurse functioning as a caregiver. When teaching, the nurse helps the patient learn about health and health-care practices and it is only one aspect of caregiving.

15. 1. **The patient is the center of the health team and has primary responsibility for making health-care decisions. Consumers are more knowledgeable than ever before, have a greater awareness of health issues, and have a desire to be responsible for health-care decisions. In addition, more knowledgeable consumers (patients and families) have made a major impact on the delivery of health-care services in the United States because they have made their opinions and preferences known.**
2. Educated consumers, not health-care providers, control the direction and development of health-care services. Citizens are active members of the Boards of Trustees of health-care agencies in all settings, community organizations have political action committees that lobby government representatives to shape the political agenda, and the consumer movement with its demands and expectations all impact the direction of health-care reform.
3. Although some people strive to sustain life at any cost, most people prefer to seek ways to support and maintain quality, over longevity, of life. The hospice movement, which is increasing, is based on the concept of maintaining quality of life by caring for dying people in their homes surrounded by family and friends and making remaining days as comfortable and meaningful as possible.
4. Social issues are taking a front, not back, seat as a result of advances in technology. Technological advances and specialized treatments are extremely expensive. Social issues include who will pay for health-care costs, who has access to health care, and who will care for older adults and the uninsured (both of whom are increasing in numbers). In addition, ethical issues are becoming prominent in response to advances in areas such as transplant and beginning of life technology.

16. 1. **Screening surveys and diagnostic procedures are examples of Secondary Prevention. Secondary Prevention is associated with early detection, early and quick intervention, health maintenance, and prevention of complications. The Levels of Prevention identify three levels of prevention that focus on health-care activities, such as Primary Prevention (avoiding disease through health promotion and disease prevention), Secondary Prevention (early detection and treatment), and Tertiary Prevention (reducing complications, rehabilitation, restoration and maintenance of optimal function).**
2. This is not an example of Tertiary Prevention. Tertiary Prevention begins after a situation is stabilized and the focus is on rehabilitation and restoration within the limits of the disability.
3. This is not an example of Primary Prevention. Primary Prevention is associated with activities that promote health and protect against disease.
4. Acute is not one of the Levels of Prevention. The word acute refers to the type of care that is provided on the Secondary Care Level of the health-care delivery system.

17. 1. Rehabilitation interventions begin whether the patient is conscious or unconscious.
2. **As soon as a patient is diagnosed with a problem, rehabilitation interventions begin. Care should be present and future oriented.**
3. This is too late to begin rehabilitation interventions.
4. Rehabilitation interventions begin whether the patient is ambulatory or nonambulatory.

18. 1. Although this is a true statement, it does not explain why nurses need to be role models for healthy living.
2. Although this is a true statement, it does not explain why nurses need to be role models for healthy living.
3. **Congruity must exist between what nurses say and what they do. For nurses**

to be credible and attentive to the health needs of patients, nurses must work at maintaining their own health. By caring for themselves, nurses demonstrate values that they believe in and behaviors that support health and wellness. Actions speak louder than words.

4. Although this is a true statement, it does not explain why nurses need to be role models for healthy living.

19. **1. Virtually everyone in the United States over 65 years of age is protected by hospital, post-hospital extended care, and home health benefit insurance under Part A of Medicare. Patients pay a coinsurance of 20% and the other 80% is paid by the government.**

2. Medicaid is not a program that pays for the majority of health-care costs of people over 65 years of age. Medicaid is a United States federal program, that is state operated, that provides medical assistance for people with low incomes.
3. Blue Cross is a not-for-profit medical insurance plan that pays for hospital services for people of all ages, not just people over 65 years of age.
4. Blue Shield is a not-for-profit medical insurance plan that pays for care provided by health-care professionals for all age groups, not just for people over 65 years of age.

20. 1. Reengineering has not reduced hospital occupancy rates. Decreased hospital occupancy rates are related directly to Diagnostic Related Groups and the resultant decrease in lengths of stay. The concerns about a decrease in occupancy rates are not related to patient safety, but rather fiscal issues.

2. Reengineering has not increased patient acuity in the hospital setting. Although the increased acuity of hospitalized patients is a real concern when providing for patient safety, safety should not be an issue if a unit is adequately staffed with the appropriate mix of nurses to ancillary staff.
3. Reengineering does not precipitate hospital mergers. Hospital mergers and the resulting reengineering should not impact on patient safety if professional practice standards are maintained.
4. **Reengineering is concerned with training a less educationally prepared nursing assistant to implement nursing tasks that were formerly associated with the practice of nursing. This trend poses a serious threat to the safety and welfare of patients because tasks requiring the complex skills of a nurse are being delegated to minimally prepared individuals. This is dangerous in the present health-care environment where hospitalized patients are more acutely ill than ever before.**

21. **1. Providing for continuity of care is the major concern with early discharge as a result of DRGs. It requires careful planning to ensure that services, personnel, and equipment are provided in a timely and comprehensive manner and care is not fragmented and disorganized.**

2. Although this is a concern for some individuals, if the discharge planner plans early for the patient's discharge, all equipment should be in place before the patient is discharged.
3. Although this is a concern for some individuals, if patients receive supportive emotional intervention and are prepared for discharge from the first day of admission, patients will generally rather be at home than in the hospital.
4. Hospitals are pleased when they are able to discharge a person earlier than the designated length of stay indicated by the DRGs because the hospital keeps the unused portion of the DRG reimbursement.

22. **1. Change almost always causes anxiety because it requires one to move from that which is comfortable and familiar to that which is uncomfortable, unfamiliar, unpredictable, and threatening.**

2. A belief is an opinion or a conclusion that one accepts as true and may be based on either faith and/or facts and should not generate anxiety. People generally set health-care goals that do not conflict with their beliefs.
3. A value is an enduring attitude about something that is cherished and held dear to one's heart and should not generate anxiety. People generally set health-care goals that do not conflict with their values.
4. A role is a set of expectations about how one should behave. Although a health-care goal may conflict with a role one sets for oneself, another option has greater ability to contribute to anxiety than one's role.

23. **1. This is an example of an integrated health-care service network. Hospitals are joining networks to decrease costs and increase reimbursement. This is accomplished by expanding the breadth of services while avoiding duplication of services, keeping clients within the network, negotiating**

the price of supplies and equipment, and centralizing departments which results in fewer personnel (i.e., administration, staff education, and human resource departments, etc.).

2. This is not an example of a third-party reimbursement system. Third-party reimbursement refers to when someone other than the receiver of health care (generally an insurance company) pays for the services provided.
3. This is not an example of a Health Maintenance Organization (HMO). An HMO is an organization that provides primary health care for a preset fee.
4. The DRGs are pretreatment diagnoses reimbursement categories designed to decrease the average length of a hospital stay, reducing costs.

24. 1. There is no clear separation between health and illness on the Health-Illness Continuum. Each individual's personal perceptions of multiple factors determine where a person places himself/herself on the Health-Illness Continuum.
2. **Demographics are changing rapidly in the United States as we become a heterogeneous, multicultural, multiethnic society. Because of the increasing diversity of the population of the United States, nurses need to use transcultural knowledge in a skillful way to provide culturally appropriate, competent care.**
3. Internal as well as external factors are the cause of illness.
4. Most people do not view health as the absence of disease. There is no one definition of health because there are so many different factors that impact on one's definition of health. Therefore, a definition of health depends on each individual person's own perspective.

25. 1. Approximately only 4.5% of adults 65 years or older live in a nursing home. Ninty-one percent of adults 65 years or older live alone or with a spouse.
2. **Studies report that one-third of older adults 75 years of age and older experience at least 1 fall each year; falls have become the leading cause of injury deaths for older adults.**
3. Although older adults may take more time to process and respond to information, only approximately 5% to 7% of adults over 65 years of age experience dementia.
4. The percentage of older adults below the designated poverty level is less than 9.8% and is declining.

26. 1. This is an example of care associated with the Tertiary Level of Health-Care Delivery. Tertiary care is associated with long-term, chronic, and hospice care and specialized services.
2. This is an example of care on the Secondary Level of Health-Care Delivery. Secondary care (acute care) includes emergency treatment, critical care, and care associated with intensive and elaborate diagnosis and treatment.
3. This is an example of care on the Secondary Level of Health-Care Delivery. Secondary care (acute care) includes emergency treatment, critical care, and care associated with intensive and elaborate diagnosis and treatment.
4. **This is an example of the Primary Level of Health-Care Delivery. Primary care is associated with activities that promote health and protect against disease. The health-care system has three Levels of Health-Care Delivery that describe the scope of services and settings, which includes Primary, Secondary, and Tertiary.**

27. 1. Only nursing management positions contain an administrative component.
2. **Nurses work in a variety of settings; however, a component that is common to all settings is the use of the nursing process to develop patient plans of care.**
3. Not all Registered Nurse positions include direct physical care of patients. For example, many positions in home care, clinics, industry, and schools focus on case finding, ongoing monitoring of progress, and teaching rather than direct physical care.
4. The majority of nurses' time is concerned with implementing independent and dependent functions within the scope of nursing practice, not spent assisting the physician. In most settings, the nurse and physician work in a collaborative relationship to help patients cope with human responses to illness and disease.

28. 1. This is not the largest group of health-care professionals in the United States.
2. Nurse aides are not health-care professionals.
3. This is not the largest group of health-care professionals in the United States.
4. **Nurses comprise the largest group of health-care professionals in the United States. There are not enough Registered Nurses to meet the present demand. It is predicted that if the demand for nurses**

continues at the present rate and even if the present rate of graduating nurses increases slightly each year, by the year 2020 the nation's supply of Registered Nurses will only meet 72% of the demand.

29. 1. This is not a major factor that prevents an overhaul of the health-care delivery system of the United States. Most elected officials recognize the need for health-care reform and the need to respond to the desires of their political constituencies if they are to be reelected.
2. This is not a major factor that prevents an overhaul of the health-care delivery system of the United States.
3. Health-care delivery in the United States is an extremely complex service industry consisting of public, voluntary, and proprietary businesses with multiple disciplines of health-care workers represented. The system is influenced by federal, state, and local social, economic, ethical, and consumer driven issues.
4. Physician input is only one factor that may prevent an overhaul of the health-care delivery system of the United States. Although the American Medical Association has a strong political action committee, it was unable to prevent the institution of prospective reimbursement systems that in many ways dramatically changed the work world of the physician as well as placing limits on financial compensation for medical services provided.

30. 1. Health promotion is not emphasized in the traditional health-care delivery system in the United States. However, in 1992, the National League for Nursing predicted that, in the future, health care in the United States will move from the traditional hospital setting to the community with an emphasis on health promotion.
2. Illness prevention is not emphasized in the traditional health-care delivery system in the United States. In 1992, the National League for Nursing predicted that in the future health care in the United States will move from the traditional hospital setting to the community with an emphasis on illness prevention.
3. Traditional health-care delivery has always centered on activities associated with diagnosing, treating, and curing illness and disease. In addition, hospitals account for the largest proportion of money spent on health care and employs the largest number of health-care workers.
4. Rehabilitation and long-term care are not emphasized in the traditional health-care delivery system in the United States.

31. 1. This is not the purpose of a patient classification system.
2. A Patient Classification System, or Acuity Reports, are designed to rate patients in terms of high or low acuity; the level of acuity is based on the amount of time and nursing resources that are needed to care for the patient. A patient who is unstable and requires constant monitoring and nursing intervention will be rated a higher acuity score than a patient who is stable and relatively self-sufficient in activities of daily living.
3. Ongoing Quality Improvement Programs are designed to establish whether or not standards of care have been met and are not a patient classification system.
4. Standardized expected outcomes are established by professional educational and practice organizations, credentialing bodies, and critical pathways, not by a patient classification system.

32. 1. A Home Care Nurse provides and coordinates health services in the home.
2. A Primary Nurse has total responsibility for the planning and delivery of nursing care to a specific patient for the duration of the patient's hospitalization. Primary nursing is a nursing care delivery system that attempts to prevent fragmentation of care and ensure a comprehensive and consistent approach to meeting patients' needs while in the hospital.
3. A Case Manager coordinates and links health-care services to clients and their families at single levels of care (e.g., during hospitalization) and across levels of care (e.g., progression through hospitalization, extended-care facilities, and home care).
4. A Nurse Manager's job is to ensure that the objectives and goals of the organization are met appropriately, efficiently, and in a cost-effective manner.

33. 1. Studies and position papers from all segments of the health-care industry indicate the need to provide more health-care services in the community and not the institutional setting. To meet the health-care needs of older adults in the future, efforts have to begin now to provide more community-based support services so that people can remain in their own homes and not have to move to an institutional setting.

2. More services need to address the primary, not secondary, health-care needs of the community. Secondary health-care services include emergency care, acute care, diagnosis, and complex treatment. The present health-care system has an infrastructure that supports the delivery of secondary health-care services. More emphasis must be placed on providing services that meet the primary health-care needs of society, which include health promotion, illness prevention, health education, environmental protection, and early detection and treatment.
3. **Consumers are more aware than ever before that change in their own behavior and lifestyle will have a major influence on their own health status. Public health service announcements, community health education programs, and even television programs and media print materials (newspapers and magazines) have improved consumer awareness.**
4. Consumers, not health-care providers, should be charged with the primary responsibility for providing appropriate health-care services. As individuals or as groups, consumer demands and expectations will have the greatest impact on the delivery of health care.

34. 1. Although undocumented immigrants are increasing in numbers, it is not the group posing the greatest challenge to financing health care in the United States.
2. Although the medically uninsured are increasing in numbers, it is not the group posing the greatest challenge to financing health care in the United States.
3. Although the March of Dimes has identified a 35% increase in the number of preterm infants since 1981, because of an increase in multiple-gestations and the failure to receive early prenatal care in singletons, it is not the group posing the greatest challenge to financing health care in the United States.
4. **The percentage of older adults in the United States is expected to increase to 22% of the population by the year 2030. Fourteen percent of the 22% will be people over the age of 85. Because chronic illness is more prevalent among older adults, additional health-care services will be needed in the future. The need for increased services will increase costs.**

35. 1. **Medicaid is a federally funded, but state regulated, health insurance program for individuals with low incomes.**
2. This describes Medicare, not Medicaid.
3. Participation in programs providing care to people living below the designated poverty level are voluntary, not mandatory.
4. Health-care reimbursement in the hospital setting in the United States is based on a prospective, not retrospective, reimbursement formula. Diagnostic Related Groups is a predetermined hospital reimbursement rate based on a medical problem.

36. 1. When functioning as a provider, the nurse is in the caregiver, not advocate, role. Caregiving involves identifying and meeting the patient's needs by helping the patient regain health through the caring process.
2. When functioning as a nurturer, the nurse is in the caregiver, not advocate, role. Nurture means to encourage, foster, and promote, all of which are components of caregiving.
3. **Of the options offered, the word protector best describes the role of the nurse when functioning as the patient's advocate. In the role of advocate, the nurse protects and supports patients' rights and assists in asserting those rights when patients are unable to defend themselves.**
4. Evaluation does not describe patient advocacy. Evaluation is an important function, not role, of the nurse. Evaluation is the last step in the nursing process and is a determination of whether or not the patient's goals are achieved.

37. 1. **To maintain quality control and cost containment, third-party payers have preauthorization criteria for surgery that may include requirements, such as second opinions and initial conservative therapies.**
2. This is unrelated to preauthorization. A checklist summarizes the patient's preoperative preparation to ensure that all significant activities and safety precautions have been completed.
3. Diagnostic tests are not related to the concept of preauthorization. Diagnostic tests are performed to identify actual or potential health problems that may influence, or be affected by, the surgery.
4. This is unrelated to preauthorization. Informed Consent is a legal document giving permission for surgery including the procedure, surgical site, and surgeons.

38. 1. Many hospitalized patients may be emotionally fragile because of the stress of the experience. It is only when patients are a threat to themselves or others that they should not be placed with another patient and should be under constant supervision.

2. This is not a requirement for roommates. A patient does not have to converse with, or be responsible for, another patient.
3. The location of a bed within a room is insignificant. When two beds are available, the choice may be left to patient preference.
4. **One patient's physical condition should not interfere with another patient's physical condition. For example, a patient with a communicable disease should be in a private room while a patient with an incision or an open wound should not be in a room with a patient with an infection.**

39\. Answer: 2, 1, 3, 4

2. **Providing a special diet is a dependent function of the nurse. The physician's order should be verified first.**
1. **The diet manual should be reviewed to determine if the requested food is permitted on the ordered diet.**
3. **If the requested food is not indicated in the diet in the dietary manual, the nurse should collaborate with appropriate dietary resources (e.g., nutritionist, dietitian).**
4. **If the food is not permitted on the diet, the nurse can function as a patient advocate by collaborating with the practitioner to determine if an occasional concession can be made regarding a patient's food preference.**

40\.

1. **Departments of Health (state, county, city, or other local government units) are considered official agencies because primarily they are funded by tax money. They are concerned with health promotion and disease prevention.**
2. The American Heart Association is a voluntary not-for-profit organization, not an official organization.
3. The National League for Nursing (NLN) is a not-for-profit organization founded in 1952 to foster the development and improvement of nursing education and services. The NLN is not an official organization.
4. Nonprofit community hospitals are voluntary, not official, organizations.
5. **The Veterans Administration is an official organization because it comes under the umbrella of government supported/ operated and is financed by taxation.**

Community-Based Nursing

KEYWORDS

The following words include English vocabulary, nursing/medical terminology, concepts, principles, or information relevant to content specifically addressed in the chapter or associated with topics presented in it. English dictionaries, nursing textbooks, and medical dictionaries, such as *Taber's Cyclopedic Medical Dictionary*, are resources that can be used to expand your knowledge and understanding of these words and related information.

Case management
Coalition
Collaboration
Collegial
Community
Continuity
Demographics
Discharge planning
Epidemiology
Focus group
Global initiatives
Health-care settings
- Acute care – hospitals
- Adult day care
- Ambulatory care centers
- Assisted-living residence
- Clinics
- Extended care
- Home health services
- Hospice (inpatient, residential, in the home)
- Industrial or occupation settings
- Life-care community
- Long-term care – nursing homes
- Neighborhood community health center
- Physician's offices
- Psychiatric facilities
- Rehabilitation centers
- School settings
- Urgent visit centers

Health-care reform
Healthy People 2000
Holistic
Initiatives
Levels of health-care delivery
- Primary
- Secondary
- Tertiary

Levels of Prevention
- Primary prevention
- Health promotion
- Health protection
- Preventive health services
- Secondary prevention
- Tertiary prevention

Managed care
Metropolitan
Nursing's Agenda for Health Care Reform
Occupational nurse
Outreach
Population
Primary care
Public health nurse
Public policy
Quality improvement, quality management
Referral
Respite care
Rural
Self-help group
Suburban
Urban
Vulnerable populations
Wellness

QUESTIONS

1. The nurse understands that a need that falls within the category of Tertiary Health-Care Delivery is:
   1. Critical care
   2. Long-term care
   3. Diagnostic care
   4. Preventive care

2. A person at home is recovering from an illness that has caused functional deficits. Which support service identified by the nurse will provide the most benefit for this person?
   1. Meals on Wheels program
   2. Church outreach program
   3. Home health-care agency
   4. Hospice services

3. The major role of the nurse in the community setting is:
   1. Advisor
   2. Educator
   3. Surrogate
   4. Counselor

4. Which statement accurately reflects a concept about a healthy community?
   1. Health of a community is based on the sum of the health of its individuals
   2. The primary focus in community health is on the health of each member of society
   3. The focus of community health mainly is on healing the sick and preventing disease
   4. Promotion of health is one of the most important components of community health practice

5. The nurse understands that a feature common to most containers for prescription medications that are used in the home is:
   1. Drip-proof tops
   2. Unit dose packages
   3. Sun repellent plastic
   4. Child-resistant covers

6. The nurse must initiate nursing services in the home setting. Which is the most important factor that the nurse must consider to ensure third-party reimbursement?
   1. The patient must be able to perform some self-care
   2. The family has the financial resources to pay for the care
   3. Additional family members need to be available for support
   4. Intervention must be ordered by a provider with a license to prescribe

7. The home care nurse is assessing a patient and family members from a cultural perspective. It is most important for the nurse to:
   1. Use the patient as the main source of data
   2. Interview the members of the patient's family
   3. Recognize beliefs common to the patient's ethnic group
   4. Recall experiences of caring for patients with a similar background

8. In which setting do nurses most often need to *wear many hats*?
   1. Urban centers
   2. Rural communities
   3. Acute care hospitals
   4. Rehabilitation facilities

9. Which factor is essential to promote healthy lifestyles and behaviors within the community setting?
   1. The entire family must be committed to making changes
   2. A practitioner's order is necessary before care can be provided
   3. There must be resources available to support the desired changes
   4. The focus must be on the community as a whole, not on individuals

10. When attending a national professional convention, a group of nurses agree that in the United States there has been a noticeable decline in:
    1. Public health services
    2. At-risk patient groups
    3. Costs of health care
    4. Self-help groups

11. The community health nurse identifies that an example of an intervention associated with Secondary Prevention is:
 1. Conducting a cardiac risk assessment for people over forty years of age
 2. Teaching a low-fat diet to a person with high cholesterol
 3. Immunization of a child during the first year of life
 4. Monthly self-breast examinations by women

12. A family member requests relief from caring for a relative who has a rapidly debilitating malignancy. To which agency should the nurse refer the family member for respite care?
 1. Hospice program
 2. Meals on Wheels
 3. Ambulatory care center
 4. Alcohol treatment center

13. An important role of the nurse that takes on more emphasis in the delivery of health care in the home than in the acute care setting is:
 1. Modifying the environment
 2. Providing for healthy meals
 3. Delivering skilled nursing care
 4. Coordinating the efforts of the health team

14. The difference between the acute and home care settings is that in the home care setting the:
 1. Patient is the center of the health team
 2. Nurse functions as an advocate for the patient
 3. Nurse is responsible for coordinating the efforts of the health team
 4. Patient is not discharged until teaching regarding self-care is completed

15. The action related to advocacy that reflects the nurse's attempt to work with families to explore the nature and consequences of their choices is:
 1. Affirming
 2. Informing
 3. Mediating
 4. Interviewing

16. Nursing activities related to the concept of community nursing begin:
 1. On the first contact with the patient
 2. After the patient is admitted to the hospital
 3. When the practitioner writes discharge orders
 4. At the time referrals are made to community resources

17. The nurse must collect information about a community to identify its needs. The most significant assessment by the nurse is:
 1. The demographics of the community
 2. What the community thinks is important
 3. How many support services are available
 4. Environmental data as it relates to public safety

18. The home care nurse is caring for a variety of patients in their homes. The nurse identifies that the individual who will have the most difficult time adjusting to a prescribed regimen of long-term home health care is the:
 1. Middle school–aged child
 2. Preschool-aged child
 3. Adolescent
 4. Older adult

19. A factor that differentiates nursing care in the home from care in the acute setting is that in the home:
 1. Nurses work more independently
 2. Nurses need excellent communication skills
 3. Patients need to be taught how to care for themselves
 4. Patients have needs that require less technical nursing skills

20. A woman is concerned about her children accidentally ingesting her husband's prescription medications. The home care nurse should teach the mother to keep medications:
    1. On a high shelf
    2. In a locked cabinet
    3. In a medicine cabinet in the bathroom
    4. On a shelf in the back of the refrigerator

21. The most important health team member in an assisted-living facility is the:
    1. Occupational Therapist
    2. Nurse Aide
    3. Patient
    4. Nurse

22. A patient's contract for home care services is about to end but the patient still requires care. The home care nurse understands that continuation of services mainly depends on which factor?
    1. Presence of a physician's order
    2. Nursing documentation of the need for care
    3. Retrospective audits of quality management
    4. Patient satisfaction with the care being provided

23. Which factor is essential to the health of a community?
    1. Availability of medical specialists
    2. Consumers having health insurance
    3. Everyone having access to health care
    4. Public Health Nurses working in the community

24. According to the document, *Healthy People 2000*, an activity associated with Health Protection is:
    1. Teaching a program about alcohol abuse
    2. Encouraging children to be physically fit
    3. Administering immunizations to children
    4. Working as an occupational nurse in a factory

25. The nurse identifies the health-care needs of the members of a community. The nurse's most efficient initial approach to meet these needs is to:
    1. Involve community leaders to work within the political arena to obtain funding for programs
    2. Write research grants to explore the community's health needs in more detail
    3. Design educational programs that address the identified needs
    4. Make residents aware of the resources in the community

26. The home care nurse is performing an initial patient and home assessment. Which is the most essential assessment that must be made by the nurse?
    1. Can the home environment support the safety of the patient?
    2. Is the family willing to participate in the patient's recovery?
    3. Does the patient have the potential for self-care?
    4. Can the patient participate in the plan of care?

27. During the process of performing a community assessment, the nurse invites members of the community to come to a meeting and share opinions and concerns about a particular issue. This method of data collection is called:
    1. An opinion survey
    2. A community forum
    3. A demographic assessment
    4. An observation of participants

28. A significant role of the nurse in the home care setting is:
    1. Case management
    2. Discharge planning
    3. Enlisting family support
    4. Modifying patient values

29. The nurse is preparing a patient for discharge from the hospital. Which is designed primarily to provide for a continuum of comprehensive health care after discharge?
1. Home care agencies
2. Urgent visit centers
3. Physicians' offices
4. Respite programs

30. The nurse must conduct a community assessment. The nurse should first collect data about the:
1. General health of community members
2. Characteristics of community members
3. Physical environment of the community
4. Social services available in the community

31. A nursing supervisor in a home care agency is providing an orientation program to a group of newly hired patient companions. The nurse should teach them that in the United States families:
1. Are groups of people related by blood, marriage, adoption, or birth
2. Are made up of fathers, mothers, and their children
3. Vary based on their structural composition
4. Live in the same household

32. The major role of the nurse in the home associated with infection control is the role of:
1. Counselor
2. Caregiver
3. Advocate
4. Teacher

33. The home care nurse is providing care for a family supporting a patient with a chronic illness. The most important factor the nurse can convey to caregivers who care for family members in the home who have a stable but chronic illness is to:
1. Have extra equipment and supplies in the home for emergencies
2. Plan a daily and monthly schedule of caregiving activities
3. Care for themselves as well as the family member
4. Keep a daily journal of the patient's status

34. Which statements most reflect hospice care in the health-care delivery system? Check all that apply.
1. _____ Patients must have less than six months to live to receive services
2. _____ It assists families to care for their dying relatives at home
3. _____ Care is more expensive than in the acute care setting
4. _____ It provides mainly physical care to the dying person
5. _____ Hospice is a method of care rather than a location

35. Identify the nursing interventions that reflect Tertiary Health-Care Delivery. Check all that apply.
1. _____ Providing emotional support to family members after the death of a relative
2. _____ Teaching a patient how to use a wheelchair after a stroke
3. _____ Conducting a smoking cessation class
4. _____ Administering an influenza vaccine
5. _____ Changing a dressing after surgery

ANSWERS AND RATIONALES

1. 1. Critical care lies in the category of Secondary, not Tertiary, Level of Health-Care Delivery. The Secondary Level of Health-Care Delivery is associated with acute care, complex diagnosis, treatment of disease and illness, and emergency care.
   2. Long-term care lies in the category of Tertiary Level of Health-Care Delivery. The Tertiary Level of Health-Care Delivery is associated with rehabilitation, care of the dying, and long-term care.
   3. Diagnostic care lies in the category of Secondary, not Tertiary, Level of Health-Care Delivery.
   4. Preventive care lies in the category of Primary, not Tertiary, Level of Health-Care Delivery. Primary Health-Care Delivery is concerned with promoting health and preventing disease.

2. 1. Meals on Wheels provides for only the nutritional needs of a patient.
   2. Although church outreach programs may be able to provide some support services, generally they are not as effective an agency as another option to provide the multiple services needed or to coordinate the continuum of comprehensive services that a person with functional deficits will need. Many church outreach programs generally serve as a source of information about services and programs available in the community, and they provide additional support that augments home care services.
   3. A home health-care agency is designed to coordinate the comprehensive services that a patient may need to recover from an illness that has caused functional deficits. This person may need help in areas such as assistance with activities of daily living, physical and occupational rehabilitation, direct nursing care, counseling, etc.
   4. Hospice services are designed to assist patients who have less than six months to live and who have chosen to forego additional curative treatment for palliative care and support of quality of life. Hospice programs also provide support services to members of the patient's family as well as bereavement care after the death of the patient.

3. 1. Nurses should not advise or tell patients what to do. Patients need to make their own choices based on information and their own values, beliefs, and goals.
   2. Of the roles presented in the options, the role of educator is most important in the home care setting. As a teacher, the nurse helps patients manage, maintain or restore their health; identifies the patient's learning needs, readiness, and motivation to learn; formulates a teaching plan in conjunction with the patient; employs appropriate teaching strategies; and evaluates outcomes of learning.
   3. The surrogate role is not a professional role of the nurse. A surrogate role is assigned to a nurse when patients believe that the nurse reminds them of another person and projects that role and the feelings patients have for the other person onto the nurse.
   4. Although nurses function as counselors, a role in another option is more frequently employed in the home care setting.

4. 1. A healthy community seeks to provide infrastructure, resources, and activities that support a healthy community and is not just reflective of the health of its members.
   2. Community health focuses on families, groups, and the community, not just individuals.
   3. This statement focuses on illness and is too limited in relation to community health.
   4. Health promotion has taken on new meaning as consumers take more and more responsibility for their health status. Teaching about promoting health is a more positive perspective than teaching about preventing illness, which is a negative perspective.

5. 1. This is not common to all medication containers. Only medications in liquid form need to have drip-proof tops.
   2. Most prescriptions filled for home use are in multidose containers.
   3. Not all medications need to be protected from the sun.
   4. All prescriptions filled for home use are dispensed in containers with child-resistant tops, as required by law. If a person has a physical limitation such as arthritis that interferes with one's ability to open a medication container, the person can request that a nonsafety top be provided. The pharmacy generally will document the request in its computer and may even require that a waiver be signed and witnessed for the record.

6. 1. This is not necessary. In some instances, the family members provide total care with no help from the patient.
2. A person does not have to be wealthy to receive nursing services in the home. For example, Medicare, Medicaid, or private health-care insurance plans assume some of the costs of care provided in the home.
3. The presence of family members is not a requirement for home care services. However, if it is unsafe for the patient to be home alone or unattended for long periods, the home may not be the most appropriate setting. In addition, patients who have no family support may rely on a friend, neighbor, or volunteers from a neighborhood outreach group to help in a supportive way.
4. **Health-care professionals who have prescriptive licenses (e.g., physicians, nurse practitioners, physician's assistants) must order home care nursing services. An order from a provider with a prescriptive license is required if a home care agency is to receive reimbursement from third-party sources (i.e., government, medical insurance plans, etc.). Orders written by these professionals direct the medical plan of care.**

7. 1. **The patient is the center of the health team and is the most important source of information about his/her perspective.**
2. Family members provide only their own views, which are not the most important when assessing variables that affect a patient from a cultural perspective.
3. Each patient is an individual, and generalizations should not be made based on a person's ethnic or cultural group. Generalizations often are based on stereotypes that are preconceived and untested beliefs about people based on their culture, race, and/or ethnic backgrounds.
4. This denies the individuality of the patient. Generalizations often are based on stereotypes, which are preconceived and untested beliefs about people based on their culture, race, and/or ethnic backgrounds. Stereotyping a patient can lead to inaccurate assessments and result in inappropriate or potentially harmful actions or omission of care.

8. 1. Of the options presented, nurses working in urban centers are less likely to wear many hats. Urban centers refer to cities with a population of more than 50,000 individuals. Urban areas tend to have a concentration of specialized services where nurses have specific roles and responsibilities.
2. **Nurses working in rural communities wear many hats. The adage *wear many hats* refers to someone with many different roles and responsibilities. Rural refers to *the country* or *the farm* where communities are less populated and are a great distance from physicians and health-care services. Because of the uneven distribution of health-care professionals and services in rural areas versus urban areas, nurses working in a rural area will assume many different roles and perform multiple tasks.**
3. Of the options presented, nurses working in the acute care setting are less likely to wear many hats. Generally, nurses working in acute care settings have specific roles and responsibilities.
4. Of the options presented, nurses working in a rehabilitation setting are less likely to wear many hats. Generally, nurses working in a rehabilitation setting have specific roles and responsibilities.

9. 1. Each individual person is responsible for his/her own health seeking actions and behavior. It is ideal if all members of a family are interested and motivated to promote a healthy lifestyle; however, not all members of a family are committed to this value.
2. Educational intervention is an independent function of the nurse and does not require a practitioner's order. Education is the key in relation to recognizing and understanding the importance of behaviors that support a healthy lifestyle.
3. **Resources that support *health promotion*, *health protection*, and *preventive health services* are essential if one expects members of the community to engage in healthy lifestyles and behaviors. Resources, such as availability of health professionals, sites for *primary health prevention* programs for meetings and provision of services, consumables in the form of equipment and medications (immunizations), etc., must be available to promote and support health.**
4. Although programs are designed to meet the needs of groups in a community, each individual must be reached and influenced when promoting healthy lifestyles and behaviors.

10. 1. **The services of public health agencies established at the federal, state, and**

local levels to safeguard and improve the physical, mental and social well-being of an entire community are on the decline. In an effort to reduce the escalating rise in the budgets of public health agencies, programs and services have been reduced or terminated.

2. Patient groups at risk are on the rise; for example, groups such as older adults, the homeless, the uninsured, people living below the poverty level, single-parent families, and immigrants.
3. The cost of health care is dramatically on the rise. More than 15.5% of the Gross Domestic Product is spent on health-care costs and is still rising.
4. Self-help groups are on the rise. More than 500 self-help groups represent almost all the major health problems, life events, or crises. The National Self-Help Clearinghouse provides information about existing groups and guidelines on how to begin a new group. Consumer access to The World Wide Web and the Internet has disseminated information about self-help groups.

11. 1. This is Primary, not Secondary, prevention. Primary prevention is concerned with generalized health promotion and specific protection against disease. Risk assessments for specific diseases are included in Primary prevention.
2. A low-fat diet generally is part of a medical management program for a person who is overweight or who has high cholesterol. This is Tertiary, not Secondary, prevention. Tertiary prevention is associated with attempts to reduce the extent and severity of a health problem in an effort to limit disability as well as restore and maintain function.
3. This is Primary, not Secondary, prevention. Primary prevention includes protecting people from disease.
4. **Secondary prevention is associated with early detection of disease and prompt intervention.**

12. 1. **A hospice program is an example of an agency that might provide respite care in an inpatient setting or in the home. The caregiving role is physically and emotionally grueling and family members may need relief from the caregiving role or a break to attend a family function or go on vacation.**
2. Meals on Wheels does not provide respite care. It provides nutritious, low-cost meals for homebound people so that they can remain in their own homes.
3. Ambulatory care centers do not provide respite care. Ambulatory care centers provide care for people with conditions that do not require hospitalization. Services may include diagnosis and treatment of disease and illness, as well as simple surgical procedures in which the patient returns home the same day.
4. An alcohol treatment center does not provide respite care. It provides a specialized service in the care and treatment of individuals who abuse alcohol.

13. 1. **The hospital environment rarely requires modification because it is designed to provide for the safety needs of patients. However, in the home setting, a home hazard assessment needs to be implemented to identify potential problems with walkways, stairways, floors, furniture, bathrooms, kitchens, electrical and fire protection, toxic substances, communication devices and issues associated with medications and asepsis. Although the nurse may not be able to change a patient's living space and lifestyle, recommendations can be made that will eliminate or minimize risks.**
2. Ensuring that patients receive healthy meals is an important responsibility of the nurse in all settings in which nurses work.
3. Delivering skilled nursing care is an important responsibility of the nurse in all settings in which nurses work.
4. Coordinating the efforts of the health team is an important responsibility of the nurse in all settings in which nurses work.

14. 1. The patient is the center of the health team in all settings.
2. The nurse functions as an advocate for the patient in both the acute care and home care settings. The role of advocate is important in all settings because in this role the nurse protects and supports patients' rights.
3. The nurse is responsible for coordinating the efforts of the members of the health team in both the acute care and home care settings.
4. **Because of the shorter length of hospital stays, patients are being discharged before all teaching and counseling are completed. However, in the home care setting, patients are provided with appropriate care until they are able to care for themselves without needing ongoing home care intervention.**

15. 1. Affirm means to state positively, to declare firmly, to ratify, and to assert. Exploring the nature and consequences of choices is not affirming.
    2. To inform is an important role of the nurse when functioning as a patient advocate. Inform means to give information, to enlighten, and to give knowledge. When working with families to explore the nature and consequences of their choices, the nurse can provide information so that people understand the ramifications of their choices. An informed decision is a decision based on an understanding of the facts and ramifications associated with the choice.
    3. Mediate means to negotiate or intercede. Exploring the nature and consequences of choices is not mediating.
    4. Interview means to meet and talk for the purpose of collecting information. Exploring the nature and consequences of choices is not interviewing. However, interviewing skills may be employed when the nurse explores with the patient the nature and consequences of choices.

16. **1. As soon as contact with the patient is made, planning and teaching should begin so the patient is prepared for discharge and returned to the community.**
    2. The nurse does not have to wait until the patient is admitted to the hospital to begin preparing for the patient's return to the community.
    3. This is too late to prepare the patient for the return to the community.
    4. This is too late. Referrals can be anticipated before admission in most situations.

17. 1. This is not as important as an assessment presented in another option. The demographics of a community are only one component of a community assessment.
    2. The members in the community are the primary source of data about the community and their needs. Just as the patient is the center of the health team when caring for an individual, the collective membership of a community is the center of the health team when caring for the health-care needs of a community.
    3. This does not help to identify the needs of a community. After the needs of the community are identified, then the ability of the health-care system to deliver the necessary services is assessed.
    4. This is not as important as an assessment presented in another option. Environmental data is only one component of a community assessment.

18. 1. A middle school–aged child has to deal with the developmental conflict of Industry versus Inferiority. Tasks associated with this age, deriving pleasure from accomplishments and developing a sense of competence, can be facilitated in the home setting. Although a middle school–aged child will have to adjust to the need for long-term home health care, there are fewer crises occurring during the middle school years that impact on development than the number of crises occurring in a group in another option.
    2. A preschool-aged child is dependent on a parent to provide for basic human needs and coping with the developmental conflict of Initiative versus Guilt. Tasks associated with this age, the development of confidence in ability and having direction and purpose, can be facilitated in the home setting. Although a preschool-aged child will have to adjust to the need for long-term home health care, there are fewer crises occurring during the preschool years that impact on development than the number of crises occurring in a group in another option.
    3. The adolescent generally will have the hardest time adjusting to the need for long-term home health care than any other stage of development. Adolescents experience multiple and complex physiological, psychological, and social developmental milestones. Adolescents want to be attractive to others, similar to their peers, and accepted within a group. It is common for adolescents to experience mood swings, make decisions without having all the facts, challenge authority, and assert the self. Being relatively isolated in the home for an extended period will pose serious stressors associated with adjustment, which can dramatically influence the outcome of the developmental tasks of adolescence.
    4. The developmental conflict of Ego Integrity versus Despair challenges older adults to understand their worth and accept the end of life. Although older adults will have the second-hardest time adjusting to the need for long-term home health care of the options offered, there are fewer crises occurring during the older adult years that impact

on development than the number of crises occurring in a group in another option.

19. **1. In the home setting, patients tend to have less physicians' orders and therefore nurses work more independently. In addition, the roles of the nurse in community-based practice today are expanding dramatically. In 1991, the American Nurses Association published *Nursing's Agenda for Health Care Reform*, which made recommendations for health-care reform. The major predictions influencing nurse accountability included: nurses will become community leaders; community-nursing centers will expand and focus on preventing disease and promoting health; and the center of health care will shift to the home setting. Nurses already work independently in such programs as community outreach, nursing centers, nurse-sponsored wellness and health promotion programs, and independent practice. These roles require the nurse to utilize nursing theory and skills that are in the scope of the legal definition of nursing practice and do not require dependence upon physician's orders.**

2. Excellent communication skills are essential in both the acute care and community-based settings.
3. Teaching occurs in both the acute care and community-based settings. In addition, some patients may never be able to care for themselves.
4. Excellent technical skills are essential in both the acute care and community-based settings. Patients at home receive highly technical therapy such as hemodialysis, intravenous therapy, wound care, and ventilator support.

20. 1. This is not a safe place to keep medications. Children have natural curiosity, problem-solving abilities, and the agility to climb to a top shelf.

2. A locked area is the safest place to store prescription as well as over-the-counter medications to prevent accidental ingestion by children.

3. This is not a safe place to keep medications. Children have natural curiosity, problem-solving abilities, and the agility to climb up to a medicine cabinet.
4. This is not a safe place to keep medications. Children have natural curiosity and problem-solving abilities, and could get to the back of a shelf in a refrigerator.

21. 1. The Occupational Therapist (OT) is not the most important member of the health team. An Occupational Therapist generally is not a member of the health team in an assisted-living residence. On occasion, a physician may order occupational therapy and the resident will either go to an Occupational Therapist to receive therapy or one will come to the person and provide therapy.

2. Although Nurse Aides are the people who provide the bulk of the assistance needed by residents in an assisted-living residence, they are not as important as another member of the health team.

3. The patient is always the center of the health team in every setting and is the most important member.

4. The nurse is not the most important health team member in an assisted-living facility. An assisted-living residence (i.e., apartment, villa, or condominium) provides limited assistance with activities of daily living, meal preparation, laundry services, transportation, and opportunities for socialization, not extensive nursing services.

22. 1. The physician generally is not the health-care professional making the decision whether a patient is eligible for continuation of services or is ready for discharge from the home care program. In the home care setting a physician's order is necessary to initiate home care services as well as orders directing the nurse in the dependent functions of the nurse.

2. Case management by the nurse in the home care setting includes determining when the patient is ready for discharge. After the nurse determines that the patient is ready for discharge, it is conveyed to the physician and the physician discharges the patient. Nursing documentation supports the decision. Often the nurse needs to document objectively the status of the patient to convince the health-care provider and the insurer that the patient needs a continuation of services.

3. Quality Management activities are unrelated to whether a patient is to receive a continuation of services or is to be discharged from a home health-care program. Ongoing Quality Management Programs are designed to monitor the quality of care being delivered and identify problem areas so that efforts can be employed to improve care.
4. Dissatisfaction with the services of a home health agency may influence whether or not the patient and/or family wants a continuation

of services. However, satisfaction or dissatisfaction should not influence whether the patient still needs the services of the home health-care agency.

23. 1. Although it is important to have access to medical specialists, another option has priority. In addition, the availability of primary care practitioners, not specialists, is more essential because Primary Health Care addresses health promotion, illness prevention and entry into Secondary Health Care (diagnosis and treatment of illness and disease).
 2. Although individuals with health insurance have better access to health-care services, it is not essential to have health insurance to receive health care. People can pay privately or, if indigent, they can apply for various government and nonprofit-supported programs that provide basic care. In addition, hospital emergency departments, by law, cannot turn away patients who need emergency care.
 3. For a healthy community, all members of the community must have access to health care. The health of a community depends on each member of the community having appropriate and comprehensive health care.
 4. Public Health Nurses work for only the federal, state, or local governments implementing programs supported by taxes. These programs are only a small percentage of the multitude of programs and services that are designed to support community health.

24. 1. According to the document *Healthy People 2000*, this is a Health Promotion, not Health Protection, activity.
 2. According to the document *Healthy People 2000*, this is a Health Promotion, not Health Protection, activity.
 3. According to the document *Healthy People 2000*, this is a Preventive Health Service, not an activity associated with Health Protection.
 4. In 1990, *Healthy People 2000*, a document prepared by the United States Department of Health and Human Services with input from 24 national nursing organizations, outlined 298 health-related objectives. This document differentiated the Primary Prevention Level of Health Care into three areas: Health Promotion, Health Protection, and Preventive Health Services. Health Protection was defined as actions by the government and industry to reduce environmental factors that are a threat to health. It included activities, such as controlling factors that maintain occupational safety, preventing accidents and infectious diseases, and controlling environmental toxic agents and radiation.

25. 1. This is not the most efficient approach. This may be necessary if present resources are not available to meet the needs of the community.
 2. The health needs of the members of the community are identified already. Further study at this time does not appear to be appropriate.
 3. This is not the most efficient approach. This may eventually be done after an action in another option is implemented first.
 4. This is the most efficient initial approach to meeting the identified needs of the members of the community. The use of presently available resources is more efficient than the other options presented.

26. **1. The first and most important assessment made by the home care nurse focuses on determining whether the patient's home environment is safe. Safety and security are basic needs identified by Maslow's Hierarchy of Needs.**
 2. Although it is often helpful when family members participate in a home care patient's recovery, it is not necessary.
 3. A patient's potential for self-care is not a criterion for receiving home care services. Patients who have little or no potential for self-care receive home care services.
 4. Patients who are unable to participate in the plan of care because they are mentally, emotionally, or physically disabled are still eligible for home care.

27. 1. This is not an example of an opinion survey. An opinion survey is designed to collect each individual person's perspective about the problem being studied. Results are tallied to identify the major concerns. Opinion surveys generally are questionnaires.
 2. A forum is defined as an opportunity for open discussion. Inviting people from the community to share opinions and concerns about a particular issue for the purpose of collecting data is called a community forum.
 3. This is not an example of a demographic assessment. A demographic assessment is the quantitative study of the characteristics of a population. A demographic assessment might include information such as distribution of the population by gender, size, growth, density, and ethnicity.

4. This is not an example of an observation of participants. Direct observation is a method of data collection that might be used to determine whether individuals follow a specific procedure or behave in an expected manner.

28. 1. **Case management is a major role of the nurse in the home care setting. The nurse engages in activities, such as assessing, planning, coordinating nursing care and professional services, making referrals, monitoring medical progress, maintaining documentation, evaluating and monitoring outcomes, determining closure and discharging the patient after goal achievement.**
2. Although discharge planning is a component of the role of the nurse in the home care setting, it is not the role with the highest priority. Traditionally, discharge planning is focused on moving a person from the hospital to the home. However, in the present health-care environment, discharge planning is conducted when moving a patient from one level of care to another and occurs in many settings.
3. Although family support is helpful, it is the patient's interest and motivation in achieving expected outcomes that is the most important contributing factor to success.
4. The role of the nurse is to help the patient achieve expected outcomes that are within the patient's present value and belief systems. Although a patient might be healthier if other behaviors were adopted, it is difficult, and sometimes impossible, to change or modify a person's values and beliefs.

29. 1. **Home care agencies are responsible for coordinating and providing for a continuum of comprehensive health-care services after a patient is discharged from the hospital. Because of the decreased length of stay in the hospital setting, patients are being discharged sooner than ever before and are in need of home care services.**
2. Urgent visit centers are designed to deal with the treatment of noncritical emergencies, such as infections, minor injuries, and physical responses to disease or illness as well as primary care services.
3. Physicians' offices are the traditional primary care setting for ambulatory care. Patients go to physicians' offices for routine physicals and the diagnosis and treatment of routine illnesses or diseases. Follow-up visits to the physician are only one aspect of comprehensive health care.
4. Respite programs provide for short stay, intermittent, inpatient or day-care services to patients who generally are cared for at home. This service provides a rest period for family members who have the responsibility of sustained caregiving.

30. 1. Although the general health of the members of a community is important, it is not the first data that the nurse should collect when assessing a community.
2. **Acquiring core information about the people in the community is the first stage in assessing a community. Core characteristics about the members of a community include information such as vital statistics, values and beliefs, demographics, religious groups, etc.**
3. Although a community's physical environment (including information such as whether it is rural, suburban, or urban, physical boundaries, density, size, types of lodgings, incidence of crime, etc.) is important to know, it is not the first data that the nurse should collect when assessing a community.
4. Although it is important to know information such as agencies and services provided, the accessibility to health-care services, sources of health information, transportation services, routine caseloads, etc., it is not the first data that the nurse should collect when assessing a community.

31. 1. Families are not limited to individuals who are related by blood, marriage, adoption, or birth.
2. This is an example of a nuclear family and is only one example of a family structure.
3. **A family is defined as a social group whose members are closely related by blood, marriage, or friendship. Today, family structure is diverse and includes families, such as traditional nuclear families, single-parent families, blended families, cohabitating families, gay and lesbian families, families with foster children, and single people living alone but who are part of an extended family.**
4. Family members remain connected by their relationships, not because they all live in the same household.

32. 1. Counseling is related to helping a patient recognize and cope with emotional stressors, improve relationships, and promote personal growth, not dealing with infection control issues.

2. Although the term caregiver is broad and could include many different roles of the nurse, caregiver generally refers to direct *laying on of the hands* when providing direct care. This is not the major role of the nurse when dealing with infection control issues in the home setting.
3. The role of advocate is not the most appropriate role presented in the options when dealing with infection control issues in the home setting. In the role of advocate, the nurse protects and supports patients' rights and assists in asserting those rights when patients are unable to defend themselves, not dealing with infection control issues.
4. **Of the roles presented in the options, the role of teacher is most important in the home care setting when addressing infection control issues. Nurses need to teach patients and their family members how to maintain a clean environment, make modifications to the environment to support asepsis, and perform procedures associated with aseptic and sterile technique to prevent infection. Nurses also can teach patients and their family members about the steps in the Chain of Infection and actions that they can implement to reduce the risk of infection. Because the nurse is in the home only for a limited amount of time at each visit, it is important that the nurse teach the patient and family members how to best reduce the risk of infection on a daily basis.**

33\. 1. Although this is a good idea, it is not the most important factor a home care nurse can convey to a person caring for a family member in the home.
2. Although this might contribute to efficiency as well as gaining a feeling of control over the activities that must be accomplished, it is not the most important factor a home care nurse can convey to a person caring for a family member in the home.
3. **Caregiver role strain experienced by a family member is a serious concern of home care nurses. Caregivers often fail to address their own health needs because of the extraordinary burden of the caregiver role, which can jeopardize their own health and well-being. Caregivers should be encouraged to delegate responsibilities to other family members, to get adequate sleep, rest and nutritional intake, to seek assistance from agencies that provide respite services, to take time for leisure activities and a vacation, and to join a caregiver support group.**
4. A daily journal of the patient's status is unnecessary when a patient is in stable condition. If the patient experienced an acute episode, then a record of the patient's daily status could be helpful in monitoring progress or lack of progress.

34\. 1. **To be eligible for hospice services, an individual must be diagnosed as having less than 6 months to live. It is a service to support patients and their families through the process of dying.**
2. **Most hospice care is delivered in patients' homes supported by a team of health-care providers and volunteers. However, there are inpatient hospice programs, palliative care units in hospitals, and residential hospice settings.**
3. The home is a less expensive setting than other health-care settings because family members provide most of the care supported by a team of professionals, nonprofessionals, and volunteers.
4. Hospice services include not only palliative care and support of quality of life for the terminally ill patient but emotional support to patients and family members. In addition, it includes services that assist family members with bereavement and adjustment after the death of the patient.
5. **Hospice is not a setting but a movement. It provides supportive, palliative services that focus on managing pain, treatment of symptoms and helping patients maintain their quality of life so they can live the remainder of their lives to the fullest.**

35\. 1. **Providing bereavement services is an example of Tertiary Health-Care Delivery. Tertiary care is associated with rehabilitation, long-term care, and care of the dying. The Levels of Health-Care Delivery, which describe the scope of services and settings where health care is provided, includes Primary, Secondary, and Tertiary. The Levels of Health-Care Delivery should not be confused with Levels of Prevention.**
2. **Teaching a patient how to use a wheelchair after a stroke is an example of Tertiary Health-Care Delivery. It provides services related to rehabilitation.**

3. This is an example of a service provided on the Primary, not Tertiary, Level of Health-Care Delivery. Primary Health Care is associated with illness prevention, health promotion, early detection and routine treatment, environmental protection and health education.
4. Immunizations are an example of Primary, not Tertiary, Health-Care Delivery. Primary Health Care is concerned with promoting health, preventing disease, early and basic detection and treatment of disease, environmental protection, and health education.
5. Changing a dressing after surgery is care associated with the Secondary, not Tertiary, Level of Health-Care Delivery. Secondary Health Care is associated with acute care, complex diagnosis and treatment of disease and illness, and emergency care.

3 Psychosociocultural Nursing Care

Nursing Care Across the Life Span

KEYWORDS

The following words include English vocabulary, nursing/medical terminology, concepts, principles, or information relevant to content specifically addressed in the chapter or associated with topics presented in it. English dictionaries, nursing textbooks, and medical dictionaries, such as *Taber's Cyclopedic Medical Dictionary*, are resources that can be used to expand your knowledge and understanding of these words and related information.

Accommodation
Adolescent (teenager)
Agism, ageism
Assimilation
Bonding
Brazelton, Berry–Neonatal Behavioral Assessment Scale
Cephalocaudal
Child abuse
Congenital anomalies
Critical time
Developmental
- Milestones
- Stressor
- Task

Developmental tasks
Differentiated development
Egocentrism
Embryo
Erikson, Erik–Theory of Personality Development
Failure to thrive
Fetal alcohol syndrome
Fetus
Fowler, James–Theory of Faith Development
Freud, Sigmund–Psychoanalytical Theory
Gender-role development
Genetics
Growth
Havighurst, Robert–Developmental Task Theory of Development
Infancy, infant
Intellect, intellectual
Kohlberg, Lawrence–Theory of Moral Development
Latchkey children
Learning disability
Life cycle
Life events
Low birth weight
Maslow, Abraham—Hierarchy of Basic Human Needs
Menarche
Menopause
Middle adulthood
Middle school–aged child
Midlife crisis
Moral reasoning
Newborn
Nocturnal emission
Organogenesis
Older adult
Physique
Piaget, Jean—Cognitive Development Theory
Polypharmacy
Pre/postmenopausal
Preschool-aged child
Preschooler
Preterm
Proximodistal
Puberty
Regression
Reminiscence
Retirement
Role reversal
Sandwich generation

Senescence
Short stature
Sibling
Sibling rivalry
Substance abuse
Teratogenic
Toddler
Young Adulthood

QUESTIONS

1. When the nurse cares for individuals across the life span, which age group generally demonstrates an inefficiency of adaptation?
   1. 60 plus years
   2. 40 to 60 years
   3. 12 to 19 years
   4. 3 to 11 years
2. The nurse is caring for children with a variety of ages. At what age do children first recognize that death is irreversible, universal, and natural?
   1. 6
   2. 9
   3. 12
   4. 15
3. The nurse identifies that the behavior in an adult that indicates an unresolved developmental conflict associated with adolescence is:
   1. Being overly concerned about following daily routines
   2. Requiring excessive attention from others
   3. Relying on oneself rather than others
   4. Failing to set goals in life
4. The nurse identifies that an individual who nurtures, teaches, and gives to others reflects which stage of Erikson's Stages of Development?
   1. Generativity versus Stagnation
   2. Ego Integrity versus Despair
   3. Industry versus Inferiority
   4. Initiative versus Guilt
5. Which comment best demonstrates agism? "He is 75 years old and:
   1. Has outlived his usefulness."
   2. Reads the newspaper with difficulty."
   3. Reminisces about his past work experience."
   4. Is most happy when working in his home workshop."
6. When planning nursing care, the nurse needs to remember that energy expenditure and nutrient requirements are higher during the:
   1. First year of life
   2. Early adult years
   3. Middle adult years
   4. End of the life cycle
7. The nurse understands that according to Erikson, establishing relationships based on commitment mainly occurs in which stage of psychosocial development?
   1. Generativity versus Stagnation
   2. Identity versus Role Confusion
   3. Intimacy versus Isolation
   4. Trust versus Mistrust
8. Which age group should the nurse identify is reflected in the following statement? "More time is spent in bed but less time is spent asleep."
   1. Two-year-olds
   2. Forty-year-olds
   3. Seventy-year-olds
   4. Fourteen-year-olds

9. A common stressor identified by the nurse that is associated with the developmental stage of early childhood (1–3 years) is:
   1. Accepting limited dietary choices
   2. Adjusting to a change in physique
   3. Responding to life-threatening illness
   4. Resolving conflicts associated with independence

10. The nurse is providing dietary teaching to a group of adolescents recently diagnosed with diabetes mellitus. The nurse understands that many foods are ingested by the adolescent because of:
    1. Taste
    2. Routine
    3. Pressure
    4. Preference

11. The nurse is administering medication to an older adult. For which response to medication that occurs most frequently in older adults should the nurse assess the patient?
    1. Toxicity
    2. Side effects
    3. Hypersensitivity
    4. Idiosyncratic effects

12. When the nurse assesses patients in the following age groups, the nurse understands that the age group that has the greatest potential to demonstrate regression when ill is:
    1. Infants
    2. Toddlers
    3. Adolescents
    4. Young adults

13. When the nurse assesses an adult, which behavior may indicate an unresolved developmental task of infancy?
    1. Avoiding assistance from others
    2. Rationalizing unacceptable behaviors
    3. Being overly concerned about cleanliness
    4. Apologizing constantly for small mistakes

14. When assessing the ability to age successfully, the nurse understands that this is based on a person's ability to:
    1. Cope with social isolation
    2. Adjust to the change in social roles
    3. Associate with members of every age groups
    4. Increase the number of meaningful relationships

15. The nurse is assessing the skin of an older adult. Which change in the patient's skin should the nurse anticipate?
    1. Increased tone
    2. Decreased dryness
    3. Increased elasticity
    4. Decreased thickness

16. Which patient should the nurse identify is at the greatest risk when taking a drug that has a high teratogenic potential?
    1. Older adult man
    2. Pregnant woman
    3. Four-year-old child
    4. One-month-old baby

17. An older adult is admitted to the intensive care unit. For which common behavioral adaptation to sensory overload should the nurse monitor the patient?
    1. Dementia
    2. Confusion
    3. Drowsiness
    4. Bradycardia

18. The nurse identifies which word as being unrelated to principles of growth and development?
    1. Unpredictable
    2. Sequential
    3. Integrated
    4. Complex

19. The nurse in the emergency department is assessing patients of various ages. The nurse understands that the age group that has the greatest individual differences in appearance and behavior is:
    1. Children
    2. Adolescents
    3. Older adults
    4. Middle-aged adults

20. A patient tells the nurse about experiencing problems with sleep and requests sleeping medication. Which concept associated with drug therapy and quality of sleep is important for the nurse to understand when planning nursing care for this patient?
    1. Sedatives are not well tolerated by older adults
    2. Antianxiety drugs are the least helpful to support sleep
    3. Effectiveness of hypnotics increases with prolonged use
    4. Melatonin is the drug of choice for long-term use in sleep disorders

21. Which concept should the nurse understand is reflective of Erikson's Theory of Personality Development?
    1. Defense mechanisms help to cope with anxiety
    2. Moral maturity is a central theme in all stages of development
    3. Achievement of developmental goals is affected by the social environment
    4. Two continual processes, assimilation and accommodation, stimulate intellectual growth

22. A resident in a nursing home reminisces about past-life events. The nurse identifies that according to Erikson, the patient is in which stage of psychosocial development?
    1. Autonomy versus Shame and Doubt
    2. Identity versus Role Confusion
    3. Generativity versus Stagnation
    4. Ego Integrity versus Despair

23. The nurse in the clinic is monitoring patients for iron deficiency anemia. Which group of individuals is considered to be at the greatest risk?
    1. Postmenopausal women
    2. Older adults
    3. Teenagers
    4. Infants

24. The nurse identifies that the age group that is at the greatest risk for constipation is:
    1. Inactive school-aged children
    2. Middle-aged adults
    3. Older-aged adults
    4. Bottle-fed infants

25. The nurse identifies that a patient in middle adulthood is experiencing a developmental crisis when there is an inability to:
1. Achieve a feeling of success
2. Develop peer relationships
3. Delay satisfaction
4. Face death

26. A 2-year-old child is trying to eat with a spoon and is making a mess. The nurse should:
1. Provide finger foods until the child is older
2. Offer praise and encouragement as the child eats
3. Feed the child along with the child's attempts at eating
4. Take the spoon and feed the child until the child is more capable

27. The nurse working in a nursing home is providing care to a group of older adults. The decline in which system in the older adult most often influences the ability to maintain safety?
1. Sensory
2. Respiratory
3. Integumentary
4. Cardiovascular

28. Which psychodynamic theorist believed that 10-year-old children gain pleasure from accomplishments?
1. Lawrence Kohlberg
2. Berry Brazelton
3. Sigmund Freud
4. Erik Erikson

29. The nurse understands that, according to Erikson, the person who becomes self-absorbed and obsessed with one's own needs is having difficulty resolving which stage of psychosocial development?
1. Industry versus Inferiority
2. Ego Integrity versus Despair
3. Generativity versus Stagnation
4. Identity versus Role Confusion

30. One of the participants attending a parenting class asks the teacher, "What is the leading cause of death during the first year of life?" Besides exploring the person's concerns, the nurse should respond:
1. Sudden infant death syndrome
2. Unintentional injuries
3. Congenital anomalies
4. Preterm birth

31. The nurse identifies that the person at greatest risk for problems with regulating body temperature is the:
1. Toddler
2. Teenager
3. Older adult
4. School-aged child

32. The nurse understands that an individual who is preoccupied with work and the drive to succeed at the expense of emotionally committing to others reflects a negative resolution of which stage of Erikson's Stages of Development?
1. Autonomy versus Shame and Doubt
2. Identify versus Role Confusion
3. Ego Integrity versus Despair
4. Intimacy versus Isolation

33. When meeting the sleep needs of patients, the nurse identifies that the group that has the most problems as a result of multiple, complex developmental factors is:
1. Infants
2. Toddlers
3. Adolescents
4. Preschoolers

34. To what is a person referring when during an interview the person says, "I am a member of the *sandwich generation*?"
1. Cares for children and aging parents at the same time
2. There is a role reversal between parents and self
3. Assists own parents and spouse's parents
4. Has both older and younger siblings

35. The nurse is planning a teaching session for an older adult about a prescribed medication regimen. An issue of major concern for the nurse is that older adults:
1. Experience an increase in absorption of drugs from the gastrointestinal tract
2. Often use alcohol to cope with the multiple stressors of aging
3. Are less motivated to follow a prescribed drug regimen
4. Have a decreased risk for adverse reactions to drugs

36. The nurse understands that the stage of development that is most unstable and challenging with regard to the development of a personal identity is:
1. Toddlerhood
2. Adolescence
3. Childhood
4. Infancy

37. The nurse in the operating room cares for patients with a variety of ages. The nurse understands that the individual at the greatest risk for complications during surgery is the:
1. Middle-aged adult
2. Pregnant woman
3. Adolescent
4. Infant

38. The nurse understands that a word that describes the process of growth and development is:
1. Fast
2. Simple
3. Limiting
4. Individual

39. For which common physiologic changes associated with aging should the nurse assess for in an older adult? Check all that apply.
1. _____ Increase in sebaceous gland activity
2. _____ Deterioration of joint cartilage
3. _____ Loss of social support system
4. _____ Decreased hearing acuity
5. _____ Increased need for sleep

40. The nurse is facilitating a mothers' class and the women begin discussing experiences that reflect the intellectual development of their children. Each woman describes a situation that reflects one of the stages of Jean Piaget's theory about logical thinking. Place the situations described in order beginning with the sensorimotor stage and ending with formal operations.
1. "My son touched the radiator and got burned. He'll never do that again."
2. "My son is learning math and is getting 100s on his tests. He is so smart."
3. "My daughter is on the debating team in school. We go to interschool meets."
4. "My daughter asked an obese lady if she had a baby in her stomach. I was so embarrassed."

Answer: _______________

ANSWERS AND RATIONALES

1. 1. **When a person reaches 60 years of age and older, all physiologic systems are less efficient, which reduces compensatory reserve.**
   2. In the 40- to 60-year-old age group a person will begin to see the earliest signs of aging. Changes are gradual and insidious and generally do not impact on function.
   3. In the 12- to 19-year-old age group the adolescent is experiencing rapid growth and a beginning transition to adulthood, not a decline in the ability to adapt.
   4. In the 3- to 11-year-old age group children are growing at a continuous pace in their ability to adapt to the world around them, not declining in their ability to adapt.

2. 1. A 6-year-old child is developing an understanding of the differences among the concepts of past, present, and future. A 6-year-old child believes that death is temporary, can be caused by bad thoughts, may be a punishment, and that magic can make the dead person alive.
   2. **A 9-year-old child has a more realistic understanding of death than a younger child and recognizes that death is universal, irreversible, and natural. A 9-year-old child has a beginning knowledge of his/her own mortality and may fear death.**
   3. Recognizing that death is irreversible, universal, and natural occurs at an earlier age than 12 years.
   4. Recognizing that death is irreversible, universal, and natural occurs at an earlier age than 15 years.

3. 1. This relates to Freud's Anal Stage of development (1 to 3 years). According to Freud, if a parent is strict, overbearing, and oppressive during toilet training, the child may develop traits of an anal retentive personality (obsessive-compulsive tendencies, rigid thought patterns, stinginess, and/or stubbornness).
   2. Seeking excessive attention from others is most likely the result of an unresolved task of the 6- to12-year-old age group (school age), Industry versus Inferiority. Seeking attention often is an attempt to increase self-esteem.
   3. People who have difficulty accepting help from others or who would rather do things themselves generally have not completely resolved the developmental task of infancy, Trust versus Mistrust.
   4. **The main developmental task of adolescence is forming a sense of personal identity as a foundation for the tasks of young adulthood, making decisions regarding career choices, and selecting a mate. An adult who has difficulty setting goals in life or who is unable to make a commitment to others indicates an unresolved conflict of Identity versus Role Confusion.**

4. 1. **The 25- to 45-year-old adult (Generativity versus Stagnation) strives to fulfill life goals associated with family, career, and society as well as being able to give to and care for others. A positive resolution of the conflict associated with this age group is often displayed in teaching, counseling, and community volunteer work.**
   2. Adults 65 years of age and older strive to resolve the conflict of Ego Integrity versus Despair. Successful resolution results in accepting one's life, recognizing the good and accepting the mistakes, willing to face death, and having a sense of integrity and wholeness.
   3. The 6- to 12-year-old child (Industry versus Inferiority) strives to gain control over the self, develop feelings of confidence and adequacy, and achieve the ability to carry out a task to completion.
   4. The 3- to 6-year-old child (Initiative versus Guilt) strives to become purposeful and self-directed.

5. 1. **This statement is a clear example of agism whereby older adults are systematically stereotyped and discriminated against because they are old. This is a form of prejudice, an unfavorable opinion without concrete information about the individual. Agism is based on the misconceptions that older adults are no longer productive, are narrow minded, are unable to learn, are dependent, experience memory loss, live in a nursing home, are ill, boring, etc.**
   2. This is not a discriminatory statement indicative of agism.
   3. This is not a discriminatory statement indicative of agism.
   4. This is not a discriminatory statement indicative of agism.

6. 1. **During the first year of life nutritional needs per unit of body weight are the greatest in comparison to any other time during the life span. Birth weight generally doubles in 4 to 6 months and triples by the end of the first year.**
   2. Although young adults tend to be active and require nutrients adequate to meet a high energy expenditure, physical growth slows and the basal metabolic rate begins to stabilize, so they require fewer calories than do other age groups.
   3. During the middle adult years energy expenditure decreases and nutritional needs stabilize. People in other age groups have greater needs for nutrients to meet physiologic demands than do those in the middle adult years.
   4. Older adults experience a decrease in basal metabolic rate, lean body mass, and physical activity, which contribute to a decrease in caloric needs.

7. 1. Middle-aged adults (25 to 45 years—Generativity versus Stagnation) strive to fulfill life goals associated with family, career, and society as well as to give to and care for others.
   2. Adolescents (12 to 20 years—Identity versus Role Confusion) strive to make the transition from childhood to adulthood with a sense of personal self.
   3. **Young adults (18 to 25 years—Intimacy versus Isolation) strive to establish mature relationships, commit to suitable partners, and develop social and work roles acceptable to society. Unsuccessful resolution results in self-absorption, egocentricity, and emotional isolation.**
   4. Infants (newborn to 18 months—Trust versus Mistrust) strive to have their needs met through interacting with others. When their needs are consistently met they develop a sense of trust in their caregivers.

8. 1. Toddlers are active once awake and rarely spend much time in bed when not sleeping. Toddlers sleep 12 to 14 hours a day, including one or two daytime naps.
   2. Middle-aged adults sleep about 6 to 8 hours a day. Although middle-aged adults spend more time in bed awake than when they were younger, they spend less time in bed awake than an age group in another option.
   3. **Older adults still need 7 to 9 hours of sleep daily but often receive less due to difficulty falling asleep and more frequent awakening. They often go to bed earlier in an effort to get more sleep and end up spending more time in bed awake. Sleeping difficulties are attributed to a decrease in melatonin, less deep sleep, a decrease in exercise, more naps, movement disorders, sleep apnea and medical and pychological problems.**
   4. Adolescents sleep 8 to10 hours a day. Adolescents generally have high activity levels and stay up late. It may seem as though adolescents are always sleeping because they sleep later in the morning, but generally they go to bed much later at night.

9. 1. More often people in the older age group need to adapt to the stress of a declining ability to ingest, digest, and/or absorb particular food. This might be required of an older adult who is learning to adjust to a therapeutic diet.
   2. This is an expected developmental task of adolescence, not early childhood. Many bodily changes occur in this transitional period, such as a growth spurt and sexual maturity.
   3. This is not an expected developmental stressor of this age group. Only a small percentage of the population of 18-month- to 3-year-old children face the challenge of a life-threatening illness.
   4. **During early childhood the child gains independence through learning right from wrong. Independence occurs with guidance from parents as the child learns self-control without feeling shame and doubt. When parents are overly protective or critical, feelings of inferiority will develop.**

10. 1. Although taste influences choices of foods ingested by the adolescent, a factor identified in another option generally has more influence over what adolescents eat.
    2. Adolescents tend to have few rigid routines because of their busy schedules. A factor identified in another option generally has more influence over what adolescents eat than do routines.
    3. **Peers often dictate the dietary choices of adolescents. Fad dieting and demands of socialization that generally involve fast food are commonly seen among adolescents.**
    4. Although personal preferences may influence choices of foods ingested by the adolescent, a factor identified in another option generally has more influence over what adolescents eat.

11. 1. **This is a serious concern because of a decrease in efficiency of hepatic metabolism and renal excretion of drugs in the older adult.**
2. Although side effects are a concern in the older adult, another option is a greater concern.
3. Although hypersensitivity is a concern in the older adult, another option is a greater concern.
4. Although idiosyncratic effects are a concern in the older adult, another option is a greater concern.

12. 1. Infants already demonstrate behavior on the most basic level.
2. **Toddlers are less able to understand and interpret what is happening to them when ill; therefore, they commonly regress to a previous level of development in an attempt to reduce anxiety.**
3. Adolescents generally want to behave in an adult manner and, therefore, demonstrate a controlled behavioral response to illness.
4. Although some young adults may regress to an earlier level of development as a coping strategy, regression commonly is not used as a defense mechanism when coping with illness.

13. 1. **People who avoid help from others and who would rather do things themselves generally have not completely resolved the developmental task of Trust versus Mistrust during infancy.**
2. Rationalizing unacceptable behaviors is a defense mechanism, not an indication of an unresolved developmental task of infancy. Rationalization is used to justify in some socially acceptable way ideas, feelings, or behavior through explanations that appear to be logical.
3. This behavior relates more to the Anal Stage of Freud's Psychosexual Theory of Development. Freud believed that when toilet training is approached in a rigid and demanding manner, a child develops into an adult who is overly concerned with orderliness and cleanliness.
4. This may indicate an unresolved conflict of Autonomy versus Shame and Doubt associated with the 18-month- to 3-year-old age group. One of the developmental tasks of this age group is learning right from wrong. When parents are overly critical and controlling, a child may develop an overly critical Superego and become an adult who feels the need to constantly apologize for small mistakes.

14. 1. Although social isolation is a risk for some older adults because of declining health, death of family members and friends, fear of crime or injury precipitating a desire not to leave the house, most older adults seek opportunities to maintain and build social contacts via the telephone, Internet, community groups, senior centers, life-care communities, etc.
2. **The older adult needs to adjust to multiple changes in social roles to emerge emotionally integrated with an intact ego and sense of wholeness. Changes in social roles are often dramatic as the result of retirement, death of significant others, changing responsibilities within the extended family structure, moving to different living quarters, and decreasing finances.**
3. Although older adults associate with members of all age groups, they generally establish an explicit affiliation with members of their own age group. This supports a sharing of common interests and concerns as well as meeting belonging and self-esteem needs as older adults seek status among their peers.
4. Older adults do not always have the energy or stamina needed to invest in increasing the number of new meaningful relationships. In addition, they tend to experience a decrease, not increase, in meaningful relationships because of the death of members of their circle of friends and relatives.

15. 1. As a person's skin ages it decreases, not increases, in tone because of loss of dermal mass. This occurs because of flattening of the dermal-epidermal junction, reduced thickness and vascularity of the dermis, and slowing of epidermal proliferation.
2. As a person's skin ages it increases, not decreases, in dryness because of a reduction in moisture content, sebaceous gland activity, and circulation to the skin.
3. As a person's skin ages it decreases, not increases, in elasticity because collagen fibers become coarser and more random, and there is a degeneration of elastic fibers in the dermal connective tissue.
4. **The skin of the older adult decreases in thickness because of loss of dermal and subcutaneous mass. This occurs in response to a flattening of the dermal-epidermal junction, reduced thickness and vascularity of the dermis, and slowing of epidermal proliferation.**

16. 1. An older adult man is not at risk when receiving a medication that has a teratogenic effect.
    2. **A pregnant woman is at risk. Teratogenic refers to a substance that can cross the placental barrier and interfere with growth and development of the fetus.**
    3. A 4-year-old child is not at risk when receiving a medication that has a teratogenic effect.
    4. A newborn is not at risk when receiving a medication that has a teratogenic effect.

17. 1. Dementia is a progressive irreversible decline in mental function that is not caused by sensory overload.
    2. **Confusion is a common response to sensory overload. Because of excessive sensory stimulation a person is unable to perceive the environment accurately or respond appropriately.**
    3. Sensory overload generally precipitates anxiety, agitation, and restlessness, not drowsiness.
    4. If sensory overload precipitates anxiety and the autonomic nervous system is stimulated by the *fight or flight* mechanism, tachycardia, not bradycardia, will occur.

18. 1. **Growth and development is an orderly process that follows a predictable, not unpredictable, path. There are three predictable patterns: cephalocaudal—proceeding from head to toe; proximodistal—progressing from gross motor to fine motor movements; and symmetrical—both sides developing equally. Growth is marked by measurable changes in the physical aspects of the life cycle and development is marked by behavioral changes that occur because of achievement of developmental tasks and their resulting functional abilities and skills.**
    2. Growth and development follow a sequential timetable whereby multiple dynamic changes occur in a systematic and orderly manner.
    3. Individuals grow and develop in the physiologic, cognitive, psychosocial, moral and spiritual realms in an integrated way, with each one influencing the others.
    4. Growth and development is a complex process that involves multiple influencing variables, such as genetics, experience, health, culture, and environment.

19. 1. School-aged children (6 to 12 years) tend to have fewer differences in appearance and behavior from their peers. These children begin to be involved with formalized groups where conformity is expected.
    2. Although adolescents may be viewed as different from the norms of their parents, they are similar to their peers. In their search for self-identity, adolescents experience role confusion. To control anxiety with role confusion, they are attracted to and conform with peer groups, which provide a sense of security.
    3. Although there is diversity in this age group, individuals have to adjust to common experiences such as physical decline, retirement, multiple losses, and changes in social roles. Older adults commonly seek out people of the same age to share similar interests and find status among their peers.
    4. **Middle-aged adults (40 to 60 years) are in a time of transition between young adulthood and older adulthood. Therefore, individuals in this group, more so than in any other age group, have the greatest individual differences in appearance and behavior as they span the norms seen in young adulthood, middle adulthood, and older adulthood.**

20. 1. **Sedatives are not well tolerated by older adults because a decrease in the absorption, metabolism, and excretion of the drug can result in toxicity. In addition, they may experience idiosyncratic (unexpected or opposite) effects.**
    2. Antianxiety drugs depress the central nervous system and therefore are helpful in supporting sleep.
    3. The effectiveness of hypnotics decreases, not increases, with prolonged use. They should be used only as a short-term intervention because tolerance and rebound insomnia occur in approximately 4 weeks.
    4. Although melatonin demonstrates promise as a drug to support sleep, it is not the drug of choice because its safety and efficacy are not yet established.

21. 1. Sigmund Freud, not Erikson, identified that defense mechanisms are used to reduce anxiety by preventing conscious awareness of threatening thoughts or feelings.
    2. Lawrence Kohlberg, not Erikson, established a framework for understanding the development of moral maturity, which is the ability to independently recognize what is right and what is wrong.

3. **Erikson expanded on Freud's Theory of Personality Development by giving equal emphasis to the influence of a person's social and cultural environment. Erikson stressed that psychosocial development depends on an interactive process between the physical and emotional variables during a person's life at eight distinct stages. Each stage requires resolution of a developmental conflict that has opposite outcomes and that requires interaction within the self and with others in the environment.**
4. Assimilation and accommodation of new information necessary to stimulate intellectual growth is a concept basic to Jean Piaget's Theory of Cognitive Development, not Erikson's Theory of Personality Development. Assimilation involves the process of organizing new information into one's present body of knowledge, and accommodation involves rearranging and restructuring thought processes to deal with the imbalance caused by new information and thereby increase understanding.

22. 1. The 18-month- to 3-year-old child (Autonomy versus Shame and Doubt) strives for independence.
2. The 12- to 20-year-old adolescent (Identity versus Role Confusion) strives to make the transition from childhood to adulthood with a sense of personal self.
3. The 25- to 65-year-old adult (Generativity versus Stagnation) strives to fulfill life goals associated with family, career, and society as well as being able to give to and care for others.
4. **The adult 65 years and older (Ego Integrity versus Despair) conducts a review of life events and seeks to come to terms with and accept responsibility for one's own life, including what it was in light of what one had hoped it would be.**

23. 1. Cessation of estrogen and progesterone production during menopause does not contribute to iron deficiency anemia.
2. Although older adults are at risk for iron deficiency anemia because of decreased intake and less efficient absorption of nutrients, they are not at as high a risk as an age group in another option.
3. Although teenagers are at risk for iron deficiency anemia because of rapid growth and diets high in fat and low in vitamins, they are not at as high a risk as an age group in another option.
4. **This age group is at the highest risk for iron deficiency anemia because of the increased physiological demand for blood production during growth, inadequate solid food intake after 6 months of age, and formula not fortified with iron. In addition, premature or multiple-birth infants are at special risk because of inadequate stores of iron during the end of fetal development.**

24. 1. Although inactivity may promote constipation, there are no physiological changes in school-aged children that will compound the risk for constipation.
2. Although middle-aged adults experience a slower gastrointestinal motility than when they were younger, they are not at as great a risk for constipation as an age group in another option.
3. **Older adults are at the greatest risk for constipation because of decreases in: activity levels, intake of high-fiber foods, peristalsis, digestive enzymes, and fluid intake.**
4. Constipation in infants is uncommon except when they are weaned from formula to cow's milk or when their diet is mismanaged.

25. 1. **The major task of middle adulthood is successfully fulfilling lifelong goals that involve family, career, and society. If these goals are not achieved, a crisis is often precipitated.**
2. Developing peer relationships is one of the developmental tasks of the 6- to 12-year-old child and adolescent, not the middle-aged adult.
3. Delaying satisfaction is one of the developmental tasks of the 18-month- to 3-year-old child, not the middle-aged adult.
4. Facing death is one of the developmental tasks of the 65-year-old and older adult, not the middle-aged adult.

26. 1. Although finger foods help to avoid a mess during mealtime, the child needs to learn how to use utensils when eating. This intervention interferes with the achievement of the task associated with this age group.
2. **From 18 months to 3 years of age (Autonomy versus Shame and Doubt) the child strives for independence. Attempts to feed oneself should be encouraged and enthusiastically praised even though the child may make a mess. It allows the child to practice and perfect new skills, helps to develop fine motor skills,**

and supports control of the self and the environment.

3. This should be avoided. When children are made to feel that the job they are doing is not good enough, it conveys a sense of shame and doubt and will make them feel inadequate.
4. This is discouraging to the child and may precipitate feelings of inadequacy, shame, and doubt. When caregivers always do what children should be learning, children are not permitted to learn for themselves.

27. 1. **A decline in vision, hearing, tactile sensation to pain and pressure, and a slower response time have the greatest impact on an older adult's ability to maintain safety over all of the systems offered in the other options.**
2. Although there is a decline in respiratory functioning, it does not pose as great a threat to safety when compared to a decline in another system of the body.
3. Alterations in the integumentary (skin) system generally do not pose a threat to safety when compared to a decline in another system of the body.
4. Although a decline in cardiovascular functioning can contribute to decreased physical activity, endurance, and balance and orthostatic hypotension, it does not pose as great a threat to safety as a decline in another system of the body.

28. 1. Kohlberg is best known for his Theory of Moral Development. People move through 6 stages of moral reasoning where the concepts about what is right and what is wrong progressively become more complex.
2. Brazelton is known for his Neonatal Assessment Scale, which is used to assess an infant's integrative behavioral processes in relation to various stimuli.
3. Freud identified the 6- to 12-year-old age group to be a period of latency during which sexual development lies dormant and emotional tension is reduced.
4. **Erik Erikson believed that 6- to 12-year-old children are in conflict over the developmental task of Industry versus Inferiority. Ten-year-old children strive to work or produce, compete and cooperate, and be competent.**

29. 1. The 6- to 12-year-old child strives to resolve the conflict of Industry versus Inferiority. Unsuccessful resolution results in lack of motivation and feelings of inadequacy, inferiority, and guilt. Successful resolution results in a positive control over the self, feelings of confidence and adequacy, and the ability to carry a task to completion.
2. Adults 65 years of age and older strive to resolve the conflict of Ego Integrity versus Despair. Unsuccessful resolution results in a fear of death and dissatisfaction with one's life. Successful resolution results in accepting one's life (recognizing the good and accepting the mistakes), having a sense of integrity and wholeness, and being willing to face death.
3. **The 25- to 65-year-old adult who is unable to successfully resolve the conflict of Generativity versus Stagnation becomes egocentric, disinterested in others, and self-absorbed. Successful resolution results in the ability to give to and care for others.**
4. The 12- to 20-year-old adolescent strives to resolve the conflict of Identity versus Role Confusion. Unsuccessful resolution results in self-doubt, dysfunctional relationships, and even antisocial behavior. Successful resolution results in personal integration of a self-identity.

30. 1. The most recent CDC statistics available at the time of this book's publication indicate that 8% of all infant deaths are caused by SIDS.
2. The most recent CDC statistics available at the time of this book's publication indicate that 3.8% of all infant deaths are caused by unintentional injury.
3. **The most recent CDC statistics available at the time of this book's publication indicate that 20.1% of all infant deaths are caused by congenital anomalies.**
4. The most recent CDC statistics available at the time of this book's publication indicate that 16.6% of all infant deaths are cause by preterm births.

31. 1. Toddlers generally are able to regulate body temperature as long as they are basically healthy.
2. Adolescents generally are able to regulate body temperature as long as there are no coexisting health problems.
3. **Regulation of body temperature depends on the ability to dilate or constrict blood vessels and control the activity of sweat glands. In the older adult: the production of sweat glands decreases, reducing a person's ability to perspire and resulting in risk for heat exhaustion; there are decreased amounts of muscle mass and subcutaneous fat, which lead to increased**

susceptibility to cold; there is inefficient vasoconstriction in response to cold and inefficient vasodilation in response to heat; and there is a diminished ability to shiver, which increases body temperature.

4. School-aged children generally are able to regulate temperature as long as there are no other underlying medical conditions.

32. 1. The 18-month- to 3-year-old child who has feelings of self-doubt, low self-control and self-esteem reflects difficulty in resolving the conflict of Autonomy versus Shame and Doubt. Successful resolution results in independence, displays of emerging willpower, and a sense of control.
2. The 12- to 20-year-old adolescent who has self-doubt, dysfunctional relationships, and even antisocial behavior reflects a negative resolution of the conflict of Identity versus Role Confusion. Successful resolution results in an integration of a personal self.
3. The adult 65 years and older who is preoccupied with reliving life because of dissatisfaction with the past reflects a negative resolution of the task of Ego Integrity versus Despair. Conducting a review of life events, seeking to come to terms with and accepting responsibility for one's own life, and accepting what it was in light of what one had hoped it would be reflects successful resolution of the conflict of Ego Integrity versus Despair.
4. **Young adults 18 to 25 years of age who are self-absorbed, egocentric, and emotionally isolated reflect a negative resolution of the conflict of Intimacy versus Isolation. Successful resolution results in the ability to establish mature relationships, commit to a suitable partner, and develop social and work roles acceptable to society.**

33. 1. Infants initially sleep 17 to 20 hours a day and by the end of the first year are sleeping 12 to 16 hours a day. Frequent awakening for feeding is expected and not a sleep problem for the infant.
2. Toddlers (18 months to 3 years) generally sleep 12 to 15 hours a day with one or two naps. Toddlers occasionally will awaken during the night because of teething pains, illness, separation anxiety, and loneliness; awakening during the night is not unusual in the toddler. If caregivers establish regular bedtime routines and provide emotional comfort, sleep problems are minimal during this age group.
3. **Adolescents (12 to 20 years) have more multiple and complex physiological (e.g., puberty), psychological (e.g., self-identity and independence issues), and social (e.g., peer pressure, altered roles, and maturing relationships) milestones than any other stage of development. Anxiety associated with all of these stressors contributes to altered sleep patterns and sleep deprivation. Adolescents generally need 8 to 10 hours of sleep a day; however, adolescents' sleep needs vary widely.**
4. Preschoolers (3 to 5 years) have well established sleep-wake cycles, they sleep 10 to 12 hours a day, and daytime napping decreases. Dreams and nightmares, which can awaken the child, are common but are not considered abnormal. Establishing consistent rituals that include quiet time helps to minimize nighttime awakening.

34. 1. **When middle-aged adults are caring for their children and their aging, dependent parents at the same time, they are referred to as the *sandwich generation*. Their parents and children represent the bread and they are the meat in between.**
2. Role reversal is not a definition of *sandwich generation*.
3. Assisting both sets of parents is not a definition of *sandwich generation*.
4. Being a middle child between older and younger siblings is not the definition of *sandwich generation*.

35. 1. Older adults experience a decreased, not increased, absorption of drugs from the GI tract.
2. Although approximately 10% of older adults have some problem with alcohol use late in life, the literature supports the fact that there is a decrease, not increase, in the incidence of alcoholism with the aged.
3. **The literature documents that 75% of older adults are to some degree intentionally noncompliant with drug therapy because of inconvenience, side effects, and/or perceived ineffectiveness of the drugs.**
4. Older adults have an increased, not decreased, risk for adverse reactions to drugs. Adverse effects are any effects that are not therapeutic. Side effects are minor adverse effects that in most cases can be tolerated.

36. 1. Although toddlers (18 months to 3 years; early childhood—Autonomy versus Shame and Doubt) experience a number of developmental milestones, it is not as unstable or complex as another stage of development. Toddlers explore and test the environment, develop independence, and have a beginning ability to control the self.

2. **Adolescents (12 to 20 years—Identity versus Role Confusion) have multiple and complex physiological (e.g., puberty), psychological (e.g., self identity and independence), and social (e.g., peer pressure, altered roles, and maturing relationships) milestones than any other stage of development. The multiplicity of these stressors can have a major impact on the development of the adolescent's personal identity and sense of self.**
3. Although children in early childhood or toddlerhood (18 months to 3 years—Autonomy versus Shame and Doubt) and late childhood (3 to 6 years—Initiative versus Guilt) experience a number of developmental milestones, they are not as unstable or complex as another age group. The main tasks of childhood are achievement of self-control, initiation of one's own activities, and development of purpose and competence.
4. Although infants (birth to 18 months—Trust versus Mistrust) experience a number of developmental milestones, it is not as unstable or complex as another age group. The main tasks of infancy are to adjust to living in and responding to the environment and the development of trust.

37.
1. Middle-aged adults usually are safe candidates for surgery.
2. Although a pregnant woman has unique needs during surgery, as long as the mother's cardiovascular and fluid and electrolyte status are maintained the fetus is supported and safe.
3. Although the adolescent has needs related to body image and separation from friends, the physiologic risk of surgery is not increased.
4. **Infants are at risk for volume depletion because of a small blood volume and limited fluid reserves. In addition, immature liver and kidneys affect the ability to metabolize and eliminate drugs, an undeveloped immune system increases the risk of infection, and immature temperature regulating mechanisms increase the risk of hyperthermia and hypothermia.**

38.
1. Some stages are faster and some are slower depending on the person and the developmental level.
2. The growth and development process is very complex and influenced by many different factors.
3. Just the opposite is true; the growth and development process helps people to extend themselves to be the most that they can be.
4. **Although people follow a general pattern, they do not grow and develop at exactly the same rate or extent.**

39.
1. Although sebaceous glands increase in size with age, the amount of sebum produced decreases, hastening the evaporation of water from the stratum corneum resulting in cracked, dry skin.
2. **Older adults generally experience a deterioration of the hyaline cartilage surface of joints which tears, allowing bones to be in direct contact with each other. Often this results in the formation of spurs or projecting points that limit joint motion.**
3. Loss of a social support system is a psychosocial, not physiologic, change commonly experienced by older adults.
4. **Hearing acuity decreases, particularly in relation to high-pitched sounds, because of atrophy in the organ of Corti and cochlear neurons, loss of the sensory hair cells, and degeneration of the stria vascularis.**
5. Older adults have the same need for sleep as younger individuals. However, it is more difficult for older adults to obtain the quality and quantity of sleep desired. Chemical, structural, and functional changes in the nervous system disrupt circadian rhythms and sleep.

40. **Answer: 1, 4, 2, 3**

1. **The *sensorimotor* stage (birth to 2 years) is governed by sensations in which simple learning takes place. It progresses from reflex activity, through repetitive behaviors, to imitative behavior. They are curious, experiment, and learn primarily through trial and error.**
4. **The *preoperational* stage (2 to 7 years) involves thinking that is concrete and tangible; they cannot reason beyond the observable. Also, their thinking is *transductive*; that is, knowledge of one characteristic is transferred to another.**
2. **The *concrete-operational* stage (7 to 11 years) reflects an increasing ability to use symbols and understand relationships between things and ideas. Judgments are made based on what they reason (conceptual thinking) rather than just**

what they see (preoperational thinking). Also, they develop the concept of *conservation*; that is, physical factors (e.g., volume, weight, and number) remain the same even though outward appearances may change.

3. The *formal operational* stage (11 to 15 years) involves thinking that is abstract, theoretical, philosophical, and hypothetical. Thinking is characterized by flexibility, adaptability, and drawing logical conclusions.

Communication

KEYWORDS

The following words include English vocabulary, nursing/medical terminology, concepts, principles, or information relevant to content specifically addressed in the chapter or associated with topics presented in it. English dictionaries, nursing textbooks, and medical dictionaries, such as *Taber's Cyclopedic Medical Dictionary*, are resources that can be used to expand your knowledge and understanding of these words and related information.

- Active listening
- Assertive skills
- Barriers to communication
  - Advising
  - Direct questions
  - Disapproving
  - False reassurance
  - Moralizing
  - Patronizing
  - Probing
- Body language
- Cliché
- Communication process
  - Encoding by sender
  - Message
  - Channel of communication
    - Auditory
    - Kinesthetic
    - Visual
  - Decoding by receiver
  - Feedback
- Confidential
- Confidentiality
- Confrontation
- Congruence
- Content themes
- Conversation
- Empathy, empathetic, empathic
- Exploring
- Focus
- Formal interview
- Gossip
- Group dynamics
- Inference
- Informal interview
- Interaction
- Interpersonal communication
- Intrapersonal communication
- Listening skills
- Nonverbal
- Organizational communication
- Rapport
- Response
- Space
  - Intimate
  - Personal
  - Social
  - Public
- Territoriality
- Therapeutic communication skills
  - Clarifying
  - Focusing
  - General leads
  - Indirect question
  - Open-ended question
  - Paraphrasing
  - Reflection
  - Responding
  - Silence
  - Summarizing
  - Touching
  - Validating
- Therapeutic relationship, phases
  - Orientation
  - Working
  - Termination
- Verbal
- Verbalization
- Visual cues

QUESTIONS

1. A patient states, "Do you think I could have cancer?" The nurse responds, "What did the doctor tell you?" What interviewing approach did the nurse use?
   1. Paraphrasing
   2. Confrontation
   3. Reflective technique
   4. Open-ended question
2. The main purpose of the working phase of a therapeutic nurse-patient relationship is to:
   1. Establish a formal or informal contract that addresses the patient's problems
   2. Implement nursing interventions that are designed to achieve expected patient outcomes
   3. Develop rapport and trust so the patient feels protected and an initial plan can be identified
   4. Clearly identify the role of the nurse and establish the parameters of the professional relationship
3. The nurse uses reflective technique when communicating with an anxious patient. The nurse uses reflective technique in this situation because it focuses on:
   1. Feelings
   2. Content themes
   3. Clarification of information
   4. Summarization of the topics discussed
4. A patient says, "I don't know if I'll make it through this surgery." Which response by the nurse may block further communication by the patient?
   1. "You sound scared."
   2. "You think you will die."
   3. "Surgery can be frightening."
   4. "Everything will be all right."
5. The patient states, "My wife is going to be very upset that my prostate surgery probably is going to leave me impotent." What is the best response by the nurse?
   1. "I'm sure your wife will be willing to make this sacrifice in exchange for your well-being."
   2. "The doctors are getting great results with nerve-sparing surgery today."
   3. "Your wife may not put as much emphasis on sex as you think."
   4. "Let's talk about how you feel about this surgery."
6. The patient states, "I think that I am dying." The nurse responds, "You feel as though you are dying?" What interviewing approach did the nurse use?
   1. Focusing
   2. Reflecting
   3. Validating
   4. Paraphrasing
7. The nurse plans to foster a therapeutic relationship with a patient. It is most important that the nurse:
   1. Work on establishing a friendship with the patient
   2. Use humor to defuse emotionally charged topics of discussion
   3. Sympathize with the patient when the patient shares sad feelings
   4. Demonstrate respect when discussing emotionally charged topics
8. A patient who is to receive nothing by mouth (NPO) in preparation for a bronchoscopy says, "I'm worried about the test and I can't even have a drink of water." What is the best response by the nurse?
   1. "Let's talk about your concerns regarding the test."
   2. "I'll see if the doctor will let you have some ice chips."
   3. "The doctor will review the results of the test as soon as possible."
   4. "As soon as the test is over I'll get you whatever you would like to drink."

9. A patient verbally communicates with the nurse while exhibiting nonverbal behavior. To confirm the meaning of the nonverbal behavior, the nurse should:
   1. Look for similarity in meaning between the patient's verbal and nonverbal behavior
   2. Ask family members to help interpret the patient's behavior
   3. Validate inferences by asking the patient direct questions
   4. Recognize that what a patient says is most important

10. The patient appears tearful and is quiet and withdrawn. The nurse says, "You seem very sad today." What interviewing approach did the nurse use?
    1. Examining
    2. Reflecting
    3. Clarifying
    4. Orienting

11. Which nursing action best reflects the concept of therapeutic communication?
    1. Using interviewing skills to discuss the patient's concerns
    2. Letting the patient control the focus of conversation
    3. Setting time aside to talk with the patient
    4. Agreeing with a patient's statements

12. The nurse is attempting to develop a helping relationship with a patient who was recently diagnosed with cancer. The nurse understands that a factor that is unique to this helping relationship is that it is:
    1. Characterized by allowing the patient to assume the dominant role
    2. Distinguished by an equal sharing of information
    3. Specific to a person while guided by a purpose
    4. Based on the needs of both participants

13. The nurse is collecting data for an admission nursing history. Which question by the nurse is best to open the discussion?
    1. "What brought you to the hospital?"
    2. "Would it help to discuss your feelings?"
    3. "Do you want to talk about your concerns?"
    4. "Would you like to talk about why you are here?"

14. The nurse must conduct a focused interview to complete an admission history. Which interviewing technique should the nurse use?
    1. Probing
    2. Clarification
    3. Direct questions
    4. Paraphrasing statements

15. An agitated 80-year-old patient states, "I'm having trouble with my bowels." Which response by the nurse incorporates the interviewing skill of reflection?
    1. "You seem distressed about your bowels."
    2. "You're having trouble with your bowels?"
    3. "It's common to have problems with the bowels at your age."
    4. "When did you first notice having trouble with your bowels?"

16. The nurse understands that the statement that is most accurate about communication is:
    1. Communication is inevitable
    2. Behavior clearly reflects feelings
    3. Hands are the most expressive part of the body
    4. Verbal communication is essential for human relationships

17. The patient is upset and crying and mentions something about her job that the nurse cannot understand. The nurse's best response is:
    1. "It's natural to be worried about your job."
    2. "Your job must be very important to you."
    3. "Calm down so that I can understand what you are saying."
    4. "I'm not quite sure I heard what you were saying about your work."

18. When providing nursing care, humor should be used to:
   1. Diminish feelings of anger
   2. Refocus the patient's attention
   3. Maintain a balanced perspective
   4. Delay dealing with the inevitable

19. The nurse evaluates that therapeutic communication is effective when:
   1. Verbal and nonverbal communication is congruent
   2. Interaction is conducted in a professional manner
   3. Common understanding is achieved
   4. Thoughts can be put into words

20. A patient is admitted to the hospital with cirrhosis of the liver caused by long-term alcohol abuse. What is the best response by the nurse when the patient says, "I really don't believe that my drinking a couple of beers a day has anything to do with my liver problem?"
   1. "You find it hard to believe that beer can damage the liver?"
   2. "How long have you been drinking a couple of beers a day?"
   3. "Each beer is equivalent to one shot of liquor so it's just as damaging to the liver as hard liquor."
   4. "You may believe that beer is not harmful but research shows that it is just as bad for you as hard liquor."

21. The patient states, "I can't believe that I couldn't even eat half my breakfast." Which statement by the nurse uses the interviewing skill of reflection?
   1. "Let's talk about your inability to eat."
   2. "What part of your breakfast were you able to eat?"
   3. "How long have you been unable to eat most of your breakfast?"
   4. "You seem surprised that you were unable to eat all your breakfast."

22. What is the best response by the nurse when the patient's husband says, "I just don't know what to say to my wife if she asks how I feel about her breast cancer."
   1. "How do you feel about your wife's diagnosis?"
   2. "This is a difficult topic. However, let's talk about it."
   3. "Do you think you could be as supportive as you can possibly be?"
   4. "Men don't always understand what women are going through. Ask her about how she feels."

23. What is being communicated when the nurse leans forward during a patient interview?
   1. Interest
   2. Privacy
   3. Anxiety
   4. Aggression

24. What best describes the following proverb? *What you do speaks so loudly I cannot hear what you say.*
   1. Nonverbal messages are often more meaningful than words
   2. Hearing ability is an important factor in the communication process
   3. Listening to what people say requires attention to what is being said
   4. When people talk too loudly it is hard to understand what is being said

25. A mother whose young daughter has died of leukemia is crying, and is unable to talk about her feelings. What is the best response by the nurse?
   1. "Everyone will remember her because she was so cute. She was one of our favorites."
   2. "As hard as this is, it is probably for the best because she was in a lot of pain."
   3. "She put up the good fight but now she is out of pain and in heaven."
   4. "I feel so sad. It can be hard to deal with such a precious loss."

26. The goals of therapeutic communication mainly should depend on the:
    1. Environment in which communication takes place
    2. Role of the nurse in the particular clinical setting
    3. Skill level of the nurse in the situation
    4. Concerns of the patient

27. A young man who had a leg amputated because of trauma says, "No one will ever choose to love a person with one leg." What is the best response by the nurse?
    1. "You are a good looking young man, and you will have no trouble meeting someone who cares."
    2. "You may feel that way now, but you will feel differently as time passes."
    3. "Do you feel that no one will marry you because you have one leg?"
    4. "How do you see your situation at this point?"

28. The nurse is changing a patient's dressing over an abdominal wound. Which level of space around the patient is entered during the dressing change?
    1. Personal
    2. Intimate
    3. Social
    4. Public

29. The stage of an interview that establishes the relationship between the nurse and the patient is the:
    1. Opening stage
    2. Working stage
    3. Surrogate stage
    4. Examining stage

30. The patient is exhibiting anxious behavior and states, "I just found out that I have cancer everywhere and I don't have very long to live. My life is over." What is the best response by the nurse?
    1. "It might be good if your wife were here right now. Shall I call her?"
    2. "What might be the best way to approach this terrible news?"
    3. "That is so sad. You must feel like crying."
    4. "It sounds like you feel hopeless."

31. Which interviewing skill is being used when the nurse says, "You mentioned before that you are having a problem with your colostomy?"
    1. Focusing
    2. Clarifying
    3. Paraphrasing
    4. Acknowledging

32. The patient says, "I am really nervous about having a spinal tap tomorrow." The best response by the nurse is:
    1. "I'll ask the doctor for a little medication to help you relax."
    2. "Patients who have had a spinal tap say it is not that uncomfortable."
    3. "The doctor is excellent and is very careful when spinal taps are done."
    4. "It's all right to be nervous, and I don't remember anyone who wasn't."

33. A patient with chest pain is being admitted to the Emergency Department. When asked about next of kin the patient states, "Don't bother calling my daughter, she is always too busy." What is the best response by the nurse?
    1. "She might be upset if you don't call her."
    2. "What does your daughter do that makes her so busy?"
    3. "Is there someone else that you would like me to call for you?"
    4. "I can't imagine that your daughter wouldn't want to know that you are sick."

34. Effective therapeutic communication mainly depends on the nurse's ability to:
    1. Send a verbal message
    2. Use interviewing skills
    3. Be assertive when collecting data
    4. Display sympathy when communicating

35. *Active listening* by a nurse means:
    1. Identifying the patient's concerns and exploring them with why questions
    2. Determining the content and feeling of the patient's message
    3. Employing silence to encourage the patient to talk
    4. Using nonverbal skills to display interest

36. A patient who has had a number of postoperative complications appears upset and agitated, yet withdrawn. The most appropriate statement by the nurse should be:
    1. "You seem agitated. Tell me why you are upset."
    2. "You've been having a pretty rough time of it since surgery."
    3. "It's not uncommon to have complications after the kind of surgery that you had."
    4. "I'm not sure that I know everything that has been happening. Tell me what has happened to you since surgery."

37. The nurse is admitting a patient to the unit who was transferred from the Emergency Department. When facilitating communication, the nurse should:
    1. Ensure that the patient has an effective way to communicate with health-team members
    2. Use interviewing techniques to control the direction of the patient's communication
    3. Minimize energy spent by the patient on negative feelings and concerns
    4. Refocus to the positive aspects of the patient's situation and prognosis

38. The nurse is assisting a confused patient with a diagnosis of Alzheimer's dementia to eat. What should the nurse say?
    1. "Please eat your meat."
    2. "It's important that you eat."
    3. "What would you like to eat?"
    4. "If you don't eat, you can't have dessert."

39. Which are the most important nursing actions when speaking with an older adult who is hearing-impaired? Check all that apply.
    1. _____ Limit background noise
    2. _____ Exaggerate lip movements
    3. _____ Raise the pitch of your voice
    4. _____ Stand directly in front of the patient when speaking
    5. _____ Raise the volume of your voice while speaking directly toward the patient's good ear

40. A patient with a colostomy wants to learn how to irrigate a newly created colostomy. The nurse provides this teaching by developing a therapeutic nurse-patient relationship and implementing teaching strategies. Identify the statements that are included in the working phase of this therapeutic relationship. Check all those that apply.
    1. _____ "How do you feel about doing this procedure?"
    2. _____ "Would you like to try to insert the cone yourself today?"
    3. _____ "You did a great job managing the instillation of fluid today."
    4. _____ "I am here to help you learn how to irrigate your colostomy."
    5. _____ "I'll arrange for a home care nurse to visit you in your home when you are dischaged."

ANSWERS AND RATIONALES

1. 1. The nurse's response is not an example of paraphrasing, which is restating the patient's basic message in similar words.
   2. This is not an example of confrontation. A confronting or challenging statement fails to consider feelings, puts the patient on the defensive, and is a barrier to communication.
   3. The nurse's response is not an example of reflective technique, which is referring back the basic feelings underlying the patient's statement.
   4. **This open-ended statement invites the patient to elaborate on the expressed thoughts with more than a one- or two-word response.**

2. 1. Formal or informal contracts are established during the introductory (orientation), not working, phase of a therapeutic relationship.
   2. **During the working phase of the therapeutic relationship, nursing interventions have a twofold purpose: assisting patients to explore and understand their thoughts and feelings, and facilitating and supporting patient decisions and actions.**
   3. The development of trust is the primary goal of the introductory (orientation), not working, phase of a therapeutic relationship. Trust is achieved through respect, concern, credibility, and reliability.
   4. These tasks are achieved during the introductory (orientation), not working, phase of a therapeutic relationship.

3. 1. **The reflective technique requires active listening to identify the underlying emotional concerns or feelings contained in patients' messages. These feelings are then referred back to patients to promote a clearer understanding of what they have said.**
   2. Content themes are referred back to patients through paraphrasing, which is a restatement of what was said in similar words.
   3. When seeking clarification, the nurse can indicate confusion, restate the message, or ask the patient to elaborate in an attempt to make the patient's message more understood.
   4. Summarization reviews the significant points of discussion to reiterate or clarify information.

4. 1. This example of reflective technique identifies feelings, which promotes communication.
   2. This example of paraphrasing restates the content of the patient's message, which promotes communication.
   3. This example of reflective technique focuses on feelings, which promotes communication.
   4. **This response is false reassurance. It denies the patient's concerns about survival and does not invite the patient to elaborate.**

5. 1. This response is false reassurance. Only the wife can make this statement.
   2. Although a true statement, this response negates the patient's concerns and cuts off communication.
   3. This may or may not be a true statement. Only the wife can make this statement.
   4. **The patient may be using projection to cope with the potential for impotence. This response indicates that it is acceptable to talk about sexuality and invites the patient to verbalize concerns.**

6. 1. This is not an example of focusing, which centers on the key elements of the patient's message in an attempt to eliminate vagueness. It keeps a rambling conversation on target to explore the major concern. The patient was not rambling.
   2. This is not an example of reflecting, which focuses on feelings. The use of the word "feel" does not make the nurse's statement an example of reflection.
   3. This is not an example of validating. Consensual validation, a form of clarification, verifies the meaning of specific words rather than the overall meaning of the message. This ensures that both patient and nurse agree on the meaning of the words used.
   4. **The nurse's response is an example of paraphrasing because it uses similar words to restate the patient's message.**

7. 1. The nurse should maintain a professional relationship with the patient. Nurses may be "friendly" toward patients, but should not establish a "friendship" with a patient.
   2. Humor with emotionally charged issues may be viewed as minimizing concerns or frivolous, and could be a barrier to communication.

3. Sympathy denotes pity, which should be avoided. The nurse should empathize, not sympathize, with the patient.
4. **Emotionally charged topics should be approached with respectful, sincere interactions that are accepting and nonjudgmental, which will promote further verbalizations.**

8. 1. **This response encourages the patient to explore concerns. Verbalization of concerns, validation of feelings, and patient teaching may help reduce anxiety.**
2. This intervention bypasses data collection. In addition, ice chips are composed of water, which is contraindicated before and initially after a bronchoscopy because of the risk for aspiration.
3. This response ignores both of the patient's concerns and addresses a completely different issue.
4. Fluid and food are not permitted after a bronchoscopy until the gag reflex returns.

9. 1. **The patient is the primary source of information. When nonverbal communication reinforces the verbal message, the message reflects the true feelings of the patient because nonverbal behavior is under less conscious control than verbal statements.**
2. This abdicates the nurse's responsibility to others and obtains a response that is influenced by emotion and subjectivity.
3. Direct questions are too specific. Open-ended questions or gently pointing out the incongruence between actions and words are more effective techniques than direct questions in this situation.
4. Nonverbal behaviors, rather than verbal statements, better reflect true feelings. Actions speak louder than words!

10. 1. Examining is not an interviewing technique.
2. **Reflective technique refers to feelings implied in the content of verbal communication or in exhibited nonverbal behaviors. Patients who are crying, quiet, and withdrawn often are sad.**
3. This is not an example of clarifying, which is the use of a statement to better understand a message when communication is unclear, rambling, or garbled.
4. This is not an example of orienting. Reality orientation is a nursing technique used to assist patients in restoring an awareness of what is actual, authentic, or real.

11. 1. **Therapeutic communication is patient-centered and goal-directed. It facilitates the exploration of the patient's thoughts and feelings and helps to establish a constructive relationship between the nurse and patient.**
2. Although this often is done, there are many times when the patient may ramble and need to be refocused by the nurse.
3. Although this often is done, therapeutic communication can occur at any time, such as when providing physical hygiene or performing a procedure.
4. Although this often is done, there are many times when this response is inappropriate.

12. 1. There are times that the nurse must assume a dominant role; examples include when the patient is unconscious, out of touch with reality, in a crisis, or experiencing panic.
2. In a therapeutic relationship, the focus is on the patient, not the nurse.
3. **The helping relationship (interpersonal relationship, therapeutic relationship) is a personal, client-focused, goal-oriented process whereby the nurse assists a person to problem-solve and meet needs.**
4. The purpose of a therapeutic relationship is to focus on and meet the needs of the patient, not the nurse.

13. 1. **This is a focused open-ended statement that invites the patient to communicate while centering on the reason for seeking health care.**
2. This direct question can be answered with a "yes" or "no" response. If the response is "no" then communication will be cut off.
3. This direct question can be answered with a "yes" or "no" response which may limit communication.
4. The desire to talk and the need to talk are different issues. It is helpful if health-care providers collect as much significant data as possible.

14. 1. Probing questions violate the patient's privacy, may cut off communication, and are inappropriate even in a focused interview. Probing interviewing occurs when the nurse persistently attempts to obtain information even after the patient indicates an unwillingness to discuss the topic or pursues information out of curiosity, rather than because the information is significant.
2. Although clarification may be used during a focused interview to understand what the patient is saying, it is not the primary

technique utilized for seeking specific information.

3. **A focused interview explores a particular topic or obtains specific information. Direct questions meet these objectives and avoid extraneous information.**
4. Paraphrasing may be used during a focused interview to redirect ideas back to the patient so that the patient can verify that the nurse received the message accurately or to allow the patient to hear what was said. However, it is not a technique that obtains specific information quickly.

15. 1. **This response recognizes and reflects back the underlying feeling in the patient's message (reflective technique). When people consider themselves in trouble, they usually feel threatened or stressed.**
2. This restates the patient's comment and is an example of paraphrasing, not reflection.
3. This negates the patient's concerns and shuts off communication.
4. This is not an example of reflection; it is a direct question that collects specific information.

16. 1. **Theory indicates that all behavior has meaning, people are always behaving, and we cannot stop behaving or communicating; therefore, communication is inevitable.**
2. Behavior may imply, not clearly reflect, feelings. The nurse should obtain verbal feedback from the patient regarding assumptions about behavior.
3. The face, not the hands, is the most expressive part of the body.
4. All communication, not just verbal communication, is essential for human relationships.

17. 1. This may or may not be an accurate assumption.
2. This makes an assumption that may be erroneous.
3. This patronizing response treats the patient in a condescending manner. The patient cannot calm down.
4. **This response requests additional information in an attempt to clarify an unclear message.**

18. 1. Humor used inappropriately can cause anger to be increased, suppressed or repressed. Anger should be expressed safely.
2. The focus should be on the patient's concerns.
3. **Humor is an interpersonal tool and a healing strategy. It releases physical and psychic energy, enhances well-being, reduces anxiety, increases pain tolerance, and places experiences within the context of life.**
4. Coping strategies should not be delayed because delay increases stress and anxiety and prolongs the process.

19. 1. This just ensures that the message probably reflects the true feelings of the patient.
2. Interactions, even if conducted in a professional manner, may or may not be effective.
3. **Understanding is the foundation of therapeutic communication. When the nurse comprehends, appreciates, and empathizes with the patient, therapeutic communication is effective. The working phase of the helping relationship can then move forward and is productive.**
4. This just ensures that ideas or feelings are communicated. Sending a message is communication occurring in just one direction.

20. 1. **This is an example of paraphrasing. It repeats the content in the patient's message in similar words to provide feedback to let the patient know whether the message was understood and to prompt further communication.**
2. This response does not address the content or emotional theme of the patient's statement. In addition, this probing question may be a barrier to further communication.
3. This response is confrontational, which may put the patient on the defensive and inhibit further communication.
4. This assertive, confronting, judgmental response will put the patient on the defensive and cut off communication.

21. 1. This statement does not employ reflective technique.
2. This direct question elicits a minimal amount of information about only one aspect of eating.
3. This direct question focuses on just one aspect of the problem, duration.
4. **This question is an example of reflective technique because it focuses on the feeling of surprise.**

22. 1. This question is too direct. The husband may not be in touch with his feelings and will be unable to answer the question.
2. **This response acknowledges that the patient is in a dilemma and it offers an opportunity to explore the situation.**

Validation and an invitation to talk provide emotional support, even if the opportunity to talk is declined.

3. This response focuses on the patient's needs and ignores the husband's concerns.
4. This response is condescending and focuses on the patient's, not the husband's, needs.

23. 1. **Leaning forward is a nonverbal behavior that conveys involvement. It is a form of physical attending, which is being present to another.**

2. Privacy is not reflected by leaning forward during an interview. Privacy is facilitated by pulling a patient's curtain or finding a separate room or quiet space to talk.
3. A closed posture, avoidance of eye contact, increased muscle tension, and increased motor activity convey anxiety.
4. Piercing eye contact, increased voice volume, challenging or confrontational conversation, invasion of personal space, and inappropriate touching convey aggression, which is a hostile, injurious, or destructive action or outlook.

24. 1. **Nonverbal communication (body language) conveys messages without words and is under less conscious control than verbal statements. When a person's words and behavior are incongruent, nonverbal behavior most likely reflects the person's true feelings.**

2. Although hearing, one aspect of decoding a message, is an important factor in the communication process, it is unrelated to the stated proverb.
3. Although this true statement reflects *active listening*, it is unrelated to the stated proverb.
4. This statement is unrelated to the stated proverb. The volume of a message may or may not influence understanding of the message. The volume of a message occurs on the physiologic level, while understanding a message occurs on the cognitive level.

25. 1. This response is not therapeutic because it focuses on the nurses rather than on the mother.

2. The first part of this response minimizes the loss. The second part of the response focuses on the pain experienced by the child, which may increase the mother's grief.
3. This response minimizes the loss and focuses on the pain experienced by the child, which may increase the mother's grief. Also, the mother may not believe in heaven.
4. **The first sentence communicates empathy. The second sentence focuses on the feelings surrounding loss and provides an opportunity for the patient to verbalize. Both of these are therapeutic responses to the situation.**

26. 1. Although the environment may enhance or be a barrier to communication, it does not determine the goals of communication.

2. The role of a nurse in a particular setting does not dictate the goals of communication.
3. Although the interviewing skills of the nurse may determine the effectiveness of communication, it does not set the goals of communication.
4. **The patient and significant others and their needs are always the focus of nursing interventions, including the goals of communication.**

27. 1. This negates the patient's concerns. The patient needs to focus on the "negative" before focusing on the "positive." In addition, only the future will tell if the patient meets someone who cares.

2. This is false reassurance. There is no way the nurse can ensure that his belief will change.
3. **This is an example of paraphrasing, which restates the patient's message in similar words. It promotes communication.**
4. This statement is unnecessary. The patient has already stated his point of view.

28. 1. "Laying on of the hands" does not occur with personal distance. Personal space ($1^1/_2$ to 4 feet) is effective for communicating with another. It is close enough to imply caring and is not extended to the distance that implies lack of involvement.

2. **Physically caring for a patient involves inspection and touch that invades the instinctual, protective distance immediately surrounding an individual. Intimate space (physical contact to $1^1/_2$ feet) is characterized by body contact and visual exposure.**
3. Invasive touching does not occur with social distance. Social space (4 to 12 feet) is effective for more formal interactions or group conversations.
4. Touching is not used with public distance. Public space (12 feet and beyond) is effective for communicating with groups or the community. Individuality is lost.

29. 1. **The purposes of the opening stage of an interview are to establish rapport and orient the interviewee. A relationship is**

established through a process of creating goodwill and trust. The orientation focuses on explaining the purpose and nature of the interview and what is expected of the patient.

2. This is not the purpose of the working stage. In the working stage, also called the body stage, of an interview patients communicate how they think, feel, know, and perceive in response to questions by the nurse.
3. There is no stage called the surrogate stage in an interview. Hildegard Peplau identified six roles that nurses assume during therapeutic relationships, and one of these is the surrogate role. The nurse may be assigned a surrogate role by a patient to help resolve problems that need to be worked out in a supportive environment.
4. There is no stage called the examining stage in an interview. Examining takes place during a physical assessment, when specific skills are used to collect data systematically to identify health problems.

30. 1. This response abdicates the nurse's responsibility to explore the patient's concerns immediately. In addition, it could be an erroneous assumption.
2. The patient is in the shock and disbelief mode of coping and will not be able to explore approaches to coping. In addition, using the words "terrible news" may increase anxiety and hopelessness.
3. This response imposes the nurse's feelings and own coping skills into the situation.
4. This is an example of reflective technique. When no solutions to a problem are evident, a person becomes hopeless (i.e., despairing, despondent).

31. 1. This example of focusing helps the patient explore a topic of importance. The nurse selects one topic for further discussion from among several topics presented by the patient.
2. This is not an example of clarifying, which lets the patient know that a message was unclear and seeks specific information to make the message clearer.
3. This is not an example of paraphrasing, which is restating the patient's message in similar words.
4. This is not an example of acknowledging, which is providing nonjudgmental recognition for a contribution to the conversation, a change in behavior, or an effort by the patient.

32. 1. This statement avoids the patient's feelings and fails to respond to the patient's need to talk about concerns. It cuts off communication.
2. This is a generalization that minimizes the patient's concern and should be avoided.
3. This is false reassurance, which discourages discussion of feelings and should be avoided.
4. This statement is therapeutic. It recognizes the patient's feelings, gives the patient permission to feel nervous, and reassures the patient that one's behavior is not unusual. This statement sets the groundwork for the next statement, such as, "Let's talk a little bit about the spinal tap and the concerns you may have."

33. 1. This response will put the patient on the defensive and jeopardize the nurse-patient relationship.
2. This response requires the patient to rationalize the daughter's behavior and focuses on information that is not significant at this time.
3. This response lets the patient know that the message has been heard and moves forward to meet the need to notify a significant other of the patient's situation.
4. This provides false reassurance. Only the daughter can convey this message.

34. 1. Communication involves both verbal and nonverbal messages.
2. Communication is facilitated by interviewing techniques that involve attitudes, behaviors, and verbal messages. Interviewing skills promote therapeutic communication because they are patient-centered and goal-directed.
3. Assertiveness when collecting data may be perceived by the patient as aggression, which is a barrier to communication.
4. A therapeutic relationship should avoid sympathy because it implies pity. The nurse should empathize, not sympathize, with patients.

35. 1. "Why" statements are direct questions that tend to put the patient on the defensive and cut off communication.
2. Active listening is the use of all the senses to comprehend and appreciate the patient's verbal and nonverbal thoughts and feelings.
3. Silence is passive, not active. Silence allows the patient time for quiet contemplation of what has been discussed.
4. When talking with patients, verbal and nonverbal cues are used to indicate

care and concern, which promote communication.

36. 1. The first part of this statement uses the therapeutic interviewing technique of reflection, which identifies the underlying feelings of the patient and is appropriate. However, the second half of the statement is asking for an explanation, which is inappropriate. Patients often interpret *why* questions as accusations, which can cause resentment and mistrust and should be avoided.

2. This is an example of the therapeutic interviewing skill of an open-ended statement. It demonstrates that the nurse recognizes what the patient is going through, and the broad opening encourages free verbalization by the patient. At the very least, it demonstrates caring and concern.

3. This statement minimizes the patient's feelings and is not supportive.

4. This statement will not inspire confidence in the nurse. Nurses should know what is happening if care is to be comprehensive and patient-centered.

37. **1. Communication between the patient and health-care providers is essential, particularly for obtaining subjective data and feedback. Speech, pantomime, writing, touch, and picture boards are examples of channels of transmission (e.g., mediums used to convey a message).**

2. The patient, not the nurse, should direct the flow of communication.

3. Negative feelings or concerns must be addressed. Both physical and psychic energy are used when coping with stress.

4. The focus must be on the patient's present concerns before refocusing to other issues because anxiety increases if immediate concerns are not addressed. Focusing on the negative sometimes is necessary before focusing on the positive.

38. **1. Confused patients more easily understand simple words and sentences.**

2. This may not be understood by the confused patient.

3. A confused patient may not be able to make a decision.

4. This is a threat and should be avoided when talking with patients.

39. **1. Limiting competing stiumuli promotes reception of verbal messages.**

2. This may be demeaning and ineffective because the patient may not be able to read lips.

3. This is not helpful. Hearing loss in the older adult typically involves a decreased perception of high-pitched sounds.

4. This focuses the patient's attention on the nurse. A hearing-impaired receiver must be aware that a message is being sent before the message can be received and decoded.

5. This is demeaning and may be viewed by the patient as aggressive behavior.

40. 1. This statement reflects the orientation phase of a therapeutic relationship. Although exploration of feelings is done throughout the phases, the primary goal of the orientation phase is the establishment of trust. Trust is promoted when the nurse focuses on the patient's emotional needs, is respectful, and individualizes care.

2. This statement reflects the working phase of a therapeutic relationship. It involves completing interventions that address expected outcomes, such as learning how to perform a colostomy irrigation.

3. This statement reflects the working phase of a therapeutic relationship. It includes providing feedback and encouragement.

4. This statement reflects the orientation phase of a therapeutic relationship. The nurse and patient make a verbal agreement to work together to assist the patient to achieve a goal.

5. This statement reflects the termination phase of a therapeutic relationship. It focuses on summarizing what has transpired and been accomplished and looks to the future.

Psychological Support

KEYWORDS

The following words include English vocabulary, nursing/medical terminology, concepts, principles, or information relevant to content specifically addressed in the chapter or associated with topics presented in it. English dictionaries, nursing textbooks, and medical dictionaries, such as *Taber's Cyclopedic Medical Dictionary*, are resources that can be used to expand your knowledge and understanding of these words and related information.

- Acceptance
- Agitation
- Anticipatory grieving
- Anxiety
  - Mild
  - Moderate
  - Severe
  - Panic
- Autonomy
- Behavior modification
- Beliefs
- Bereavement
- Body image
- Confrontational
- Confusion
- Conscious, unconscious, subconscious
- Coping
- Crisis
  - Adventitious/unpredictable events
  - Developmental/maturational
  - Situational
- Crisis intervention
- Defense mechanisms
  - Compensation
  - Conversion
  - Denial
  - Depersonalization
  - Dissociation
  - Identification
  - Intellectualization
  - Introjection
  - Minimization
  - Projection
  - Rationalization
  - Reaction formation
  - Regression
  - Repression
  - Sublimation
  - Substitution
  - Suppression
- Delirium
- Delusions
- Dementia
- Dependence
- Depression
- Desensitization
- Dysfunctional grieving
- Ego integrity
- Egocentric (self-absorbed)
- Empathy, empathetic, empathic
- Endorphin
- Fantasy
- Freudian terms
  - Ego
  - Id
  - Superego
- Frustration
- Gratification
- Grief, grieving
- Guided imagery
- Hallucinations
- Hopelessness
- Identity
- Loss
- Meditation
- Memory
- Midlife crisis
- Mourning
- Orientation
- Panic attack
- Perception
- Personal identity
- Positive mental attitude
- Powerlessness
- Progressive relaxation
- Psyche
- Psychodynamic
- Psychosocial development
- Psychotherapy
- Relocation stress syndrome
- Resilience
- Respect
- Role
- Role ambiguity

Role conflict
Role strain
Self-concept
Self-esteem
Social isolation
Somatic responses
Spiritual distress
Spirituality
Suicidal
Sympathy
Transference/Counter Transference
Trust
Values
Withdrawn

QUESTIONS

1. After being hospitalized for a surgical procedure, a man who was impressed with the care he received from the nurses decides to change careers and become a nurse. This is an example of:
1. Fantasy
2. Projection
3. Identification
4. Intellectualization

2. The nurse can anticipate that anxiety occurs in response to:
1. Identifiable fears
2. Unexpected events
3. Threats to ego integrity
4. Anticipated dependence

3. Which situation identified by the nurse reflects the defense mechanism of displacement?
1. A woman is very nice to her mother-in-law whom she secretly dislikes
2. A man says that he is not so bad, so don't believe what they say about him
3. An adolescent puts a poor grade on a test out of his mind when at his after-school job
4. An older man gets angry with friends after family members attempt to talk with him about his illness

4. Which is the best way for the nurse to support patients' self-esteem needs across the life span?
1. Employing a positive mental attitude
2. Providing a nonjudgmental environment
3. Encouraging social interaction with others
4. Supporting the use of defense mechanisms

5. The nurse identifies that a patient is mildly anxious. The nurse understands that when a patient is mildly anxious the patient may appear:
1. Alert
2. Fearful
3. Forgetful
4. Preoccupied

6. The nurse understands that the underlying basis of all the defense mechanisms is:
1. Compensation
2. Suppression
3. Regression
4. Repression

7. When assessing a patient, it is important for the nurse to understand that fear most commonly is experienced when the precipitating cause is:
1. Life-threatening
2. Unexpected
3. Recurrent
4. Unknown

8. A patient expresses a sense of hopelessness. Which nursing diagnosis identified by the nurse is the priority?
1. Risk for Self-Directed Violence
2. Ineffective Individual Coping
3. Powerlessness
4. Fatigue

9. When assessing a patient for anxiety, the nurse recognizes that anxiety is a:
1. Reaction triggered by a known stressor
2. Response that is avoidable
3. Universal experience
4. Threat to the Id

10. A woman with diabetes does not follow her prescribed diet and states, "Everyone with diabetes cheats on their diet." The nurse identifies this response as an example of:
1. Rationalization
2. Sublimation
3. Undoing
4. Denial

11. Which is a defining characteristic of the nursing diagnosis Powerlessness?
1. Inability to communicate
2. Experiencing multiple losses
3. Inability to control prognosis
4. Progressive debilitating disease

12. Which word reflects a concept that is nonessential for the nurse to establish a therapeutic relationship?
1. Trust
2. Caring
3. Control
4. Empathy

13. A man with a heart condition continues to perform strenuous sports against medical advice. The nurse identifies that the patient is using the defense mechanism known as:
1. Denial
2. Repression
3. Introjection
4. Dissociation

14. The nurse is caring for a patient with a comprehension deficit. To best support this patient the nurse should:
1. Ask that unclear words be repeated
2. Speak directly in front of the patient
3. Make a referral for a hearing evaluation
4. Establish structured activities of daily living

15. An important concept to understand about anxiety in order to provide appropriate nursing care is that:
1. Panic attacks generally have a slow onset that can be prevented if identified early
2. One can conceptualize anxiety as being similar to the health-illness continuum
3. People who lead healthy lifestyles rarely experience anxiety
4. Anxiety is an abnormal reaction to realistic danger

16. Which word reflects the ability of a person to perceive another person's emotions accurately?
1. Trust
2. Empathy
3. Sympathy
4. Autonomy

17. Which patient adaptation identified by the nurse is unrelated to clinically depressed older adults?
    1. Fatigue
    2. Stress incontinence
    3. Activity intolerance
    4. Disturbed sleep pattern

18. When considering the concepts regarding the defense mechanism of projection, the nurse identifies that the person who fears being taken advantage of usually is:
    1. In denial
    2. An opportunist
    3. Depersonalizing
    4. Eager to please others

19. When the nurse denies a patient the use of a defense mechanism, this action will:
    1. Damage the Id
    2. Cause more anxiety
    3. Facilitate effective coping
    4. Encourage emotional growth

20. Which nursing intervention best supports a patient's sense of self?
    1. Maintaining respectful interactions
    2. Verbalizing realistic expectations
    3. Exploring maladaptive responses
    4. Referring to counseling services

21. Which defense mechanism is being used when a patient who has just been diagnosed with terminal cancer calmly says to the nurse, "I'll have to get on the Internet to assess my options?"
    1. Intellectualization
    2. Introjection
    3. Depression
    4. Denial

22. A person addicted to alcohol says to the nurse, "I just drink a little to help me relax after a hard day at work." Which defense mechanism is the patient using?
    1. Substitution
    2. Suppression
    3. Rationalization
    4. Intellectualization

23. A patient is told that surgery is necessary and the patient begins to experience elevations in pulse, respirations, and blood pressure. What stage of anxiety is indicated by these nursing assessments?
    1. Mild
    2. Moderate
    3. Severe
    4. Panic

24. The nurse identifies which defense mechanism is being used when an adolescent who is a poor student excels in sports?
    1. Projection
    2. Sublimation
    3. Displacement
    4. Compensation

25. Which nursing action best demonstrates support of human dignity in the practice of nursing?
    1. Maintaining confidentiality of information about clients
    2. Supporting the rights of others to refuse treatment
    3. Obtaining sufficient data to make inferences
    4. Staying at the scene of an accident

26. The nurse identifies that a patient who has diabetes and continues to eat foods with a high glycemic index is using the defense mechanism of:
1. Intellectualization
2. Introjection
3. Regression
4. Denial

27. To provide the most effective psychosocial support, which data are the most helpful to the nurse?
1. Progress notes
2. Medical history
3. Patient concerns
4. Family contributions

28. A preoperative patient is anxious about pending elective surgery. Which is the best way for the nurse to help the patient reduce the anxiety?
1. Involve significant others
2. Use distraction techniques
3. Foster verbalization of feelings
4. Use progressive desensitization strategies

29. The nurse concludes that a woman who remembers only the good times after the death of her husband is using the defense mechanism of:
1. Compensation
2. Minimization
3. Repression
4. Regression

30. A patient strongly states the desire to go to the hospital coffee shop for lunch regardless of hospital policy. The nurse identifies that this behavior most likely reflects:
1. The need to regain some measure of control
2. Anger with the policies of the hospital
3. Disappointment with hospital food
4. A desire for a change of scenery

31. The nurse understands that physical exercise reduces anxiety by:
1. Reducing metabolism of adrenaline
2. Stimulating endorphin production
3. Interfering with concentration
4. Decreasing acidity of blood

32. The nurse has been caring for a female patient for several days while diagnotic tests are being completed. The physician informs the patient that she has inoperable cancer and her prognosis is poor. After the physician leaves, the patient begins to cry. The nurse should:
1. Touch the patient's hand to provide support
2. Leave the room to give the patient privacy to cry
3. Telephone the patient's family to inform them of the diagnosis
4. Ask the patient how she feels to encourage ventilation of feelings

33. Which might a patient be at risk for in the psychosocial domain when the nursing assessment indicates that the patient is almost completely paralyzed?
1. Infection
2. Self-harm
3. Constipation
4. Powerlessness

34. The nurse understands that the situation that stimulates the greatest anxiety for most people is:
1. Accepting assistance from nonfamily members
2. Arranging for home care before discharge
3. Carrying out self-care activities when ill
4. Managing uncertainty about an illness

35. The nurse is caring for a patient who is scheduled for intravenous chemotherapy for cancer. Which defense mechanism is being used when the patient says to the daughter, "Be brave"?
1. Rationalization
2. Minimization
3. Substitution
4. Projection

36. Which is the most appropriate inference made by the nurse when a patient says, "I'm the same age as my father when he died. Am I going to die of my cancer?" The patient is experiencing:
1. Grieving associated with perceived impending death
2. Powerlessness associated with feelings of loss of control
3. Fear associated with perceived threat to biological integrity
4. Ineffective coping associated with inadequate psychological resources

37. A patient who is withdrawn says, "When I have the opportunity, I am going to commit suicide." The best response by the nurse is:
1. "You have a lovely family. They need you."
2. "Let's explore the reasons you have for living."
3. "You must feel overwhelmed to want to kill yourself."
4. "Suicide does not solve problems. Tell me what is wrong."

38. A dying patient is withdrawn and depressed. The nursing action that is most therapeutic is:
1. Assisting the patient to focus on positive thoughts daily
2. Explaining that the patient still can accomplish goals
3. Accepting the patient's behavioral adaptation
4. Offering the patient advice when appropriate

39. When the nurse analyzes a patient's statements, which statements best reflect the dimensions of self-esteem? Check all that apply.
1. _____ "I really like the me that I see."
2. _____ "What do I want to achieve?"
3. _____ "How do I appear to others?"
4. _____ "I like to do things my way."
5. _____ "I'm OK, you're OK."

40. Anxiety can progress through levels of severity from mild to panic. The patient's level of anxiety will influence how the nurse approaches the patient situation. Place these patient statements in order as anxiety progresses from mild, to moderate, to severe and finally to panic.
1. "I want to know more about the surgery I am having tomorrow."
2. "I don't think I am going to make it through the surgery tomorrow."
3. "I can't concentrate and all I think about is the pain I may have tomorrow."
4. "I get butterflies in my stomach when I think about the surgery tomorrow."

Answer: _______________

ANSWERS AND RATIONALES

1. 1. This scenario is not an example of fantasy. Fantasy is an imagined situation that provides for wish-fulfillment.
2. This scenario is not an example of projection. Projection is attributing to others unacceptable thoughts, emotions, motives, or characteristics that are within oneself.
3. This scenario is an example of identification. Identification helps a person avoid self-deprecation. The person reduces anxiety by emulating the behavior of someone respected.
4. This scenario is not an example of intellectualization. Intellectualization is the use of reasoning to avoid facing unacceptable stimuli in an effort to protect the Ego from anxiety.

2. 1. Anxiety is triggered by an unknown stressor, whereas identifiable stressors contribute to a fear response.
2. An unexpected event may, or may not, contribute to anxiety.
3. Anxiety is a psychological adaptation to a threat to the self or self-esteem. The Ego is the *self*. Therefore, whenever the Ego is threatened, a person will become anxious.
4. When a person feels a disruption to an identifiable source that is perceived as dangerous, as with an anticipated dependence, the individual may experience fear, not anxiety.

3. 1. This is an example of reaction formation, not displacement. Reaction formation is when a person develops conscious attitudes, behaviors, interests, and feelings that are the exact opposite to unconscious attitudes, interests, and feelings.
2. This is an example of minimization. Minimization allows a person to decrease responsibility for one's own behavior.
3. This is an example of suppression, not displacement. Suppression is a conscious attempt to put unpleasant thoughts out of the conscious mind to be dealt with at a later time.
4. This is an example of displacement. Displacement is the transfer of emotion from one person or object to a person or an object that is more acceptable and less threatening.

4. 1. The nurse's personal attitudes should not be imposed on the patient. An attitude is a mental position or feeling toward a person, an object, or an idea.
2. When the nurse establishes a nonjudgmental environment and functions without biases, preconceptions, or stereotypes and avoids challenging a patient's values and beliefs, a patient's self-esteem is supported.
3. This may or may not support self-esteem needs. The benefit of this intervention depends on the relationships that develop and whether they promote self-worth.
4. This should be avoided because support of defense mechanisms results in reality distortion. The nurse just should recognize when defense mechanisms are being used because all behavior has meaning. The use of defense mechnaisms should be accepted, not supported.

5. 1. Increased alertness occurs when one is mildly anxious. Alertness and vigilance are the result of an increase in one's perceptual field and state of arousal in response to the stimulation of the autonomic nervous system when one feels threatened.
2. Fearfulness is not a response to anxiety. Fearfulness is an adaptation to an identifiable source, while anxiety is caused by an unidentifiable source.
3. Forgetfullness reflects moderate, not mild, anxiety. With mild anxiety, the person increases arousal and perceptual fields and is motivated to learn. With moderate anxiety, the person has a narrowed focus of attention and may become forgetful because of an inability to focus attention.
4. Preoccupation reflects moderate, not mild, anxiety.

6. 1. Compensation is not the underlying basis of all defense mechanisms. Compensation is used to overcome a perceived weakness by emphasizing a more desirable trait.
2. Suppression is not the underlying basis of all defense mechanisms. Suppression is a conscious attempt to put unpleasant thoughts out of the conscious mind to be dealt with at a later time.
3. Regression is not the underlying basis of all defense mechanisms. Regression is resorting to an earlier, more comfortable pattern of

behavior that was successful in earlier years and is now inappropriate.
4. **Repression is the basis of all defense mechanisms. All defense mechanisms contain an element of the need to unconsciously exclude upsetting or painful emotions, thoughts, or experiences.**

7. 1. **Life-threatening events that intimidate one's safety and security generally precipitate fear in most people.**
2. An unexpected event may or may not cause fear. A surprise party may be unexpected, yet be pleasant and fun, posing no threat.
3. A recurrent event may or may not cause fear. A recurrent event may be a pleasant event, posing no threat.
4. The unknown usually precipitates anxiety, not fear.

8. 1. **Risk for Self-Directed Violence takes priority over the other three nursing diagnoses because of the potential for suicide.**
2. Although a person who expresses hopelessness may also demonstrate an inability to manage stressors because of inadequate physical, psychologic, behavioral, or cognitive resources, another option identifies a nursing diagnosis that has a higher priority.
3. Although a person who expresses hopelessness may also perceive a lack of personal control over events or situations, another option identifies a nursing diagnosis that has a higher priority.
4. Although a person who expressess hopelessness may also experience an overwhelming sense of exhaustion unrelieved by rest, another option identifies a nursing diagnosis that has a higher priority.

9. 1. Anxiety is triggered by an unknown stressor, whereas, fear is a response to a known stressor.
2. Anxiety cannot be avoided. It is an expected aspect of everyday living. Every time someone experiences something new, it is a threat to the identity or self-esteem; therefore, people feel anxious.
3. **Anxiety is a common and universal response to a threat. Every time people experience something new that is a threat to the identity or self-esteem, they may feel anxious. Anxiety is a psychosocial response to an unknown stress; it may be a vague sense of apprehension at one extreme to impending doom at the other extreme.**
4. Anxiety is a response to a threat to the Ego, not the Id.

10. 1. **This is an example of rationalization. Rationalization is used to justify in some socially acceptable way ideas, feelings, or behavior through explanations that appear to be logical.**
2. This is not an example of sublimation. Sublimation is the channeling of primitive sexual or aggressive drives into activities or behaviors that are more socially acceptable, such as sports or creative work.
3. This is not an example of undoing. Undoing is use of actions or words in an attempt to cancel unacceptable thoughts, impulses, or acts. This reduces feelings of guilt through reparation (atonement, retribution).
4. This is not an example of denial. Denial is an unconscious protective response that involves a person's ignoring or refusing to acknowledge something unacceptable or unpleasant to reduce anxiety.

11. 1. An inability to communicate is a *related to* factor, not a defining characteristic.
2. Experiencing multiple losses is a *related to* factor, not a defining characteristic.
3. **A *defining characteristic* of the nursing diagnosis Powerlessness is an expression of dissatisfaction about an inability to control a situation that is negatively affecting outlook, goals, and lifestyle.**
4. A progressive debilitating disease is a *related to* factor, not a defining characteristic.

12. 1. Trust is essential to the therapeutic relationship. A reliance on someone without doubt helps make the patient feel comfortable, rather than anxious.
2. Caring is essential to the therapeutic relationship. Caring conveys emotional closeness and is demonstrated through compassion, interest, and concern.
3. **Control is nonessential to a therapeutic relationship. The purpose is not to have control over the patient, but to identify and meet the needs of the patient.**
4. Empathy is essential to the therapeutic relationship. It is important for the nurse to understand the patient's emotional state and point of view, which can be accomplished through empathetic listening and responding.

13. 1. **This scenario is an example of denial. Denial is being used when a person ignores or refuses to acknowledge something unacceptable or unpleasant.**

2. This scenario is not an example of repression. Repression is an unconscious mechanism whereby painful or unpleasant ideas are kept from conscious awareness.
3. This scenario is not an example of introjection. Introjection is the taking into one's personality the norms and values of another as a means of reducing anxiety.
4. This scenario is not an example of dissociation. Dissociation occurs when a person segregates a group of thoughts from consciousness or when an object or idea is segregated from its emotional significance in an effort to avoid emotional distress.

14. 1. It is the patient who is having difficulty with comprehension who may need words repeated, not the nurse.
2. This action does not facilitate comprehension. It helps a patient with a hearing deficit recognize that someone is speaking, and it facilitates lip reading if the patient has the ability to read lips.
3. The patient's problem is a decreased ability to process and understand information, not a hearing loss.
4. **New experiences require a person to process information and problem-solve, which is difficult to do for the person with a comprehension deficit. Lack of understanding is threatening to feelings of safety and security. Structure and routines provide predictability, which limits confusion, disorientation, and anxiety.**

15. 1. Panic attacks cannot be prevented if identified early, and they do not have a slow onset. Panic attacks usually occur suddenly and spontaneously, build to a peak in ten minutes or less, and last from several minutes to as long as an hour.
2. **People can experience anxiety along a continuum from no anxiety to mild, moderate, severe, or panic, just as health is viewed along a continuum from illness to health.**
3. Healthy people experience anxiety when the Ego is threatened. Anxiety is a universal response to a threat. People will feel anxious when exposed to something new that is a threat to self-identity or self-esteem.
4. A realistic danger triggers a fear response, which is an expected reaction.

16. 1. Trust is not the nurse's perceiving the patient's emotions accurately. Trust is established when a patient has confidence in the nurse because the nurse demonstrates competence, respect for the patient, and behaves in a predictable way.
2. **Empathy is the nurse's ability to have insight into the feelings, emotions, and behavior of the patient.**
3. Sympathy is more than expressing concern and sorrow for a patient, but also contains an element of pity. When sympathetic, the nurse may let one's own feelings interfere with the therapeutic relationship, which can impair judgment and limit the ability to identify realistic solutions to problems. Although sympathy is a caring response, it is not therapeutic, as is empathy.
4. Autonomy is being self-directed, not being able to perceive another person's emotions.

17. 1. Fatigue is often associated with depression. A depressed person may become inactive and sedentary, which may cause deconditioning that contributes to fatigue.
2. **Stress incontinence is unrelated to depression. Stress incontinence is a physiologic, not psychologic, problem caused by an involuntary loss of small amounts of urine in response to a rise in intra-abdominal pressure.**
3. Activity intolerance is often associated with depression. A depressed person may become inactive and sedentary, which can cause deconditioning that contributes to activity intolerance.
4. A disturbed sleep pattern is often a response to depression. Anxiety and depression can elevate epinephrine blood levels, which can result in less REM and Stage IV NREM sleep, as well as contribute to frequent awakening.

18. 1. The person who fears being taken advantage of is not in denial. When in denial, a person ignores or refuses to acknowledge something unacceptable or unpleasant.
2. **Projection is attributing unacceptable thoughts, emotions, motives, or characteristics within oneself to others. In projection, a person who fears being taken advantage of usually is a person who is an opportunist.**
3. The person who fears being taken advantage of is not depersonalizing. Depersonalization is treating a person as an object instead of as a person.
4. A person who fears being taken advantage of usually is *not* eager, rather than eager, to please others.

19. 1. Denying the use of defense mechanisms will stress the Ego, not the Id. Id impulses are physiologic, body processes that are dominated by the pleasure principle, not by psychologic or social processes as seen in the Ego.
    2. Defense mechanisms are used to reduce anxiety and achieve or maintain emotional balance. If a nurse identifies reality and does not recognize the patient's need to use defense mechanisms, the patient will become more anxious, even to the point of panic.
    3. Denying a patient the use of a defense mechanism will contribute to ineffective coping, not facilitate effective coping.
    4. Denying the use of defense mechanisms will not encourage emotional growth. Emotional growth develops as a result of gaining insight into behavior, recognizing reality, and addressing problems constructively.

20. **1. Respectful interaction demonstrates to patients that they are valuable and important and lays the foundation on which trust can be built between the nurse and patient.**
    2. Verbalizing realistic expectations may challenge a patient who is not ready to face reality, which may increase anxiety and result in a decrease in a sense of self.
    3. Defense mechanisms are adaptive, not maladaptive, unless carried to the extreme. Confronting maladaptive responses before the patient is capable of dealing with reality will cause anxiety to increase and self-esteem to decrease.
    4. Although counseling services are an excellent way for a patient to support the Ego and to increase self-esteem, another option offers a better strategy to support a patient's sense of self.

21. **1. This is an example of intellectualization. Intellectualization is the use of reasoning to avoid facing unacceptable stimuli in an effort to protect the Ego from anxiety.**
    2. This is not an example of introjection. Introjection is the taking into one's personality the norms and values of another as a means of reducing anxiety.
    3. This is not an example of depression. Depression is not a defense mechanism, it is an altered mood indicated by feelings of sadness, discouragement, and loss of interest in usual pleasurable activities.
    4. This is not an example of denial. Denial is ignoring or refusing to acknowledge something unacceptable or unpleasant.

22. 1. This scenario is not an example of substitution. Substitution is the replacement of an unattainable, unavailable, or unacceptable goal, emotion, or motive with one that is attainable, available, or acceptable in an effort to reduce anxiety, frustration or disappointment.
    2. This scenario is not an example of suppression. Suppression is a conscious attempt to put unpleasant thoughts out of the conscious mind to be dealt with at a later time.
    3. This scenario is an example of rationalization. Rationalization is used to justify in some socially acceptable way ideas, feelings, or behaviors through explanations that appear to be logical.
    4. This scenario is not an example of intellectualization. Intellectualization is the use of reasoning to avoid facing unacceptable stimuli in an effort to protect the Ego from anxiety.

23. 1. During mild anxiety, the pulse, respirations, and blood pressure remain at the resting rate.
    2. During moderate anxiety, the pulse, respirations, and blood pressure are noticeably elevated in response to the stimulation of the autonomic nervous system.
    3. During severe anxiety, the pulse, respirations, and blood pressure are more than just noticeably elevated. The pulse and respirations are rapid and may be irregular, and the blood pressure is high, not just noticeably elevated.
    4. During a panic attack, the pulse and respirations are very rapid and may be irregular, the blood pressure will be high, and the patient may hyperventilate. If a panic attack is extreme, the blood pressure may suddenly drop and cause fainting.

24. 1. This scenario is not an example of projection. Projection is attributing unacceptable thoughts, emotions, motives, or characteristics within oneself to others.
    2. This scenario is not an example of sublimation. Sublimation is diversion of unacceptable instinctive urges or the libido to socially acceptable and personally approved outlets.
    3. This scenario is not an example of displacement. Displacement is when emotion is transferred from one person or object

to another person or object that is more acceptable and safe.

4. **This scenario is an example of compensation. Compensation is an attempt to achieve respect in one area as a substitute for a weakness in another area.**

25. 1. **Confidentiality respects the patient's right to privacy, which is a component of human dignity.**
2. This supports the right of a patient to self-determination, which is based on the concept of freedom, not human dignity.
3. This reflects the nurse's attempt to seek the truth, not support human dignity.
4. This reflects a nurse's attempt to be responsible and accountable, not support human dignity.

26. 1. This scenario is not an example of intellectualization. Intellectualization is the use of reasoning to avoid facing unacceptable stimuli in an effort to protect the Ego from anxiety.
2. This scenario is not an example of introjection. Introjection is the taking into one's personality the norms and values of another as a means of reducing anxiety.
3. This scenario is not an example of regression. Regression is resorting to an earlier, more comfortable pattern of behavior that was successful in earlier years but is now inappropriate.
4. **This scenario is an example of denial. Denial is the ignoring of or refusal to acknowledge something unacceptable or unpleasant.**

27. 1. Progress notes, while helpful, are history and may not reflect the current needs of the patient.
2. A medical history, while helpful, is history and may not reflect the current needs of the patient.
3. **The patient is the center of the health team and is the primary source of data. The patient generally can provide subjective data about feelings and concerns regarding her/his illness and its impact that no one else can provide.**
4. Family members' contributions generally supplement, clarify, and validate data collected from the patient. Only patients can give first-hand descriptions of how they feel and what concerns them. If a patient is confused, mentally or emotional disabled, unconscious, unable to communicate due to pain or critical illness, or is too young, the family can be a helpful secondary source of data.

28. 1. Significant others generally are as anxious as the patient because anxiety is contagious. Anxious significant others bring to the discussion their own emotional problems that can misdirect the focus from the patient as well as compound the problem.
2. Although distraction techniques, such as guided imagery, can help manage stress, another option offers a more effective intervention to reduce anxiety.
3. **Using interviewing techniques encourages the patient to verbalize feelings and explore concerns, which reduce anxiety. Verbalization uses energy, makes concerns recognizable, and promotes problem solving. Talking about one's feelings was called *catharsis* by Freud.**
4. Anxiety is not something one can desensitize oneself to by increasing exposure to the stressor. With anxiety, the stressor is unknown.

29. 1. This scenario is not an example of compensation. Compensation is making an attempt to achieve respect in one area as a substitute for a weakness in another area.
2. This scenario not an example of minimization. Minimization is not admitting to the significance of one's own behavior, thereby reducing one's responsibility.
3. **This is an example of repression. Repression is an unconscious mechanism whereby painful or unpleasant ideas are kept from conscious awareness.**
4. This scenario is not an example of regression. Regression is resorting to an earlier, more comfortable pattern of behavior that was successful in earlier years but is now inappropriate.

30. 1. **Acting-out behaviors that reflect attempts to control events often are covert expressions of feeling powerless.**
2. All behavior has meaning. Patients generally follow hospital policies because they recognize that they are designed to keep patients safe. When they do not follow rules, usually it is an attempt to control events, not because they are angry.
3. Patients have an opportunity to choose foods they like from the menu, request alternative meals if they are unhappy with the food that arrives, and to ask family members to bring in food as long as the food is permitted on the ordered diet. Wanting to go to the hospital coffee shop against hospital policy

is an inappropriate strategy to deal with the disappointment with hospital food.
4. Most hospital units have a lounge that supports patients' needs to have a change of scenery from their rooms.

31. 1. Exercise promotes, not reduces, metabolism of adrenaline and thyroxine thereby minimizing autonomic arousal and decreasing vigilance associated with the anxious response.
2. Exercise stimulates endorphin production, which promotes a sense of well-being and euphoria. Also, endorphins act as opiates and produce analgesia by modulating the transmission of pain perception.
3. Endorphins improve one's ability to concentrate and problem-solve by increasing circulation, which facilitates oxygenation of brain cells.
4. Endorphins increase, not decrease, the acidity of blood. This improves digestion and metabolism and thereby increase one's energy level.

32. **1. Touching the patient conveys concern and caring and is supportive.**
2. Leaving abandons the patient at a time when the patient needs emotional support.
3. Conveying this information to the patient's family is a violation of confidentiality.
4. Crying is a way to express sad feelings and needs to be supported before the nurse uses open-ended, not direct, questions to encourage ventilation of feelings.

33. 1. The risk for infection is a concern in the physiologic, not the psychosocial, domain.
2. Data do not support the concern that the patient will cause self-harm. The data related to the risk for self-harm is an expression of a desire to harm oneself, commit suicide, or die.
3. The risk for constipation is a concern in the physiologic, not the psychosocial, domain.
4. People who are unable to care for themselves independently often perceive a lack of control over events, and the nurse should be alert to the presence of data that support powerlessness.

34. 1. Generally, attendance by educated health-care professionals provides a patient with a sense of security and safety; this reduces, not increases, anxiety.
2. Home care commonly empowers a person, which in turn reduces, not increases, anxiety. The patient is reassured that daily needs will be addressed in the home environment, where patients generally are most comfortable.
3. Carrying out one's own activities of daily living supports one's self-esteem and self-identity and most commonly reduces, not increases, anxiety.
4. Uncertainty about an illness or the unknown is a threat to one's life, self-identify, self-esteem, and/or significant relationships. Uncertainty causes the greatest anxiety for most people.

35. 1. This is not an example of rationalization. Rationalization is used to justify in some socially acceptable way ideas, feelings, or behavior through explanations that appear to be logical.
2. This is not an example of minimization. Minimization is not admitting to the significance of one's own behavior, thereby reducing one's responsibility.
3. This is not an example of substitution. Substitution is replacement of an unattainable, unavailable, or unacceptable goal, emotion, or motive with one that is attainable, available, or acceptable in an effort to reduce anxiety, frustration or disappointment.
4. This is an example of projection. Projection is attributing unacceptable thoughts, emotions, motives, or characteristics within oneself to others.

36. 1. This statement does not indicate that the patient perceives that his death is imminent. A characteristic of grieving is that the person must express distress regarding a loss or potential loss. This patient is asking questions, not displaying distress related to a perceived impending death.
2. This statement does not reflect powerlessness. People who are powerless usually do not ask questions.
3. This statement supports the fact that the patient is experiencing fear. A characteristic of fear is the verbalization of feelings of apprehension and alarm related to an identifiable source.
4. This statement does not indicate that the patient is ineffectively coping or that he has inadequate psychological resources. He is gathering data by appropriately asking questions, which is an effective, task-oriented action in the coping process.

37. 1. This statement is inappropriate; the patient is unable to cope, is selecting the ultimate escape, and is not capable of meeting the needs

of others; this response also may precipitate feelings such as guilt.
2. This denies the patient's feelings; the patient must focus on the negatives before exploring the positives.
3. **This statement identifies feelings and invites further communication.**
4. This is a judgmental response that may cut off communication. This response is too direct, and the patient may not consciously know what is wrong.

38. 1. Focusing on positive thoughts is inappropriate because it denies the patient's feelings; the patient needs to focus on the future loss.
2. Focusing on positive thoughts is inappropriate because it denies the patient's feelings; the patient needs to focus on the future loss.
3. **Depression is the fourth stage of dying according to Kübler-Ross; patients become withdrawn and non-communicative when feeling a loss of control and recognizing future losses. The nurse should accept the behavior and be available if the patient wants to verbalize feelings.**
4. It is never appropriate to offer advice; people must explore their alternatives and come to their own conclusions.

39. 1. **This statement best reflects the dimension of self-esteem. Self-esteem is a person's self-evaluation of one's own worth or value. A person whose self-concept comes close to one's ideal self generally will have a high self-esteem.**
2. This statement reflects one's self-expectations, not self-esteem. Establishing expectations contributes to the composition of the ideal self.
3. This statement reflects self-concept, not self-esteem. Self-concept is an individual's knowledge about oneself. Self-concept is derived from all the collective beliefs and images about oneself as a result of interaction with the environment, society, and feedback from others.
4. This statement is a reflection of a patient's need to be autonomous and self-reliant. Having confidence in one's ability to complete a task is only one component of self-concept.
5. **This statement reflects the dimension of self-esteem. By stating "I'm OK" the person demonstrates self-acceptance.**

40. Answer: 1, 4, 3, 2
1. **Mild anxiety is a slightly aroused state that enhances perception, learning, and performance of activities.**
4. **Moderate anxiety increases the arousal state that precipitates feelings of tension and nervousness. The heart and respiratory rates increase and the person may have mild gastrointestinal symptoms, such as a feeling of butterflies in the stomach.**
3. **Severe anxiety consumes the person's physical and emotional energy. Perceptions are decreased and the person focuses on limited aspects of what is precipitating the anxiety.**
2. **Panic is an overwhelming state where the person feels out of control. Perceptions may be distorted and exaggerated, and the person may have feelings of impending doom.**

Teaching and Learning

KEYWORDS

The following words include English vocabulary, nursing/medical terminology, concepts, principles, or information relevant to content specifically addressed in the chapter or associated with topics presented in it. English dictionaries, nursing textbooks, and medical dictionaries, such as *Taber's Cyclopedic Medical Dictionary*, are resources that can be used to expand your knowledge and understanding of these words and related information.

- Accredited
- Active participation
- Assumption
- Behavior modification
- Certified
- Compliance
- Comprehension
- Continuing education program
- Culturally competent
- Expectation
- Experiential
- Explain
- Focus group
- Formal teaching
- Identify
- Illiteracy
- Informal teaching
- Inservice education program
- Intelligence
- Interpret
- Knowledge
- Knowledge deficit
- Learning domains
  - Affective
    - Receiving
    - Responding
    - Valuing
    - Organizing
    - Characterizing
  - Cognitive
    - Acquisition
    - Comprehension
    - Application
    - Analysis
    - Synthesis
    - Evaluation
  - Psychomotor
    - Set
    - Guided response
    - Mechanism
    - Complex overt response
    - Adaptation
    - Origination
- Learning styles
- Literacy
- Locus of control
  - External
  - Internal
- Maturity
- Motivation
- Orientation program
- Pedagogy
- Positive feedback
- Post-test
- Predict
- Pre-test
- Readiness
- Reading level
- Reinforcement
- Relevant
- Repetition
- Reward
- Self-actualized
- Survey
- Teaching/learning contract
- Teaching methods
  - Active learning
  - Audiovisual aids
  - Case study
  - Computer-assisted instruction
  - Demonstration
  - Discussion
  - Lecture
  - Programmed instruction
  - Return demonstration
  - Role-playing
  - Simulation
  - Written material

QUESTIONS

1. The nurse must implement a teaching plan for a patient recently diagnosed with heart failure. What should the nurse do first?
   1. Identify the patient's level of recognition of the need for learning
   2. Frame the goal within the patient's value system
   3. Assess the patient's personal support system
   4. Determine how the patient prefers to learn

2. A teaching-learning concept basic to all teaching plans is to present content from the:
   1. Cognitive to the affective domain
   2. Formal to the informal
   3. Simple to the complex
   4. Broad to the specific

3. The nurse is planning a teaching plan for an older adult. Which common factor among older adult patients must be considered by the nurse?
   1. Learning may require more energy
   2. Intelligence decreases as people age
   3. Older adults rely more on visual rather than auditory learning
   4. Older adult patients are more resistant to change that accompanies new learning

4. The nurse is teaching a postoperative patient deep breathing and coughing exercises. Which method of instruction is most appropriate in this situation?
   1. Explanation
   2. Demonstration
   3. Video presentation
   4. Brochure with pictures

5. The nurse is teaching a patient colostomy care in relation to the affective domain. Which teaching method is most effective for this situation?
   1. Discussing a pamphlet about colostomy care from the American Cancer Society
   2. Exploring how the patient feels about having a colostomy
   3. Providing a demonstration on how to do colostomy care
   4. Showing a videotape demonstrating colostomy care

6. The nurse understands that role-playing is a more effective and creative learning activity than other methods of learning because it:
   1. Eliminates the need for a teacher
   2. Provides more fun than other methods
   3. Requires active participation by the learner
   4. Gives the learner the opportunity to be another person

7. To be culturally competent when implementing a teaching plan, the nurse first should assess the patient's:
   1. Religious affiliation
   2. Support system
   3. National origin
   4. Health beliefs

8. The nurse is assessing a patient to determine educational needs. Which is most important for the nurse to consider?
   1. Make no assumptions about the patient
   2. Teaching may be informal or formal in nature
   3. The teaching plan should be documented on appropriate records
   4. A copy of the teaching/learning contract should be given to the patient

9. The nurse identifies that learning in the psychomotor domain is demonstrated when a patient:
   1. Accepts the need to have a colostomy
   2. Understands why certain foods should be avoided
   3. Verbalizes the rationale for daily colostomy irrigations
   4. Changes a colostomy bag without contaminating the hands

10. Which word best describes the nurse's role when functioning as a teacher?
    1. Provide
    2. Comfort
    3. Empower
    4. Collaborate

11. The nurse is evaluating a patient's learning regarding nutrition. Which behavior reflects the highest level of learning in the cognitive domain?
    1. Modifies favorite recipes by eliminating foods that have to be avoided
    2. Evaluates the benefits associated with avoidance of certain foods
    3. States why a mother's diet may affect breast-feeding
    4. Identifies a list of foods to be avoided

12. The nurse understands that the main purpose of continuing education programs is to:
    1. Update professional knowledge
    2. Network within the nursing profession
    3. Fulfill requirements for an advanced degree
    4. Graduate from an accredited nursing program

13. The nurse is designing a teaching-learning program for a patient who is to be discharged from the hospital. What should the nurse do first?
    1. Identify the patient's locus of control
    2. Use a variety of teaching methods appropriate for the patient
    3. Formulate an achievable, measurable, and realistic patient goal
    4. Assess the patient's current understanding of the content to be taught

14. The nurse is to provide nutritional counseling for an older adult. What should the nurse do first?
    1. Plan educational sessions in the late afternoon
    2. Speak louder when talking
    3. Provide large-print books
    4. Assess for readiness

15. The nurse is teaching an older adult how to perform a dressing change. Which nursing action is most important to address a developmental stress of aging?
    1. Speak louder when talking to the patient
    2. Use terminology understandable to the patient
    3. Have the patient provide a return demonstration
    4. Allow more time for the patient to process information

16. A nursing instructor is evaluating a student nurse's knowledge. The highest level of learning in the cognitive domain is demonstrated when the student nurse:
    1. Identifies the expected properties of urine
    2. Explains the importance of producing urine
    3. Recognizes when something is contaminated
    4. Interprets laboratory results of diagnostic urine testing

17. A patient asks the nurse, "What does 96 indicate when my blood pressure is 140 over 96?" What is the best response by the nurse?
    1. "The 96 is the pressure within an artery when the heart is resting between beats."
    2. "The 96 reflects the lowest pressure within a vein when blood moves through it."
    3. "Everyone is different so it's really relative to each individual what it means."
    4. "Let's talk about the concerns you may have about your blood pressure."

18. The nurse is planning a weight reduction program with an obese patient. The nurse understands that an important component that can determine the success or failure of this plan is:
1. Using an eight-hundred-calorie daily dietary regimen
2. Rewarding compliant behavior with favorite foods
3. Encouraging at least one hour of exercise daily
4. Setting realistic goals

19. The nurse is providing health teaching for a patient with a comprehension deficit. Which is the best intervention by the nurse that supports this patient's learning?
1. Establishing a structured environment
2. Asking that unclear words be repeated
3. Speaking directly in front of the patient
4. Making a referral for a hearing evaluation

20. The nurse is teaching a patient recently diagnosed with diabetes mellitus the step-by-step procedure of administering an insulin injection. However, after two sessions the patient is still reluctant to self-administer the insulin. The nurse should:
1. Have the patient administer the injection to an orange
2. Keep reinforcing the principles that have been presented
3. Give the patient an opportunity to explore concerns about the injection
4. Determine if a member of the family is willing to administer the insulin

21. Every person who attended a smoking cessation educational program completed a questionnaire. This type of evaluation is called a:
1. Survey
2. Post-test
3. Case study
4. Focus group

22. A patient is readmitted to the hospital because of nonadherence to the prescribed health-care regimen. What should the nurse do first?
1. Encourage healthy behaviors
2. Develop a trusting relationship
3. Use educational aids to reinforce teaching
4. Establish why the client is not following the regimen

23. The nurse is teaching a patient with a hearing impairment. The nurse should:
1. Limit educational sessions to ten minutes
2. Provide information in written format
3. Use multiple teaching methods
4. Teach in group settings

24. When assessing the results of dietary teaching for a patient with diabetes mellitus, the nurse identifies that learning occurred in the affective domain when the patient:
1. Discusses which food on the ordered diet must be avoided
2. Eats the food on the special diet ordered by the physician
3. Compiles a list of foods that are permitted on the diet
4. Asks about which foods can be eaten

25. The nurse educator in the hospital's Community Outreach Department understands that the group that benefits the most from role-playing is:
1. Older adults who are preparing to retire from the workforce
2. Middle-aged adults preparing for total knee replacement surgery
3. Men who are unwilling to admit that they have a drinking problem
4. Adolescents who are learning to abstain from recreational drug use

26. To be most effective, the nurse should prepare educational medical material at what grade reading level?
 1. Fourth-grade
 2. Sixth-grade
 3. Eighth-grade
 4. Tenth-grade

27. The nurse uses computer-assisted instruction as a strategy when providing preoperative teaching. The nurse understands that the greatest advantage of computer-assisted instruction is that:
 1. Learners can progress at their own rate
 2. It is the least expensive teaching strategy
 3. There are opportunities for pre- and post-testing
 4. Information is presented in a well-organized format

28. Which behavior identified by the nurse indicates the highest level of learning in the psychomotor domain?
 1. Demonstrating a well-balanced stance with crutches
 2. Identifying the correct equipment that is needed for a colostomy irrigation
 3. Performing a dry sterile dressing change without contaminating the equipment
 4. Recognizing the difference between systolic and diastolic blood pressure sounds

29. The nurse is assessing a patient's readiness to learn about smoking cessation. The nurse understands that the most important factor that determines that a teaching program is needed by the patient is the patient's:
 1. Previous experience
 2. Perceived need
 3. Expectations
 4. Flexibility

30. The nurse is teaching a preschool-age child. The teaching method most appropriate for the nurse to use is:
 1. Demonstrations
 2. Coloring books
 3. Small groups
 4. Videos

31. Which type of program is the nurse attending when participating in a program about a new intravenous pump provided by the hospital staff education department?
 1. Continuing education program
 2. Inservice education program
 3. Certification program
 4. Orientation program

32. The nurse is planning teaching about weight reduction strategies to an obese patient. Before implementing the teaching plan, the nurse first should assess the patient's:
 1. Intelligence
 2. Experience
 3. Motivation
 4. Strengths

33. The nurse is planning to engage a patient in a program to learn about a newly diagnosed illness. Which psychosocial adaptation to the illness has the greatest impact on the patient's future success with learning?
 1. Fear
 2. Denial
 3. Fatigue
 4. Anxiety

34. The unit secretary tells the nurse that the physician has just ordered a low-calorie diet for a patient who is overweight. Place these nursing interventions in the order in which they should be implemented.

1. Verify the dietary order
2. Determine food preferences
3. Teach specifics about a low calorie diet
4. Review a meal plan designed by the patient
5. Assess the patient's motivation to follow the diet

Answer: ______________

35. Which best describes a patient with an external locus of control? Check all that apply.

1. _____ Behaving appropriately to obtain the right to watch a television program
2. _____ Is self-motivated when implementing health promotion behaviors
3. _____ Wants to please family members with efforts to get well
4. _____ Understands the expected outcome of therapy
5. _____ Is a self-actualized adult

ANSWERS AND RATIONALES

1. **1. The learner must recognize that the need exists and that the material to be learned is valuable. Motivation is the most important factor influencing learning.**
   2. Although this is important, it is not the first thing the nurse should do before implementing a teaching plan.
   3. Although supportive individuals (family members, friends, neighbors, etc.) can assist in helping the patient maintain a positive mental attitude and reinforce learning, another option has a higher priority.
   4. Although the teacher should identify a patient's learning style, a variety of teaching methods, not just the patient's preference, should be used. This ensures that as many senses as possible are stimulated when learning, thereby increasing the probability of a successful outcome to the learning.

2. 1. Teaching and learning involve one or all domains of learning and do not move from one to the other in progressive order. *Cognitive* learning involves the intellect and requires thinking. *Cognitive* learning increases in complexity from *knowledge* to *comprehension*, *application*, *analysis*, *synthesis*, and *evaluation* of information. *Affective* learning involves the expression of feelings and the changing of beliefs, attitudes, or values. *Affective* learning increases in complexity from *receiving* to *responding*, *valuing*, *organizing*, and *characterizing*. In addition, there is the *psychomotor domain*, which is related to mastering a skill and requires motor activity. Learning in this domain increases in complexity from *readiness to take action* to a *guided response*, *mechanism*, *complex-overt response*, *adaptation*, and *origination*.
   2. Teaching methods that are formal or informal are equally effective. The key is to select the approach that is most likely to be effective for the individual learner. This depends on a variety of factors, such as intelligence, content to be taught, learning style preferences, available resources, reading level, etc.
   3. Complex material is best learned when easily understood aspects of the topic are presented first as a foundation for the more complex aspects. When moving from the simple to the complex, a person works at integrating and incorporating the less complex, new learning into one's body of knowledge and understanding before moving on to more complex information.
   4. There is no documented principle that supports the need to present content in the direction of broad to specific rather than specific to broad. Each individual patient and the information to be taught will influence the direction in which content is taught.

3. **1. Various physiological changes of aging impact on the rate of learning (declines in sensory perception and speed of mental processing, and more time needed for recall) requiring the use of multisensory teaching strategies and a slower approach. In addition, older adults may have less physical and emotional stamina because of more chronic illnesses, so they may require shorter and more frequent learning sessions.**
   2. Although some older adults may experience a decline in short-term memory, they are not less intelligent. When older adults experience a decline in sensory function (vision, hearing), they may feel ashamed or frustrated, causing withdrawal. Behaviors reflective of withdrawal may be misperceived as a decline in intelligence.
   3. This is not necessarily true. Individuals usually have learning preferences that persist throughout life.
   4. Older adults generally are not resistant to change. Some older adults may be less motivated to learn if they believe that death is near. However, in this situation when older adults are shown how learning will improve quality of life and independence, they are motivated to learn.

4. 1. This is not the best approach to teach a psychomotor skill. An explanation uses words to describe a behavior that the learner then has to attempt to perform.
   2. A demonstration is the best strategy for teaching a psychomotor skill. A demonstration is an actual performance of the skill by the teacher who is acting as a role model. A demonstration usually is followed by a return demonstration. The learner can imitate the teacher during a return demonstration, ask questions, and receive feedback from the instructor.

3. Although a video provides a realistic performance of the skill, it does not allow for questions or feedback.
4. A brochure with pictures is too static and unidimensional for teaching a psychomotor skill.

5. 1. This option reflects learning in the *cognitive domain*. *Cognitive* learning involves the intellect and requires thinking.
2. **This option reflects learning in the *affective domain*. *Affective* learning is concerned with feelings, emotions, values, beliefs, and attitudes about the colostomy.**
3. Providing a demonstration on colostomy care is an example of a teaching strategy in the *psychomotor domain*. The *psychomotor domain* is related to mastering a skill and requires the use of physical and motor activity.
4. Showing a videotape demonstrating colostomy care is an example of a teaching strategy in the *psychomotor domain*. It reflects a beginning awareness of the objects needed and steps to be implemented in a skill.

6. 1. A teacher is always needed to facilitate learning. With role-playing the teacher offers guidance and feedback while providing a safe, supportive environment.
2. Role-playing is no more or less fun than many other active and creative learning strategies.
3. **Learning activities that actively engage the learner have been shown to be more effective as well as more fun than methods that do not actively engage the learner. When learners are actively involved, they assume more responsibility for their own learning and develop more self-interest in learning the content.**
4. Role-playing is designed to support rehearsing a desired behavior in a safe environment. Although it may involve an opportunity to play another person, which allows one to view a situation from another vantage point, it is not the most important reason why role-playing is effective.

7. 1. Although religious affiliation may be important to know, it is only one part of a patient's sociocultural makeup. Another option has a higher priority.
2. Although the level of support is important to know, it is only one part of a patient's sociocultural makeup. Another option has a higher priority.
3. Although national origin is important to know, it is only one part of a patient's sociocultural makeup. In addition, nurses have to be careful not to make generalizations and stereotype an individual because of national origin, because each person is an individual.
4. **Individuals have their own beliefs associated with cultural health practices, faith beliefs, diet, illness, death and dying, and lifestyle which all have a major impact on health beliefs.**

8. 1. **Many variables influence an individual's willingness and ability to learn (readiness, motivation, physical and emotional abilities, education, age, cultural and health beliefs, cognitive abilities, etc.). Since everyone is unique with individual needs, the nurse must avoid making assumptions and generalizations.**
2. The patient's needs must be identified before teaching formats and strategies are designed.
3. The patient's needs must be identified before the teaching plan is designed, implemented, and documented.
4. The patient's needs must be identified before a plan is designed and a contract is written.

9. 1. Accepting the need to have a colostomy indicates learning on the *valuing level* in the *affective*, not *psychomotor*, *domain*. *Valuing* is demonstrated when learning is incorporated into the learner's behavior because it is perceived as important.
2. Understanding why certain foods should be avoided indicates learning on the *comprehension level* in the *cognitive*, not *psychomotor*, *domain*. Learning on the *comprehension level* is reflected in the ability to understand the meaning of learned content.
3. Understanding the rationale for daily colostomy irrigation indicates learning on the *comprehension level* in the *cognitive*, not *psychomotor*, *domain*. Learning on the *comprehension level* is reflected in the ability to understand the meaning of learned content.
4. **Changing a colostomy bag without contaminating the hands is an example of learning in the *psychomotor domain*. Learning in the *psychomotor domain* is related to mastering a skill and requires motor activity.**

10. 1. Although a teacher may *provide* opportunities for learning, it is not the best word to describe the goal of the nurse when functioning as a teacher.
2. Although a teacher may *comfort* the patient when teaching, it is not the best word

to describe the goal of the nurse when functioning as a teacher.

3. **The purpose of teaching patients is to ensure that they have the knowledge and authority (empower) to respond most effectively to their own situation.**
4. Although a teacher may *collaborate* with other health team members to provide the best learning opportunities for the patient, it does not describe the relationship with a patient in a teaching/learning relationship and is not the primary role of the nurse when teaching.

11. 1. This reflects learning on the *characterizing level* and is the highest level out of 5 levels of learning in the *affective*, not *cognitive*, *domain*.
2. **This is an appropriate example of learning on the *evaluation level* and is the highest level of learning out of the 6 levels of learning in the *cognitive domain*.**
3. This reflects learning on the *comprehension level*, which is the second out of 6 levels of learning in the *cognitive domain*.
4. Identifying a list of foods to avoid reflects learning on the *knowledge level*, which is the first of 6 levels of complexity in the *cognitive domain* of learning.

12. 1. **Continuing education programs are formal learning experiences designed to update and enhance professional knowledge or skills. This is necessary because of the explosion in information and technology within health care. Some states require evidence of continuing education units (CEUs) for license renewal.**
2. Although nurses who attend continuing education programs have the opportunity to professionally network with other nurses, it is not the main purpose of attending a continuing education program.
3. Continuing education programs do not fulfill requirements for an advanced degree. Master's and doctoral programs grant advanced degrees in specialty areas (i.e., parent-child health, psychiatry, medical-surgical nursing, gerontology, etc.) and practice roles (i.e., nurse practitioner, education, administration, etc.).
4. Continuing education programs do not prepare a person to graduate from an accredited nursing degree program. Associate degree programs, baccalaureate degree programs, and diploma schools of nursing prepare graduates to take the NCLEX-RN examination.

13. 1. Although this may be done to determine if the patient has an internal locus of control (those who do are more likely to take responsibility for their own learning), it is not the first thing the nurse should do of the options offered.
2. Although a variety of teaching methods should be used so that all the senses are engaged in learning, it is not the first thing the nurse should do of the options offered.
3. Goal setting is accomplished after the nurse gathers essential information that will influence the goal, particularly in relation to the achievable and realistic factors of a goal.
4. **Learners bring their own lifetimes of learning to the learning situation. The nurse needs to customize each teaching plan, capitalize on the patient's previous experience and knowledge, and identify what the patient still needs to know before teaching can begin.**

14. 1. Late in the afternoon is not the best time to schedule teaching sessions for older adults. They may tire from the energy and effort required to perform daily activities, and therefore may be too tired to concentrate.
2. Speaking in a lower-pitch tone rather than speaking louder is more effective. Older adults often experience a decline in the ability to hear high-pitch tones.
3. Not all older adults have vision problems. This should be done only for the patient who has visual problems.
4. **If the patient does not recognize the need to learn or value the information to be learned, the patient will not be ready to learn.**

15. 1. This is not only unnecessary but contraindicated in some older adults who have hearing loss with recruitment. Recruitment occurs when a slight increase in sound intensity causes discomfort or pain. In addition, although hearing acuity declines in older adults, they often wear hearing aids that correct hearing to a functional level. High-pitch hearing loss is the most common hearing loss in the older adult and can be addressed by the teacher lowering the pitch of the voice, not by speaking louder.
2. This teaching principle is common to all age groups, not just older adults.
3. This teaching principle is common to all age groups, not just older adults. This ensures that the learner has learned all the critical elements associated with the skill.
4. **Reaction time will slow with aging; therefore, older adults need more time to process and respond to information or perform a skill. In addition, some older**

adults may have less energy, experience more fatigue, and may need shorter, frequent learning sessions.

16. 1. Identifying the expected properties of urine reflects learning on the *knowledge level*, which is the first of 6 levels of complexity in the *cognitive domain*.

2. Explaining the importance of producing urine reflects learning on the *comprehension level*, which is the second of 6 levels of complexity in the *cognitive domain*.

3. Recognizing when something is contaminated reflects learning on the *comprehension level*, which is the second level of 6 levels of complexity within the *cognitive domain*.

4. This is the highest level of learning in the *cognitive domain* of the choices offered. Interpretation of laboratory results of urine testing reflects learning on the *analysis level*, which is the fourth of 6 levels of learning in the *cognitive domain*.

17. 1. This response is simple, direct, and uses language that is easily understood.

2. 96 is the pressure in the artery, not the vein.

3. This does not answer the question, which can be frustrating to the patient. When a question receives a meaningless response, the patient may perceive that the nurse is not interested in taking the time to explain the concept.

4. The patient is requesting simple information. The question has to be answered first, and then any concerns can be addressed.

18. 1. This is a dependent function of the nurse and requires a physician's order. In addition, an 800-calorie diet is too few calories to acquire basic nutrients to maintain adequate health. Weight loss diets should be between 1200 and 1500 calories for women and between 1500 and 1800 for men.

2. Learning is encouraged when positive behaviors are reinforced with a reward. However, food in this scenario should be avoided as a reward because it may foster old habits that contributed to the original weight gain. For people with an internal locus of control, rewards should center on recognition of personal achievement such as pleasing oneself, returning to a usual lifestyle, avoiding complications, and in this scenario losing weight. For the person with an external locus of control, rewards might center on privileges or praise received from pleasing significant others or members of the health team.

3. Although exercise is an important component of any weight loss program, exercise alone will not determine the success or failure of a weight loss program.

4. Setting realistic goals is important to the success of a weight loss plan. Since achieving success is dependent largely upon motivation, the teacher should design goals that demonstrate immediate progress or growth. One strategy is to design numerous realistic short-term intermediary goals that are achieved more easily than one long-term goal.

19. 1. For people who have difficulty with comprehension, participating in a learning program often makes them feel overwhelmed and threatened. The teacher needs to provide a structured environment where variables are controlled to reduce anxiety and support comprehension. The nurse should minimize ambiguity, provide a familiar environment, teach at the same time each day, limit environmental distractions, and provide simple learning materials.

2. This action helps the nurse understand what the patient is saying; it does not help the patient with a comprehension deficit to understand.

3. This helps the patient who is hearing-impaired, not the patient who has a comprehension deficit.

4. The patient does not need a hearing evaluation. The patient's problem is a diminished capacity to understand, not a hearing loss.

20. 1. The patient already knows the technique of how to administer the injection. The issue is the patient is reluctant to self-administer the injection.

2. The nurse has been doing this and it has not been effective. A reassessment is necessary.

3. When a teaching plan is ineffective, the nurse must gather more data and revise the teaching plan to achieve the desired goal.

4. This promotes dependency and prevents the patient from becoming self-sufficient.

21. 1. The terms *questionnaire* and *survey* are used interchangeably to describe a type of evaluation tool designed to gather data about a topic.

2. A post-test is not a questionnaire. A post-test is an examination given to assess cognitive learning after an educational program is completed.

3. A case study is not a questionnaire. A case study is a teaching tool that presents a scenario and a sequence of data to which the learner is required to analyze and respond.
4. A focus group is not a questionnaire. A focus group is designed to gather opinions and suggestions from a group of people about a particular topic using a discussion, not survey, format.

22. 1. Several other important factors that support adherence to a health-care regimen come before encouraging healthy behaviors.
2. A trusting relationship between the patient and the nurse is essential. Patients have to be confident that the nurse will maintain confidentiality, has credibility, and is genuinely interested in their success.
3. Although using educational aids to reinforce teaching supports adherence to a health-care regimen, an action in another option has priority.
4. This is not the first thing the nurse should do to facilitate adherence to a health-care regimen. After it is determined that the patient is not following the health-care regimen, then the nurse can assess the factors contributing to noncompliance.

23. 1. This is unnecessary. Hearing is the problem, not fatigue.
2. It is not necessary to limit teaching methods to print material for the hearing impaired. Print material lends itself mainly to learning in the *cognitive domain*. Print material is not as effective in facilitating learning in the *affective* and *psychomotor domains*, which require different teaching strategies.
3. Varieties of teaching methods facilitate learning because multiple senses are stimulated. When we see, hear, and touch, learning is more effective than when we see or hear alone. In addition, research demonstrates that we remember only 10% of what we read, 20% of what we hear, 30% of what we see, 50% of what we see and hear, and 80% of what we say and do.
4. A group setting is the least desirable teaching format for hearing-impaired individuals. One-on-one learning sessions limit background noise and distractions that hinder learning. In addition, a one-on-one session allows for individual feedback that ensures that the message is received as intended.

24. 1. This is an example of learning on the *knowledge level* in the *cognitive*, not *affective*, *domain*. *Cognitive* learning involves the intellect and requires thinking. It increases in complexity from *knowledge* to *comprehension*, *application*, *analysis*, *synthesis*, and *evaluation* of information.
2. This is an example of learning on the *valuing level* in the *affective domain*. Valuing is demonstrated when learning is incorporated into the learner's behavior because it is perceived as important. *Affective* learning involves the expression of feelings and the changing of beliefs, attitudes, or values.
3. This is an example of learning on the *knowledge level* in the *cognitive*, not *affective*, *domain*. *Cognitive* learning involves the intellect and requires thinking.
4. This is not an outcome demonstrating learning. This is an example of a question a learner might ask when learning content on the *knowledge level* in the *cognitive domain*. *Cognitive* learning involves the intellect and requires thinking.

25. 1. This technique is least likely to be used by adults preparing to retire. Role-playing is most often used when learning parenting and other interpersonal skills, such as interviewing.
2. This technique is least likely to be used by adults preparing for knee replacement surgery. Role-playing is most often used when learning parenting and other interpersonal skills, such as interviewing.
3. Men who are unwilling to admit that they have a drinking problem are not demonstrating readiness to learn. In addition, role-playing requires a person to assume a role for the purpose of learning a new behavior. These men are demonstrating an unwillingness to learn new behavior.
4. This group should benefit most from role-playing. Role-playing provides a safe environment in which to practice interpersonal skills. It enables the adolescent to rehearse what should be said, learn to respond to the emotional environment, and experience the pressures of the person playing the peer using drugs.

26. 1. Twenty percent of Americans read at or below the fifth-grade reading level and are considered functionally illiterate. Studies demonstrate that people generally read 3 to 5 grades below their highest grade of education.
2. Randomized studies demonstrate that the average reading level of individuals who need health teaching is 6.8 grades of schooling.

3. The eighth-grade reading level is too high a reading level for educational medical material. Randomized studies demonstrate that only 22% of individuals needing health teaching are able to profit from written health materials on the eighth-grade reading level.
4. The tenth-grade reading level is too high a reading level for educational medical material. Twenty percent of Americans read at or below the fifth-grade reading level and are considered functionally illiterate.

27. **1. Learners progress through a program at their own pace viewing informational material, answering questions, and receiving immediate feedback. Some programs feature simulated situations that require critical thinking and a response. Correct responses are rationalized, praise is offered, and incorrect responses trigger an explanation of why the wrong answer is wrong and offer encouragement to try again. This is a superior teaching strategy for the learner who may find that group lessons are paced either too fast or too slow for effective learning.**
2. Computer-assisted instruction (CAI) is not the least inexpensive teaching strategy. CAI requires a computer, keyboard and station, software, technical support to install, maintain, and repair equipment, and a computer-literate teaching staff to preview, select, and implement CAI programs.
3. Although individual computer-assisted programs (CAI) often include pre- and post-testing components, it is not the greatest advantage of CAI as a teaching strategy.
4. Although computer-assisted programs (CAI) generally are well organized in a programmed instruction (step-by-step) format, it is not the greatest advantage of using CAI as a teaching strategy.

28. 1. When a person achieves the ability to perform a behavior with confidence (demonstrates a well-balanced stance with crutches), learning has been achieved on the *mechanism level* of the *psychomotor domain*.
2. When the patient is able to identify the correct equipment for a colostomy irrigation, a readiness for action has been demonstrated. This example indicates learning on the *set level* of the *psychomotor domain*.
3. This option reflects the highest level of learning of the options offered. When a person achieves the ability to perform a behavior that requires a complex movement pattern with confidence, learning has been achieved on the *complex-overt response level* of learning in the *psychomotor domain*.
4. When a person achieves the ability to perform a behavior with confidence (recognize the difference between systolic and diastolic blood pressure sounds), learning has been achieved on the *mechanism level* of the *psychomotor domain*.

29. 1. Although previous experience is important to know when designing a teaching program, it is not as important as another option when determining whether a teaching program is needed.
2. Readiness to learn and motivation, which are closely tied together, are the two most important factors contributing to the success of any learning program. The learner must recognize that the learning need exists and that the material to be learned is valuable.
3. Although expectations are important to know so the teacher can incorporate them into the teaching plan, particularly when goal-setting, it is not as important as another option when determining whether a teaching program is needed.
4. Although it is important to know how flexible a patient is when designing a teaching plan, particularly when goal-setting, it is not as important as another option when determining whether a teaching program is needed.

30. 1. Demonstrations generally are used for teaching a skill. Skills involve learning about equipment, rationales, and sequencing multiple steps and are too cognitively complex for the developmental abilities of a preschooler. A teaching method in another option is more age-appropriate for a preschooler.
2. This is the best approach because it requires preschoolers to be active participants in their own learning. In addition, the child has a product to take home and be proud of, it reduces anxiety associated with learning because coloring is an activity most preschoolers are familiar with, and it is within a preschooler's cognitive level.
3. Preschoolers are just beginning to interact with peers, have a short attention span, and get distracted easily, and therefore need a one-on-one relationship with the teacher. The teacher facilitates the learning specifically for the individual, keeps the

learner focused, and provides reinforcement on the learner's cognitive level. Other age-specific strategies include games, storybooks, the use of dolls, puppets or toys, and role-playing.

4. A video requires concentration and an attention span that may be beyond the developmental abilities of a preschooler.

31. 1. This is not an example of a continuing education program. Continuing education (CE) refers to formal professional development experiences designed to enhance the knowledge or skills of practitioners.

2. Inservice programs generally are provided by health-care agencies to reinforce current knowledge and skills or provide new information about such things as policies, theory, skills, practice or equipment.

3. This is not an example of a certification program. The American Nurses Association has a certification program where nurses can demonstrate minimum competence in specialty areas. Achievement of certification demonstrates advanced expertise and a commitment to ensuring competence.

4. This is not an example of an orientation program. An orientation program is provided by a health-care agency to introduce new employees to the policies, procedures, departments, services, table of organization, expectations, equipment, etc., within the agency.

32. 1. This is a subjective assessment that is difficult to perform. Declining functional abilities, debilitating diseases, pain, and stress may impair the intellectual functioning of some individuals.

2. Although it is important to assess a patient's experience before implementing a teaching plan, of the options offered, it is not the first thing the nurse should do.

3. If the patient does not recognize the need to learn or value the information to be learned, the patient will not be ready to learn.

4. Although it is important to assess a patient's strengths before implementing a teaching plan, of the options offered, it is not the first thing the nurse should do.

33. 1. Although fear will affect the success of a teaching program and will need to be assessed and modification employed, it is not the factor that will have the greatest impact on the future success of a teaching program. Fear initially causes change; however, as fear subsides a person usually returns to the previous behavior.

2. Of all the options presented, the patient in denial is the person least ready and motivated to learn. The patient in denial is unable to recognize the need for the learning.

3. Fatigue is a physiologic, not psychosocial, adaptation to an illness. When teaching, the nurse needs to assess the patient's stamina and modify the teaching program so as not to unduly strain the patient, and yet meet the objectives.

4. Although anxiety is important, it is not the factor that has the greatest impact on the future success of a teaching program. Mild anxiety is motivating. Moderate anxiety will motivate a patient to learn but may require the nurse to keep concepts and approaches simple. The person with moderate anxiety may need to be focused, and distractions minimized to facilitate learning. If severe anxiety or panic are present, the teaching program will have to be postponed until the patient is less anxious.

34. **Answer: 1, 5, 2, 3, 4**

1. This should be done first because a diet requires a practitioner's order; following a sepecific diet is a dependent function of the nurse.

5. Assessing motivation is one of the most important factors influencing learning. The learner must recognize that the need exists and that the need will be addressed through the learning.

2. Determining food preferences is part of nursing assessment. Food preferences can then be included in the teaching plan about the low-calorie diet.

3. Details of the diet can be taught after the order is verified, motivation is determined, and preferences identified.

4. Evaluation is the final step of teaching. A meal plan designed by the patient requires not just an understanding of the information but an ability to apply the information.

35. **1. The person with an external locus of control is motivated by rewards that center on privileges, incentives, or praise received from pleasing significant others or members of the health team. Watching television is a privilege in this situation.**

2. This behavior indicates an internal, not external, locus of control. People with an

internal locus of control are motivated by personal internal rewards such as achieving a personal goal, pleasing oneself, returning to a usual lifestyle, and avoiding complications.

3. **Pleasing others precipitates feedback that is often viewed as positive by the recipient. Positive verbal or nonverbal communication from another is an external reward.**
4. Understanding the expected outcome of therapy is associated with recognizing the goal one is working to achieve; it does not describe an external locus of control.
5. A self-actualized adult is motivated by an internal locus of control. According to Maslow, the self-actualized person is an individual who has a need to develop to one's maximum potential and personally realize one's qualities and abilities.

Essential Components of Nursing Care

4

Nursing Process

KEYWORDS

The following words include English vocabulary, nursing/medical terminology, concepts, principles, or information relevant to content specifically addressed in the chapter or associated with topics presented in it. English dictionaries, nursing textbooks, and medical dictionaries, such as *Taber's Cyclopedic Medical Dictionary*, are resources that can be used to expand your knowledge and understanding of these words and related information.

Achievement
Actual outcome
Analyze
Assessment
Care plan conferences
Care plan types
  Individualized
  Standardized
  Computerized
  Case management
  Clinical pathway
Cluster of data
Collaborative problem
Conclusion
Contributing factor
Corrective action
Database
Data collection methods
  Interview
  Inspection
  Observation
  Palpation
  Percussion
  Examination
  Auscultation
Decision-making process
Deductive reasoning
Defining characteristic
Diagnostic label
Diagnostic reasoning process
Discharge planning
Documentation of care
Dynamic
Effective
Etiology
Evaluation
Expected outcome
Formulate
Functions of the nurse
  Dependent
  Independent
  Interdependent
Goal—components
  Achievable
  Measurable
  Realistic
  Time frame
Gordon's Functional Health Patterns
Holistic Identity
Implementation
Inductive reasoning
Inference
Information-processing theory
Interpret
Intervention skills
  Teaching
  Collaborating
  Managing
  Coordinating
  Monitoring
  Assisting
  Supporting
  Protecting
  Sustaining
Medical diagnosis
Medical record, parts of
History and Physical
  Admission sheet

Progress notes
Flow sheets
Doctor's orders
Consents
Laboratory results
Medication administration record
Nursing care plan
Nursing Diagnosis
Nursing Process
Objective data
Organize
Policy
Primary source
Priority
Problem statement
Procedure
Protocols
Rationale
Related to factor
Risk factors
Secondary source
Secondary to factor
Significance
Signs
Standards of practice
Subjective data
Symptoms
Taxonomy
Variance

QUESTIONS

1. When two nursing diagnoses appear closely related, what should the nurse do first to determine which diagnosis most accurately reflects the needs of the patient?
   1. Reassess the patient
   2. Examine the *related to* factors
   3. Analyze the *secondary to* factors
   4. Review the defining characteristics
2. The nurse performs an assessment of a newly admitted patient. The nurse understands that this admission assessment is conducted primarily to:
   1. Diagnose if the patient is at risk for falls
   2. Ensure that the patient's skin is intact
   3. Establish a therapeutic relationship
   4. Identify important data
3. The nurse identifies that the patient statement that provides subjective data is:
   1. "I'm not sure that I am going to be able to manage at home by myself."
   2. "I can call a home-care agency if I feel I need help at home."
   3. "What should I do if I have uncontrollable pain at home?"
   4. "Will a home health aide help me with my care at home?"
4. The nurse understands that evaluation most directly relates to which aspect of the Nursing Process?
   1. Goal
   2. Problem
   3. Etiology
   4. Implementation
5. The nurse comes to the conclusion that a patient's elevated temperature, pulse, and respirations are significant. What step of the Nursing Process is being used when the nurse comes to this conclusion?
   1. Implementation
   2. Assessment
   3. Evaluation
   4. Diagnosis
6. When the nurse considers the Nursing Process, the word "identify" is to "recognize" as the word "do" is to:
   1. Plan
   2. Evaluate
   3. Diagnose
   4. Implement

7. The nurse is collecting subjective data associated with a patient's anxiety. Which assessment method should be used to collect this information?
   1. Observing
   2. Inspecting
   3. Auscultation
   4. Interviewing

8. Which nursing action reflects an activity associated with the diagnosis step of the Nursing Process?
   1. Formulating a plan of care
   2. Identifying the patient's potential risks
   3. Designing ways to minimize a patient's stressors
   4. Making decisions about the effectiveness of patient care

9. The nurse collects objective data when a hospitalized patient states:
   1. "I am hungry."
   2. "I feel very warm."
   3. "I ate half my lunch."
   4. "I have the urge to urinate."

10. The nurse understands that subjective data has been obtained when the patient states:
    1. "I just went in the urinal and it needs to be emptied."
    2. "My pain feels like a 5 on a scale of 1 to 5."
    3. "The doctor said I can go home today."
    4. "I only ate half my breakfast."

11. During which of the five steps in the Nursing Process does the nurse determine whether outcomes of care are achieved?
    1. Implementation
    2. Evaluation
    3. Diagnosis
    4. Planning

12. When considering the Nursing Process, the nurse understands that the word "observe" is to "assess" as the word "determine" is to:
    1. Plan
    2. Analyze
    3. Diagnose
    4. Implement

13. An essential concept related to understanding the Nursing Process is that it:
    1. Is dynamic rather than static
    2. Focuses on the role of the nurse
    3. Moves from the simple to the complex
    4. Is based on the patient's medical problem

14. The nurse is caring for a male patient with a urinary elimination problem. Which is the most accurately stated goal? "The patient will:
    1. Be taught how to use a urinal when on bed rest."
    2. Experience fewer incontinence episodes at night."
    3. Be assisted to the toilet every two hours and whenever necessary."
    4. Transfer independently and safely to a commode before discharge."

15. Which word best describes the role of the nurse when using the Nursing Process to meet the needs of the patient holistically?
    1. Teacher
    2. Advocate
    3. Surrogate
    4. Counselor

16. The nurse understands that the word most closely associated with scientific principles is:
    1. Data
    2. Problem
    3. Rationale
    4. Evaluation

17. A pebble dropped into a pond causes ripples on the surface of the water. Which part of the nursing diagnosis is most directly related to this concept?
    1. Defining characteristics
    2. Outcome criteria
    3. Etiology
    4. Goal

18. The nurse teaches a patient to use visualization to cope with chronic pain. This action reflects which step of the Nursing Process?
    1. Planning
    2. Diagnosis
    3. Evaluation
    4. Implementation

19. A patient has multiple diagnostic tests performed. Where in the patient's chart can the nurse find documentation about the current medical diagnosis after the diagnostic tests results are reported?
    1. Physician's History and Physical
    2. Social Service Record
    3. Admission Sheet
    4. Progress Notes

20. During which of the five steps in the Nursing Process does the nurse analyze data critically?
    1. Diagnosis
    2. Clustering
    3. Collection
    4. Assessment

21. The nurse is caring for a patient with a fever. Which is a well-designed goal for this patient? The patient will:
    1. Have a lower temperature
    2. Be given aspirin every eight hours prn
    3. Be taught how to take an accurate temperature
    4. Maintain fluid intake sufficient to prevent dehydration

22. During the evaluation step of the Nursing Process, the nurse must:
    1. Establish outcomes
    2. Determine priorities
    3. Take corrective action
    4. Set the time frames for goals

23. Determining what nursing actions will be employed occurs in which step of the Nursing Process?
    1. Implementation
    2. Assessment
    3. Diagnosis
    4. Planning

24. The nurse understands that the appropriateness of a Nursing Diagnosis is supported by its:
    1. Defining characteristics
    2. Planned interventions
    3. Diagnostic statement
    4. Related risk factors

25. The nurse understands that the primary goal of the assessment phase of the Nursing Process is to:
 1. Build trust and rapport
 2. Collect and cluster data
 3. Establish goals and outcomes
 4. Identify and validate the medical diagnosis

26. Which human response identified by the nurse is an example of objective data?
 1. Pain of 5 on a 1 to 10 pain scale
 2. Irregular radial pulse of 50 bpm
 3. Shortness of breath
 4. Dizziness

27. The Planning step of the Nursing Process is influenced most directly by the:
 1. Related factors
 2. Diagnostic label
 3. Secondary factors
 4. Medical diagnosis

28. The nurse collects data about a patient. Next, the nurse should:
 1. Write a patient-centered goal
 2. Formulate a nursing diagnosis
 3. Design a plan of nursing interventions
 4. Determine the significance of the information

29. The nurse understands that human responses can be classified as objective or subjective. Identify all those that are subjective.
 1. _____ Nausea S
 2. _____ Jaundice O
 3. _____ Dizziness S
 4. _____ Diaphoresis O
 5. _____ Hypotension O

30. Nurses use the Nursing Process to provide nursing care. These statements reflect nursing care being provided to a variety of patients. Place the statements in order as the nurse progresses through the steps of the Nursing Process starting with assessment and ending with evaluation.
 1. "I am going to give you an enema."
 2. "What brought you to the hospital today?"
 3. "The patient's adaptations indicate that he is dehydrated."
 4. "The patient will have a bowel movement in the morning."
 5. "Did you sleep last night after I gave you the sleeping medication?"
 Answer: _______________

ANSWERS AND RATIONALES

1. 1. If a thorough assessment is completed initially, a reassessment should not be necessary.
   2. To establish which of two nursing diagnoses is most appropriate is not dependent upon identifying the factors that *contributed to* (also known as *related to* or *etiology of*) the nursing diagnosis. These factors are identified after the problem statement is identified.
   3. To establish which of two nursing diagnoses is more appropriate is not dependent upon analyzing the *secondary to* factors. *Secondary to* factors generally are medical conditions that precipitate the *related to* factors. The *secondary to* factors are identified after the *related to* factors of the problem are identified.
   4. **The first thing the nurse should do to differentiate between two closely associated nursing diagnoses is to compare the data collected to the major and minor defining characteristics of each of the nursing diagnoses being considered.**

2. 1. Although completing a nursing admission assessment includes an assessment of the risk for falls, it is only one component of the assessment.
   2. Although completing a nursing admission assessment includes an assessment of the skin, it is only one component of the assessment.
   3. Although completing a nursing admission assessment helps to initiate the nurse–patient relationship, it is not the primary purpose of completing a nursing admission assessment.
   4. **This is the primary purpose of a nursing admission assessment. Data must be collected and then analyzed to determine significance, and grouped in meaningful clusters before a nursing diagnosis can be made.**

3. 1. **This is subjective information because it is the patient's perception and can be verified only by the patient. Subjective data are those adaptations, feelings, beliefs, preferences, and information that only the patient can confirm.**
   2. This is neither subjective nor objective. It is a statement indicating an understanding of how to seek home care services after discharge.
   3. This is neither subjective nor objective. It is a question indicating that the patient wants more information about how to control pain when at home.
   4. This is neither subjective nor objective. It is a statement exploring who will provide assistance with care once the patient goes home.

4. 1. **To evaluate the effectiveness of a nursing action, the nurse needs to compare the *actual* patient outcome with the *expected* patient outcome. The expected outcomes are the measurable data that reflect goal achievement, and the actual outcomes are what really happened.**
   2. The problem is associated with the first half (problem statement) of the Nursing Diagnosis, not the Evaluation, step of the Nursing Process.
   3. Etiology is a term used to identify the factors that *relate to* or *contribute to* the problem statement of the Nursing Diagnosis, not the Evaluation, step of the Nursing Process.
   4. Implementation is a step separate from Evaluation in the Nursing Process. Nursing care must be implemented before it can be evaluated.

5. 1. This is not an example of the Implementation step of the Nursing Process. During the Implementation step, planned nursing care is delivered.
   2. This is not an example of the Assessment step of the Nursing Process. Although data may be gathered during the Assessment step, the manipulation of the data is conducted in a different step of the Nursing Process.
   3. This is not an example of the Evaluation step of the Nursing Process. Evaluation occurs when actual outcomes are compared with expected outcomes, which reflect attainment or nonattainment of the goal.
   4. **During the Diagnosis step of the Nursing Process, data are critically analyzed and interpreted; significance of data is determined; inferences are made and validated; cues and clusters of cues are compared with the defining characteristics of nursing diagnoses; contributing factors are identified; and nursing diagnoses are identified and organized in order of priority.**

6. 1. The words *identify* and *recognize* have the same definition. They both mean the same as that which is known. The word *plan* does not fit the analogy because the definitions of *plan* and *do* are different. The word *plan* means a method

of proceeding. The word *do* means to carry into effect or to accomplish.

2. The words *identify* and *recognize* have the same definition. They both mean the same as that which is known. The word *evaluate* does not fit the analogy because the definitions of *evaluate* and *do* are different. The word *evaluate* means to determine the worth of something, whereas the word *do* means to carry into effect or to accomplish.
3. The words *identify* and *recognize* have the same definition. They both mean the same as that which is known. The word *diagnose* does not fit the analogy because the definitions of *diagnose* and *do* are different. The word *diagnose* means to identify the patient's human response to an actual or potential health problem. The word *do* means to carry into effect or to accomplish.
4. **This is the correct analogy. The words *identify* and *recognize* have the same definition. They both mean the same as that which is known. The words *do* and *implement* both have the same definition. They both mean to carry out some action.**

7. 1. Observation is the deliberate use of all the senses, and involves more than just inspection and examination. It includes surveying, looking, scanning, scrutinizing, and appraising. Although the nurse makes inferences based on data collected by observation, this is not as effective as another data collection method to identify subjective data associated with a patient's anxiety.
2. Inspection involves the act of making observations of physical features and behavior. Although the nurse observes behaviors and makes inferences based on their perceived meaning, another data collection method is more effective in identifying subjective data associated with a patient's anxiety.
3. Auscultation is listening for sounds within the body. This collects objective, not subjective, data, which are measurable.
4. **Interviewing a patient is the most effective data collection method when collecting subjective data associated with a patient's anxiety. The patient is the primary source for subjective data about beliefs, values, feelings, perceptions, fears and concerns.**

8. 1. This occurs during the Planning, not Diagnosis, step of the Nursing Process.
2. **Potential risk factors are identified during the Diagnosis step of the Nursing Process. Risk diagnoses are designed to address situations where patients have a particular vulnerability to health problems.**
3. This occurs during the Planning, not Diagnosis, step of the Nursing Process.
4. This occurs during the Evaluation, not Diagnosis, step of the Nursing Process.

9. 1. Hunger is an example of subjective, not objective, data. Subjective data are those adaptations, feelings, beliefs, preferences, and information that only the patient can confirm.
2. Feeling warm is an example of subjective, not objective, data. Subjective data are those adaptations, feelings, beliefs, preferences, and information that only the patient can confirm.
3. **The amount of food eaten by a patient can be objectively verified. The nurse measures and documents the percentage of a meal ingested by a patient to quantify the amount of food consumed.**
4. Having the urge to void is an example of subjective, not objective, data. Subjective data are those adaptations, feelings, beliefs, preferences, and information that only the patient can confirm.

10. 1. This is an objective, not subjective, statement indicating something that is checkable and measurable. Objective data can be verified.
2. **A patient's perception about a pain level is subjective information. Subjective data are those adaptations, feelings, beliefs, preferences, and information that only the patient can confirm.**
3. This is an objective, not subjective, statement indicating something that is checkable and measurable. Objective data can be verified.
4. This is an objective, not subjective, statement indicating something that is checkable and measurable. Objective data can be verified.

11. 1. During the Implementation step of the Nursing Process, outcomes are not determined, but rather planned nursing care is delivered.
2. **Evaluation occurs when actual outcomes are compared with expected outcomes that reflect goal achievement. If the goal is achieved, the patient's needs are met.**
3. During the Diagnosis step of the Nursing Process, outcomes are not determined; rather, the nurse diagnoses human responses to actual or potential health problems.
4. During the Planning step of the Nursing Process, expected outcomes are determined, but their achievement is measured in another step of the Nursing Process.

12. 1. The definitions of the words *observe* and *assess* are similar. Observe means to examine something scientifically, and assess means to determine the significance of something. The word *plan* does not fit the analogy because the definitions of the words *plan* and *determine* are not similar. *Determine* means to reach a decision. *Plan* means to carry into effect or to accomplish.

2. The definitions of the words *observe* and *assess* are similar. *Observe* means to examine something scientifically, and *assess* means to determine the significance of something. The word *analyze* does not fit the analogy because *analyze* is not a step in the Nursing Process. The steps in the Nursing Process are Assessment, Diagnosis, Planning, Implementation, and Evaluation.

3. The definitions of the words *observe* and *assess* are similar. *Observe* means to examine something scientifically, and *assess* means to determine the significance of something. The word *diagnose* appropriately completes the analogy because the definitions of *determine* and *diagnose* are similar. *Determine* means to reach a decision about something and *diagnose* means to make a decision based on the assessment and analysis of a human response.

4. The definitions of the words *observe* and *assess* are similar. *Observe* means to examine something scientifically, and *assess* means to determine the significance of something. The word *implement* does not fit the analogy because the definitions of *determine* and *implement* are not similar. *Determine* means to reach a decision about something and *implement* means to carry out some action.

13. 1. The Nursing Process is a dynamic five-step problem-solving process (Assessment, Diagnosis, Planning, Implementation, and Evaluation) designed to diagnose and treat human responses to health problems. The nurse moves among the steps in response to the changing needs of the patient.

2. The Nursing Process focuses on the needs of the patient, not the role of the nurse.

3. Moving from the simple to the complex is a principle of teaching, not the Nursing Process. The Nursing Process is a complex interactive five-step problem-solving process designed to meet a patient's needs. It requires an understanding of systems and information-processing theory, and the critical-thinking, problem-solving, decision-making, and diagnostic-reasoning processes.

4. The Nursing Process is concerned with a person's human responses to actual or potential health problems, not the patient's medical problem.

14. 1. This is not a goal. This is an action the nurse plans to implement to help a patient achieve a goal.

2. This goal is inappropriate because the word *fewer* is not specific, measurable, or objective.

3. This is not a goal. This is an action the nurse plans to implement to help a patient achieve a goal.

4. This is a correctly worded goal. Goals must be patient-centered, measurable, realistic, and include the time frame in which the expected goal is to be achieved. The word *independently* indicates that no help is needed, and the word *safely* indicates that no injury will occur. The time frame is before discharge.

15. 1. Although functioning as a teacher is an important role of the nurse, it is a limited role compared to another option. As a teacher, the nurse helps the patient gain new knowledge about health and health care to maintain or restore health.

2. When the nurse supports, protects, and defends a patient from a holistic perspective, the nurse functions as an advocate. Advocacy includes exploring, informing, mediating, and affirming in all areas to help a patient navigate the health-care system, maintain autonomy, and achieve the best possible health outcomes.

3. The word surrogate is not the word that best describes this scenario. The nurse is placed in the surrogate role when a patient projects onto the nurse the image of another and then responds to the nurse with the feelings for the other person's image.

4. Although functioning as a counselor is an important role of the nurse, it is a limited role compared to another option. As counselor, the nurse helps the patient improve interpersonal relationships, recognize and deal with stressful psychosocial problems, and promote achievement of self-actualization.

16. 1. The word *data* (evidence or information) is not associated with the term *scientific principles* (established rules of action).

2. The word *problem* (difficulty or crisis) is not associated with the term *scientific principles* (established rules of action).
3. The word *rationale* (justification based on reasoning) is closely associated with the term *scientific principles* (established rules of action). Scientific principles are based on rationales.
4. The word *evaluation* (determining the value or worth of something) is not associated with the term *scientific principles* (established rules of action).

17. 1. Defining characteristics do not contribute to the problem statement but support or indicate the presence of the nursing diagnosis. Defining characteristics are the major and minor signs and symptoms that support the presence of a nursing diagnosis.
2. Outcome criteria are not a part of the nursing diagnosis. Outcome criteria (goals) are part of the Planning step of the Nursing Process.
3. The etiology (also known as *related to* or *contributing factors*) are the conditions, situations, or circumstances that add to the development of the human response identified in the problem statement of the nursing diagnosis. The etiology precipitates the problem just as a pebble dropped in a pond causes ripples on the surface of water.
4. Goals are not part of the nursing diagnosis. Goals are the expected outcomes or what is hoped that the patient will achieve in response to nursing intervention.

18. 1. This is not an example of the Planning step of the Nursing Process. During the Planning step, the nurse identifies and plans the nursing interventions that seem most likely to be effective.
2. This is not an example of the Diagnosis step of the Nursing Process. During the Diagnosis step of the Nursing Process, data are critically analyzed and interpreted; significance of data are determined; inferences are made and validated; signs and symptoms and clusters of signs and symptoms are compared with the defining characteristics of nursing diagnoses; contributing factors are identified; and nursing diagnoses are identified and organized in order of priority.
3. This is not an example of the Evaluation step of the Nursing Process. Evaluation occurs when actual outcomes are compared with expected outcomes that reflect goal achievement.
4. This is an example of the Implementation step of the Nursing Process. During the Implementation step, planned nursing care is delivered.

19. 1. The Physician's History and Physical contains a history of the patient, a physical, and the medical problems on the day of admission to the hospital. The admission medical diagnosis may be different after diagnostic tests are completed.
2. Although the patient's medical diagnosis might be documented on the patient's Social Service Record, it is not the major source for this information.
3. This is the best source for identifying the patient's admitting medical diagnosis, but it will not contain the current medical diagnosis if the diagnosis changed after completion of diagnostic tests.
4. Generally the Progress Notes contain documentation by all members of the health team. After a patient is admitted and diagnostic tests completed, the patient's medical diagnosis may change. The ongoing changes and current status of the patient are documented in the Progress Notes.

20. **1. During the Diagnosis step of the Nursing Process, data are critically analyzed and interpreted; significance of data is determined; inferences are made and validated; signs and symptoms and clusters of signs and symptoms are compared with the defining characteristics of nursing diagnoses; contributing factors are identified; and nursing diagnoses are identified and organized in order of priority.**
2. Clustering data is not a step in the Nursing Process. Clustering data occurs during the Diagnosis step.
3. Collection is not a step in the Nursing Process. During the Assessment step data are collected from different sources using various methods.
4. During the Assessment step of the Nursing Process data are collected from different sources using various methods.

21. 1. This goal is inappropriate because the word *lower* is not specific, measurable, or objective.
2. This is not a goal. This is an action the nurse plans to implement to help a patient achieve a goal.
3. This is not a goal. This is an action the nurse plans to implement to help a patient achieve a goal.

4. This is a well written goal. Goals must be patient-centered, specific, measurable, realistic, and have a time frame in which the expected outcome is to be achieved. The words *sufficient* and *dehydration* are based on generally accepted criteria against which to measure the patient's actual outcome. The word *maintain* connotes continuously, which is a time frame.

22\. 1. Establishing outcomes is part of the Planning, not Evaluation, step of the Nursing Process.
2. Determining priorities is part of the Diagnosis, not Evaluation, step of the Nursing Process. Priority setting is a decision-making process that ranks a patient's nursing diagnoses in order of importance.
3. Corrective action takes place in the Evaluation step of the Nursing Process. If during evaluation it is determined that the goal was not met, the reasons for failure have to be identified and the plan modified.
4. Setting time frames for goals to be achieved is part of the Planning, not Evaluation, step of the Nursing Process.

23\. 1. This does not occur during the Implementation step of the Nursing Process. During the Implementation step, the nurse puts the plan of care into action. Nursing interventions include actions that are dependent (requiring a physician's order), independent (autonomous actions within the nurse's scope of practice), and interdependent (interventions that require a physician's order but that permit the nurse to use clinical judgment in their implementation).
2. This does not occur during the Assessment step of the Nursing Process. During the Assessment step, the nurse uses various skills such as observation, interviewing, and physical examination to collect data from various sources.
3. This does not occur during the Diagnosis step of the Nursing Process. A nursing Diagnosis is made when the nurse identifies the patient's human responses to actual or potential health problems.
4. The identification of nursing actions designed to help a patient achieve a goal occurs during the Planning step of the Nursing Process.

24\. **1. The defining characteristics are the major and minor cues that form a cluster that support or validate the presence of a Nursing Diagnosis. At least one major defining characteristic must be present for a nursing diagnosis to be considered appropriate for the patient.**
2. Planned interventions do not support the Nursing Diagnosis. They are the nursing actions designed to help resolve the *related to* or *contributing to* factors and achieve expected patient outcomes that reflect goal achievement.
3. The diagnostic statement cannot support the Nursing Diagnosis because it is the first part of the Nursing Diagnosis. A Nursing Diagnosis is made up of two parts, the *diagnostic statement* (also known as *the problem statement)* and the *related to* factors (also known as factors that *contribute to* the problem or *the etiology)*.
4. Related risk factors cannot support the Nursing Diagnosis because they are the second part of the nursing diagnosis. A nursing diagnosis is made up of two parts, the diagnostic statement (also known as *the problem statement*) and the *related to* factors (also known as factors that *contribute to* the problem or *the etiology*).

25\. 1. Although trust and rapport may be established during the assessment phase of the Nursing Process, they are not the primary purpose. The development of trust and rapport generally takes time.
2. The primary purpose of the Assessment step of the Nursing Process is to collect data from various sources using a variety of approaches. After data are collected, they are clustered into meaningful categories and interpreted during the Diagnosis step of the Nursing Process.
3. When a five-step Nursing Process is followed, identifying goals and outcomes occur during the Planning, not Assessment, step of the Nursing Process.
4. Identifying and validating the medical diagnosis are not within a Registered Nurse's legal scope of nursing practice.

26\. 1. A patient's perception about a pain level is an example of subjective, not objective, data. Subjective data are those adaptations, feelings, beliefs, preferences and information that only the patient can confirm.
2. A radial pulse is objective, not subjective, information. Objective data are measurable and checkable.
3. A patient's complaint about shortness of breath is an example of subjective, not objective, data.

Subjective data are those adaptations, feelings, beliefs, preferences, and information that only the patient can confirm.

4. A patient's complaint about dizziness is an example of subjective, not objective, data. Subjective data are those adaptations, feelings, beliefs, preferences, and information that only the patient can confirm.

27. 1. **Related factors (i.e., contrbuting to factors, etiology) contribute to the problem statement of the Nursing Diagnosis and directly impact on the Planning step of the Nursing Process. Nursing interventions are selected to minimize or relieve the effects of the related factors. If nursing interventions are appropriate and effective, the human response identified in the problem statement part of the Nursing Diagnosis will be resolved.**
2. The Planning step of the Nursing Process includes setting a goal, identifying the outcomes that will reflect goal achievement, and planning nursing interventions. Although the wording of the goal is directly influenced by the diagnostic label (problem statement of the Nursing Diagnosis), the selection of nursing interventions is not.
3. Secondary factors generally have only a minor influence on the Planning step of the Nursing Process.
4. The medical diagnosis does not influence the Planning step of the Nursing Process. The nurse is concerned with *human responses* to actual or potential health problems, not the medical diagnosis.

28. 1. Goals are designed after a Nursing Diagnosis is identified, not after data are collected.
2. Once data are collected, the nurse must first organize and cluster the data to determine significance and make inferences. After all this is accomplished, then the nurse can formulate a Nursing Diagnosis.
3. Nursing care is planned after Nursing Diagnoses and goals are identified, not immediately after data are collected.
4. **After data are collected, they are clustered to determine their significance.**

29. 1. **Nausea is an unpleasant, wavelike sensation in the back of the throat, epigastrium, or abdomen that may lead to vomiting. It is considered subjective data because it cannot be measured by the nurse objectively. It is experienced only by the patient.**
2. A yellow color of the skin, whites of the eyes, and mucous membranes (jaundice) because of deposition of bile pigments from excess bilirubin in the blood is objective, not subjective, information. Objective data are measurable and checkable.
3. **This is subjective information because it is the patient's perception and can be verified only by the patient. Subjective data are those adaptations, feelings, beliefs, preferences, and information that only the patient can confirm.**
4. Excessive sweating (diaphoresis) is objective, not subjective, information. Objective data are measurable and checkable.
5. Abnormally low systolic and diastolic blood pressure levels (hypotension) can be measured and verified and therefore are objective data.

30. **Answer: 2, 3, 4, 1, 5**
2. **Objective and subjective data must be collected, verified, and communicated during the Assessment step of the Nursing Process.**
3. **Data is clustered, analyzed, and their significance determined (which all lead to a conclusion about the patient's condition) during the Diagnosis step of the Nursing Process.**
4. **Identifying goals, projecting outcomes, setting priorities, and identifying interventions are all part of the Planning step of the Nursing Process.**
1. **Planned actions are initiated and completed during the Implementation step of the Nursing Process.**
5. **Identifying responses to care, comparing actual outcomes to expected outcomes, analyzing factors that affected outcomes, and modifying the plan of care if necessary are all part of the Evaluation step of the Nursing Process.**

Physical Assessment

KEYWORDS

The following words include English vocabulary, nursing/medical terminology, concepts, principles, or information relevant to content specifically addressed in the chapter or associated with topics presented in it. English dictionaries, nursing textbooks, and medical dictionaries, such as *Taber's Cyclopedic Medical Dictionary*, are resources that can be used to expand your knowledge and understanding of these words and related information.

Afebrile
Affect
Aneroid manometer
Anterior
Apnea
Asymptomatic
Attention span
Auscultation
Auscultatory gap
Autonomic nervous system
Balance
Barrel chest
Blood pressure
Blood viscosity
Body weight
Borborygmi
Bowel sounds
Bradycardia
Bradypnea
Breast examination
Breathing
- Costal (thoracic)
- Diaphragmatic (abdominal)

Breath sounds
- Expected
  - Bronchial
  - Bronchovesicular
  - Vesicular
- Adventitious
  - Crackles (rales)
  - Gurgles (rhonchi)
  - Pleural friction rub
  - Stridor
  - Wheeze

Capillary refill
Cardiac output
Chills
Circadian rhythms
Clubbing
Comatose
Core temperature
Data
- Objective
- Primary source of
- Secondary source of
- Subjective

Defervescence
Deformities
Delirium
Dental caries
Dependent edema
Diastolic
Diplopia
Diurnal variations
Doppler
Drowsiness
Ecchymosis
Edema
- Dependent edema
- Sacral edema

Erythema
Erythrocytes
Eupnea
Exacerbation
Examination
Exhalation
External respiration
Febrile
Fever
Functional health patterns
Gait
General Adaptation Syndrome
Health history
Hirsutism
Hyperemia
Hypertension

Hypotension
Hypovolemic shock
Inhalation
Inspection
Internal respiration
Jaundice
Korotkoff's sounds
Lateral
Lesion
Lethargy
Leukocytes
Level of consciousness
Local Adaptation Syndrome
Malaise
Memory
Mental status
Mobility
Mood
Neuro-checks
Neutrophils
Night blindness
Observation
Orientation
Orthostatic hypotension
Pain assessment scale
Palpation
Pap smear
Papillae on the tongue
Parasympathetic nervous system
Partial thromboplastin time
Percussion
Peripheral vascular resistance
Physical
Plaque
Platelets
Posterior
Posture
Prostate specific antigens (PSA)
Pruritus
Pulse deficit
Pulse pressure
Pulse sites
- Apical
- Brachial
- Carotid
- Femoral
- Pedal
- Popliteal
- Posterior tibial
- Temporal
- Tibial

Pyrexia
Rash
Red blood cell count
Reflexes
Remission
Respirations
- Biot's
- Cheyne-Stokes
- Kussmaul

Sagittal plane
Sensation
Shivering
Sigmoidoscopy
Sordes
Sphygmomanometer
Spinal tap
Stance
Stethoscope
Strength
Superior
Symmetry
Sympathetic nervous system
Systolic
Tachycardia
Tachypnea
Tartar
Texture
Thermometers
- Disposable
- Electronic
- Glass
- Intravenous catheter
- Temperature-sensitive strips
- Tympanic

Thrombocytes
Transverse plane
Tremor
Temperature sites
- Axillary
- Oral
- Rectal

Turgor
Urticaria
Variance

QUESTIONS

1. The nurse is assessing a postoperative patient for signs of hemorrhage. Which adaptation is most indicative of shock?
   1. Hyperemia
   2. Hypotension
   3. Irregular pulse
   4. Slow respirations

2. The nurse is monitoring the vital signs of a group of patients. When reviewing these results, the nurse must remember that body temperature usually is at its highest at:
   1. 12 AM–2 AM
   2. 6 AM–8 AM
   3. 4 PM–6 PM
   4. 8 PM–10 PM

3. When assessing for borborygmi, which physical examination method should the nurse use?
   1. Auscultation
   2. Percussion
   3. Inspection
   4. Palpation

4. The nurse plans to take a patient's radial pulse. Which method of examination should be used by the nurse?
   1. Palpation
   2. Inspection
   3. Percussion
   4. Auscultation

5. Which nursing action is common to all instruments when taking a temperature?
   1. Identify that the reading is below 96°F before insertion
   2. Wash with cool soap and water after use
   3. Place a disposable sheath over the probe
   4. Ensure that the instrument is clean

6. The nurse concludes that a patient is experiencing hyperthermia. Which assessment precipitated this conclusion?
   1. Mental confusion
   2. Increased appetite
   3. Decreased heart rate
   4. Rectal temperature of 101°F

7. The nurse in the Emergency Department is engaging in an initial assessment of a patient. Which assessment takes priority?
   1. Blood pressure
   2. Airway clearance
   3. Breathing pattern
   4. Circulatory status

8. The nurse is obtaining a patient's blood pressure. Which information is most important for the nurse to document?
   1. Staff member who took the blood pressure
   2. Patient's tolerance to having the blood pressure taken
   3. Position of the patient if the patient is not in a sitting position
   4. Difference between the palpated and auscultated systolic readings

9. The nurse is teaching a cancer prevention community health class. Which recommended cancer screening guideline for asymptomatic nonrisk people should the nurse include?
   1. Pap smears annually for females 13 years of age and older
   2. Mammograms annually for women 30 years of age and older
   3. Prostate-specific antigens yearly for men 30 years of age and older
   4. Sigmoidoscopies every 5 years for patients 50 years of age and older

10. The nurse understands that body heat production is increased by:
    1. Vasodilation
    2. Evaporation
    3. Shivering
    4. Radiation

11. The nurse is assessing a patient's bilateral pulses for symmetry. However, the nurse should not assess which pulse sites on both sides of the body at the same time?
    1. Radial
    2. Carotid
    3. Femoral
    4. Brachial

12. The nurse is caring for a patient who is experiencing an increase in symptoms associated with multiple sclerosis. Which term best describes a recurrence of symptoms associated with a chronic disease?
    1. Variance
    2. Remission
    3. Adaptation
    4. Exacerbation

13. The nurse in the clinic must obtain the vital signs of each patient before each patient is assessed by the practitioner. The nurse should obtain a temperature via the rectal route for a patient:
    1. Who is a mouth breather
    2. With a history of vomiting
    3. With an intelligence of a seven-year-old child
    4. Who cannot tolerate a semi-Fowler's position

14. A patient with hypertension is given discharge instructions to take the blood pressure every day. The nurse is evaluating a family member taking the patient's blood pressure as part of the patient's discharge teaching plan. The nurse identifies that further teaching is necessary when the family member:
    1. Places the diaphragm of the stethoscope over the brachial artery
    2. Applies the center of the bladder of the cuff directly over an artery
    3. Releases the valve on the manometer so that the gauge drops 10 mm Hg per heartbeat
    4. Inserts the 2 earpieces of the stethoscope into the ears so that they tilt slightly forward

15. A patient has a serious vitamin K deficiency. For which adaptation should the nurse assess this patient?
    1. Skin lesions
    2. Bleeding gums
    3. Night blindness
    4. Muscle weakness

16. The nurse identifies that a patient with a fever has warm skin. An additional adaptation that confirms the defervescence (flush) phase of a fever is:
    1. Sweating
    2. Shivering
    3. Cyanotic nail beds
    4. Goosebumps on the skin

17. When evaluating a patient's temperature, the nurse recalls that people usually have the lowest body temperature at:
    1. 4 AM–6 AM
    2. 8 AM–10 AM
    3. 4 PM–6 PM
    4. 8 PM–10 PM

18. Which method of examination is being used when the nurse's hands are used to assess the temperature of a patient's skin?
    1. Palpation
    2. Inspection
    3. Percussion
    4. Observation

19. The nurse must assess for the presence of bowel sounds in a postoperative patient. The nurse should auscultate the patient's abdomen:
    1. Prior to palpation
    2. Using a warmed stethoscope
    3. Starting at the left lower quadrant
    4. For at least three minutes in each quadrant

20. Which assessment requires the nurse to assess the patient further?
    1. 18-year-old woman with a pulse rate of 140 after riding 2 miles on an exercise bike
    2. 50-year-old man with a BP of 112/60 upon awakening in the morning
    3. 65-year-old man with a respiratory rate of 10
    4. 40-year-old woman with a pulse of 88

21. The nurse is interviewing a newly admitted patient. Which patient statement indicates the onset of a fever? "I feel:
    1. Cold."
    2. Warm."
    3. Sweaty."
    4. Thirsty."

22. The nurse is monitoring the status of postoperative patients. The vital sign that changes first indicating that a postoperative patient has internal bleeding is the:
    1. Body temperature
    2. Blood pressure
    3. Pulse pressure
    4. Heart rate

23. A patient has had a 101°F fever for the last 24 hours. How often should the nurse monitor this patient's temperature?
    1. Every 2 hours
    2. Every 4 hours
    3. Every 6 hours
    4. Every 8 hours

24. The nurse is unable to palpate a patient's brachial pulse. Which pulse should the nurse assess to determine adequate brachial blood flow in this patient?
    1. Radial
    2. Carotid
    3. Femoral
    4. Popliteal

25. Which can cause urine to appear red?
    1. Beets
    2. Strawberries
    3. Cherry Jell-O
    4. Red food dye

26. The nurse is assessing a patient's heart rate by palpating the carotid artery. What is the most important thing the nurse should do when assessing a pulse at this site?
 1. Monitor for a full minute
 2. Palpate just below the ear
 3. Press gently when palpating the site
 4. Massage the site before assessing for rate

27. The nurse obtains the blood pressure of several adults. What blood pressure result causes the most concern?
 1. 102/70
 2. 140/90
 3. 125/85
 4. 118/75

28. The nurse is planning care for a patient who has an intolerance to activity. What is the first assessment that should be made by the nurse?
 1. Influence on the other family members
 2. Impact on functional health patterns
 3. Pattern of vital signs
 4. Range of motion

29. The nurse concludes that a patient has inadequate nutrition. Which patient adaptation supports this conclusion?
 1. Presence of surface papillae on the tongue
 2. Reddish-pink mucous membranes
 3. Cachectic appearance
 4. Shiny eyes

30. The nurse must take a patient's rectal temperature. The nurse should:
 1. Take the temperature for 5 minutes
 2. Wear gloves throughout the procedure
 3. Place the patient in the right lateral position
 4. Insert the thermometer 2 inches into the rectum

31. Which usually is unrelated to a nursing physical assessment?
 1. Posture and gait
 2. Balance and strength
 3. Hygiene and grooming
 4. Blood and urine values

32. The patient has a temperature of 102°F and complains of feeling thirsty. Which additional adaptation should the nurse expect during this febrile stage of a fever?
 1. Restlessness with confusion
 2. Decreased respiratory rate
 3. Profuse perspiration
 4. Pale, cold skin

33. The nurse is performing a psychosocial assessment. Which assessment should be identified as a subtle indicator of depression?
 1. Unkempt appearance
 2. Anxious behavior
 3. Tense posture
 4. Crying

34. The nurse in the Emergency Department is caring for a patient who has been diagnosed with hypothermia. The presence of which factor in the patient's history may have precipitated this condition?
 1. Heat stroke
 2. Inability to sweat
 3. Excessive exercise
 4. High alcohol intake

35. A patient has lost approximately 2 units of blood during a vaginal delivery. For which response to this blood loss should the nurse assess this patient?
 1. Rapid, shallow breathing
 2. Increased urinary output
 3. Hypertension
 4. Bradypnea

36. The nurse understands that a concern that is common to the collection of specimens for culture and sensitivity tests, regardless of their source, is:
 1. A preservative media must be used
 2. Two specimens should be obtained
 3. Surgical asepsis must be maintained
 4. A morning specimen should be collected

37. A patient's vital signs are: oral temperature 99°F, pulse 88 beats per minute with a regular rhythm, respirations 16 breaths per minute and deep, and blood pressure 180/110 mm Hg. The sign that should cause the most concern is the:
 1. Pulse
 2. Respirations
 3. Temperature
 4. Blood pressure

38. A patient is admitted to the Emergency Department with difficulty breathing. Which patient response identified by the nurse causes the most concern?
 1. Low pulse oximetry
 2. Wheezing on expiration
 3. Shortness of breath on exertion
 4. Using accessory muscles of respiration

39. A patient is admitted with a tentative diagnosis of myasthenia gravis. The physician orders edrophonium chloride (Tensilon) 2 mg to be administered intravenously. After no reaction the physician orders 8 mg to be administered intravenously. The expected response is an improvement in muscle weakness confirming the diagnosis of myasthenia gravis. However, within 30 seconds after administration of the 8 mg of Tensilon, the patient experiences a cholinergic reaction with increased muscle weakness, bradycardia, diaphoresis, and hypotension. The physician orders atropine sulfate 1 mg to be administered intravenously stat. The vial of atropine sulfate indicates 0.5 mg/mL. Calculate how many mLs of atropine sulfate the nurse should administer intravenously.

Answer:____________ **mL.**

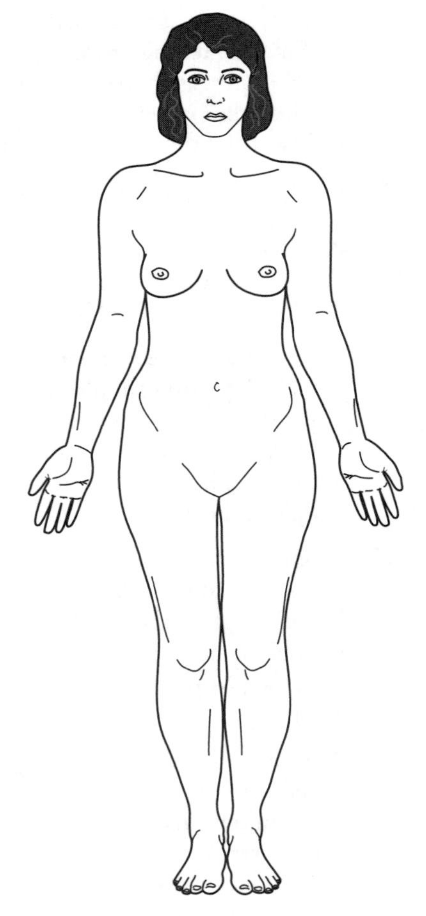

40. Place an X (on the figure to the right) over the site that is used most often by the nurse for assessing a patient's heart rate.

ANSWERS AND RATIONALES

1. 1. During the compensatory stage of shock, blood is shunted away from, not toward, the periphery. Hyperemia is an increase in blood flow to an area where the overlying skin becomes reddened and warm.
   2. **The circulating blood volume is reduced by 25% to 35% during the compensatory stage of shock and 35% to 50% during the progressive stage of shock as the peripheral vessels constrict to increase blood flow to vital organs. This shunting of blood causes hypotension.**
   3. With shock, the heart rate increases (tachycardia); it is not irregular. The heart rate increases during the compensatory stage of shock to maintain adequate blood flow to body tissues.
   4. During the compensatory stage of shock, the respiratory rate increases, not decreases, to maintain adequate oxygenation of body cells.

2. 1. The body temperature is on the decline during this time.
   2. The body temperature is just beginning to rise from its lowest level, which occurs between 4 AM and 6 AM.
   3. Although the body temperature is rising, it has not reached its peak at this time.
   4. **Diurnal variations (circadian rhythms) vary throughout the day with the highest body temperature usually occurring between 8 PM and midnight.**

3. 1. **Auscultation is the process of listening to sounds produced in the body. It is performed directly by just listening with the ears or indirectly by using a stethoscope that amplifies the sounds and conveys them to the nurse's ears. Active intestinal peristalsis causes rumbling, gurgling, and tinkling abdominal sounds known as bowel sounds (borborygmi).**
   2. Percussion may stimulate intestinal motility, which increases bowel sounds, but it is not the assessment method used to hear bowel sounds. Percussion is the act of striking the body's surface to elicit sounds that provide information about the size and shape of internal organs or whether tissue is air-filled, fluid-filled, or solid.
   3. Inspection cannot assess bowel sounds. Inspection uses the naked eye to perform a visual assessment of the body.
   4. Palpation may stimulate intestinal motility, which increases bowel sounds, but it is not the assessment method used to hear bowel sounds. Palpation is the examination of the body using the sense of touch.

4. 1. **Palpation, the examination of the body using the sense of touch, is used to obtain the heart rate at a pulse site. When measuring a pulse, an artery is compressed slightly by the fingers so that the pulsating artery is held between the fingers and a bone or firm structure.**
   2. A pulse is not measured by using the sense of sight. Inspection uses the naked eye to perform a visual assessment of the body.
   3. Percussion cannot measure a pulse. Percussion is the act of striking the body's surface to elicit sounds that provide information about the size and shape of internal organs or whether tissue is air-filled, fluid-filled, or solid.
   4. Auscultation is used to obtain an apical, not radial, pulse. Auscultation is the process of listening to sounds produced in the body. It is performed directly by just listening with the ears or indirectly by using a stethoscope that amplifies the sounds and conveys them to the nurse's ears.

5. 1. This is not true for all thermometers, such as chemical disposable thermometers, temperature-sensitive tape, and electronic thermometers. This is true for glass/plastic thermometers.
   2. This is true only for glass/plastic thermometers.
   3. This is true only for electronic thermometers and sometimes used for glass/plastic thermometers.
   4. **This is an acceptable medical asepsis practice. All instruments, regardless of their type, must be clean before use with a patient.**

6. 1. Mental confusion is a not a common human response to hyperthermia.
   2. Loss of appetite (anorexia), not an increased appetite, is a common human response to hyperthermia.
   3. An increased heart rate (tachycardia), not a decreased heart rate (bradycardia), is a common human response to hyperthermia.
   4. **A rectal temperature of 101°F (38.8°C) or oral temperature of 100°F (37.8°C) is**

a common human response that indicates hyperthermia.

7. 1. Although important, blood pressure is related to circulation, which is not the priority.
   2. **Patient assessment must always be conducted in order of priority of needs. In an emergency, the ABCs of assessment are airway, breathing, and circulation. A clear airway is essential for life and, therefore, has priority.**
   3. Although important, breathing is not the priority.
   4. Although important, circulation is not the priority.

8. 1. Although this should be done, it is not the most important information that should be documented.
   2. This is necessary only if the patient did not tolerate the procedure.
   3. **The patient's position when the blood pressure is measured may influence results. Generally, systolic and diastolic readings are lower in the horizontal than in the sitting position. There is a lower reading in the uppermost arm when a person is in a lateral recumbent position. A change from the horizontal to an upright position may result in a temporary decrease (5 to 10 mm Hg) in blood pressure; when it exceeds 25 mm Hg systolic or 10 mm Hg diastolic, it is called orthostatic hypotension.**
   4. This is unnecessary because they are approximately the same.

9. 1. A Pap smear should be performed at age 18 and yearly thereafter. If the person is sexually active, has a sexually transmitted disease, has a mother who took diethylstilbestrol during pregnancy, or has a family history of cervical or uterine cancer, a Pap smear should be performed before age 18 and then every subsequent year.
   2. The American Cancer Society recommends a mammography every 12 to 18 months when a woman is between 40 and 49 years of age and annually when 50 years of age or older.
   3. Prostate-specific antigen (PSA) should be performed at age 50 and yearly thereafter.
   4. **A sigmoidoscopy should be performed at age 50 and every 5 years thereafter.**

10. 1. Vasodilation brings warm blood to the peripheral circulation where it is lost through the skin via radiation.
    2. Evaporation (vaporization) is the conversion of a liquid into a vapor. When perspiration on the skin evaporates, it promotes heat loss.
    3. **Shivering generates heat by causing muscle contraction, which increases the metabolic rate by 100% to 200%.**
    4. Radiation is the transfer of heat from the surface of one object to the surface of another without direct contact.

11. 1. There are no contraindications for palpating both radial arteries at the same time.
    2. **It is unsafe to palpate both carotid arteries at the same time. Slight compression of both carotid arteries can interfere with blood flow to the brain. In addition, compression of the carotid arteries can stimulate the carotid sinuses, which causes a reflex drop in the heart rate.**
    3. There are no contraindications for palpating both femoral arteries at the same time.
    4. There are no contraindications for palpating both brachial arteries at the same time.

12. 1. Variance occurs when there is a variation or deviation from a critical pathway. This occurs when goals are not met or interventions are not performed according to the stipulated time period.
    2. A remission is a period during a chronic illness of lessened severity or cessation of symptoms.
    3. An adaptation is a physical or emotional response to an internal or external stimulus.
    4. **An exacerbation is the period during a chronic illness when symptoms reappear after a remission or absence of symptoms.**

13. 1. **Mouth breathing allows environmental air to enter the mouth, which results in an inaccurately low reading. To take an oral temperature the instrument must remain under the tongue of a closed mouth until the reading is obtained. This can take as little as several seconds (electronic thermometers) or as long as 3 to 4 minutes (glass/plastic thermometers).**
    2. A history of vomiting does not negate the use of an oral thermometer. If the patient should begin to vomit, the nurse can remove the thermometer.
    3. A 7-year-old child understands cause and effect and can follow directions regarding the use of an oral thermometer.
    4. An oral thermometer can be used with a patient maintained in any position.

14. 1. This is a correct action when obtaining a blood pressure reading. The brachial

artery is close to the skin's surface, and the diaphragm of the stethoscope is used for low-pitched sounds of a blood pressure reading.
2. This ensures an accurate reading because it provides uniform and complete compression of the brachial artery.
3. **This may result in an inaccurate reading. The valve on the manometer should be opened to allow the gauge to drop 2 to 3 mm Hg per heartbeat.**
4. This ensures that the openings in the earpieces of the stethoscope are facing toward the ear canal for uninterrupted transmission of sounds.

15. 1. Vitamin K deficiency is not associated with skin lesions. Vitamin C causes small skin hemorrhages and delays wound healing. Riboflavin deficiency causes lip lesions, seborrheic dermatitis, and scrotal and vulval skin changes.
2. **A disruption in the clotting mechanism of the body can result in bleeding. Vitamin K plays an essential role in the production of the clotting factors II (prothrombin), VII, IX, and X.**
3. A deficiency in vitamin A, not K, results in night blindness.
4. A deficiency in thiamin, not vitamin K, causes muscle weakness.

16. 1. **Profuse diaphoresis (sweating) occurs during the defervescence (flush) stage of a fever. During this stage, the fever abates and body temperature returns to the expected range.**
2. Shivering is an adaptation associated with the onset (chill) stage of a fever. During this stage, the body responds to pyrogens by conserving heat to raise body temperature and reset the body's thermostat.
3. Cyanosis of the nail beds occurs during the onset (chill) stage of a fever. Vasoconstriction and shivering are the body's attempt to conserve heat.
4. Contraction of the arrector pili muscles (goosebumps), an attempt by the body to trap air around body hairs, is associated with the onset (chill, initiation) stage of a fever. During this stage, the body responds to pyrogens by conserving heat to raise body temperature and reset the body's thermostat.

17. 1. **Diurnal variations (circadian rhythms) vary throughout the day with the lowest body temperature usually occurring between 4 AM and 6 AM. The metabolic rate is at its lowest while the person is sleeping.**
2. The body temperature is rising between 8 AM and 10 AM.
3. The body temperature is rising between 4 PM and 6 PM.
4. The body temperature is at its highest between 8 PM and 10 PM.

18. 1. **Gross temperature assessments (cold, cool, warm, hot) can be obtained by palpation. Palpation is the examination of the body using the sense of touch. Sensory nerves in the fingers transmit messages through the spinal cord to the cerebral cortex, where they are interpreted.**
2. Inspection cannot assess skin temperature. Inspection uses the naked eye to perform a visual assessment of the body.
3. Percussion cannot assess skin temperature. Percussion is the act of striking the body's surface to elicit sounds that provide information about the size and shape of internal organs or whether tissue is air-filled, fluid-filled, or solid.
4. Observation cannot assess skin temperature. Observation uses the naked eye to perform a visual assessment of the body.

19. 1. **Bowel sounds are auscultated before palpation and percussion because these techniques stimulate the intestines and thus cause an increase in peristalsis and a false increase in bowel sounds.**
2. This is done for patient comfort, not to influence the accuracy of the assessment.
3. This is not necessary. Many people begin the systematic 4-quadrant assessment in the lower right quadrant over the ileocecal valve where the digestive contents from the small intestine empty through a valve into the large intestine.
4. This is unnecessary. Bowel sounds may be hyperactive (1 every 3 seconds) or hypoactive (1 every minute). After a sound is heard, the stethoscope is moved to the next site. For sounds to be considered absent there must be no sounds for 3 to 5 minutes.

20. 1. This is an acceptable increase in heart rate with strenuous aerobic exercise.
2. This is an acceptable blood pressure with the body at rest. The expected blood pressure in an adult is a systolic of 90–119 mm Hg and a diastolic of 60–79 mm Hg.
3. **A respiratory rate of 10 is below the expected respiratory rate for an adult and should be assessed further. The expected respiratory rate for an adult is 12 to 20 breaths per minute.**

4. This is within the expected range of 60 to 100 beats per minute.

21. 1. **Feeling cold occurs during the onset (chill) stage of a fever because of vasoconstriction, cool skin, and shivering.**
2. Feeling warm is associated with the defervescence (flush) stage of a fever because of sudden vasodilation.
3. Feeling sweaty occurs during the defervescence (flush) stage of a fever because of the body's heat loss response.
4. Feeling thirsty is associated with the febrile (fever) stage of a fever because of mild to severe dehydration.

22. 1. Although the body temperature decreases as shock progresses because of a decreased metabolic rate, it is not one of the first signs of shock.
2. Two other vital signs will alter before blood pressure as the heart attempts to compensate for a decreased circulating blood volume.
3. Although during shock the pulse pressure will narrow, other vital signs will reflect compensation first. Pulse pressure is the difference between the systolic and diastolic pressures.
4. **The initial stage of shock begins when baroreceptors in the aortic arch and the carotid sinus detect a drop in the mean arterial pressure. The sympathetic nervous system responds by constricting peripheral vessels and increasing the heart and respiratory rates. During the compensatory stage of shock, the effects of epinephrine and norepinephrine continue with stimulation of alpha-adrenergic fibers causing vasoconstriction of vessels supplying the skin and abdominal viscera and beta-adrenergic fibers causing vasodilation of vessels supplying the heart, skeletal muscles, and respiratory system.**

23. 1. This is too frequent for routine monitoring of body temperature. Although the set point for body temperature changes rapidly, it takes several hours for the core body temperature to change.
2. **This is an appropriate interval of time for routine monitoring of body temperature. It is frequent enough to identify trends in changes in body temperature while limiting unnecessary assessments.**
3. Every 6 hours is too long an interval for monitoring a patient with a fever and is unsafe.
4. Every 8 hours is too long an interval for monitoring a patient with a fever and is unsafe.

24. 1. **The brachial artery splits (bifurcates) into the radial and ulnar arteries. When there is an adequate radial pulse, the brachial artery must be patent.**
2. This information is useless. The carotid arteries are in the neck while the brachial arteries are in the arms. A carotid pulse site is located on the neck at the side of the larynx, between the trachea and the sternomastoid muscle.
3. This information is useless. The femoral arteries are in the legs while the brachial arteries are in the arms. A femoral pulse site is in the groin in the femoral triangle. It is in the anterior, medial aspect of the thigh, just below the inguinal ligament, halfway between the anterior superior iliac spine and the symphysis pubis.
4. This information is useless. The popliteal arteries are in the legs while the brachial arteries are in the arms. A popliteal pulse site is in the lateral aspect of the hollow area at the back of the knee (popliteal fossa).

25. 1. **Betacyanin, a pigment that gives beets their purplish-red color, is excreted in the urine and feces of some people when it is nonmetabolized (a genetically determined trait). This bright red pigment turns the urine and feces red for several days after eating beets.**
2. Strawberries will not turn the urine red. However, they can cause an allergic reaction (reason is unknown), producing the cellular release of histamine and hives.
3. Many gelatin desserts contain red dye number 3 but it does not turn the urine red. Red dye number 3 found in foods, such as maraschino cherries and gelatin desserts, is a suspected carcinogen.
4. Red food dye does not turn the urine red. Red dye number 3 found in foods, such as maraschino cherries and gelatin desserts, is a suspected carcinogen.

26. 1. This is unnecessarily long, and even slight compression can interfere with blood flow to the brain.
2. This is not the site to access the carotid artery. A carotid pulse site is located on the neck at the side of the larynx, between the trachea and the sternomastoid muscle.
3. **The carotid artery should be palpated with a light touch to prevent an interference**

in blood flow to the brain and stimulation of the carotid sinus that can cause a reflex drop in the heart rate.

4. This is contraindicated. Massage can stimulate the carotid sinus located at the level of the bifurcation of the carotid artery, which results in a reflex drop in the heart rate.

27. 1. This blood pressure reading is acceptable for an adult which is a systolic of 90–119 mm Hg and a diastolic of 60–79 mm Hg.
    2. This blood pressure is within the parameters of Stage I hypertension and is the blood pressure that should cause the most concern. A systolic reading of 140–159 mm Hg or a diastolic reading of 90–99 mm Hg indicates Stage I hypertension.
    3. Although this blood pressure is within the parameters of prehypertension and should cause concern, it is not the highest blood presssure of the options offered. Prehypertension is indicated by a systolic reading in the range of 120–139 mm Hg or a diastolic reading in the range of 80–89 mm Hg.
    4. This blood pressure reading is within the expected range for an adult which is a systolic of 90–119 mm Hg and a diastolic of 60–79 mm Hg.

28. 1. Although the influence on the other family members might eventually be assessed, it is not the main priority.
    2. Although the impact on functional health patterns might eventually be assessed, it is not the main priority.
    3. Activity intolerance is related to the inability to maintain adequate oxygenation to body cells, which is associated with respiratory and cardiovascular problems. Obtaining the vital signs (pulse, respirations, and blood pressure) will provide valuable information about these systems.
    4. Activity intolerance is related to the cardiovascular and respiratory systems, not the nervous and musculoskeletal systems.

29. 1. The tongue usually is pink, moist, and smooth, with papillae and fissures present. A beefy red or magenta color, smooth appearance, and an increase or decrease in size indicates nutritional problems.
    2. This is the usual color of mucous membranes because of their rich vascular supply. Pale mucous membranes or the presence of lesions indicates nutritional problems.
    3. Cachexia is general ill health and malnutrition marked by weakness and excessive leanness (emaciation).
    4. The eyes are always moist and shiny because lacrimal fluid continually washes the eyes. Pale or red conjunctivae, dryness, and soft or dull corneas are signs of nutritional problems.

30. 1. A glass or plastic rectal thermometer must remain in place 2 to 4, not 5, minutes to obtain an accurate reading. An electronic thermometer usually will obtain a reading within several seconds.
    2. Gloves, personal protective pieces of equipment, are the best way the nurse is protected from contracting or transmitting a pathogen.
    3. The left, not right, lateral position is the best position to place a patient when obtaining a rectal temperature because it utilizes the anatomical position of the anus and rectum for safe, easy insertion of the thermometer.
    4. This is too far and can cause damage to the mucous membranes. A lubricated thermometer should be inserted 1.5 inches into the rectum to ensure a safe, accurate reading.

31. 1. Assessing posture and gait are within the scope of nursing practice because they reflect human responses.
    2. Assessing balance and strength are within the scope of nursing practice because they reflect human responses.
    3. Assessing hygiene and grooming are within the scope of nursing practice because they reflect human responses.
    4. Ordering and assessing urine and blood values are not in the independent practice of nursing. These assessments are dependent or interdependent functions of the nurse and are covered by specific orders or standing orders respectively.

32. **1. Restlessness with confusion may indicate the beginning of delirium associated with high fevers that alter cerebral functioning. Delirium is associated with the febrile (fever, flush) stage of a fever.**
    2. During the febrile (fever) stage of a fever the pulse and respiratory rates will increase, because of an increase in the basal metabolic rate, in an attempt to pump oxygenated blood to the tissues.
    3. Profuse diaphoresis (sweating) occurs during the defervescence (flush), not the febrile, stage of a fever.

4. Pale, cold skin occurs during the onset stage of a fever because of vasoconstriction, which is an attempt to conserve body heat.

33. 1. **When people are depressed, they frequently do not have the physical or psychic energy to perform the activities of daily living and often exhibit an unkempt appearance. A disheveled, untidy appearance is a covert, subtle indication of depression.**
2. Anxious behavior is overt, not covert and subtle.
3. Tense posture is overt, not covert and subtle.
4. Crying is overt, not covert and subtle.

34. 1. Hyperthermia, not hypothermia, is associated with this condition. Heat stroke (heat hyperpyrexia) is failure of the heat regulating capacity of the body, resulting in extremely high body temperatures (105°F).
2. Hyperthermia, not hypothermia, can result from the lack of sweat. The inability to perspire does not allow the body to cool by the evaporation of sweat (vaporization).
3. Hyperthermia, not hypothermia, can result from excessive exercise. Exercise increases heat production as carbohydrates and fats break down to provide energy. Body temperature temporarily can rise as high as 104°F.
4. **Excessive alcohol intake interferes with thermoregulation by providing a false sense of warmth, inhibiting shivering and causing vasodilation, which promotes heat loss. In addition, it impairs judgment, which increases the risk of making inappropriate self-care decisions.**

35. 1. **With a decrease in circulating red blood cells, the respiratory rate will increase to meet oxygen needs.**
2. With a reduction in blood volume, there will be less blood circulating through the kidneys, resulting in a decreased (not increased) urinary output.
3. With a reduction in blood volume, the blood pressure will be decreased, not elevated.
4. The respiratory rate will increase, not decrease, with blood loss.

36. 1. This is not necessary for all specimens.
2. Generally, if a specimen is collected using proper technique, one specimen is sufficient for testing for culture and sensitivity.
3. **The results of a culture and sensitivity are faulty and erroneous if the collection container or inappropriate collection technique introduces extraneous microorganisms that falsify and misrepresent results. Surgical asepsis (sterile technique) must be maintained.**
4. This is not necessary for any culture and sensitivity specimen.

37. 1. This is within the expected pulse rate of 60 to 100 beats per minute, the rhythm is regular; the patient should be assessed further and the information compared to the patient's baseline data.
2. This is within the expected respiratory rate of 14 to 20 breaths per minute.
3. This is within the expected temperature range of 97.6°F to 99.6°F for an oral temperature.
4. **The blood pressure is above the expected systolic of less than 120 mm Hg and a diastolic of less than 80 mm Hg and, of the options presented, should cause the most concern. A blood pressure with a systolic reading greater than 160 or a diastolic reading greater than 100 indicates stage II hypertension.**

38. 1. **Pulse oximetry is a noninvasive procedure to measure the oxygen saturation of the blood. The expected value is ≥ 95%. If a patient's pulse oximetry result is low, the patient is hypoxic and needs medical intervention.**
2. Although wheezing on expiration, which is associated with asthma, requires continuous monitoring, it is not as critical an assessment as a low pulse oximetry. Wheezing on exhalation that increases in severity or wheezing on both inhalation and exhalation becomes a priority in relation to the situations presented.
3. Shortness of breath is an expected response to exertion and is not a cause for concern.
4. Although using accessory muscles of respiration requires monitoring, it is not as critical an assessment as a low pulse oximetry. Some people with chronic respiratory problems always use accessory muscles of respiration when breathing.

39. **Answer: 2 mL. Solve the question by using ratio and proportion.**

$$\frac{\text{Desired}}{\text{Have}} \quad \frac{1\text{ mg}}{0.5\text{ mg}} \times \frac{x\text{ mL}}{1\text{ mL}}$$

$$\frac{0.5x}{0.5} = \frac{1\text{ mL}}{0.5}$$

$$x = 2\text{ mL}$$

40. **The radial pulse is the most easily found and accessible site for routine monitoring of the pulse, and it provides accurate information when the heart rate is regular. The radial pulse site is where the radial artery runs along the radial bone, on the thumb side of the inner aspect of the wrist.**

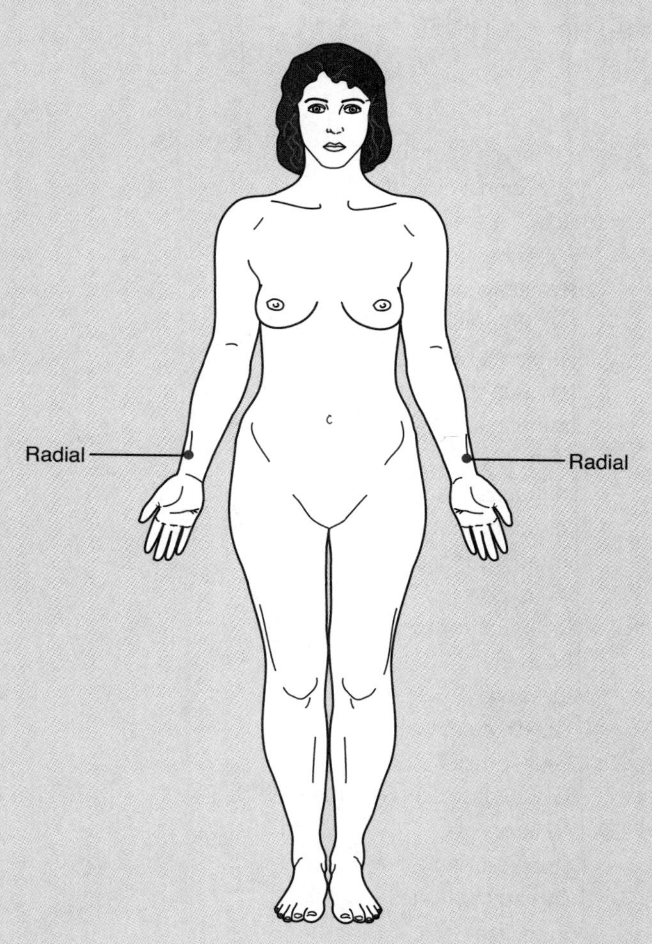

Infection Control

KEYWORDS

The following words include English vocabulary, nursing/medical terminology, concepts, principles, or information relevant to content specifically addressed in the chapter or associated with topics presented in it. English dictionaries, nursing textbooks, and medical dictionaries, such as *Taber's Cyclopedic Medical Dictionary*, are resources that can be used to expand your knowledge and understanding of these words and related information.

- Abrasion
- Afebrile
- Anaerobes
- Antibiotics
- Antibody
- Antigen
- Antimicrobial
- Antipyretic
- Aseptic technique
- Bacteria
- Biohazardous
- Chain of infection
  - Characteristics of pathogen
  - Portal of entry
  - Reservoir
  - Portal of exit
  - Mode of transmission
  - Characteristics of the host
- Colonization
- Communicable disease
- Contamination
- Culture and sensitivity
- Debridement
- Discharge
- Drainage, exudate
  - Purulent, pus
  - Sanguineous
  - Serosanguineous
  - Serous
- Endogenous
- Erythema
- Erythrocyte Sedimentation Rate (ESR)
- Excoriated
- Exogenous
- Exudate
- Febrile
- Fever
- Flora
- Fungi
- General Adaptation Syndrome (GAS)
- Granulocytes
- Harbor
- Healing
  - Primary intention
  - Secondary intention
- Host
- Hyperthermia
- Hypothalamus
- Hypothermia blanket
- Iatrogenic
- Immune response
- Immune system
- Immunity
- Immunization
- Immunocompromised
- Immunosuppression
- Incubation
- Inflammatory response
- Interferon
- Invasion
- Leukocyte migration
- Leukocytosis
- Local Adaptation Syndrome (LAS)
- Neutropenia
- Opportunistic
- Ova and parasites
- Pathogen
- Pediculosis
- Phagocytosis
- Pneumonia
- Pressure ulcer
- Primary line of defense
- Pyrogens
- Resistance
- Risk
- Scabies
- Secondary line of defense
- Septicemia
- Specimen
- Standard precautions
- Subclinical
- Surgical asepsis
- Susceptible
- Systemic

Transmission
Transmission-based precautions
  Airborne precautions
  Contact precautions
  Droplet precautions
Virulence
Virus
Wet to damp dressing
White blood cell count

QUESTIONS

1. The nurse is caring for a group of hospitalized patients. What should the nurse do first to prevent patient infections?
   1. Provide small bedside bags to dispose of used tissues
   2. Encourage staff to avoid coughing near patients
   3. Administer antibiotics as ordered
   4. Identify patients at risk
2. The nurse identifies that a patient has an inflammatory response. Which local patient adaptation supports this conclusion?
   1. Fever
   2. Erythema
   3. Bradypnea
   4. Tachycardia
3. A patient has a wound that is healing by secondary intention. To best support healing of the wound, the nurse should expect the practitioner's order to state, "Clean wound with:
   1. Betadine and apply a dry sterile dressing."
   2. Normal saline and cover with a gauze dressing."
   3. Normal saline and apply a wet-to-damp dressing."
   4. Half peroxide and half normal saline and apply a wet to dry dressing."
4. The nurse identifies that the greatest risk for a wound infection exists for a patient with a:
   1. Surgical creation of a colostomy
   2. First-degree burn on the back
   3. Puncture of the foot by a nail
   4. Paper cut on the finger
5. The nurse understands that the skin protects the body from infections because the:
   1. Cells of the skin are constantly being replaced, thereby eliminating external pathogens
   2. Epithelial cells are loosely compacted on skin, providing a barrier against pathogens
   3. Moisture on the skin surface prevents colonization of pathogens
   4. Alkalinity of the skin limits the growth of pathogens
6. The nurse must collect the following specimens. Which specimen collection does not require the use of surgical aseptic technique?
   1. Stool for ova and parasites
   2. Specimen for a throat culture
   3. Urine from a retention catheter
   4. Exudate from a wound for culture and sensitivity
7. A patient is positive for *Clostridium difficile.* The nurse should institute the isolation precaution known as:
   1. Droplet
   2. Contact
   3. Reverse
   4. Airborne
8. Which patient information collected by the nurse reflects a systemic adaptation to a wound infection?
   1. Hyperthermia
   2. Exudate
   3. Edema
   4. Pain

9. To interrupt the transmission link in the chain of infection, the nurse should:
1. Wash the hands before and after providing care to a patient
2. Position a commode next to a patient's bed
3. Provide education about a balanced diet
4. Change a dressing when it is soiled

10. The nurse is providing for the nutrition needs of several patients. The nurse identifies the need for an increase in caloric intake above average requirements for the patient who has:
1. Nausea
2. Dysphagia
3. Pneumonia
4. Depression

11. The nurse is caring for patients with a variety of wounds. The nurse understands that healing by primary intention most likely occurs with:
1. Cuts in the skin from a kitchen knife
2. Excoriated perianal areas
3. Abrasions of the skin
4. Pressure ulcers

12. The primary reason why the nurse should avoid glued-on artificial nails is because they:
1. Interfere with dexterity of the fingers
2. Could fall off in a patient's bed
3. Harbor microorganisms
4. Can scratch a patient

13. The nurse understands that subclinical infections most commonly occur in:
1. Infants
2. Adolescents
3. Older adults
4. Children of school age

14. The nurse understands that the factor that places a patient at the greatest risk for developing an infection is:
1. Implantation of a prosthetic device
2. Presence of an indwelling urinary catheter
3. Burns more than twenty percent of the body
4. Multiple puncture sites from laparoscopic surgery

15. The nurse understands that a secondary line of defense against infection is the:
1. Mucous membranes of the respiratory tract
2. Urinary tract environment
3. Integumentary system
4. Immune response

16. Which nursing action protects the patient as a susceptible host in the chain of infection?
1. Wearing personal protective equipment
2. Administering childhood immunizations
3. Recapping a used needle before discarding
4. Disposing of soiled gloves in a waste container

17. A patient tells the nurse, "I think I have an ear infection." The nurse should assess this patient for which objective human response to an ear infection?
1. Throbbing pain
2. Purulent drainage
3. Dizziness when moving
4. Hearing a buzzing sound

18. The nurse is concerned about a patient's ability to withstand exposure to pathogens. What blood component should the nurse monitor?
 1. Platelets
 2. Neutrophils
 3. Hemoglobin
 4. Erythrocytes

19. The nurse understands which primary (nonspecific) defense protects the body from infection?
 1. Tears in the eyes
 2. Alkalinity of gastric secretions
 3. Bile in the gastrointestinal system
 4. Moist environment of the epidermis

20. When brushing a patient's hair, the nurse notes white oval particles attached to the hair behind the ears. The nurse should assess the patient further for signs of:
 1. Scabies
 2. Dandruff
 3. Hirsutism
 4. Pediculosis

21. The nurse understands that a rise in body temperature is associated with the presence of infection because:
 1. Pain activates the sympathetic nervous system
 2. Erythema increases the flow of blood throughout the body
 3. Leukocyte migration precipitates the inflammatory response
 4. Phagocytic cells release pyrogens that stimulate the hypothalamus

22. The nurse understands that an example of an iatrogenic infection is a:
 1. Vaginal infection in a postmenopausal woman
 2. Respiratory infection contracted from a grandchild
 3. Urinary tract infection in a patient who is sedentary
 4. Wound infection caused by unwashed hands of a caregiver

23. The physician orders a wound to be packed with a wet-to-damp gauze dressing. The nurse understands that this is done primarily to:
 1. Minimize the loss of protein
 2. Facilitate the healing process
 3. Increase resistance to infection
 4. Prevent the entry of microorganisms

24. The nurse understands that a primary (nonspecific) defense that protects the body from infection is:
 1. Antibiotic therapy
 2. The high pH of the skin
 3. Cilia in the respiratory tract
 4. The alkaline environment of the vagina

25. A patient has a wound infection. Which local human response should the nurse expect to identify?
 1. Hyperthermia
 2. Neutropenia
 3. Malaise
 4. Edema

26. The nurse is caring for a patient with a high fever secondary to septicemia. When the physician orders a cooling blanket, the nurse understands that it is used to achieve heat loss via:
 1. Radiation
 2. Convection
 3. Conduction
 4. Evaporation

27. The nurse identifies that a patient condition unrelated to infection is:
    1. Catabolism
    2. Hyperglycemia
    3. Ketones in the urine
    4. Decreased metabolic activity

28. Which nursing action protects the patient from infection at the portal of entry?
    1. Positioning an indwelling urine collection bag below the level of the patient's pelvis
    2. Enclosing a urine specimen in a biohazardous transport bag
    3. Wearing clean gloves when handling a patient's excretions
    4. Handwashing after removal of soiled protective gloves

29. Which patient statements indicate that further teaching by the nurse is necessary regarding how to ensure protection from food contamination? Check all that apply.
    1. _____ "I should stuff a turkey an hour before putting it in the oven."
    2. _____ "I love juicy rare hamburgers with onion and tomato."
    3. _____ "I prefer chicken salad sandwiches with mayonnaise."
    4. _____ "I know to spit out food that doesn't taste good."
    5. _____ "I should defrost frozen food in the refrigerator."

30. A patient is admitted to the ambulatory surgery unit for an elective procedure. When performing a physical assessment, the nurse identifies that the patient has *Pediculus capitis* (head lice). Place the nurse's interventions in priority order.
    1. Establish contact isolation
    2. Comb the hair with a fine tooth comb
    3. Obtain an order for a pediculocidal shampoo
    4. Notify the physician of the patient's condition
    5. Wash the patient's hair with a pediculocidal shampoo

    Answer: _______________

TFEE erythyma

ANSWERS AND RATIONALES

1. 1. Although this is something the nurse may provide to contain soiled tissues, it is not the first action the nurse should implement to prevent infection.
   2. Although this is something the nurse may do to limit airborne or droplet transmission of microorganisms, it is not the first action the nurse should implement to prevent infection.
   3. Antibiotics generally are ordered by a practitioner for patients who have infections. Antibiotics rarely are ordered prophylactically to prevent the development of resistant strains of microorganisms.
   4. **This is the most important first step in the prevention of infection. A patient who is at high risk may need to receive special protective precautions as well as transmission-based precautions to protect others.**

2. 1. A fever is a systemic, not local, response to inflammation.
   2. **Local trauma or infection stimulates the release of kinins, which increases capillary permeability and blood flow to the local area. The increase of blood flow to the area causes erythema (redness).**
   3. Bradypnea is a regular but excessively slow rate of breathing (less than 12 breaths per minute) and is not an adaptation to the local or general inflammatory syndromes.
   4. Tachycardia is an elevated heart rate higher than 100 beats per minute and is unrelated to the Local Adaptation Syndrome.

3. 1. Betadine is cytotoxic and should not be used on clean granulating wounds.
   2. Although normal saline is appropriate for cleansing a wound, a moist, not dry, environment facilitates epithelialization and minimizes scar formation.
   3. **Cleaning with normal saline will not damage fibroblasts. Wet-to-damp dressings allow epidermal cells to migrate more rapidly across the wound surface than dry dressings, thereby facilitating wound healing.**
   4. Hydrogen peroxide is cytotoxic and should not be used on clean granulating wounds.

4. 1. Surgery is conducted using sterile technique. In addition, preoperative preparation of the bowel helps to reduce the presence of organisms that have the potential to cause infection.
   2. There is no break in the skin in a first-degree burn; therefore, there is less of a risk for a wound infection than an example in another option.
   3. **Of all the options, puncture of the foot by a nail has the greatest risk for a wound infection. A nail is a soiled object that has the potential of introducing pathogens into a deep wound that can trap them under the surface of the skin, a favorable environment for multiplication.**
   4. Paper generally is not heavily soiled and the wound edges are approximated. This is less of a risk than an example in another option.

5. 1. **Epithelial cells of the skin are regularly shed along with potentially dangerous microorganisms that adhere to the skin's outer layers, thereby reducing the risk of infection.**
   2. Epithelial cells on the skin are closely, not loosely, compacted providing a barrier against pathogens.
   3. Moisture on the skin surface facilitates, not prevents, colonization of pathogens.
   4. Acidity, not alkalinity, of the skin limits the growth of pathogens.

6. 1. **Stool for ova and parasites does not have to be sterile because test results for the presence of parasitic eggs and parasites are not altered if the specimen is contaminated with exogenous organisms.**
   2. Sterile technique is used to collect a throat culture, to avoid contaminating the specimen with exogenous organisms that may alter the accuracy of test results.
   3. The bladder is a sterile cavity and the nurse must use sterile technique to collect urine from the port of a retention catheter (Foley) so as not to introduce any pathogens. In addition, it is important not to introduce exogenous organisms that may contaminate the specimen and alter the accuracy of test results.
   4. Sterile technique is used to collect exudate from a wound to avoid contaminating the specimen with exogenous organisms that may alter the accuracy of test results.

7. 1. Droplet precautions are used for patients who have an illness transmitted by particle droplets larger than 5 microns; for example, mumps, rubella, pharyngeal diphtheria, Mycoplasma

pneumonia, pertussis, streptococcal pharyngitis, and pneumonic plague.

2. **Contact precautions are used for patients who have an illness transmitted by direct contact or with items contaminated by the patient; for example, gastrointestinal, respiratory, skin, or wound infections or colonization with drug-resistant bacteria including *C. difficile*, *E. coli*, *Shigella* as well as other infections/infestations, such as hepatitis A, herpes simplex virus, impetigo, pediculosis, scabies, syncytial virus, and parainfluenza.**
3. Reverse precautions, also known as neutropenic precautions, are used for patients who are immunocompromised; isolation practices are employed and personal protective equipment is worn by the caregiver to protect the patient from the caregiver.
4. Airborne precautions are used for patients who have an illness transmitted by airborne droplet nuclei smaller than 5 microns; for example, varicella, rubeola, and tuberculosis.

8\. 1. **Hyperthermia is a common systemic adaptation to infection. With hyperthermia, microorganisms or endotoxins stimulate phagocytic cells that release pyrogens, which stimulate the hypothalamic thermoregulatory center and cause fever.**
2. Exudate is a local, not systemic, response to an injury or inflammation. Exudate is cleared away through lymphatic drainage or exits from the body via a wound.
3. Edema is a local, not systemic, adaptation to infection. Chemical mediators increase the permeability of small blood vessels, thereby causing fluid to enter the interstitial compartment resulting in local edema.
4. Pain is a local, not systemic, adaptation to inflammation because swelling of inflamed tissue exerts pressure on nerve endings.

9\. 1. **This is an example of controlling the mode of transmission. Direct transmission of microorganisms from one person to another is interrupted when microorganisms are removed from the skin surface by handwashing. Handwashing is part of hand hygiene, which also includes nail care, skin lubrication, and wearing of minimal jewelry in a health-care environment.**
2. This is an example of controlling the reservoir and the portal of exit from the reservoir, not the mode of transmission, link in the chain of infection.
3. This is an example of reducing the susceptibility of the host, not the mode of transmission, link in the chain of infection.
4. This is an example of controlling the reservoir (source) and portal of exit from the reservoir, not the mode of transmission, link in the chain of infection.

10\. 1. Nausea does not precipitate a need for an increase in caloric intake above average requirements. However, frequent small dry feedings and medications to limit nausea may be used.
2. Dysphagia, difficulty swallowing, does not precipitate a need for an increase in caloric intake above average requirements. However, the texture of foods and the rate of feeding may have to be adjusted.
3. **The individual with pneumonia requires an increase in caloric requirements because of an increased resting energy expenditure and hypermetabolic state. With an infection, more energy is needed to regulate an elevated body temperature and extra protein is needed to produce antibodies and white blood cells.**
4. Depression does not precipitate a need for an increase in caloric intake above average requirements. If a depressed patient becomes withdrawn and sedentary, caloric requirements may decrease.

11\. 1. **A cut in the skin caused by a sharp instrument with minimal tissue loss can heal by primary intention when the wound edges are lightly pulled together (approximated).**
2. Excoriation heals by secondary intention, not primary intention. Excoriation is an injury to the surface of the skin. It can be caused by friction, scratching, and chemical or thermal burns.
3. An abrasion heals by secondary intention, not by primary intention. In an abrasion, friction scrapes away the epithelial layer exposing the underlying tissue.
4. A pressure ulcer heals by secondary intention, not primary intention. Secondary intention healing occurs when wound edges are not approximated because of full thickness tissue loss and the wound is left open until it fills with new tissue.

12\. 1. Artificial nails do not interfere with finger dexterity if kept at a reasonable length (not longer than ¼ inch beyond the end of the finger).

2. Although this is a concern, it is not the main reason they should be avoided.
3. **Studies have demonstrated that artificial nails, especially when cracked, broken, or split, provide crevices in which microorganisms can grow and multiply, and therefore should be avoided by direct care providers.**
4. When artificial nails are cared for so that they remain intact and free of cracks or breaks, they should not scratch the skin.

13. 1. Infants generally respond to infections with acute symptoms that are identified easier and earlier than in an age group in another option.
2. Adolescents generally respond to infections with acute symptoms that are identified easier and earlier than in an age group in another option.
3. **Infections are more difficult to identify in the older adult because the symptoms are not as acute and obvious as in other age groups because of the decline in all body systems related to aging.**
4. School-aged children generally respond to infections with acute symptoms that are identified easier and earlier than in an age group in another option.

14. 1. Although wound infections can occur when prosthetic devices are implanted, they are surgically implanted under sterile conditions to minimize this risk.
2. Although urinary tract infections can occur with an indwelling urinary catheter, even though generally it is a closed system, an example in another option places a person at a greater risk for infection.
3. **Burns more than 20% of a person's total body surface generally are considered major burn injuries. When the skin is damaged by a burn, the underlying tissue is left unprotected and the individual is at risk for infection. The greater the extent and the deeper the depth of the burn, the higher the risk for infection.**
4. Laparoscopic surgery is performed using sterile technique to minimize the risk of infection. An example in another option places a person at a greater risk for infection.

15. 1. Protective mechanisms in the respiratory tract provide a primary, not secondary, line of defense against pathogenic microorganisms. Primary defenses are nonspecific immune defenses that are anatomical, mechanical, or chemical barriers. In the respiratory tract they include intact mucous membranes, mucus, bactericidal enzymes, cilia, sneezing, and coughing.
2. Protective mechanisms in the urinary tract environment provide a primary, not secondary, line of defense against pathogenic microorganisms. These defenses include intact mucous membranes, urine flowing out of the body, and urine acidity.
3. Skin provides a primary, not secondary, line of defense against pathogenic microorganisms. These defenses include intact skin, surface acidity, and the usual flora that is found on the skin.
4. **The immune response is a specific, secondary line of defense against pathogenic microorganisms. The production of antibodies to neutralize and eliminate pathogens and their toxins (immune response) is activated when phagocytes fail to completely destroy invading microorganisms. The primary, nonspecific defenses (anatomical, mechanical, chemical, and inflammatory) work in harmony with the secondary defense (immune response) to defend the body from pathogenic microorganisms.**

16. 1. This is an example of controlling the mode of transmission, not the susceptible host, link in the chain of infection.
2. **This is an example of an action designed to interrupt the susceptible host link in the chain of infection by increasing the resistance of the host to an infectious agent.**
3. Discarding uncapped, used syringes in a sharps container disrupts the chain of infection at the reservoir link in the chain of infection. The nurse should never recap a used needle because of the risk of a needle-stick injury.
4. This is an example of controlling the mode of transmission, not the susceptible host, link in the chain of infection.

17. 1. Throbbing pain is subjective, not objective, information because pain cannot be observed; it is felt and described only by the patient.
2. **Purulent drainage from the ear is objective information because it can be observed and measured.**
3. Dizziness is subjective, not objective, information because it cannot be measured; dizziness is experienced and described only by the patient.
4. Hearing a buzzing sound (tinnitus) is subjective, not objective, information because

it cannot be observed; a buzzing sound is perceived and described only by the patient.

18. 1. Platelets are essential for blood clotting and are unrelated to an individual's ability to withstand exposure to pathogens.

2. Neutrophils, the most numerous leukocytes (white blood cells), are a primary defense against infection because they ingest and destroy microorganisms (phagocytosis). When the leukocyte count is low, it indicates a compromised ability to fight infection.

3. Hemoglobin is the part of the red blood cell that carries oxygen from the lungs to the tissues and is unrelated to the assessment of an individual's ability to withstand exposure to pathogens.

4. Red blood cells (erythrocytes) do not reflect an individual's ability to withstand exposure to pathogens. Erythrocytes transport oxygen via hemoglobin molecules.

19. 1. Tears flush the eyes of microorganisms and debris and are a primary (nonspecific) defense that protects the body from infection.

2. Acidity, not alkalinity, of gastric secretions is a primary (nonspecific) defense mechanism that protects the body from infection.

3. Bile helps emulsify fats; it does not protect the body from infection.

4. A dry, not moist, epidermis is a primary (nonspecific) defense mechanism that protects the body from infection.

20. 1. This adaptation is not indicative of scabies. Scabies is a communicable skin disease caused by an itch mite (*Sarcoptes scabiei*) and is characterized by skin lesions (small papules, pustules, excoriations, and burrows ending in a vesicle) with intense itching.

2. This adaptation is not indicative of dandruff. Dandruff is the excessive shedding of dry white scales as a result of the expected exfoliation of the epidermis of the scalp. Dandruff scales do not attach to the hair and can be easily brushed away from the hair shaft.

3. This adaptation is not indicative of hirsutism. Hirsutism is the excessive growth of hair or hair growth in unusual places, particularly in females. In females, usually it is caused by excessive androgen production or metabolic abnormalities.

4. Pediculosis (*Pediculus humanus capitis*) is characterized by white oval particles attached to the hair. When identified, the nurse needs to assess the patient further for the presence of scratch marks on the scalp and by asking the patient if the head feels itchy. In addition, the nurse must assess the extent of infestation and if any other areas of the body are infested with other types of lice (*P. humanus corporis*—body, and *Phthirus pubis*—pubic and axillary hair).

21. 1. Pain does not cause a rise in body temperature directly.

2. Erythema does not increase the flow of blood throughout the body. Increased blood flow to a localized area causes erythema.

3. Leukocyte migration does not precipitate the inflammatory response but is a phase of the inflammatory response. White blood cells reach a wound within a few hours to ingest bacteria and clean a wound of debris through the process of phagocytosis.

4. Microorganisms or endotoxins stimulate phagocytic cells, which release pyrogens that stimulate the hypothalamic thermoregulatory center causing fever.

22. 1. This is not an example of an iatrogenic infection.

2. This is not an example of an iatrogenic infection.

3. This infection is caused by a decrease in bladder tone and urinary residual as a result of inactivity and is unrelated to an iatrogenic infection.

4. Iatrogenic refers to a disease or adaptation caused by the effects of some medical treatment. When a caregiver does not wash his/her hands, thereby transmitting a pathogen that causes a wound infection, the result is an iatrogenic infection.

23. 1. Wet-to-damp packing of a wound is not done to minimize the loss of protein from a wound. Protein loss occurs until the wound heals.

2. Packing a wound with wet-to-damp dressings allows epidermal cells to migrate more rapidly across the bed of the wound surface than dry dressings, thereby facilitating wound healing.

3. Although packing a wound with wet-to-damp dressings will wick exudate up and away from the base of the wound and therefore help to increase resistance to a wound infection, it is not the primary reason for its use.

4. This is not the primary purpose of a wet-to-damp gauze dressing. Dry sterile dressings are used to prevent the entry of microorganisms into a wound.

24. 1. Antibiotic therapy is the use of chemotherapeutic agents to control or eliminate bacterial infections. It is not a primary (nonspecific) defense that protects the body from infection. The inappropriate use of antibiotics destroys the usual flora of the body and can predispose an individual to additional infections.
2. The low, not high, pH of the skin protects the body from infection.
3. **Cilia in the respiratory tract are a primary (nonspecific) defense mechanism that protects the body from infection. Mucus, produced by the respiratory tract, traps microorganisms, which are then propelled away from the lungs by cilia.**
4. The acidic, not alkaline, environment of the vagina protects it from the growth of pathogens.

25. 1. Hyperthermia is a systemic, not local, adaptation to a wound infection. Microorganisms, or endotoxins, stimulate phagocytic cells that release pyrogens, which stimulate the hypothalamic thermoregulatory center to produce fever.
2. An increase in white blood cells (leukocytosis), not a decrease in white blood cells (neutropenia), occurs in response to both local and systemic infections.
3. Discomfort, uneasiness, or indisposition (malaise) is a systemic, not local, response to infection.
4. **Chemical mediators increase the permeability of small blood vessels, thereby causing fluid to move into the interstitial compartment, resulting in local edema.**

26. 1. Radiation is not related to heat loss via a cooling (hypothermia) blanket. Radiation is heat loss from one surface to another without direct contact.
2. Convection is not related to heat loss via a cooling (hypothermia) blanket. Convection is the loss of heat as a result of the motion of cool air flowing over a warm body. The heat is carried away by air currents that are cooler than the warm body.
3. **Conduction is the transfer of heat from a warm object (skin) to a cooler object (cooling blanket) during direct contact.**
4. Evaporation is unrelated to heat loss via a cooling (hypothermia) blanket. Evaporation is the conversion of a liquid to a vapor, which occurs when perspiration on the skin is vaporized. For each gram of water that evaporates from the skin, approximately 0.6 of a calorie of heat is lost.

27. 1. Catabolism, the destructive phase of metabolism with its resultant release of energy, is related to infection.
2. Serum glucose is elevated (hyperglycemia) in the presence of an infection because of the release of glucocorticoids in the General Adaptation Syndrome.
3. The presence of ketones in the urine, a sign that the body is using fat as a source of energy, is related to infection because of the associated increased need for calories for fighting the infection.
4. **Metabolic activity increases, not decreases, with an infection as the body increases its activity and mounts a defense to fight invading pathogenic microorganisms.**

28. 1. **This is an action designed to interrupt the portal of entry link in the chain of infection. By keeping the collection bag below the level of the patient's pelvis backflow is prevented, which reduces the risk of introducing pathogens into the bladder.**
2. This is an example of controlling the reservoir and mode of transmission links in the chain of infection.
3. This is an example of controlling the mode of transmission, not the portal of entry, link in the chain of infection.
4. This is an example of controlling the mode of transmission, not the portal of entry, link in the chain of infection.

29. 1. **Placing stuffing inside a turkey and letting it stand at room temperature is not advisable because it promotes the multiplication of microorganism.**
2. **Hamburger meat should be thoroughly cooked so that disease-producing microorganisms within the meat are destroyed.**
3. This statement does not indicate a lack of knowledge about the use or storage of mayonnaise.
4. This statement does not indicate a lack of knowledge about what to do when it is determined that something does not taste right.
5. This is the correct way to defrost frozen food. Food should not be defrosted in an environment between 45°F to 140°F because bacteria will rapidly grow in this temperature range.

30. Answer: 1, 4, 3, 5, 2

1. **Medical aseptic techniques must be instituted to protect others from being exposed to the infestation.**
4. **The physician must be notified because the surgery must be cancelled and treatment instituted.**
3. **Treatment with a pediculocidal shampoo requires a practitioner's order; it is a dependent function of the nurse.**
5. **The patient's hair should be washed as soon as possible with a medicated shampoo (gamma benzene hexachloride [Lindane], malathion, or pyrethrin).**
2. **After the hair is washed with a pediculocidal shampoo, it should be combed with a fine-toothed comb to remove the nits (eggs).**

Safety

KEYWORDS

The following words include English vocabulary, nursing/medical terminology, concepts, principles, or information relevant to content specifically addressed in the chapter or usually associated with topics presented in it. English dictionaries, nursing textbooks, and medical dictionaries, such as *Taber's Cyclopedic Medical Dictionary*, are resources that can be used to expand your knowledge and understanding of these words and related information.

Abdominal thrust (Heimlich maneuver)
Asphyxiation
Aspiration
Burns
Call bell
Cardiopulmonary resuscitation
Child-proof devices
Disaster plan
Drowning
Dysphagia
Electrical grounding
Electrical hazards
Electrical surge
Falls
Fire evacuation protocol
Fire extinguishers—A, B, C
Fire safety
Functional alignment
Incident Report
Injury
Knots
  Clove hitch
  Half bow
  Slip-knot
Latex allergy
Physical hazards
Poisoning
Pollution
RACE—response to a fire
Restraints
  Belt
  Elbow
  Jacket
  Mitt
  Mummy
  Poncho
  Vest
Side rails
Smother
Strangulation
Suffocation
Supervision
Three-pronged plug
Trauma

QUESTIONS

1. A patient has dysphagia. Which common nursing action takes priority when feeding this patient?
   1. Ensuring that dentures are in place
   2. Medicating for pain before providing meals
   3. Providing verbal cueing to swallow each bite
   4. Checking the mouth for emptying between every bite

2. A 3-year-old child is admitted to the pediatric unit. The best way for the nurse to maintain the safety of this preschool-aged child is by:
   1. Teaching the child how to use the call bell
   2. Placing the child in a crib with high side rails
   3. Keeping the child under constant supervision
   4. Having the child stay in the playroom most of the day

3. Which time of day is of most concern for the nurse when trying to protect a patient with dementia from injury?
   1. Afternoon
   2. Morning
   3. Evening
   4. Night

4. A patient consistently tries to pull out a urinary retention catheter. As a last resort to maintain integrity of the catheter and patient safety, the nurse obtains an order for a restraint. Which type of restraint is most appropriate in this situation?
   1. Mummy restraint
   2. Elbow restraint
   3. Jacket restraint
   4. Mitt restraint

5. The nurse is orienting a newly admitted patient to the hospital. It is most important for the nurse to teach the patient how to:
   1. Notify the nurse when help is needed
   2. Get out of the bed to use the bathroom
   3. Raise and lower the head and foot of the bed
   4. Use the telephone system to call family members

6. Profuse smoke is coming out of the heating unit in a patient's room. The nurse should first:
   1. Open the window
   2. Activate the fire alarm
   3. Move the patient out of the room
   4. Close the door to the patient's room

7. The nurse must apply a hospital gown to a patient receiving an intravenous infusion in the forearm. The nurse should:
   1. Insert the IV bag and tubing through the sleeve from inside of the gown first
   2. Disconnect the IV at the insertion site, apply the gown, and then reconnect the IV
   3. Close the clamp on the IV tubing no more than 15 seconds while putting on the gown
   4. Don the gown on the arm without the IV, drape the gown over the other shoulder, and adjust the closure behind the neck

8. The nurse is planning care for a patient with a wrist restraint. The restraint should be removed, the area massaged, and the joints moved through their full range every:
   1. Shift
   2. Hour
   3. Two hours
   4. Four hours

9. Which is the first action the home care nurse should employ to prevent falls by an older adult living at home?
   1. Conduct a comprehensive risk assessment
   2. Encourage the patient to remove throw rugs in the home
   3. Suggest installation of adequate lighting throughout the home
   4. Discuss with the patient the expected changes of aging that place one at risk

10. The nurse is preparing a bed to receive a newly admitted patient. Which action is most important?
    1. Place the patient's name on the end of the bed
    2. Ensure that the bed wheels are locked
    3. Position the call bell in reach
    4. Make an open bed

11. An appropriately worded goal associated with the nursing diagnosis Risk for Injury is, "The patient will be:
    1. Taught how to call for help to ambulate."
    2. Kept on bed rest when dizzy."
    3. Restrained when agitated."
    4. Free from trauma."

12. The nurse understands that in the hospital setting an electrical appliance should have a three-pronged plug because it:
1. Controls stray electrical currents
2. Promotes efficient use of electricity
3. Shuts off the appliance if there is an electrical surge
4. Divides the electricity among the appliances in the room

13. A patient with Parkinson's disease is experiencing difficulty swallowing. The nurse understands that the most serious risk associated with dysphagia is:
1. Anorexia
2. Aspiration
3. Self-care deficit
4. Inadequate intake

14. The nurse is caring for a confused patient. To prevent this patient from falling, the nurse should:
1. Encourage the patient to use the corridor handrails
2. Place the patient in a room near the nurses' station
3. Reinforce how to use the call bell
4. Maintain close supervision

15. When teaching children about fire safety procedures, the school nurse should teach them that if their clothes catch on fire they should:
1. Yell for help
2. Roll on the ground
3. Take their clothes off
4. Pour water on their clothes

16. The physician orders a vest restraint for a patient. What should the nurse do first when applying this restraint?
1. Ensure that the back of the vest is positioned on the patient's back
2. Permit four fingers to slide between the patient and the restraint
3. Inspect the patient's skin where the restraint is to be placed
4. Secure the restraint to the bed frame using a slipknot

17. An unconscious patient begins vomiting. In which position should the nurse place the patient?
1. Supine
2. Side-lying
3. Orthopneic
4. Low-Fowler's

18. The nurse is assisting a patient to use a bedpan. What is the most important nursing intervention?
1. Dusting powder on the rim before placing the bedpan under the patient
2. Positioning the rounded rim of the bedpan toward the front of the patient
3. Ensuring that the bedside rails are raised once the patient is on the bedpan
4. Encouraging the patient to help as much as possible when using the bedpan

19. A toaster is on fire in the pantry of a hospital unit. The nurse should first:
1. Unplug the toaster
2. Activate the fire alarm
3. Put out the fire with an extinguisher
4. Evacuate patients from the room next to the kitchen

20. The nurse understands that the most common factor that contributes to falls in the hospital setting is:
1. Wet floors
2. Frequent seizures
3. Advanced age of patients
4. Misuse of equipment by nurses

21. An adaptation that indicates that a further nursing assessment is necessary to determine if the patient has difficulty swallowing is:
   1. Abdominal cramping
   2. Epigastric pain
   3. Constipation
   4. Drooling

22. The nurse is assessing a patient who is being admitted to the hospital. Which is the most important information collected by the nurse that indicates whether the patient is at risk for physical injury?
   1. Weakness experienced during a prior admission
   2. Medication that increases intestinal motility
   3. Two recent falls that occurred at home
   4. The need for corrective eyeglasses

23. To best prevent a patient from falling, the nurse should:
   1. Provide a cane
   2. Keep walkways clear of obstacles
   3. Assist the patient with ambulation
   4. Encourage the patient to use the handrails in the hall

24. The nurse teaches a nursing assistant that the last step in making an occupied bed is:
   1. Raising both side rails on the bed
   2. Lowering the height of the bed toward the floor
   3. Ensuring that the patient is in a comfortable position
   4. Elevating the head of the bed to a semi-Fowler's position

25. The nurse is caring for a patient with a nasogastric tube for gastric decompression. Which nursing action takes priority?
   1. Positioning the patient in the semi-Fowler's position
   2. Instilling the tube with 30 mL of air every 2 hours
   3. Providing care to the nares at least every 8 hours
   4. Discontinuing wall suction when providing care

26. A patient states that when turning on an electric radio a strong electrical shock was felt. What should the nurse do first?
   1. Arrange for the maintenance department to examine the radio
   2. Disconnect the radio from the source of energy
   3. Check the skin for electrical burns
   4. Take the patient's apical pulse

27. The nurse identifies that the hospitalized patient at the greatest risk for injury is a:
   1. Young child
   2. Comatose teenager
   3. Postmenopausal woman
   4. Confused middle-aged man

28. The nurse is planning care for a patient who requires bilateral arm restraints. Which information is important to understand when planning care for this patient?
   1. Their use adequately prevents injuries
   2. They require a physician's order to be applied
   3. Reasons for their use must be clearly documented
   4. Most patients recognize that they contribute to their safety

29. The nurse understands that injuries in hospitalized patients are caused most commonly by:
   1. Malfunctioning equipment
   2. Failure to use restraints
   3. Visitors
   4. Falls

30. When caring for patients, which is the first thing the nurse should do to prevent problems associated with latex allergies?
1. Use nonlatex gloves
2. Identify persons at risk
3. Keep a latex-safe supply cart available
4. Administer an antihistamine prophylactically

31. Which nursing intervention enhances an older adult's sensory perception and thereby helps prevent injury when walking from the bed to the bathroom?
1. Providing adequate lighting
2. Raising the pitch of the voice
3. Holding onto the patient's arm
4. Removing environmental hazards

32. Which human response to illness alerts the nurse that a patient has the greatest risk for aspiration during meals?
1. Bulimia
2. Lethargy
3. Anorexia
4. Stomatitis

33. The nurse is preparing a patient for a physical examination. In this situation it is most important for the nurse to:
1. Identify positions that may be contraindicated for the patient during the examination
2. Explore the patient's attitude toward health-care providers
3. Inquire about the other professionals caring for the patient
4. Ask when the patient last had a physical examination

34. The nurse identifies the presence of a fire in the dirty utility room. Place the nurse's actions in order of priority.
1. Pull the fire alarm
2. Close unit doors and windows
3. Shut the door to the utility room
4. Provide emotional support to agitated patients

Answer: ______________

35. Which actions are important when the nurse uses a stretcher? Check all that apply.
1. _____ Lowering the bed below the level of the stretcher when transferring a patient from the stretcher to a bed
2. _____ Guiding the stretcher around a turn leading with the end with the patient's head
3. _____ Ensuring the patient's head is at the end with the swivel wheels
4. _____ Pulling the stretcher on the elevator with the patient's feet first
5. _____ Pushing the stretcher from the end with the patient's head

ANSWERS AND RATIONALES

1. 1. Although this should be done if a patient has dentures, it is not the priority.
   2. Although an analgesic may be administered, it can cause drowsiness that may increase the potential for aspiration in a patient with dysphagia.
   3. Although this should be done, the patient may be physically incapable of following this direction.
   4. **This is the safest way to ensure that a bolus of food is not left in the mouth where it can be aspirated and cause an airway obstruction.**

2. 1. A preschool-aged child does not have the cognitive and emotional maturity to use a call bell.
   2. A preschool-aged child might attempt to climb over the side rails. A crib with high side rails is more appropriate for an infant.
   3. **Constant supervision ensures that an adult can monitor the preschool-aged child's activity and environment so that safety needs are met. Preschool-aged children are active, curious, and fearless and have immature musculoskeletal and neurological systems, narrow life experiences, and a limited ability to understand cause and effect. All of these factors place preschool-aged children at risk for injury unless supervised.**
   4. This is inappropriate because most preschoolers still take 1 or 2 naps daily, the child may be on bed rest, and periods of activity and rest should be alternated to conserve the child's energy.

3. 1. The sunlight and usual afternoon activities generally help keep patients with dementia more oriented and safe.
   2. The sunlight and the routine morning activities of hygiene, grooming, dressing, and eating generally help keep patients with dementia more oriented and safe.
   3. As the day progresses and the sun sets, the concern for safety increases because of altered cognition (sundowner sydrome). However, in the evening there are activities of daily living and available caregivers to distract the patient and provide for safety.
   4. **At night, patients with dementia often continue to experience confusion and agitation. At night there is less light, less activity, and fewer caregivers, so there are fewer orienting stimuli. Patients who are confused or agitated are at an increased risk for injury because they may not comprehend cause and effect and, therefore, lack the ability to make safe judgments.**

4. 1. A mummy restraint usually is used to immobilize an infant or very young child during a procedure.
   2. An elbow restraint usually is used to prevent flexion of the elbow in an infant or young child to prevent the pulling out of tubes.
   3. A jacket restraint usually is used to keep a person from falling out of bed while not immobilizing the extremities.
   4. **A mitt restraint covers the hand to prevent the fingers from grasping and pulling out tubes.**

5. 1. **Explaining how to use a call bell meets safety and security needs. It reinforces that help is immediately available at a time when the patient may feel physically or emotionally vulnerable in an unfamiliar environment.**
   2. Patients generally do not need teaching about how to get out of bed to go to the bathroom. This instruction depends on the individual needs of a patient.
   3. Although this is part of orienting a patient to the hospital environment, it is not the most important point to emphasize with a patient.
   4. Although this is part of orienting a patient to the hospital environment, it is not the most important point to emphasize with a patient.

6. 1. This is contraindicated because environmental air will feed the fire, causing it to increase in severity.
   2. Although this will be done, it is not the priority at this point in time.
   3. **The patient's physical safety is the priority. The patient must be removed from direct danger before the alarm is activated and the fire contained.**
   4. Although this will be done eventually, it is not the priority at this point in time.

7. 1. **This ensures that the IV bag and tubing are safely passed through the armhole of the gown before the patient puts the arm with the insertion site through the gown. This prevents tension on the**

tubing and insertion site, which limits the possibility of the catheter dislodging from the vein.

2. Disconnecting the IV tubing at the catheter insertion site is unsafe. This opens a closed system unnecessarily, increasing the potential for infection.
3. This is unsafe. This stops the flow of the IV solution, which can result in blood coagulating at the end of the catheter in the vein and compromising the patency of the IV tubing.
4. This leaves the patient exposed unnecessarily. It interferes with privacy, and the patient may feel cold.

8. 1. This is unsafe because it is too long a period, which promotes the development of contractures.
2. This generally is too often and unnecessary.
3. **Restraints should be removed every 2 hours. The extremities must be moved through their full range of motion to prevent muscle shortening and contractures. The area must be massaged to promote circulation and prevent pressure injuries.**
4. This is too long a period between activity and promotes the development of contractures.

9. 1. **Assessment is the first step of the Nursing Process. The best way to prevent falls is by instituting extra fall precautions for those patients at the highest risk. Most agencies have policies and procedures designed to identify, monitor, and support patients at risk.**
2. Although this is advisable, it is not the priority at this time.
3. Although this is advisable, it is not the priority at this time.
4. Although this is advisable, it is not the priority at this time.

10. 1. This violates the patient's right to privacy. An identification wristband must be worn for patient identification.
2. **Locked bed wheels are an important safety precaution. The bed must be an immovable object because the patient may touch the bed for support, lean against it when getting in or out of bed, or move around when in bed. If the bed wheels are unlocked during these maneuvers, the bed may move and the patient can fall.**
3. Although this is done, it is not the most important action in this situation to ensure patient safety.
4. Although this is done, it meets comfort, not safety, needs.

11. 1. This is a planned intervention, not a goal.
2. This is a planned intervention, not a goal.
3. This is a planned intervention, not a goal. In addition, it is inappropriate to restrain a person automatically for agitation. A restraint should be used as a last resort to prevent the patient from self-injury or injuring others.
4. **This is an appropriate goal. It is realistic, specific, measurable, and has a time frame. It is realistic to expect that all patients be safe. It is specific and measurable because safety from trauma can be compared to standards of care within the profession of nursing. It has a time frame because the words *free from* reflect the time frames of *always*, *constantly*, and *continuously*.**

12. 1. **A three-pronged plug functions as a ground to dissipate stray electrical currents.**
2. This is not the purpose of a three-pronged plug.
3. A surge protector performs this function.
4. A multiple outlet plug performs this function.

13. 1. Although lack of an appetite (anorexia) can occur with dysphagia, it is not the most serious associated risk.
2. **When a person has difficulty with swallowing (dysphagia), food or fluid can pass into the trachea and be inhaled into the lungs (aspiration) rather than swallowed down the esophagus. This can result in choking, partial or total airway obstruction, or aspiration pneumonia.**
3. Dysphagia is unrelated to self-care deficit. Feeding self-care deficit occurs when a person is unable to cut food, open food packages, or bring food to the mouth.
4. Inadequate intake of food and fluid can result with dysphagia because of fear of choking. However, it is not the most serious associated risk.

14. 1. A confused patient may not be able to follow directions or understand cause and effect.
2. This may be impossible and impractical.
3. A confused patient may not be able to follow directions or understand cause and effect.
4. **Maintaining safety of the confused patient is best accomplished through close or direct supervision. Confused patients cannot be left on their own because they may not have the cognitive ability to understand cause and effect, and therefore their actions can result in harm.**

15. 1. This may eventually be done, but the child must do something immediately without waiting for help to arrive.

2. Rolling on the ground will smother the flames and put the fire out. Children should be taught to: "Stop, drop, and roll."

3. This may be impossible. In addition, it will take time and the clothing and skin will continue to burn.

4. Finding and obtaining water will take too much time and the clothing and skin will continue to burn. Something must be done immediately.

16. 1. Although this is done, it is not the first intervention.

2. This will result in the jacket being too loose. The jacket should be applied so that 2, not 4, fingers can slide between the patient and the restraint.

3. Even when applied correctly, restraints can cause pressure and friction. A baseline assessment of the skin under the restraint should be made. In addition, the presence of a dressing, pacemaker, or subclavian catheter may influence the type of restraint to use.

4. Although this is done, it is the last, not the first, intervention of the options offered.

17. 1. The supine position will promote aspiration and should be avoided in this situation.

2. The side-lying position prevents the tongue from falling to the back of the oropharynx, allowing the vomitus to flow out of the mouth by gravity and thus preventing aspiration.

3. The orthopneic is an unsafe, impossible position in which to maintain an unconscious patient.

4. The low-Fowler's position will allow the tongue to fall to the back of the oropharynx, promoting aspiration. This position should be avoided in this situation.

18. 1. The use of powder should be avoided because it is a respiratory irritant.

2. The rounded rim of a bedpan should be placed under the patient's buttocks, not toward the front of the patient.

3. Patient safety is a priority. A bedpan is not a stable base of support and the effort of elimination may require movements that alter balance. Side rails provide a solid object to hold while balancing on the bedpan and supply a barrier to prevent falling out of bed.

4. Although this is done to promote independence and limit strain on the nurse, it is not the most important factor to consider when assisting a patient with a bedpan.

19. 1. This is unsafe because it places the nurse in jeopardy. The nurse may be exposed to an electrical charge or become burned.

2. Because no patient is in jeopardy, the nurse's initial action should be to activate the alarm. The sooner the alarm is set, the sooner professional firefighters will reach the scene of the fire.

3. The nurse may not be capable of containing or fighting the fire. Not calling for professional firefighting help first places the nurse, staff, and patients in jeopardy.

4. This is premature at this time, but it may become necessary eventually.

20. 1. Although wet floors can contribute to falls, they are not the most common factor that contributes to falls in the hospital setting.

2. Although seizures can contribute to falls, most patients do not experience seizures.

3. Older adults who are hospitalized frequently have multiple health problems, are frail, and lack stamina. All of these contribute to the inability to maintain balance and ambulate safely.

4. Although this occasionally happens and is negligence, it is not the most common factor that contributes to falls in the hospital setting.

21. 1. Abdominal cramping is related to problems such as flatus, malabsorption, and increased intestinal motility, not difficulty swallowing.

2. Epigastric pain is related to problems, such as gastritis, cholecystitis, and angina, not difficulty swallowing.

3. Although constipation may result from not eating foods high in fiber because of difficulty with chewing and swallowing, this adaptation is not as directly related to difficulty swallowing as another option.

4. The body continuously secretes saliva (approximately 1000 mL a day) that usually is swallowed. When saliva accumulates and is not swallowed, it dribbles out of the mouth (drooling). This indicates the need to assess swallowing ability.

22. 1. Although this is important information, it is not the most important factor of the options offered in this question. In addition, the prior admission may have been too long ago to have any current relevance.

2. A patient with increased intestinal motility may experience diarrhea, which may place the patient at risk for a fluid and electrolyte imbalance, not a physical injury. Although a person with diarrhea may need to use the toilet more frequently, a bedside commode or bedpan can be used to reduce the risk of falls.
3. **This is significant information that must be considered because if falls occurred before, they are likely to occur again. When a risk is identified, additional injury prevention precautions can be implemented.**
4. Although this is important information, it is not the most important factor of the options offered in this question.

23. 1. The patient may or may not need a cane. An unnecessary cane may actually increase the risk of a fall.
2. Although this should be done, it is not the best intervention of the options presented.
3. **This widens the patient's base of support, which improves balance and decreases the risk of a fall.**
4. Although this should be done, it is not the best intervention of the options presented.

24. 1. This may or may not be necessary. This action should be based on the individual needs of the patient.
2. **It is safer if the bed is in the lowest position and the patient's feet are flat on the floor when getting in or out of bed. A greater risk for injury to a patient occurs when the mattress of the bed is further from the floor.**
3. This should be done while the bed is at a comfortable working height for the caregiver.
4. This may or may not be necessary. This action should be based on the individual needs of the patient.

25. 1. **A nasogastric (NG) tube for gastric decompression passes down the esophagus, through the cardiac sphincter, and into the stomach. The cardiac sphincter remains slightly open because of the presence of the NG tube. The semi-Fowler's position keeps gastric secretions in the stomach via gravity (preventing reflux and aspiration) and allows the gastric contents to be suctioned out by the NG tube.**
2. This is not done routinely every 2 hours. This may be done to identify the presence of the tube in the stomach and help re-establish patency of the tube when it is clogged.
3. This should be done more frequently to prevent irritation and pressure.
4. This is unnecessary and can result in vomiting and aspiration.

26. 1. Although this may be done eventually, it is not the priority at this time.
2. This action is contraindicated because it may place the nurse in jeopardy.
3. This is not the priority, and electrical burns may or may not be evident.
4. **An electric shock can interfere with the electrical conduction system within the heart and result in dysrhythmias. An electric shock can be transmitted through the body because body fluids (consisting of sodium chloride) are an excellent conductor of electricity.**

27. 1. Although a young child is at risk for injury in a hospital setting, age-related precautions are always instituted. More nurses generally are assigned to pediatric units and frequently family members are at the bedside.
2. This patient is not at as high a risk for injury as a patient in another option. A comatose patient demonstrates less response to painful stimuli, generally has an absence of muscle tone and reflexes in the extremities, and appears to be in a deep sleep.
3. A postmenopausal woman is not at a high risk for injury.
4. **A confused patient is at an increased risk for injury because of the inability to comprehend cause and effect and, therefore, lacks the ability to make safe decisions.**

28. 1. This is not true. Injuries and falls can occur if restraints are not applied appropriately. In addition, research indicates that patients incur less severe injuries if left unrestrained.
2. Restraints are applied in emergencies to protect patients from harming themselves or others. A physician's order must be obtained for the original restraint within 12 hours. Agencies have protocols concerning how often restraints need to be reordered by the physician (many require reorders every 24 hours).
3. **All patient care, including the use of restraints, should adhere to standards of care. The reason for the use of restraints must adhere to standards of care and be documented on the patient's hospital record to create a legal record that protects the patient as well as the health-care providers.**

4. The opposite is true. Patients resist the use of restraints and usually are mentally or emotionally incompetent to understand their necessity or benefits.

29. 1. Malfunctioning equipment is not a common cause of injuries in a hospital.
2. The use of restraints has declined dramatically and now is used only when patients may harm themselves or others.
3. Visitors are not the main cause of injuies in a hospital.
4. Research demonstrates that most injuries experienced by hospitalized patients occur from falls. Failing to call for assistance, inadequate lighting, and the physical condition of the patient all contribute to falls.

30. 1. This may or may not be necessary depending on the needs of the patient.
2. Patient allergies must be identified (e.g., latex, food, medication, etc.) before any care is provided, documented in the patient's hospital record, and appear on an allergy-alert wristband. After a risk is identified, additional safety precautions can be implemented to prevent exposure to the offending allergen. Assessment is the first step of the Nursing Process.
3. This may be available but is useless unless the supplies are used appropriately.
4. This is unnecessary. A person with a latex allergy should not be exposed to latex products.

31. 1. This provides for the safety of patients, staff, and visitors within a hospital. Inadequate lighting causes shadows, a dark environment, and the potential for misinterpreting stimuli (illusions), and is a major cause of accidents in the hospital setting.
2. When talking with older adults it is better to lower, not raise, the pitch of the voice. As people age they are more likely to have impaired hearing with higher pitch sounds.
3. This is not always necessary and therefore could be degrading or promote regression.
4. Although this should be done, furniture and medical equipment are not the only physical hazards that contribute to falls.

32. 1. Aspiration usually is not a risk with bulimia. Bulimia is characterized by episodes of binge eating followed by purging, depression, and self-depreciation.
2. When a person is sleepy, sluggish, or stuporous (lethargic), there may be a reduced level of consciousness and diminished reflexes, including the gag and swallowing reflexes. This condition can result in aspiration of food or fluids that can compromise the person's airway and respiratory status.
3. A lack of appetite (anorexia) is unrelated to aspiration. The less food or fluid is placed in the mouth, the less the risk for aspiration.
4. An inflammation of the mucous membranes of the mouth (stomatitis) may result in dysphagia and increase the risk of aspiration. However, of the options offered, it does not place a person at the greatest risk for aspiration.

33. 1. A physical examination requires a patient to assume a variety of positions such as supine, side-lying, sitting, and standing. The nurse should inquire about any positions that are uncomfortable or contraindicated because of past or current medical conditions to prevent complications.
2. Although this information may be obtained during the course of the physical examination, it is not the priority.
3. This is not the priority during a physical examination. This might be done to prevent fragmentation of care and ensure continuity of care.
4. Although this might be done, it is not a priority during a physical examination.

34. Answer: 3, 1, 2, 4
3. Closing the door to the dirty utility room protects the patients and staff members in the immediate vacinity of the fire.
1. Pulling the fire alarm ensures that appropriate hospital personnel and the fire department are notified of the fire. Trained individuals will arrive to contain and extinguish the fire and help move patients if necessary.
2. Closing unit doors and windows provide a barrier between the patients and the fire and limit drafts that could exacerbate the fire.
4. Patients should be supported emotionally during a crisis because anxiety can be contageous.

35. 1. Keeping a bed lower than a stretcher when transferring a patient from the stretcher

to a bed utilizes gravity which places less stress and strain on both the patient and nurses.

2. It is too difficult and unsafe to maneuver a stretcher with the nonswivel wheels on the leading end of the stretcher. The end of the stretcher with the patient's head does not have swivel wheels.
3. The swivel-wheeled end of the stretcher should be the leading end of the stretcher, and it is unsafe to lead with the patient's head. In addition, the end of the stretcher with the swivel wheels moves through greater arcs; this can cause dizziness. The swivel wheels of a stretcher should be at the end under the patient's feet, not the head.
4. This is unsafe and places the patient in physical jeopardy. The elevator doors may inadvertently close by the patient's head while the nurse is pulling the feet end of the stretcher into the elevator. The patient should be moved into an elevator head, not feet, first.
5. **The swivel wheels must be under the patient's feet on the leading end of the stretcher for safe maneuverability. A stretcher should always be pushed, not pulled, so that the transporter stays at the patient's head for protection.**

Medication Administration

KEYWORDS

The following words include English vocabulary, nursing/medical terminology, concepts, principles, or information relevant to content specifically addressed in the chapter or associated with topics presented in it. English dictionaries, nursing textbooks, and medical dictionaries, such as *Taber's Cyclopedic Medical Dictionary*, are resources that can be used to expand your knowledge and understanding of these words and related information.

- Acromion process
- Aerosol
- Air-lock technique
- Ampule
- Apothecary system
- Applicator
- Asepto syringe
- Auditory canal
- Automated medication-dispensing system
- Bevel
- Blister-pack
- Bolus
- Cartridge
- Cheek
- Continuous infusion
- Dilute
- Diluent
- Dispense
- Disperse
- Dissolve
- Dosage
- Filtered needle
- Five Rights
  - Right patient
  - Right medication
  - Right route
  - Right dose
  - Right frequency
- Gauge
- Greater trochanter
- Humerus bone
- Infusion
- Inject
- Injection site grids
- Injection sites
  - Abdomen
  - Deltoid
  - Dorsogluteal
  - Lateral, anterior, and posterior
  - Rectus femoris
  - Vastus lateralis
  - Ventrogluteal
- Inner/outer canthus
- Instillation
- Insulin syringe
- Interaction
- Intermittent infusion of medication
- Label
- Lacrimal duct
- Lubricate
- Mechanism of action
- Medication orders
  - PRN orders
  - Single orders
  - Standing orders
  - Stat orders
  - Stop orders
  - Telephone orders
- Medication regimen
- Metered-dose inhaler
- Metric system
- Needle bevel
- Orifice
- Over-the-counter drugs (OTCs)
- Parenteral
- Peak level
- Pinna of the ear
- Posterior superior iliac spine
- Potent
- Reconstitution
- Routes of administration
  - Buccal
  - Ear (Otic)
  - Epidural
  - Eye (Ophthalmic)
  - Intradermal
  - Intramuscular
  - Intrathecal
  - Intravenous

IV push, piggyback
Nasal cavity
Rectal
Subcutaneous
Sublingual
Topical
Transdermal
Urinary bladder
Vaginal
Rubber seal
Sciatic nerve
Sharps container
Substance abuse
Syringe
Systemic/local effect
Therapeutic drug level
Titrate
Troche
Trough level
Tuberculin syringe
Unit-dose system
Vial
Weekly pill container
Z-track

QUESTIONS

1. The nurse teaches a patient about taking a sublingual nitroglycerin tablet. The nurse evaluates that the patient understands the teaching when the patient states, "I should place it:
1. On my skin."
2. Inside my cheek."
3. Under my tongue."
4. In the lower lid of my eye."

2. The nurse plans to administer a bolus dose of a medication via a currently running intravenous infusion. The nurse should first:
1. Ensure that it is compatible with the IV solution being infused
2. Pinch the tubing above the infusion port while instilling the bolus
3. Instill it into a fifty mL bag of NS and infuse it via a secondary line
4. Administer it via a volume-control infusion set with microdrip tubing

3. The physician orders a rectal suppository for an adult patient. When administering the rectal suppository, the nurse should:
1. Lubricate the medication before insertion
2. Warm the medication to body temperature
3. Insert the medication at least two inches into the rectum
4. Place the patient in the prone position to administer the medication

4. The nurse is administering an intradermal injection. The nurse inserts the needle at a:
1. 15-degree angle
2. 30-degree angle
3. 45-degree angle
4. 90-degree angle

5. The nurse plans to administer a 3-mL intramuscular injection. The nurse understands that the least desirable muscle for the administration of this medication is the:
1. Deltoid
2. Dorsogluteal
3. Ventrogluteal
4. Vastus lateralis

6. The nurse is preparing to administer a subcutaneous injection of insulin. The nurse knows that the best site to use to promote its absorption is the patient's:
1. Upper lateral arms
2. Anterior thighs
3. Upper chest
4. Abdomen

7. When placing a cream into a patient's vaginal canal, the nurse should use:
   1. A finger
   2. A gauze pad
   3. An applicator
   4. An irrigation kit

8. The physician orders a medication that must be administered transdermally. The nurse understands that a drug administered transdermally is:
   1. Inhaled into the respiratory tract
   2. Dissolved under the tongue
   3. Absorbed through the skin
   4. Inserted into the rectum

9. The nurse is to administer an injection. To limit discomfort, the nurse should:
   1. Test for a blood return before injecting the medication
   2. Apply ice to the area before the injection
   3. Pinch the area while inserting the needle
   4. Inject the medication slowly

10. The nurse is preparing to draw up medication from a vial. What should the nurse do first?
    1. Ensure that the needle is firmly attached to the syringe
    2. Rub vigorously back and forth over the rubber cap with an alcohol swab
    3. Inject air into the vial with the needle bevel below the surface of the medication
    4. Draw up slightly more air than the volume of medication to be withdrawn from the vial

11. The instructions with a medication states to use the Z-track technique when administering the injection. Therefore, the nurse should:
    1. Pinch the site throughout the injection
    2. Massage the site after the needle is removed
    3. Remove the needle immediately after the medication is injected
    4. Change the needle after the medication is drawn into the syringe

12. The nurse instructs a patient to close his/her eyes after the administration of eye drops. The nurse understands that this is done to:
    1. Limit corneal irritation
    2. Squeeze excess medication from the eyes
    3. Disperse the medication over the eyeballs
    4. Prevent medication from entering the lacrimal duct

13. Which route is unrelated to the parenteral administration of medications?
    1. Buccal
    2. Z-track
    3. Intravenous
    4. Intradermal

14. How often should "Colace 100 mg b.i.d." be given?
    1. Three times a day
    2. Two times a day
    3. Every other day
    4. At bed time

15. The nurse must administer an intradermal injection. The technique uniquely related to the administration of an intradermal injection is:
    1. Utilizing the air-bubble technique
    2. Pinching the skin during needle insertion
    3. Inserting the needle with the bevel upward
    4. Massaging the area after the fluid is instilled

16. The nurse is preparing to reconstitute a medication in a multiple-dose vial. The nurse understands that the most essential step in the preparation of this medication is:
    1. Instilling an accurate amount of diluent into the vial
    2. Using a filtered needle when drawing up the medication from the vial
    3. Instilling air into the vial before withdrawing the reconstituted solution
    4. Wiping the rubber seal of the vial with alcohol before and after each needle insertion

17. Which characteristic of a subcutaneous injection of 5000 units of heparin should be implemented by the nurse?
    1. 3-mL syringe
    2. 22-gauge needle
    3. 90° angle of insertion
    4. 1½-inch needle length

18. The nurse understands that a contraindication for the intake of medications via the oral route is:
    1. Difficulty swallowing
    2. Gastric suctioning
    3. Unconsciousness
    4. Nausea

19. The nurse teaches the spouse of a patient how to insert a rectal suppository. The nurse identifies that further teaching is necessary when the spouse:
    1. Lubricates the tip of the suppository
    2. Wears a glove when inserting the suppository
    3. Places the suppository two inches into the rectum
    4. Inserts the suppository while the patient bears down

20. The physician orders a medication that must be administered via the intramuscular route. When administering this medication, the nurse knows that the site that has the highest risk for injury is the:
    1. Vastus lateralis
    2. Rectus femoris
    3. Ventrogluteal
    4. Dorsogluteal

21. It is most important for the nurse to use a filtered needle when preparing a parenteral medication that:
    1. Has to be reconstituted
    2. Is supplied in an ampule
    3. Appears cloudy in the vial
    4. Is to be mixed with another medication

22. When administering a subcutaneous injection, the nurse should use a:
    1. 5-mL syringe
    2. 25-gauge needle
    3. Tuberculin syringe
    4. 1½-inch long needle

23. The physician orders nose drops to be administered twice a day. When instilling the drops, the nurse should:
    1. Place the patient in the supine position with the head tilted backward
    2. Pinch the nares of the nose together briefly after the drops are instilled
    3. Instruct the patient to blow the nose 5 minutes after the drops are instilled
    4. Insert the drop applicator 1/8 inch into the nose toward the base of the nasal cavity

24. When the nurse brings pills to a patient, the patient is unable to hold the paper cup with the medications. The nurse should:
    1. Crush the pills and mix it with applesauce
    2. Have the physician order the liquid form of the drug
    3. Use the paper cup to introduce the pills into the patient's mouth
    4. Put the pills into the patient's hand and have the patient self-administer the pills

25. The nurse teaches a patient how to self-administer a steroid via a metered dose inhaler with an extender. The nurse identifies that the teaching is understood when the patient:
1. Rinses the mouth with water after the treatment
2. Position the mouthpiece one inch in front of the mouth while inhaling
3. Rolls the canister between the hands slowly before using the inhaler
4. Assumes the semi-Fowler's position with the head supported on a pillow

26. The nurse understands that an inappropriate route for a topical medication is:
1. Intradermal
2. Bladder
3. Rectum
4. Vagina

27. The nurse adds a medication to an intravenous fluid bag. Which nursing action is the priority?
1. Attaching a completed IV additive label to the bag
2. Mixing the medication and solution by rotating the bag
3. Maintaining sterile technique throughout the procedure
4. Ensuring that the drug and the IV solution are compatible

28. The nurse holds a bottle with the label next to the palm of the hand when pouring a liquid medication. The nurse does this to:
1. Conceal the label from the curiosity of others
2. Prevent the soiling of the label by spilled liquid
3. Ensure the accuracy of the measurement of the dose
4. Guarantee the label is read before pouring the liquid

29. The nurse understands that the route of drug administration not considered parenteral is:
1. Epidural
2. Transdermal
3. Subcutaneous
4. Intramuscular

30. The physician orders a medicated powder to be applied to a patient's skin. When applying a medicated powder, it is most essential that the nurse:
1. Applies a thin layer in the direction of hair growth
2. Protects the patient's face with a towel
3. Dresses the area with dry sterile gauze
4. Ensures that the skin surface is dry

31. The nurse must administer a medication that is supplied in an ampule. What should the nurse do first to access the ampule?
1. Inject the same amount of air as the fluid to be removed
2. Wipe the constricted neck with an alcohol swab
3. Break the constricted neck using a barrier
4. Insert the needle into the rubber seal

32. The nurse must administer a medication into the ear of an adult. To limit patient discomfort when administering ear drops, the nurse should:
1. Warm the solution to body temperature
2. Place the patient in a comfortable position
3. Pull the pinna of the ear upward and backward
4. Instill the fluid in the center of the auditory canal

33. The nurse instructs a patient to inhale deeply and hold each breath for a second when using a hand-held nebulizer. The nurse provides this instruction because this action will:
1. Prolong the treatment
2. Limit hyperventilation
3. Disperse the medication
4. Prevent bronchial spasms

34. Which abbreviation indicates to the nurse that the physician wants a medication administered at bedtime?
1. p.c.
2. h.s.
3. p.o.
4. a.c.

35. When administering a suppository, the nurse understands that it is absorbed in the:
1. Ear
2. Nose
3. Mouth
4. Rectum

36. The home care nurse is helping a patient with short-term memory loss how to remember to take multiple drugs throughout the day. The nurse should:
1. Instruct the patient to put medications in a weekly organizational pill container
2. Design a chart of the medications the patient takes each day during the week
3. Ask a family member to call the patient when medications are to be taken
4. Suggest that the patient wear a watch with an alarm

37. The nurse is to administer an eye irrigation to a patient's right eye. What should the nurse do?
1. Direct the flow of solution from the inner to the outer canthus
2. Irrigate with an asepto syringe two inches from the eye
3. Don sterile gloves before beginning the procedure
4. Position the patient in a right lateral position

38. A medication is delivered by the Z-track method when the nurse:
1. Uses a special syringe designed for Z-track injections
2. Pulls laterally and downward on the skin before inserting the needle
3. Administers the injection in the muscle on the anterior lateral aspect of the thigh
4. Injects the needle in a separate spot for each dose on a Z-shaped grid on the abdomen

39. The nurse must reconstitute a powdered medication. The nurse should:
1. Keep the needle below the initial fluid level as the rest of the fluid is injected
2. Instill the solvent that is consistent with the manufacturer's directions
3. Score the neck of the ampule before breaking it
4. Shake the vial to dissolve the powder

40. The nurse is preparing to administer a tablet to a patient. The nurse should remove the p.o. medication from its unit dose package:
1. Outside the door to the patient's room
2. At the patient's bedside
3. In the medication room
4. At the medication cart

41. When administering an analgesic, which nursing action is most appropriate?
1. Follow written orders exactly for the first 24 hours
2. Reassess the patient every 8 hours for drug effectiveness
3. Ask the physician to include a medication order for breakthrough pain
4. Seek a new order after two doses that do not achieve a tolerable level of relief

42. The physician orders a troche. The nurse should administer it by placing it in the patient's:
1. Ear
2. Eye
3. Mouth
4. Rectum

43. A patient has an order for 2 puffs of a bronchodilator via a metered-dose inhaler. The nurse should teach the patient to:
    1. Start breathing in while compressing the canister
    2. Hold the inspired breath for several seconds
    3. Deliver 2 puffs with each inspiration
    4. Inhale slowly for 8–10 seconds

44. The nurse is to administer an intramuscular injection. Check all that apply to this procedure.
    1. _____ Use a 1-inch needle
    2. _____ Use a 25-gauge needle
    3. _____ Insert the needle at a 45° angle
    4. _____ Aspirate before instilling the medication
    5. _____ Massage the insertion site after needle removal

45. The physician orders 18 units of Novolog R and 26 units of Novolog N to be given at 0730 AM in the same syringe. Indicate on the syringe, by shading in the appropriate area, how many total units of Novolog N and Novolog R are to be drawn into the syringe.

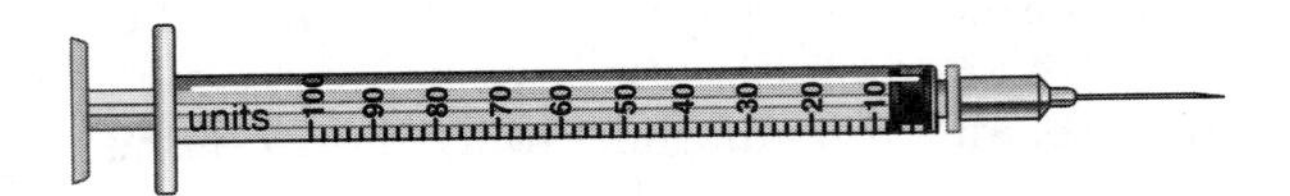

ANSWERS AND RATIONALES

1. 1. Topical medications are applied on the skin.
   2. A troche or lozenge given by the buccal route is placed between the cheek and gums.
   3. **A sublingual medication is placed under the tongue. It is absorbed quickly through the mucous membranes into the systemic circulation.**
   4. A medication placed in the lower conjunctival sac of the eye is administered for its local effect and is considered a topical medication.

2. 1. **An incompatible solution can increase, decrease, or neutralize the effects of the medication. In addition, an incompatibility may result in a compound or cause a precipitate that is harmful to the patient.**
   2. This is not the initial action. This is done immediately before and while instilling the medication to ensure that the medication flows toward the patient rather than in the opposite direction up the tubing.
   3. This is done for a medication administered via an intermittent intravenous infusion over a 30- to 90-minute period rather than an intravenous bolus (IV push) dose that is administered over 1 to 5 minutes.
   4. The volume of fluid of a bolus dose is too small to necessitate a volume-control infusion set.

3. 1. **Lubrication eases insertion by reducing friction, which limits tissue trauma and discomfort.**
   2. Warming the medication causes it to melt, making it impossible to insert. Most rectal suppositories are kept refrigerated until used.
   3. Rectal suppositories should be inserted 4 inches into the rectal canal of an adult.
   4. The patient should be placed in the left-lateral or left-Sims' position.

4. 1. **An intradermal injection is administered by inserting a needle at a 10- to 15-degree angle through the skin with the bevel of the needle facing upward toward the skin. The small volume of medication instilled just below the epidermis causes the formation of a wheal (localized area of swelling that appears like a small bubble).**
   2. This is too steep an angle for an intradermal injection and a wheal will not form.
   3. This angle is appropriate for a subcutaneous, not an intradermal, injection.
   4. This angle is appropriate for an intramuscular, not an intradermal, injection.

5. 1. **The deltoid, on the lateral aspect of the upper arm, is a small muscle that is incapable of absorbing a large medication volume. This site is more appropriate for 1 mL of solution.**
   2. The dorsogluteal site uses the gluteus maximus muscles in the buttocks, which can absorb larger medication volumes.
   3. The ventrogluteal site uses the gluteus medius and minimus muscles in the area of the hip, which can absorb larger medication volumes.
   4. The vastus lateralis muscle is located on the anterolateral aspect of the thigh, which can absorb larger medication volumes.

6. 1. Although insulin can be administered at the deltoid site, it is a small area that is not conducive to injection rotation within the site. The rate of absorption at this site is slower than at the preferred site for insulin administration.
   2. Although insulin can be administered in this site, the tissue of the thighs and buttocks have the slowest absorption rate.
   3. This site is not acceptable for the administration of insulin because of the lack of adequate subcutaneous tissue.
   4. **The abdomen is the preferred site for administration of insulin because it is a large area that promotes a systematic rotation of injections and it has the fastest rate of absorption.**

7. 1. Either a gloved finger or an applicator is used to insert a vaginal suppository, not a cream.
   2. It is impossible to insert a cream into the vaginal canal with a gauze pad. If attempted, it would traumatize the mucous membranes of the vagina.
   3. **The consistency of a cream requires that an applicator be used to ensure that the medication is deposited along the full length of the vaginal canal.**
   4. The consistency of a cream is too thick to be inserted into the vagina with an irrigating kit.

8. 1. A medication that is aerosolized is inhaled.
   2. A tablet, such as nitroglycerine, is dissolved under the tongue.
   3. **A medicated patch or disk can be applied directly to the skin where the medication is released and absorbed over time. This**

method ensures a continuous therapeutic drug level and reduces fluctuations in circulating drug levels.
4. Medications in the form of a suppository are inserted into the rectum.

9. 1. This prevents injecting medication directly into the circulatory system rather than limiting the discomfort of an injection.
2. This is contraindicated because it causes vasoconstriction, which limits absorption of the medication.
3. Pinching the skin aids in needle insertion when administering a subcutaneous injection. It does not limit the discomfort of injections.
4. Injecting slowly allows the fluid to be dispersed gradually, which limits tissue trauma and discomfort.

10. 1. This will ensure a tight seal and a closed system. If not firmly connected, the hub of the needle may disengage from the barrel of the syringe during preparation or administration of the medication when internal and external pressures are exerted on the needle and syringe.
2. The top just needs to be swiped. Rubbing back and forth is a violation of surgical asepsis because it reintroduces microorganisms to the area being cleaned.
3. This should be avoided because it causes bubbles that may interfere with the drawing up of an accurate volume of solution.
4. Excess air in the closed system raises pressure in the vial, which may cause bubbles when withdrawing the fluid and result in an inaccurate volume of solution.

11. 1. When the Z-track technique is used during an intramuscular injection, the skin and subcutaneous tissue are pulled 1 to 1½ inches to one side, not pinched.
2. Massage is contraindicated because it will force medication back up the needle track, which may result in tissue irritation or staining.
3. Removal of the needle should be delayed 10 seconds to allow the medication to begin to be dispersed and absorbed.
4. This ensures that medication is not on the outside of the needle, which prevents tracking of the medication into subcutaneous tissue during needle insertion.

12. 1. Instilling medication into the conjunctival sac prevents the trauma of drops falling on the cornea.
2. Closing the eyes gently, rather than squeezing the lids shut, prevents the loss of medication from the conjunctival sac.
3. Closing the eyes moves the medication over the conjunctiva and eyeball and helps ensure an even distribution of medication.
4. Gentle pressure over the inner canthus for one minute after administration prevents medication from entering the lacrimal duct.

13. 1. A parenteral route is one that is outside the gastrointestinal tract. A medication administered by the buccal route dissolves between the cheeks and gums, where it acts on the oral mucous membranes or is swallowed with saliva. Most troches are used for local effect.
2. Z-track is a method of administering an intramuscular injection. The intramuscular route is a parenteral route.
3. The intravenous route, a parenteral route, instills medication directly into the venous circulation.
4. The intradermal route, a parenteral route, injects medication just under the epidermis.

14. 1. The abbreviation for three times a day is t.i.d. (ter **i**n **d**ie).
2. The abbreviation b.i.d. (bis in die) represents twice a day.
3. Every other day must be written out; an abbreviation should not be used.
4. The abbreviation for hour of sleep is h.s. (**h**ora **s**omni).

15. 1. The air-bubble or air-lock technique can be used with intramuscular, not intradermal, injections. Its use is controversial particularly with disposable plastic syringes.
2. Pinching or bunching up tissue is appropriate with subcutaneous, not intradermal, injections.
3. When medication is injected with the bevel up, a small wheal will form under the skin. This technique is used only with intradermal injections.
4. Massaging the site of an intradermal injection will disperse the medication beyond the intended injection site and is contraindicated.

16. 1. The required amount of diluent must be followed exactly in a multiple-dose formulation to ensure accurate dosage preparation. The diluent for a single-dose formulation also must be exact so that the medication is diluted enough not to injure body tissues.
2. A filtered needle should be used when drawing up fluid from an ampule, not a vial. A filter

prevents shards of glass from entering the syringe.
3. Although this is an advisable practice, it is not as important as administering an accurate dose.
4. The rubber seal must be wiped with alcohol before, not after, needle insertion.

17. 1. Most doses of heparin are less than 1 mL. Three milliliters of heparin is excessive and may result in bleeding.
2. This gauge needle is too large and can cause unnecessary trauma and bleeding at the insertion site. A 25- or 26-gauge needle is adequate.
3. A ½-inch long needle inserted at a 90° angle will ensure that the heparin is inserted into subcutaneous tissue.
4. This length needle is unnecessarily long and may enter a muscle rather than subcutaneous tissue.

18. 1. Nursing interventions, such as positioning, mixing a crushed medication in applesauce, and dissolving a medication in a small amount of fluid, can be employed to facilitate the ingestion of medication.
2. Gastric suctioning can be interrupted for 20 to 30 minutes after medication has been instilled via a nasogastric tube.
3. Nothing that needs to be swallowed should ever be placed into the mouth of an unconscious patient because of the risk for aspiration.
4. Vomiting, not nausea, is a contraindication for p.o. medications.

19. 1. Lubrication is required to limit tissue trauma and ease insertion.
2. Standard precautions should be employed when there is exposure to patients' body fluids.
3. In an adult, a suppository should be inserted 4 inches to ensure it is beyond the internal sphincter.
4. Bearing down increases intraabdominal pressure which impedes the insertion of the suppository. The patient should be instructed to relax and breathe deeply and slowly while the suppository is inserted.

20. 1. The vastus lateralis site is not near large nerves or blood vessels and the muscle does not lie over a joint. It is a preferred site for infants 7 months of age and younger.
2. The rectus femoris site is not near major nerves, blood vessels, or bones. It is a preferred site for adults.
3. The ventrogluteal site is not near large nerves or blood vessels. It is a preferred site in adults and children.
4. The dorsogluteal site has the highest risk for injury because of the close proximity of the sciatic nerve, blood vessels, and bone.

21. 1. Reconstitution occurs within a closed vial and does not require a filtered needle.
2. The top of an ampule must be snapped off at its neck to access the fluid. A filtered needle prevents glass particles from being drawn into the syringe.
3. The majority of medications in vials are clear solutions. Cloudy fluid usually indicates contamination. Seek additional information from a drug guide or pharmacist.
4. It is not necessary to use a filtered needle when mixing medications.

22. 1. A subcutaneous injection should not exceed 1 mL. A 3-mL, not a 5-mL, syringe is acceptable for a subcutaneous injection.
2. A subcutaneous injection should use a 25- to 29-gauge needle, which minimizes tissue trauma. The diameter of a needle is referred to as its gauge, which ranges from 28 (small) to 14 (large).
3. The volume of a tuberculin syringe is only 1 mL. For most subcutaneous injections, a syringe that can accommodate up to 3 mL is preferred to facilitate handling of the syringe.
4. This length is appropriate for an intramuscular, not subcutaneous, injection.

23. **1. This ensures that gravity will promote the flow of medication to the posterior pharynx.**
2. This is unnecessary and can frighten the patient, who already may be having difficulty breathing.
3. Blowing the nose should be avoided because it may remove medication from the nose. Five minutes is the length of time the patient should remain in the supine position with the head tilted backward.
4. Nose drops should be directed toward the midline of the ethmoid bone with the dropper held ½ inch above the naves.

24. 1. This is done if the patient has dysphagia.
2. This is done if the patient still has difficulty swallowing a pill after it is crushed and mixed with applesauce.
3. The patient needs assistance. Keeping medication in the cup, rather than touching it with the hands, maintains medical asepsis.

4. This is unrealistic and unsafe. The patient has demonstrated the need for assistance.

25. 1. **Rinsing the mouth removes any remaining medication. This prevents irritation to the oral mucosa and tongue and prevents oral fungal infections.**
2. This promotes retention of the medication in the oropharynx, where it is swallowed rather than inhaled. This is the correct procedure if an extender (spacer) is attached to the mouthpiece.
3. This may not mix the medication adequately and result in an inadequate dose. The canister should be shaken several times before use.
4. The patient should be in an upright (standing, sitting, or high-Fowler's) position to promote lung expansion when inhaling.

26. 1. **An intradermal injection is inserted below, not on top of, the epidermis.**
2. Medications in the form of solutions can be instilled into the bladder. They are designed to work locally and are considered a topical medication.
3. Medications in the form of a suppository can be inserted into the rectum and are considered topical medications. Most are designed to work locally, although some are absorbed systemically.
4. Medications in the form of a suppository, tablet, cream, foam, or jelly can be instilled into the vagina. They are designed to work locally and are considered topical medications.

27. 1. Although this is important for safe administration of a medication administered intravenously, it is not the priority.
2. Although this should be done to ensure distribution of the medication throughout the IV solution, it is not the priority.
3. Although this is important to prevent infection, it is not the priority.
4. **An incompatibility can increase, decrease, or neutralize the effect of the medication. Also, it may cause a compound or precipitate that can harm the patient. This must be done before proceeding with subsequent steps of the procedure.**

28. 1. Although patient confidentiality should always be maintained, this is not the reason for holding the label toward the palm of the hand.
2. **Liquid medication may drip down the side of the bottle and soil the label, which may interfere with the ability to read the label accurately.**
3. Accuracy of the dose is ensured by using a calibrated cup and measuring the liquid at the base of the meniscus while positioning the cup at eye level.
4. The label should be read before holding it against the palm of the hand.

29. 1. A medication to be given via the epidural route is administered through a catheter inserted into the epidural space.
2. **Parenteral means *outside the digestive system*. However, in health care the parenteral route refers to medications given by injection or infusion. Transdermal medications are absorbed through the skin for a systemic effect.**
3. A needle is required to reach the subcutaneous tissue, the layer of fat located below the dermis and above muscle tissue.
4. A needle is required to reach the muscle layer beneath the dermis and subcutaneous tissue.

30. 1. This is done with lotions, creams, or ointments.
2. This is unnecessary. When the powder is sprinkled gently on the site, the powder should not become aerosolized.
3. This is not a universal requirement. When necessary, a dressing is applied with a practitioner's order.
4. **Moisture harbors microorganisms and when mixed with a powder will result in a paste-like substance. The site should be clean and dry before medication administration to ensure effective action of the drug.**

31. 1. This is done with a vial, not an ampule.
2. The rubber seal of a vial, not the neck of an ampule, should be wiped with alcohol.
3. **A barrier, such as a commercially manufactured ampule opener, sterile gauze, or an alcohol swab, should be used to protect the hands from broken glass.**
4. This is done with a vial, not an ampule.

32. 1. **Instilling cold medication into the ear canal is uncomfortable and can cause vertigo and nausea. Holding the bottle of medication in the hand for several minutes warms the solution to body temperature.**
2. The side-lying position with the involved ear upward must be maintained for 2 to 3 minutes for the instilled medication to disperse throughout the ear canal.
3. This straightens the ear canal and facilitates the flow of medication toward the eardrum; it does not limit discomfort.
4. This is contraindicated because the force of the fluid may injure the eardrum.

33. 1. There is no advantage in prolonging the treatment.
2. Slow, deep breathing will limit hyperventilation.
3. **A pause at the height of inspiration will promote distribution and absorption of the medication before exhalation begins.**
4. Slow inhalations and exhalations with pursed lips help prevent bronchial spasms.

34. 1. The abbreviation for after meals is p.c. (**p**ost **c**ibum).
2. **The abbreviation for hour of sleep is h.s.** (hora somni); **it is administered at bedtime.**
3. The abbreviation for by mouth is p.o. (**p**er **o**s).
4. The abbreviation for before meals is a.c. (**a**nte **c**ibum).

35. 1. Medicated solutions are administered via drops in the ear.
2. Medicated solutions are dropped or sprayed in the nose.
3. Tablets, lozenges, and troches are administered in the mouth.
4. **Suppositories—semisolid, cone-shaped, or oval-shaped masses that melt at body temperature—are inserted into the rectum.**

36. 1. **Pill distribution can be set up once a week. After the medication is taken, the empty section reminds the patient that the medication was taken, which prevents excessive doses. This is a major issue for patients with short-term memory loss.**
2. This is unrealistic. The chart may be complex, confusing, and require repeated cognitive decisions throughout the day that may be beyond the patient's ability.
3. This is unrealistic and puts an excessive burden on family members.
4. This is unrealistic. When the alarm goes off, the patient may not remember why it is ringing.

37. 1. **This prevents secretions and fluid from entering and irritating the lacrimal ducts.**
2. An asepto syringe produces a flow of fluid that is forceful and difficult to control. The irrigating piston syringe should be held 1 inch, not 2 inches, above the eye. An IV bag of solution is preferred to provide a flow of fluid by gravity that is gentle and controlable.
3. Medical, not surgical asepsis.
4. The patient should be placed in a sitting or back-lying position with the head tilted toward the affected eye.

38. 1. A special syringe is not needed for administering a medication via Z-track. The barrel of the syringe must be large enough to accommodate the volume of solution to be injected (usually 1 to 3 mL) and the needle long enough to enter a muscle (usually 1½ inches).
2. **This creates a zigzag track through the various tissue layers that prevents backflow of medication up the needle track when simultaneously removing the needle and releasing the traction on the skin.**
3. The use of the vastus lateralis muscle for a Z-track injection may cause discomfort for the patient. Z-track injections are tolerated better when the well-developed gluteal muscles are used.
4. The needle is inserted into the muscle once for a Z-track injection. The Z represents the zigzag pattern of the needle track that results when the skin traction and the needle are simultaneously removed.

39. 1. This will create excessive bubbles that can interfere with complete reconstitution or result in bubbles being drawn into the syringe. Both occurrences can result in an inaccurate dose.
2. **Compatibility is necessary so that a compound or precipitate that is harmful to a patient does not result.**
3. Reconstitution occurs in a vial (a closed system), not an ampule (an open system).
4. Shaking the vial will create excessive bubbles. The vial should be rotated between the hands to facilitate reconstitution.

40. 1. This is unsafe. This exposes the medication to the environment where it may become contaminated or grouped with other medications being administered to the patient, thus interfering with safe administration of one or more of the medications.
2. **The medication should be opened and administered immediately to the patient, limiting the potential for contamination. Reading the label immediately before opening the package is an additional safety check. Immediate administration prevents accidental disarrangement of medications that may result in a medication error.**
3. This is unsafe. It unnecessarily exposes the medication to the environment because it requires the nurse to carry the medication through the unit to the patient's room. In addition, it can become confused with the medications for other patients.

4. This is unsafe. The medication is exposed unnecessarily to the environment and it can be inadvertently confused with the medications for other patients.

41. 1. The physician's order should be followed exactly if it is a safe dose; however, if the medication is not effective, 24 hours is too long a period not to intervene.
2. The patient should be assessed every 1 to 2 hours to ensure effectiveness of the drug.
3. This is unnecessary if the drug is the appropriate dose.
4. Two doses is enough time to evaluate the effectiveness of a medication for pain. Patients should not have to endure intolerable levels of pain.

42. 1. Medications in the form of a solution are instilled into the ear.
2. Ophthalmic medications in the form of a solution or an ointment are administered in the eye.
3. A troche, a lozenge-like tablet, is dissolved slowly in the mouth in the buccal cavity to provide a localized effect.
4. Medications in the form of suppositories are inserted into the rectum.

43. **1. This ensures that a maximum amount of the drug is inhaled while the medication is still aerosolized.**
2. The breath should be held for 5 to 10 seconds, or longer, to promote distribution and absorption of the medication.
3. One puff, not 2, should be delivered with each inhalation.
4. The inhalation should start with compression of the canister and continue for another 2 to 3 seconds to ensure distribution of the medication.

44. 1. A 1.5-inch needle is required to reach muscular tissue.
2. A 22-gauge needle usually is used for an intramuscular injection; a 25-gauge needle usually is used for a subcutaneous injection.
3. The needle should be inserted at a 90° angle; a 45° angle is used for a subcutaneous injection.
4. Before instilling the medication, aspiration is done to ensure that a blood return does not occur which indicates that the needle is in a blood vessel.
5. Massage promotes dispersion of the medication.

45. **Answer: 44 units total.**
A total of 44 units of insulin should be drawn into the syringe. Eighteen units of Novolog R are drawn into the syringe first and then the 26 units of Novolog N are drawn into the syringe. It is done in this order to ensure that the Novolog N insulin, which is longer acting, does not dilute the Novolog R insulin in the vial, which is fast acting.

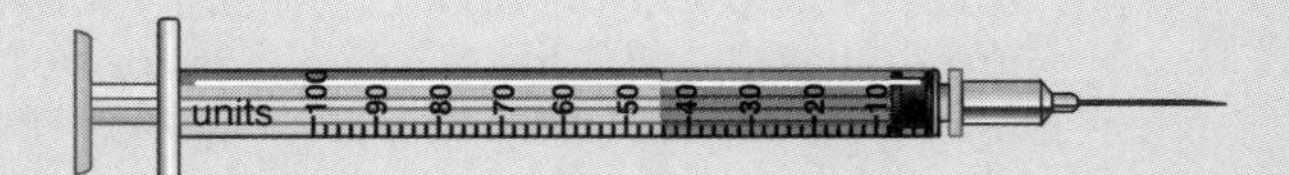

Pharmacology

KEYWORDS

The following words include English vocabulary, nursing/medical terminology, concepts, principles, or information relevant to content specifically addressed in the chapter or associated with topics presented in it. English dictionaries, nursing textbooks, and medical dictionaries, such as *Taber's Cyclopedic Medical Dictionary*, are resources that can be used to expand your knowledge and understanding of these words and related information.

Absorption
Adverse effect
Allergic/allergy
American Hospital
  Formulary Service
  Drug Information
Antagonism
Biotransformation
Blood level
Chemotherapy
Compatible
Contraindication
Controlled substance
Dependence
Drug absorption
Drug distribution
Drug effect
  Adverse
  Anaphylaxis, anaphylactic
  Idiosyncratic
  Local
  Side
  Synergistic
  Systemic
  Therapeutic
  Topical
  Toxic, toxicity
Drug Enforcement Agency (DEA)
Drug excretion
Drug levels, terms related to
  Duration
  Peak
  Onset
  Therapeutic range
  Trough
Drug metabolism
Drug name
Drug regimen
Food and Drug Administration (FDA)
Generic
Half-life
Herbal remedy
Hypersensitivity
Interaction
Megadose
Parenteral route
Pharmacist
Pharmacodynamics
Pharmacokinetics
Physician's Desk Reference (PDR)
Prescription
Prophylactic
Rash
Serum drug level
Target organ
Teratogenic
Tolerance/threshold
Trade name of drug
United States
  Pharmacopeia
  Drug Information
Urticaria

CLASSIFICATIONS OF DRUGS

Analgesic
Antacid
Antianxiety agent
Antiarrhythmic
Antibacterial
Antibiotic
Anticholinergic
Anticoagulant
Anticonvulsant/antiepeleptic
Antidepressant
Antidiabetic
Antidiarrheal
Antiemetic
Antifungal
Antihistamine
Antihypertensive

Antineoplastic
Antinflammatory
Antiparkinson
Antipsychotic
Antipyretic
Antiretroviral
Antitussive
Antiulcer
Bronchodilator
Cathartic
Diuretic
Emetic
Expectorant
Hypnotic
Laxative
Lipid-lowering agent
Mucolytic
Narcotic
Opioid
Skeletal muscle relaxant
Thyroid agent
Vasodilator
Vitamins and minerals

DRUG FORMS
Caplet
Capsule
Elixir
Emulsion
Enteric-coated
Extract
Liniment
Lotion
Metered-Dose Inhaler (MDI)
Ointment
Paste
Pill
Powder
Solution
Suppository
Suspension
Syrup
Tablet
Tincture
Transdermal
Troche, lozenge

QUESTIONS

1. The physician orders Maalox tablets, an antacid agent, for a patient with symptoms of indigestion. The most important thing the nurse needs to teach this patient is to:
1. Document the characteristics of gastric discomfort in a log
2. Notify the physician if coffee-ground vomitus occurs
3. Take the drug one hour before meals
4. Swallow the tablets whole

2. The nurse, working on an infection disease unit, routinely administers antibiotics. Which nursing action is most important in relation to the administration of most antibiotics?
1. Assessing for constipation
2. Administering between meals
3. Encouraging foods high in vitamin K
4. Monitoring the volume of urinary output

3. The nurse is preparing to administer an injection of heparin. What is the preferred site for this injection?
1. Leg
2. Arm
3. Buttock
4. Abdomen

4. Which concept associated with drug therapy and quality of sleep is important to understand to best plan nursing care?
1. Aggressive pain management intervention will reduce pain but increase insomnia
2. Abrupt discontinuation of hypnotic drugs can lead to withdrawal symptoms
3. Sedatives support restful sleep for people experiencing hypoxia
4. Barbiturates are the drugs of choice for insomnia

5. The nurse in the hospital is evaluating patient responses to medications. Which classification of drugs commonly precipitates diarrhea as an adverse effect?
1. Sedatives
2. Narcotics
3. Antibiotics
4. Antiemetics

6. After administering a drug, the nurse monitors the patient for reactions. Which reaction has the greatest potential to be life threatening?
1. Toxicity
2. Habituation
3. Anaphylaxis
4. Idiosyncratic

7. A public health nurse is planning a health class about herbal remedies for a group of older adults at the community center. The nurse should include that herbal remedies are:
1. Required to be labeled with information about their structure
2. Approved by the Food and Drug Administration
3. Natural because they are botanical in origin
4. Safe because they are organic

8. The nurse is assessing patients' responses to medications received. What must the nurse know about these drugs to best evaluate whether or not the expected outcomes of the drug therapy have been achieved?
1. Side effects
2. Therapeutic effect
3. Mechanism of action
4. Chemical composition

9. The nurse administers a variety of analgesics. It is important for the nurse to know that the drug that has a daily dose limit is:
1. Motrin
2. Codeine
3. Demerol
4. Morphine

10. A patient in pain requests the ordered pain medication, which is an opioid. Which nursing assessment is essential before administering an opioid?
1. Pulse
2. Respirations
3. Temperature
4. Blood pressure

11. The physician prescribes an antihypertensive medication to be administered twice a day. Before administering the antihypertensive medication, it is essential that the nurse assess the patient's:
1. Level of consciousness
2. Apical heart rate
3. Blood pressure
4. Respirations

12. Which is a common concern of the nurse when caring for patients taking drugs that depress the immune system?
1. Infection
2. Constipation
3. Sensory perceptual alterations
4. Inability to follow the therapeutic regimen

13. The physician tells a patient, who is receiving an antibiotic, that several blood specimens will be taken to evaluate the antibiotic therapy. The patient asks the nurse, "Why do these tests have to be done?" The nurse responds, "The ultimate purpose of determining peak and trough levels of a drug is to:
1. Maintain constant drug levels in the body."
2. Determine the half-life of a drug in the body."
3. Establish where biotransformation occurs in the body."
4. Monitor the rate of absorption of the drug in the body."

14. After the nurse administers an opioid, the patient becomes excitable. Which response should the nurse identify is being experienced by the patient?
1. Idiosyncratic
2. Synergistic
3. Allergic
4. Toxic

15. A patient experiences unrelenting neuropathic pain. Which classification of drug should the nurse anticipate that the physician will order for this patient?
1. Anticonvulsants
2. Antidepressants
3. Antihistamines
4. Anesthetics

16. A nurse is administering the 10 AM medications to all the patients on a hospital unit. The nurse identifies that the patient at the greatest risk for toxicity associated with most drugs is the patient with:
1. Liver disease
2. Kidney insufficiency
3. Respiratory difficulty
4. Malabsorption syndrome

17. When considering the variety of routes that medications can be administered, the nurse understands that drugs are absorbed most efficiently when they are given:
1. Orally
2. Rectally
3. Intravenously
4. Intramuscularly

18. A patient has been taking an antianxiety medication for a prolonged period of time. Which information is most helpful to the nurse when attempting to determine if the patient has developed a physiologic dependence on the drug?
1. Degree of tolerance
2. Strength of the dose
3. Perceived need by the patient
4. Time it takes to achieve the therapeutic effect

19. A patient with a severe upper respiratory tract infection is being treated with a bronchodilator. The nurse evaluates that the patient has achieved the therapeutic effect when the patient has less:
1. Viscous secretions
2. Difficulty breathing
3. Respiratory excursion
4. Bronchovesicular breath sounds

20. A patient admits to taking Milk of Magnesia (MOM) for its laxative effect several times a week. The most important information the nurse should teach a patient taking MOM is that it:
1. Can cause dependence and dehydration if taken for more than 2 weeks
2. Can cause an accumulation of sodium and potassium ions
3. Should be accompanied by 2 to 3 glasses of fluid
4. Should be taken at bedtime

21. A patient has an order for an antiemetic to be administered prn. When is it most appropriate for the nurse to administer this medication?
    1. After the patient vomits
    2. Thirty minutes before meals
    3. Four times a day when awake
    4. When the patient complains of nausea

22. After the ingestion of a new medication, the patient develops a rash, urticaria, and pruritus. The nurse concludes that the patient is experiencing a(n):
    1. Allergic response
    2. Idiosyncratic effect
    3. Anaphylactic reaction
    4. Synergistic interaction

23. A patient is taking hydrochlorothiazide once a day. Which fruit should the nurse encourage the patient to eat?
    1. Plum
    2. Orange
    3. Banana
    4. Tangerine

24. The nurse must administer a medication, that is a digitalis derivative. Which nursing assessment is essential before administering this medication?
    1. Pulse rate
    2. Blood pressure
    3. Respiratory rate
    4. Level of consciousness

25. The nurse teaches a patient to use a metered-dose inhaler (MDI). The patient asks, "Why do I need this instead of just taking a pill? The nurse responds, "A metered-dose inhaler is used because it:
    1. Provides you with a sense of control."
    2. Directs the medication into your upper respiratory tract."
    3. Delivers medication via positive pressure into your lungs."
    4. Releases the medication in small particles that you can inhale deeply."

26. Patients with multiple health problems often go to a variety of medical specialists. The response to medication that occurs more frequently in patients who go to several medical specialists is drug:
    1. Allergies
    2. Tolerance
    3. Habituation
    4. Interactions

27. The nurse is responsible for administering medications to a group of patients. The nurse understands which choice below is the most effective way to achieve and maintain a drug's therapeutic level?
    1. IV push
    2. Sublingual route
    3. Oral administration
    4. Large volume infusion

28. The nurse understands that the route of drug administration that is the fastest acting among the routes presented is:
    1. Buccal
    2. Transdermal
    3. Subcutaneous
    4. Intramuscular

29. While the nurse is applying a transdermal patch, the patient asks the nurse, "Why can't I just take a pill?" The nurse explains, "The advantage of administering a drug via a transdermal patch is that it:
1. Limits allergic responses."
2. Prevents drug interactions."
3. Delivers the drug over a period of time."
4. Provides a local rather than a systemic effect."

30. A patient asks the nurse why the physician ordered a lipid-lowering drug. When considering a response, the nurse understands that physicians generally order hyperlipidemia drug therapy:
1. After failure of diet therapy
2. For patients over 60 years of age
3. For those who are unable to exercise
4. After 2 consecutive months of elevated serum lipid levels

31. The nurse administers a prescribed antiemetic. The adaptation that indicates to the nurse that the patient is experiencing a therapeutic response to this medication is a reduction in:
1. Fever
2. Anxiety
3. Vomiting
4. Coughing

32. When contrasting prefilled, disposable unit-dose intramuscular drug cartridges versus multidose vials, the nurse understands that the primary purpose of unit-dose cartridges is to:
1. Ensure that the appropriate-length needle is attached
2. Limit the preparation time in emergencies
3. Reduce the incidence of drug interactions
4. Ensure the purity of the drugs

33. A presurgical patient is being weaned from long-term prescribed corticosteroids. The nurse understands that this is necessary because a sudden discontinuance of corticosteroids can contribute to:
1. Hypothermia
2. Bleeding
3. Seizures
4. Shock

34. The patient has an order for Lomotil, an antidiarrheal agent. The nurse should teach the patient to:
1. Inform the physician if diarrhea persists for more than 2 days
2. Be alert to the fact that it may cause hyperactivity
3. Limit fluid intake to 2000 mL per day
4. Avoid crushing the tablets

35. The nurse is administering an antihypertensive medication to a patient. Which patient adaptation should the nurse identify as an excessive response to the antihypertensive?
1. Heart rate of 60 beats per minute
2. Blood pressure of 80/60 mm Hg
3. Respirations of 24 per minute
4. Oral temperature of 98°F

36. The patient has an order for Zoloft, an antidepressant. It is most important that the nurse:
1. Monitors the patient for suicidal tendencies
2. Advises the patient to engage in psychotherapy
3. Encourages the patient to diet because weight gain is common
4. Teaches the patient to limit alcohol intake to one drink per day

37. A patient is receiving an antipyretic agent. When determining if the medication achieved a therapeutic response, the nurse should assess the patient's:
1. Urinary output
2. Pain tolerance
3. Temperature
4. Respirations

38. Before instituting patient-controlled analgesia (PCA) via a continuous intravenous route for the relief of pain, what is the most important action by the nurse?
1. Monitoring the patient's analgesic blood levels
2. Assessing the patient's respiratory status
3. Determining the patient's pain tolerance
4. Identifying the patient's pain threshold

39. Identify the drug classifications that are correctly associated with their expected therapeutic outcomes. check all that apply.
1. _____ Bronchodilators: relieve dyspnea
2. _____ Diuretics: increase urinary output
3. _____ Antitussives: prevent or relieve coughing
4. _____ Expectorants: decrease mucus production
5. _____ Antiemetics: prevent or treat nausea and vomiting

40. The physician orders 165 mg of cefazolin (Kefzol) IM every 8 hours. The drug is supplied in a vial that states that after reconsitution there will be 330 mg/mL. How much solution should the nurse administer?

Answer: __________ mL.

ANSWERS AND RATIONALES

1. 1. Although this might be done, it is not the priority. Characteristics include location, duration, intensity, and description of the discomfort.

2. These are symptoms of gastric bleeding and the physician should be notified immediately. Enzymes act on blood to produce coffee-ground emesis and tarry stools.

3. Maalox should be taken 1 to 3 hours after a meal and at bedtime to neutralize gastric acid.

4. This medication should be thoroughly chewed and taken with at least a half glass of water to prevent the tablet from entering the intestine undissolved.

2. 1. Most antibiotics tend to cause diarrhea, not constipation.

2. Food often interferes with the dissolution and absorption of antibiotics, delaying their action. Also, food can combine with molecules of certain drugs, changing their molecular structure and ultimately inhibiting or preventing their absorption.

3. Yogurt, not foods high in vitamin K, is encouraged for a patient receiving antibiotics. Yogurt helps to recolonize the endogenous flora of the GI tract that can be eradicated by antibiotics.

4. This is not necessary.

3. 1. The tissues in the legs are not preferred for the administration of heparin because muscle activity associated with walking increases the risk of hematoma formation.

2. The tissues in the arms are not preferred for the administration of heparin because muscle activity associated with movement of the arms increases the risk of hematoma formation.

3. The tissues associated with walking are not preferred for the administration of heparin because muscle activity increases the risk of hematoma formation.

4. The abdomen is the preferred site for the administration of heparin because it lacks major muscles and muscle activity. This site has the least risk for hematoma formation.

4. 1. Effective pain management will facilitate rest and sleep, not promote insomnia.

2. Barbiturate sedative-hypnotics depress the central nervous system and when withdrawn abruptly can cause withdrawal symptoms such as restlessness, tremors, weakness, and insomnia. Long-term use should be tapered by 25% to 30% weekly.

3. Sedatives, central nervous system depressants, are not advocated for patients with hypoxia because they depress respirations, which may exacerbate the hypoxia.

4. Barbiturates depress the central nervous system, alter REM and NREM sleep, result in daytime drowsiness, and cause rebound insomnia. For this reason, antianxiety drugs or tranquilizers are preferred.

5. 1. Sedatives, used to promote sleep, depress the central nervous system, which may cause constipation, not diarrhea.

2. Narcotics, opium derivatives used to relieve pain, depress the central nervous system, which may cause constipation, not diarrhea.

3. Antibiotics can alter the flora of the body, resulting in superinfections. Opportunistic fungal infections of the gastrointestinal system may cause a black, furred tongue, nausea, and diarrhea.

4. Antiemetics, used to prevent or alleviate nausea and vomiting, may cause constipation, not diarrhea.

6. 1. Medication toxicity results from excessive amounts of the drug in the body because of overdosage or impaired metabolism or excretion. Most drug toxicity that occurs immediately after administration is preventable through accurate ordering and administering of the medication. Toxicity that occurs through the cumulative effect occurs over time, and if recognized early, is not life threatening.

2. Drug habituation is a mild form of psychologic dependence that occurs over time.

3. Anaphylaxis, a severe allergic reaction, requires immediate intervention (i.e., epinephrine, IV fluids, steroids, and antihistamines) because it can be fatal.

4. An idiosyncratic effect is an unexpected, individualized response to a drug. The response can be an under-response, an over-response, or cause unpredictable, unexplainable symptoms. Usually, it is not life threatening.

7. 1. The Dietary Supplement Health and Education Act of 1994 stipulated that herbs must be labeled with information about their effects on the structure and

function of the body. Herbal substances officially are considered food supplements.

2. The Food and Drug Administration (FDA), a division of the United States Department of Health and Human Services, regulates the manufacture, sale, and effectiveness of prescription and nonprescription medications, not herbal remedies.
3. Herbs, considered by some to be "natural," are plants that are valued for their medicinal properties. As medicinal substances, they should be viewed by the consumer as drugs.
4. Just because herbs are organic does not ensure that they are safe. Many herbs even though organic can be toxic if ingested in unsafe amounts.

8. 1. Side effects are unintended effects other than the therapeutic effect.
2. Therapeutic effects are the desired, intended effects of the drug. They are the reason for which the drug is prescribed.
3. Although it is important to know the mechanism of action of a drug (pharmacodynamics), this knowledge is not as important as knowing the physical, mental, behavioral, or emotional responses indicating that a drug is having the desired impact on the patient.
4. Although it is important to know the chemical composition of a drug, this is not as significant as knowing the desired response to the medication.

9. 1. When administered to an adult, ibuprofen (Motrin) should not exceed 3600 mg/day when used as an anti-inflammatory or 1200 mg/day when used as an analgesic or antipyretic. Higher doses do not increase effectiveness and may cause major gastrointestinal and central nervous system adverse effects.
2. When administered to an adult under the supervision of a practitioner, codeine may exceed the recommended daily dosage of 120 mg.
3. When administered to an adult under the supervision of a practitioner, meperidine (Demerol) may exceed the recommended oral dosage of 1200 mg/day or the IV dose of 15 to 35 mg/hour.
4. Recommended daily doses for morphine vary based on weight of the patient and route of administration. Recommended dosages routinely are exceeded in pain management of patients with chronic, intractable (malignant) pain.

10. 1. An opioid analgesic can cause the side effect of bradycardia, so the pulse should be assessed before administration. However, assessment of heart rate is not as essential as another vital sign.
2. An opioid depresses the respiratory center in the medulla, which results in a decrease in the rate and depth of respirations. When a patient's respiratory functioning is below acceptable parameters, the drug should be withheld and the practitioner notified.
3. The side effects and adverse reactions to opioids do not include alterations in temperature.
4. An opioid can cause the side effect of hypotension. However, assessment of blood pressure is not as essential as another vital sign.

11. 1. This is unnecessary because antihypertensives do not alter the level of consciousness.
2. The apical heart rate should be assessed before administering cardiac glycosides and antidysrhythmics, not antihypertensives.
3. Antihypertensives such as beta-adrenergic blockers, calcium channel blockers, vasodilators, and ACE inhibitors all act to reduce blood pressure; therefore, the blood pressure should be obtained before and monitored after administration.
4. Respirations and breath sounds should be assessed before administering bronchodilators and expectorants, not antihypertensives.

12. 1. Drugs that suppress the immune system, such as antineoplastics (destroy stem cells that are precursors to WBCs), steroids (suppress function and numbers of eosinophils and monocytes), and antibiotics (destroy body flora), lower the body's ability to fight microorganisms that can cause infection.
2. These drugs are more likely to cause gastrointestinal disturbances such as anorexia, nausea, vomiting, and diarrhea, not constipation.
3. Most drugs that suppress the immune system usually do not cause sensory problems. Although some antineoplastic drugs can cause peripheral neuropathy, this response is not as common as gastrointestinal, hematologic, integumentary, and immune system adverse effects.
4. Although this is a concern for any patient who must follow a pharmacologic regimen, it is not the most common risk associated with drugs that suppress the immune system.

13. 1. **The peak serum level of a drug is the maximum concentration that the drug can reach in the blood (occurs when the elimination rate equals the absorption rate). Trough levels indicate the serum level of a drug just before the next dose is to be administered. The results of these two values determine the dose and time a drug should be administered to maintain a serum level of a drug within its therapeutic range.**
2. Although a drug's half-life, the usual amount of time needed by the body to reduce the concentration of the drug by one half, is helpful in determining how frequently a drug should be given initially, it does not reflect an individual patient's response to the drug.
3. Biotransformation, the process of inactivating and breaking down a drug, takes place primarily in the liver. Peak and trough levels may indirectly reflect the rate of biotransformation, not the place it occurs.
4. Peak and trough levels indirectly measure both the absorption and the inactivation and elimination of a drug from the body. This is not the purpose of peak and trough levels.

14. 1. **Excitability is an unexpected, unexplainable response to an opioid. Opioids are central nervous system depressants that relieve pain and promote sedation, not cause excitability.**
2. A synergistic response associated with an opioid is reflected by a lowered level of consciousness and sedation.
3. Allergic responses frequently manifest as a rash, urticaria, and pruritus.
4. Toxicity is manifested by sedation, respiratory depression and coma. The antidote naloxone (Narcan) may be necessary.

15. 1. Anticonvulsants do not relieve pain. Anticonvulsants depress abnormal neuronal discharges in the central nervous system, limiting or preventing seizures.
2. **Antidepressants, particularly amitriptylin (Elavil), potentiate the effects of opioids and have innate analgesic properties.**
3. Antihistamines do not relieve pain. Antihistamines block the effects of histamine at the H_1 receptor.
4. Although anesthetics do block pain, they generally are not used to relieve neuropathic pain. General anesthetics depress the central nervous system sufficiently to allow pain-free invasive procedures (e.g., surgery), and local anesthetics produce brief episodes of decreased nerve transmission when general anesthesia is not warranted.

16. 1. **Drug-metabolizing enzymes in the liver detoxify drugs to a less active form (biotransformation). With liver dysfunction, biotransformation is impaired and drugs accumulate, ultimately reaching toxic levels.**
2. Although decreased kidney function will adversely affect drug excretion, it does not pose the greatest risk for toxicity.
3. Most drugs are excreted through the kidneys, not the lungs.
4. Most drugs are excreted through the kidneys, not the intestines.

17. 1. Food, fluid, and gastric acidity can influence the dissolution and absorption of medications.
2. The absorption of rectal medications is influenced by the presence of fecal material and is unpredictable.
3. **Intravenous medications enter the bloodstream directly by way of a vein. Intravenous administration offers the quickest rate of absorption and it is within the circulatory system for easy distribution.**
4. The intramuscular route is not the first, most efficient route for absorption of medication.

18. 1. Tolerance is not a reliable indicator of dependence. Tolerance to a drug has occurred when increasing amounts of the drug must be administered to achieve the therapeutic effect.
2. Strength of a dose is not a reliable indicator of dependence. Factors such as age, weight, gender, and drug tolerance also influence the strength of a dose.
3. **Drug dependence, a form of drug abuse, occurs when a person has an emotional reliance on a drug because there is a craving for the effect or response that the drug produces.**
4. The length of time a drug takes to achieve its therapeutic effect is unrelated to the development of physiologic dependence on the drug.

19. 1. Mucolytic agents, not bronchodilators, liquefy thick, sticky (viscous) secretions.
2. **Bronchodilators expand the airways of the respiratory tract, which promotes air exchange and easier respirations.**
3. The ability of the chest to expand (respiratory excursion) increases, not decreases.

4. Bronchovesicular breath sounds will increase, not decrease, after the administration of a bronchodilator. Bronchovesicular sounds are expected blowing sounds heard over the main stem bronchi. They are blowing sounds that are moderate in pitch and intensity, and equal in length on inspiration and expiration.

20. 1. **Prolonged laxative use weakens the bowel's natural responses to fecal distention, resulting in chronic constipation. The osmotic action of magnesium salts in magnesium hydroxide draws water into the intestine, which can cause dehydration and electrolyte imbalances.**
2. MOM causes sodium and potassium to be lost from, rather than accumulate in, the body. The magnesium in MOM may be absorbed and result in hypermagnesemia.
3. Each dose should be followed by one full glass of water to promote a faster effect and help replenish lost fluid. Daily fluid intake should be 2000 to 3000 mL.
4. This will interrupt sleep. MOM causes bowel elimination 3 to 6 hours after its administration.

21. 1. This is too late. When an antiemetic is administered appropriately, vomiting should not occur.
2. **Antiemetics should be administered before a meal so that the peak effect of the drug occurs at the time of anticipated nausea.**
3. This will result in an excessive amount of this type of medication and does not correspond to events that precipitate nausea.
4. This is too late. Prophylactic administration of an antiemetic will prevent nausea.

22. 1. **A drug allergy is an immunologic response to a drug. In addition to integumentary responses, the patient may develop angioedema, rhinitis, lacrimal tearing, nausea, vomiting, wheezing, dyspnea, and diarrhea.**
2. An idiosyncratic effect is an unexpected, individualized response to a drug. The response can be an under-response, an over-response, or cause unpredictable, unexplainable symptoms.
3. The early signs of anaphylaxis are shortness of breath, acute hypotension, and tachycardia.
4. When a drug interaction occurs where the action of one or both drugs is potentiated, it is called a synergistic effect.

23. 1. One medium-size plum contains approximately 114 mg of potassium.
2. One medium-size orange contains approximately 237 mg of potassium.
3. **One medium-size banana contains approximately 450 mg of potassium. Hydrochlorothiazide, by its action in the distal convoluted tubule, promotes the excretion of potassium. Potassium must be replenished because of its vital role in the sodium-potassium pump.**
4. One medium-size tangerine contains approximately 132 mg of potassium.

24. 1. **Digoxin (Lanoxin) decreases conduction through the SA and AV nodes and prolongs the refractory period of the AV node, resulting in a slowing of the heart rate (negative chronotropic effect). When the heart rate is less than preset parameters (frequently 60 beats per minute), or higher than preset parameters (frequently 100 beats per minute), the medication should be held and a serum digoxin level assessed for exceeding its therapeutic range of 0.5 to 2 ng/mL.**
2. Dysrhythmias, not alterations in blood pressure, are cardiovascular signs of toxicity.
3. This assessment is unnecessary because a change in respiratory status is not a symptom of toxicity.
4. Toxicity may cause confusion and disorientation, not an altered level of consciousness.

25. 1. Although this may be a secondary benefit for some patients, it is not the reason for using an MDI.
2. The medication from an MDI is delivered to the lungs, which comprise the lower, not upper, respiratory tract.
3. Although an MDI delivers the medication via pressure to the patient's mouth, it is the act of the patient's inhalation that delivers the medication to its site of action.
4. **An MDI aerosolizes the medication so that the suspension of microscopic liquid droplets can be inhaled deep in the lung.**

26. 1. An allergic reaction results from an immunologic response to a medication to which the patient has been sensitized.
2. Tolerance occurs when a patient develops a decreased response to a medication and therefore requires an increased dose to achieve the therapeutic response.

3. Drug habituation is a mild form of psychologic dependence.
4. **A drug interaction occurs when one drug affects the action of another drug. The effect of one or both drugs increases, decreases, or is negated. The risk for drug interactions increases when multiple drugs are prescribed by multiple practitioners with inadequate communication among the practitioners.**

27. 1. An IV push (bolus) is the administration of a drug directly into the systemic circulation. Usually, it is administered as a single dose in an emergency. It achieves the desired level quickly, but does not maintain it.
2. The sublingual route is used intermittently and only when necessary. It is not used to maintain constant therapeutic drug levels.
3. Although the oral route is the safest, easiest, and most desirable way to administer medications, there are fluctuations in serum blood levels because the medication is administered intermittently one or more times throughout the day.
4. **With a large volume infusion, a drug is added to an IV container (usually 250 mL, 500 mL, or 1000 mL) and the resulting solution is administered over time. This approach maintains a constant serum drug level.**

28. 1. Medications dissolve between the teeth and gums, mix with saliva and are swallowed. This route has a slow onset of action.
2. The transdermal route is noted for its ability to sustain the absorption of medication, not because it produces a rapid response. The absorption of medications administered via the transdermal route is influenced by the condition of the skin, the presence of interstitial fluid, and the adequacy of circulation to the area.
3. The subcutaneous route is faster-acting than some routes because it is a parenteral route, but slower-acting than other parenteral routes because subcutaneous tissue does not have a large blood supply.
4. **The intramuscular route is the fastest-acting parenteral route (after intravenous) because it has a large vascular network that ensures rapid absorption into the bloodstream.**

29. 1. The composition of the drug, not the route by which it is administered, determines if an allergic response will occur.
2. The composition of a drug and its molecular reaction with another drug that is concurrently present determines if a drug interaction will occur.
3. **A transdermal patch placed on the skin gradually releases a predictable amount of medication that is absorbed into the bloodstream for a prescribed period of time. This approach maintains therapeutic blood levels and reduces fluctuations in circulating drug levels.**
4. Transdermal patches are used for their systemic, not local, effects.

30. 1. **Generally, conservative management of hyperlipidemia through dietary modifications and exercise is attempted before resorting to a medication. Lipid-lowering agents have side effects and adverse effects and may interact with other drugs.**
2. Lipid-lowering agents are ordered for patients who are over 60 years old only when necessary, not because they are over 60 years old.
3. Exercise is only one factor that influences the patient's lipid status. Factors such as diet, cigarette smoking, stress, concurrent diseases, and family history are additional factors that need to be considered when a pharmacologic regimen is prescribed.
4. Only people with chronically elevated lipid levels receive antilipidemics because of their significant side effects. Lifestyle modifications are attempted first.

31. 1. Antipyretics, not antiemetics, reduce fever.
2. Anxiolytics, not antiemetics, reduce anxiety.
3. **Antiemetics block the emetogenic receptors to prevent or treat nausea or vomiting.**
4. Antitussives, not antiemetics, reduce the frequency and intensity of coughing.

32. 1. Although generally this is true, there are times the attached needle is inappropriate for a particular patient and the nurse must transfer the medication into a standard syringe.
2. Although prefilled cartridges are convenient in an emergency, it is not the primary purpose of having prefilled cartridges.
3. Drug interactions can still occur with prefilled, disposable cartridges because the drug within the cartridge may alter or be altered by the concurrent presence of another medication in the patient's body.
4. **Single-dose cartridges prepared by a medication manufacturer or pharmacy**

ensure the purity of the drug. Ampules can be contaminated by glass debris, and multiple-dose vials can be contaminated by rubber debris and microorganisms.

33. 1. Acute adrenal insufficiency may cause hyperthermia, not hypothermia.
2. Acute adrenal insufficiency is unrelated to hemorrhage.
3. Acute adrenal insufficiency may cause dizziness and syncope, not seizures.
4. Exogenous glucocorticoids cause adrenal suppression. When exogenous steroids are withdrawn abruptly, the adrenal glands are unable to produce adequate amounts of glucocorticoids, thus causing acute adrenal insufficiency and shock.

34. 1. Diphenoxylate hydrochloride (Lomotil) depresses intestinal motility and effectively controls diarrhea within 24 to 36 hours. If diarrhea persists beyond 48 hours, the physician should be notified.
2. Lomotil may depress the central nervous system, which causes drowsiness and sedation, not hyperactivity.
3. When a patient is experiencing diarrhea, fluid should be encouraged, not restricted, to prevent dehydration and electrolyte imbalances.
4. Lomotil tablets are not enteric-coated and do not have extended-release properties, therefore they may be crushed if necessary.

35. 1. This heart rate is within the expected range of 60 to 100 beats per minute.
2. The acceptable range for the systolic pressure is 95 to less than 120 mm Hg. This patient's systolic reading is outside the expected range, which is an excessive drop when receiving an antihypertensive.
3. Antihypertensives do not directly affect respirations. Respirations may return to the expected range of 12 to 20 breaths per minute when cardiac output improves.
4. Antihypertensives do not influence body temperature. Expected oral temperatures range between 98°F and 98.6°F.

36. 1. When depression lifts during the early stages of antidepressant therapy, the individual has renewed energy that may support the implementation of suicidal ideation. Patient safety is the priority.
2. Although this should be done, it is not the priority.
3. A person will more likely lose, not gain, weight when taking sertraline hydrochloride (Zoloft) because its side effects include anorexia, nausea, and vomiting.
4. Alcohol should be avoided because it potentiates the central nervous system depressive effects of Zoloft.

37. 1. Intake and output is monitored when a patient is taking a diuretic, not an antipyretic.
2. Pain tolerance is monitored when a patient is taking an analgesic, not an antipyretic.
3. Antipyretics lower fever by affecting thermoregulation in the central nervous system and/or inhibiting the action of prostaglandins peripherally.
4. Respirations are monitored when a patient is taking a central nervous system depressant or bronchodilator, not an antipyretic.

38. 1. This is unnecessary.
2. Analgesics depress the central nervous system; therefore, the respiratory status must be monitored before and routinely throughout administration for signs of respiratory depression.
3. Although this may be done, it is not the priority. Pain tolerance is the highest intensity of pain that the person is willing to endure.
4. Although this may be done, it is not the priority. Pain threshold is the amount of pain stimulation a person requires before pain is felt.

39. 1. Bronchodilators relax smooth muscles of the bronchi and bronchioles increasing the diameter of their lumens (bronchodilation), resulting in a decrease in airway resistance.
2. Diuretics increase the urinary excretion of water and electrolytes such as sodium, potassium, calcium, and chloride.
3. Antitussives prevent or relieve coughing by depressing the cough center in the medulla.
4. Expectorants increase, not decrease, the flow of respiratory secretions; they decrease the viscosity of secretions, promoting the coughing up and removal of mucus from the lungs.
5. Antiemetics, depending on the agent (such as antihistamines, anticholinergics, neuroleptic agents, prokinetic agents, serotonin antagonists, and substance P neurokinin-1 receptor antagonist), act in a variety of ways to prevent, limit, or treat nausea and vomiting.

40. Answer: 0.5 mL. Use ratio and proportion to solve the problem.

$$\frac{\text{Desired}}{\text{Have}} \quad \frac{165 \text{ mg}}{330 \text{ mg}} \times \frac{x \text{ mL}}{1 \text{ mL}}$$

$$330x = 165$$
$$x = 165 \div 330$$
$$x = 0.5 \text{ mL}$$

Basic Human Needs and Related Nursing Care

5

Hygiene

KEYWORDS

The following words include English vocabulary, nursing/medical terminology, concepts, principles, or information relevant to content specifically addressed in the chapter or associated with topics presented in it. English dictionaries, nursing textbooks, and medical dictionaries, such as *Taber's Cyclopedic Medical Dictionary*, are resources that can be used to expand your knowledge and understanding of these words and related information.

Abrasion
Acne
Activities of daily living
Alopecia
Asepsis
Athlete's foot
Back massage
Baths
- Bag bath (towel bath)
- Bed bath (partial, complete)
- Shower (standup, shower chair)
- Sitz bath
- Tub bath

Bunions
Callus
Cerumen
Circumcised
Conduction
Convection
Corn
Cuticles
Dandruff
Debris
Dental Caries
Dental hygienist
Dentures
Dermatitis
Dermis
Distal
Effleurage
Emery board
Epidermis
Evaporation
Excoriation
Extremities
Flossing
Foot care
Foreskin
Genital
Gingivitis
Glossitis
Glycerin swabs
Grooming
Halitosis
Hard palate
Hirsutism
Integumentary
Kneading
Labia
Maceration
Matted hair
Moisturizing
Mucous membrane
Mucus
Oral hygiene
Orange stick
Outer/inner canthus
Pediculosis
Penis
Perianal area
Perineal care
Perineum
Periodontal disease
Peripheral neuropathy
Plaque
Proximal
Radiation
Scrotum

Sebaceous glands
Self-care deficit
Shampoo
Smegma
Sordes
Stomatitis
Tangles
Tartar
Toe pleat
Vasodilation

QUESTIONS

1. The nurse covers the patient with a cotton blanket during a bath. This is done to prevent heat loss via:
   1. Vasodilation
   2. Conduction
   3. Convection
   4. Diffusion

2. The nurse is planning to meet the hygiene needs of a patient. Which is the first assessment to be performed by the nurse?
   1. Determine the patient's preferences about hygiene practices
   2. Assess the patient's ability to assist in hygiene activities
   3. Collect the patient's toiletries needed for the bath
   4. Recognize the patient's developmental stage

3. The nurse gives a bed-bound patient a bed bath. The primary reason the nurse provides hygiene to this patient is to:
   1. Support a sense of well-being by increasing self-esteem
   2. Remove excess oil, perspiration, and bacteria by mechanical cleansing
   3. Promote circulation by stimulating the skin's peripheral nerve endings
   4. Exercise muscles by contraction and relaxation of muscles when bathing

4. Which human response, identified by the nurse, best supports the concern that a patient has a reduced capacity to provide for activities of daily living?
   1. Presence of joint contractures
   2. Inability to wash body parts
   3. Postoperative lethargy
   4. Visual disorders

5. The nurse is performing a physical assessment of a newly admitted patient and identifies the presence of acne. The nurse understands that acne is caused by:
   1. Dry, flaking skin
   2. An oversecretion of sebum
   3. Microorganisms on the skin
   4. Inadequate hygienic practices

6. When giving a patient a bed bath, the nurse washes the patient's extremities from distal to proximal. The nurse does this to:
   1. Decrease the chance of infection
   2. Facilitate removal of dry skin
   3. Stimulate venous return
   4. Minimize skin tears

7. During oral care the nurse softens and removes a patch of dried food and debris adhered to the hard palate of the patient's mouth. When documenting, the nurse identifies this condition as:
   1. Sordes
   2. Plaque
   3. Glossitis
   4. Stomatitis

8. The nurse teaches a patient that for brushing the teeth to be effective, it should be done:
   1. 4 times a day
   2. 6 times a day
   3. 3 times a day
   4. 2 times a day

9. The nurse is providing hygiene to a patient with peripheral neuropathy. The nurse should:
   1. Seek a physician's order for foot care
   2. File the toenails straight across the nail
   3. Wash the feet with lukewarm water and dry well
   4. Apply moisturizing lotion to the feet, especially between the toes

10. Which nursing intervention requires the nurse to consider the concept of personal space?
    1. Providing a bed bath
    2. Obtaining the vital signs
    3. Performing a health history
    4. Ambulating the patient down the hall

11. The nurse is bathing a febrile patient. The nurse should use tepid bath water to:
    1. Increase heat loss
    2. Remove surface debris
    3. Reduce surface tension of skin
    4. Stimulate peripheral circulation

12. The nurse must make the decision to give a patient a full or partial bed bath. This decision depends on the:
    1. Physician's order for the patient's activity
    2. Immediate needs of the patient
    3. Time of the patient's last bath
    4. Wishes of the patient

13. A patient has had a nasogastric tube to decompression for three days and is scheduled for intestinal surgery in the morning. The nurse understands that this patient is at the greatest risk for:
    1. Physical injury
    2. Impaired social interaction
    3. Decreased nutritional intake
    4. Altered oral mucous membranes

14. A patient is incontinent of urine and stool. For which patient response should the nurse be most concerned?
    1. Confusion
    2. Dehydration
    3. Altered sexuality
    4. Impaired skin integrity

15. The nurse is caring for a patient who wears eyeglasses. The nurse should:
    1. Encourage use of artificial tears while hospitalized
    2. Dry the glasses with a paper towel after cleaning the lenses
    3. Limit the time that glasses are worn in an effort to rest the eyes
    4. Use warm water to clean the lenses of glasses at least once a day

16. The nurse is giving a patient a bed bath. Which nursing action is most important?
    1. Lower the side rail on the working side of the bed
    2. Ensure that the bath water is at least 110°F
    3. Fold the washcloth like a mitt on the hand
    4. Raise the bed to the highest position

17. The nurse plans to give a patient a back rub. What is the best product the nurse can use for this intervention?
 1. Rubbing alcohol
 2. Betadine cream
 3. Baby powder
 4. Keri lotion

18. The nurse changes the linen of a bed while the patient sits in a chair. Which is the most important nursing action concerning this procedure?
 1. Ensuring the hem of the bottom sheet is facing the mattress
 2. Arranging the linen in the order in which it is to be used
 3. Shifting the mattress up to the headboard of the bed
 4. Checking the soiled bed linens for personal items

19. The nurse is responsible for providing hair care for a patient. To distribute oil evenly along hair shafts the nurse should:
 1. Brush from the scalp toward the hair ends
 2. Lift opened fingers through the hair
 3. Apply a conditioner to wet hair
 4. Use a fine-toothed comb

20. Which condition identified by the nurse places a person at the greatest risk for self-care toileting and elimination problems?
 1. Amputation of a foot
 2. Early dementia
 3. Fractured hip
 4. Pregnancy

21. The patient asks the nurse, "Why do I have to use mouthwash if I brush my teeth?" The nurse's best response is, "Mouthwash:
 1. Minimizes the formation of cavities."
 2. Helps reduce offensive mouth odors."
 3. Softens debris that accumulate in the mouth."
 4. Destroys pathogens that are found in the oral cavity."

22. When providing morning care for a patient, the nurse identifies crusty debris around the patient's eyes. When cleaning the patient's eyes, the nurse should:
 1. Wear sterile gloves
 2. Use a tear-free baby soap
 3. Position the client on the same side as the eye to be cleaned
 4. Wash the eyes with a cotton ball from the outer canthus to the inner canthus

23. The nurse is planning to shampoo the hair of a patient who has an order for bed rest. What should the nurse do first?
 1. Tape eye shields over both eyes
 2. Brush the hair to remove tangles
 3. Encourage the use of dry shampoo
 4. Wet hair thoroughly before applying shampoo

24. A patient has just had perineal surgery. Which type of bath should the nurse expect a physician to order for this patient?
 1. Sponge bath
 2. Tub bath
 3. Bed bath
 4. Sitz bath

25. The nurse must make an unoccupied bed. Which nursing action is most important?
 1. Position the call bell in reach
 2. Place a pull sheet on top of the draw sheet
 3. Ensure that the bottom sheet is free of wrinkles
 4. Complete one side of the bed before completing the other side

26. The nurse is evaluating a patient's oral hygiene practices. The nurse identifies that the teaching about removing dental plaque is effective when the patient:
1. Gargles with mouthwash
2. Uses an abrasive toothpaste
3. Flosses the teeth with waxed floss
4. Brushes the teeth with a toothbrush

27. The nurse is planning to assist a patient, who has impaired vision, with a bed bath. The most appropriate nursing intervention to facilitate bathing for this patient is:
1. Providing the patient with a liquid bath gel rather than a bar of soap
2. Giving the patient an adapted toothbrush to use when brushing the teeth
3. Ensuring the patient can locate bathing supplies placed on the over-bed table
4. Monitoring, through a crack in the curtain, the patient's ability to provide self-care

28. The nurse is providing for the hygiene and grooming needs of an obese patient with an activity intolerance. Which is the most important nursing intervention?
1. Maintaining the bed in a high-Fowler's position
2. Administering oxygen during provision of care
3. Providing rest periods every ten minutes
4. Assessing response to activity

29. The nurse is planning to meet the hygiene needs of a hospitalized patient who is experiencing hemiparesis because of a brain attack (cerebral vascular accident). Which is the most appropriate nursing intervention?
1. Encouraging a family member to bathe the patient
2. Providing minimal supervision during the bath
3. Giving total assistance with a complete bath
4. Assisting with the bath as needed

30. The nurse is planning to shave a male patient's facial hair. The nurse should:
1. Shave in the direction of hair growth
2. Use long, downward strokes with the razor
3. Hold the razor at a ninety-degree angle to the skin
4. Wrap the face with a hot, wet towel before shaving

31. The nurse is making an occupied bed. Which nursing action is most important?
1. Securing top linens under the foot of the mattress and mitering the corners
2. Ensuring that the patient's head is supported and is in functional alignment
3. Fan-folding soiled linens as close to the patient's body as possible
4. Positioning the bed in the horizontal position

32. The nurse must bathe the feet of a patient with diabetes. What should the nurse do before bathing this patient's feet?
1. File the nails straight across with an emery board
2. Ensure a physician's order for hygienic foot care is obtained
3. Teach the patient that daily foot care is essential to healthy feet
4. Assess for additional risk factors that may contribute to foot problems

33. The nurse is caring for a patient with an excessively dry mouth. Which nursing action is most important when providing mouth care for this patient?
1. Swabbing with a sponge-tipped applicator of lemon and glycerin
2. Cleansing four times a day with a water pick
3. Rinsing frequently with mouthwash
4. Providing oral care every two hours

34. The nurse is providing perineal care to a male patient. The nurse should wash the:
1. Genital area with hot, sudsy water
2. Scrotum before washing the glans penis
3. Shaft of the penis while moving toward the urinary meatus
4. Penis with one hand while holding it firmly with the other hand

35. The school nurse teaches an adolescent about skin care related to acne. The nurse identifies that the information is understood when the adolescent says, "I should wash my face:
 1. Every other day with a strong soap."
 2. And then apply an oil-based ointment."
 3. Thoroughly, but gently, three times a day."
 4. With cool water when I shower in the morning."

36. The nurse uses a cotton blanket when bathing a patient. A blanket is used because air currents increase the loss of heat from the body through the principle of:
 1. Osmosis
 2. Diffusion
 3. Conduction
 4. Evaporation

37. The nurse identifies that additional teaching about skin care is necessary when an older adult says, "I should:
 1. Bathe twice a week."
 2. Rinse well after using soap."
 3. Humidify my home in the winter."
 4. Use a bubble-bath preparation when I take a bath."

38. The school nurse identifies that teaching about skin care for acne has been effective when an adolescent states, "I should:
 1. Squeeze the white heads gently and apply a topical antibiotic."
 2. Wash my face several times a day with soap and water."
 3. Wash with an alcohol-based facial cleanser every day."
 4. Use an oil-based cream on my face after washing."

39. When providing fingernail care during a bath the nurse should:
 1. Push the cuticles back with the rounded end of a metal nail file
 2. Clean under the nails with an orange stick
 3. First soak the hands in hot water
 4. Cut the nails in an oval shape

40. After removing a bedpan from under a debilitated patient who has just had a bowel movement, the nurse's first intervention should be to:
 1. Document the results
 2. Provide perineal care
 3. Reposition the patient
 4. Cover the patient with the top linens

41. Which common problem with the hair should the nurse anticipate when patients are on complete bed rest?
 1. Dry hair
 2. Oily hair
 3. Split hair
 4. Matted hair

42. The nurse is helping a patient who has a right hemiparesis to get dressed. What should the nurse do?
 1. Put the right sleeve of the gown on first
 2. Keep the patient in an open-backed gown
 3. Encourage the patient to dress independently
 4. Leave the right sleeve off while adjusting the tie at the neck

43. A patient is incontinent of loose stools and is mentally impaired. What should the nurse do to help prevent skin breakdown?
 1. Wash the buttocks with strong soap and water
 2. Frequently check the rectal area for soiling
 3. Gently put a pad under the buttocks
 4. Place the call bell in easy reach

44. The nurse understands that there are actions common to both a bed bath and a tub bath. Identify all that apply.
1. _____ Helping the patient wash parts that cannot be reached
2. _____ Exposing just the part of the body being washed
3. _____ Providing for privacy throughout the bath
4. _____ Obtaining an order from the physician
5. _____ Ensuring that the call bell is in reach

45. The nurse plans to provide a patient with a partial bath. Place the steps in order in which the nurse should proceed.
1. Back
2. Face
3. Axilla
4. Both hands
5. Genital area
6. Change water

Answer: _______________

ANSWERS AND RATIONALES

1. 1. Vasodilation increases blood flow to the surface of the skin, which promotes, not prevents, heat loss.
   2. Conduction is the transfer of heat between two objects in physical contact.
   3. **Convection is the transfer of heat by movement of air along a surface. Using a bath blanket limits the amount of air flowing across the patient, which prevents heat loss.**
   4. Diffusion is the movement of molecules from a solution of higher concentration to a solution of lower concentration.

2. 1. **Hygiene is a personal matter determined by individual beliefs, values, and practices. Hygiene practices are influenced by culture, religion, environment, age, health, and personal preferences. When personal preferences are supported, the patient has a sense of control and usually is more accepting of care.**
   2. Although this information is significant in relation to the extent of self-care that may be expected, it is not the first assessment.
   3. This is done after several other considerations and just before actually beginning the bath.
   4. The patient's developmental level will influence how the nurse will proceed, but it is not the first assessment.

3. 1. Although a bath is refreshing and relaxing and may support self-esteem, this is not the primary reasons for bathing.
   2. **The removal of accumulated oil, perspiration, dead cells, and bacteria from the skin limits the environment conducive to the growth of bacteria and skin breakdown. An intact, healthy skin is one of the body's first lines of defense.**
   3. Although friction from rubbing the skin increases surface temperature, which increases circulation to the area, this is not the primary purpose of a bed bath.
   4. Although range-of-motion exercises may be performed while bathing a patient, it is not the purpose of the bath.

4. 1. Although a person may have contractures, a person may still be able to provide self-care.
   2. **Being unable to wash body parts is a human response indicating that a patient is unable to provide for one's own activities of daily living, such as meeting hygiene and grooming needs.**
   3. People who are lethargic or listless generally are still able to provide for their own basic self-care needs. However, they may require frequent rest periods or more time to complete the task.
   4. People who are legally blind are still able to provide for their own self-care needs.

5. 1. Dry skin is associated with aging, not acne. In the older adult, there is a decrease in sebaceous gland activity and tissue fluid.
   2. **During puberty the sebaceous glands, responding to the influence of androgens, enlarge and increase the production of sebum. The accumulation of sebum can become colonized by bacteria with a resulting inflammatory condition with papules and pustules (acne).**
   3. Microorganisms on the skin play a role in the development of cysts, but microorganisms are not the etiology of acne.
   4. Although inadequate hygienic practices will aggravate the condition, this is not the etiology of the condition.

6. 1. Friction, regardless of the direction of the washing strokes, in conjunction with soap and water, mechanically removes secretions, dirt, and microorganisms that decrease the potential for infection.
   2. Friction, regardless of the direction of the washing strokes, mechanically removes dry, dead skin cells.
   3. **The pressure exerted on the skin surface by long, smooth strokes moving from distal to proximal areas also presses on the veins, which promotes venous return.**
   4. Long, smooth washing strokes that avoid a shearing force, minimize skin tears.

7. 1. **The accumulation of matter, such as food, epithelial elements, dried secretions, and microorganisms (sordes) eventually can lead to dental caries and periodontal disease and therefore must be removed during oral hygiene.**
   2. Plaque is an invisible film composed of secretions, epithelial cells, leukocytes, and bacteria that adheres to the enamel surface of teeth.
   3. Glossitis is an inflammation of the tongue.

4. Stomatitis is an inflammation of the oral mucosa.

8. 1. **Brushing the teeth after each meal and at bedtime with daily flossing is recommended to stimulate the gums, clean the teeth, and flush the mouth of debris, thus preventing tooth decay and periodontal disease.**
2. Although ideal, brushing the teeth 6 times a day may be unrealistic.
3. This is not often enough to remove debris from the mouth to prevent tooth decay and periodontal disease.
4. Brushing just 2 times a day is inadequate to prevent tooth decay and periodontal disease.

9. 1. A physician's order is unnecessary because providing foot care is within the scope of nursing practice.
2. When the patient has peripheral neuropathy, this care should be provided by a podiatrist.
3. **Lukewarm water is comfortable and limits the potential for burns. Drying the feet limits moisture that promotes bacterial growth.**
4. Lotion between the toes in the dark moist environment of shoes promotes the growth of bacteria and the development of an infection.

10. 1. **Touching a patient during a bed bath invades the person's intimate space. When encroaching on a person's intimate space (physical contact to 1½ feet), the nurse should inform the patient when and why it is necessary.**
2. Although the nurse enters a patient's intimate space when obtaining vital signs, it does not usually involve touching the intimate parts of a patient's body and is therefore less intrusive than many other procedures.
3. This can be accomplished by remaining in a person's personal space (1½ to 4 feet) or social space (4 to 12 feet).
4. Although touching a patient while ambulating invades the person's intimate space it does not involve touching the intimate parts of a patient's body, and is therefore less intrusive than many other procedures.

11. 1. **Heat is transferred from the warm surface of the skin to the water that is in direct contact with the body and evaporation of the water promotes cooling. Tepid water is slightly below body temperature, and a person who is febrile has an elevated body temperature.**
2. Friction, not the temperature of the bath water, helps to remove surface debris.
3. Soap, not the temperature of the bath water, reduces surface tension of water, not the surface tension of skin.
4. Peripheral circulation is increased by warm water and by rubbing the skin with a washcloth.

12. 1. Full or partial bed baths can be administered regardless of the activity order written by the practitioner because it is an independent function of the nurse.
2. **A total patient assessment with an analysis of the data identifies the needs of the patient and the appropriate intervention to meet those needs.**
3. Time has no relevance in relation to identifying what type of bed bath to administer to a patient.
4. Although this is a consideration, patient teaching should convince a patient what should be done to meet his/her physical needs.

13. 1. Being NPO is unrelated to injury, which is the state in which an individual is at risk for harm because of a perceptual or physiologic deficit, a lack of awareness of hazards, or maturational age.
2. Being NPO is unrelated to impaired social interaction, which is the state in which an individual is at risk of experiencing negative, insufficient, or unsatisfactory responses from interactions.
3. Inadequate nutritional intake generally is not a concern. Most postoperative patients usually progress from a clear liquid to a regular diet in 2 to 3 days once bowel function returns. This is too short a time frame to be concered about inadquate nutritional intake.
4. **Not drinking anything by mouth can result in drying of the oral mucous membranes and a coated, furrowed tongue. The risk for altered oral mucous membranes applies to an individual who is NPO.**

14. 1. Although confusion may contribute to a patient experiencing incontinence, confusion is not a reaction to incontinence.
2. Incontinence is unrelated to dehydration.
3. Although incontinence may contribute to low self-esteem, which could impact on a person's sexual patterns, it is not the priority.
4. **Fecal material contains enzymes that erode the skin, and urine is an acidic fluid that macerates the skin. As a result, altered skin integrity is a serious concern.**

15. 1. This is unnecessary. Not everyone who wears eyeglasses has dry eyes.

2. A paper towel is coarse and may scratch the lenses of the eyeglasses. A soft nonabrasive cloth or chamois should be used.
3. Patient preference determines how long eyeglasses can be worn.
4. **Eyeglasses should be cleaned at least once a day because dirty lenses impair vision. Warm, not hot, water is used to prevent distortion of the lens or frame, particularly if it is made of a plastic compound.**

16. 1. Although this might be done to promote the body mechanics of the nurse, it is not a necessity.
2. **The temperature of bath water should be between 110 and 115 degrees F to promote comfort, dilate blood vessels, and prevent chilling. A lower temperature can cause chilling, and a higher temperature can cause skin trauma.**
3. Although a mitt retains water and heat and prevents loose ends from irritating the skin, it is not as essential as other factors that relate to patient safety.
4. Although the height of the bed should be adjusted to promote the nurse's body mechanics, it is not as essential as other factors that relate to patient safety.

17. 1. Rubbing alcohol causes drying of the skin and should not be used.
2. An antimicrobial cream is inappropriate for a back rub. Betadine stains, irritates, and dries the skin and eliminates the integument's natural flora.
3. Baby powder mixed with secretions of the skin forms a paste-like substance that supports antimicrobial growth and irritates the skin, which promote skin breakdown.
4. **Keri lotion lubricates the skin and reduces friction between the nurse's hands and the patient's back. Lotion facilitates smooth movement of the hands across the patient's skin, which is relaxing and prevents trauma to the skin.**

18. 1. Although it is important to provide a smooth surface, it is not the priority.
2. This is an efficient approach that permits each sheet to be accessible when needed; however, it is not a priority.
3. Although this is important to ensure that the patient is well supported when the head of the bed is elevated or the knee gatch employed, it is not the priority.
4. **A nurse must take reasonable precautions to ensure that a patient's personal belongings, especially eyeglasses, dentures, and prosthetic devices, are kept safe. Checking for personal belongings before placing soiled linen into a linen hamper is a reasonable, prudent nursing action.**

19. 1. **Brushing the hair from the scalp to the ends of the hair massages the scalp and distributes oils secreted by the scalp down along the length of the hair shaft.**
2. This will provide inadequate hair care. It might be done at the completion of hair care to style the hair.
3. Although a conditioner will make hair more supple, it will not facilitate distribution of oil along the hair shaft.
4. A fine-tooth comb has pointed ends and should not be used for daily grooming because it can injure the scalp, damage the hair shaft, and split the ends of hair.

20. 1. A patient with an amputation can still transfer to a bedside commode or ambulate with crutches to a bathroom.
2. When a person has early dementia, frequent reminders to perform self-toileting activities or declarative directions about toileting usually are adequate.
3. **Discomfort due to the proximity of the fracture to the pelvic area and the limitations placed on the positioning of, or weight bearing on, the affected leg impact on a patient's ability to use a bedpan or transfer to a commode.**
4. Although the enlarging uterus exerts pressure on the bladder causing urinary frequency and alteration of the person's center of gravity, self-toileting usually is not impaired.

21. 1. Dental caries are caused by plaque. Therefore, brushing and flossing, not the use of mouthwash, are the most efficient ways to prevent dental caries.
2. **An offensive odor to the breath (halitosis) can be caused by inadequate oral hygiene, periodontal disease, or systemic disease. Rinsing the mouth with mouthwash will flush the oral cavity of debris and microorganisms, which will reduce halitosis if it is caused by a local problem.**
3. Mouthwash flushes debris away from the teeth, it does not soften debris.
4. Only bactericidal mouthwashes can limit the amount of bacterial flora in the mouth; prolonged or excessive use can result in oral fungal infections.

22. 1. Medical, not surgical, asepsis is necessary. Clean gloves are adequate.

2. Soap is never used around the eyes. The eyes should be washed only with water.
3. **Tilting the head or turning the patient toward the same side as the eye to be washed facilitates the flow of water from the inner to the outer canthus. This limits secretions from entering the lacrimal ducts.**
4. The eye should be washed from the inner canthus to the outer canthus.

23. 1. This is unnecessary. Appropriate positioning will let the water flow by gravity away from the face, and a washcloth can be placed over the eyes.
2. **It is easier and causes less trauma to the hair to brush out tangles when the hair is dry rather then wet.**
3. Dry, powder shampoos can irritate the scalp and dry the hair.
4. Although this is done, it is not the first intervention.

24. 1. A sponge bath is given to reduce a patient's fever through heat loss via conduction and vaporization. Giving a sponge bath is an independent function of the nurse and does not require a physician's order.
2. Tub baths are effective for cleaning the skin. Tubs are used for therapeutic baths when medications are added to the water to soothe irritated skin.
3. A bed bath is indicated for patients with restricted mobility or decreased energy. Giving a bed bath is an independent function of the nurse and does not require a physician's order.
4. **A sitz bath immerses a patient from the midthighs to the iliac crests, or umbilicus, in a special tub, or the patient sits in a basin that fits onto the toilet seat, so the legs and feet remain out of the water. The moist heat to the genital area increases local circulation, cleans the skin, reduces soreness, and promotes relaxation, voiding, drainage, and healing. A sitz bath requires a physician's order because it is a method of applying local heat to the perineal area.**

25. 1. The call bell does not have to be positioned until there is a patient occupying the bed.
2. A pull sheet is not included in the procedure for an unoccupied bed. In addition, this creates too many layers of linens and wrinkles under a patient. The draw sheet can be used as a pull sheet.
3. **Wrinkles create ridges that exert additional pressure on the skin, promoting discomfort, skin irritation, and the development of pressure ulcers.**
4. Although this is advisable to conserve time and energy, it is not a priority.

26. 1. Mouthwash will not remove plaque, the forerunner to dental caries.
2. Abrasive toothpaste (dentifrice) can harm the enamel of teeth. Nonabrasive toothpaste and a soft toothbrush should be used.
3. Unwaxed floss is preferred because it is thinner, slides between the teeth more easily, and is more absorbent than waxed floss.
4. **Brushing the teeth involves several techniques: brushing back and forth strokes across the biting surface of teeth; brushing from the gum line to the crown of each tooth; and with the bristles at a 45-degree angle at the gum line vibrating the bristles while moving from under the gingival margin to the crown of each tooth.**

27. 1. Manipulating a bottle of bath gel may be more difficult than just using a bar of soap.
2. Adapted toothbrushes are intended for people who have neuromuscular problems that interfere with grasping and manipulating a toothbrush, not for people with impaired vision.
3. **Identifying the placement of supplies on the over-bed table facilitates the use of equipment by a person with impaired vision and encourages self-care.**
4. This is a violation of patient privacy. Patients have a right to know when they are being assessed.

28. 1. In the high-Fowler's position the abdominal organs press against the diaphragm in an obese patient, which limits respiratory excursion. The semi-Fowler's position is preferred.
2. Administration of oxygen is a dependent function of the nurse and requires a physician's order unless it is needed in an emergency situation. The situation in this question is not an emergency.
3. A rest period every 10 minutes may be inadequate or may unnecessarily prolong the bath. This is not individualized to the patient's needs.
4. **Evaluation of a patient's response to care allows the nurse to alter care to meet the patient's individual needs.**

29. 1. It is not the responsibility of the family to meet the physical needs of a hospitalized relative.

2. Minimal supervision may result in the completion of an inadequate bath.
3. This is unnecessary and may lower the patient's self-esteem, precipitate regression, or promote dependence.
4. **Hemiparesis is a weakness on one side of the body that can interfere with the performance of activities of daily living. Encouraging the patient to do as much as possible will support self-esteem, and assisting when necessary will ensure that hygiene needs are met.**

30. 1. **Shaving in the direction of hair growth limits skin irritation and prevents ingrown hairs.**
2. Short, firm but gentle strokes should be used when shaving a patient.
3. A safety razor should be held at a 45-, not 90-, degree angle to the skin.
4. A warm, not hot, washcloth applied to the face for several minutes before shaving helps to soften the beard.

31. 1. This will promote plantar flexion and should not be done without a toe pleat.
2. **Maintaining functional alignment of a patient's head when making an occupied bed promotes comfort and minimizes stress to the respiratory passages and vital anatomy in the neck.**
3. Although this is done, it is not the priority.
4. Although this may be done to facilitate tight sheets with minimal wrinkles, it is not the priority. In addition, there are many patients who cannot assume this position.

32. 1. A podiatrist should file or cut the toenails of a patient with diabetes. The toenails usually are thickened and hardened, and an inadvertent injury can take a long time to heal, become infected, and if gangrene occurs, can even lead to an amputation.
2. A physician's order is unnecessary. Foot care in relation to hygiene is within the scope of independent nursing practice.
3. Although this is important, it is not the priority.
4. **A thorough assessment of the patient is the first step of the nursing process. People with diabetes frequently have thick, hardened toenails, peripheral neuropathy, impaired arterial and venous circulation in the feet, and foot or leg ulcers.**

33. 1. Lemon and glycerin swabs are counterproductive because their use can lead to further dryness of the mucosa and an alteration in tooth enamel.
2. Oral hygiene 4 times a day is inadequate for a patient with a dry mouth, and a water pick is contraindicated because the force of the water can injure delicate dry mucous membranes.
3. Mouthwash contains astringents that can injure sensitive, delicate dry mucous membranes.
4. **Mouth breathing, oxygen use, unconsciousness, and debilitation, among other conditions, can lead to dry oral mucous membranes. The nurse should provide oral hygiene with saline rinses frequently to keep the oral mucosa moist.**

34. 1. Warm, not hot, water is used to clean the perineal area because the skin and mucous membranes of the genital area are sensitive, and hot water may cause harm.
2. The glans penis, foreskin, and shaft of the penis are cleaned before the scrotum. The scrotum is considered more soiled than the penis because of its proximity to the rectum.
3. When cleaning the shaft of the penis, bathing should start at the glans penis and then proceed down the shaft toward the scrotum.
4. **Stabilizing the penis and holding it firmly facilitates the bathing procedure and usually prevents an erection.**

35. 1. Strong soap may irritate fragile skin, and washing every other day is inadequate to cleanse the skin.
2. Oil-based ointments will block sebaceous gland ducts and hair follicles, which will aggravate the condition.
3. **Washing the face with soap and water 3 times a day will remove dirt and oil, which helps prevent secondary infection.**
4. Washing once a day is inadequate to cleanse the skin. Warm, not cool, water is necessary to remove the oily accumulation on the face.

36. 1. Osmosis is the movement of water across a membrane from an area of lesser concentration to an area of greater concentration.
2. Diffusion is a process whereby molecules move through a membrane from an area of higher concentration to an area of lower concentration without the expenditure of energy.
3. Conduction is the transfer of heat from one molecule to another while in direct physical contact.
4. **Evaporation (vaporization) is the transfer of heat through the conversion of water to a gas. This occurs through perspiration**

and insensible losses through the skin and lungs.

37. 1. This is an acceptable practice. Excessive exposure to warm water and soap exacerbates dry skin associated with aging.
 2. This is an acceptable practice. Soap removes the protective oils on the skin and soap residue irritates and dries the skin.
 3. A humidified environment limits the amount of insensible loss of moisture through the skin, which helps the skin retain fluid and remain supple.
 4. **Bubble-bath preparations cause irritation and dryness of the skin because they remove essential skin surface oils. Showers are preferable to baths because baths require submersion in warm water, which is detrimental to skin hydration and resiliency.**

38. 1. This is contraindicated because it can cause permanent scarring. In addition, infected material within a pustule can spread if squeezed.
 2. **This is an acceptable practice because it removes surface oils from sebaceous glands that plug pores, which aggravate the condition.**
 3. Alcohol is caustic and drying. Washing the face with soap and warm water several times a day is adequate.
 4. This is contraindicated. Oil-based creams will accumulate in pores and aggravate the condition.

39. 1. The cuticles should be pushed back with a washcloth or an orange stick.
 2. **An orange stick is an implement that is shaped to facilitate removal of debris from under the nails without causing tissue injury. Removal of dirt and debris decreases the risk of infection.**
 3. Hot water can cause tissue injury and should be avoided. Warm, not hot, water should be used.
 4. Cutting the corners of the nails can cause tissue trauma and promote the development of ingrown nails. The nails should be cut or filed straight across.

40. 1. This is done after the patient's immediate needs are met.
 2. **When rolling a debilitated patient off a bedpan the perianal area is exposed, which permits the nurse to provide immediate perineal hygiene. A bed-bound, debilitated patient is incapable of providing self-hygiene after having a bowel movement on a bedpan.**
 3. This is not the priority after removing a debilitated patient from a bedpan.
 4. The top linens should not have been removed during this procedure because they provide privacy and maintain dignity.

41. 1. Bed rest does not cause dry hair. Malnutrition, aging, and excessive shampooing cause dry hair.
 2. Bed rest does not cause oily hair. Infrequent shampooing causes oily hair.
 3. Bed rest does not cause hair to split. Excessive brushing, blow drying, and coloring cause hair to split.
 4. **Bed rest causes matted, tangled hair because of friction and pressure related to the movement of the head on a pillow.**

42. 1. **This puts less stress on weak muscles; the stronger side can stretch more easily to dress.**
 2. Although this is helpful, the nurse still needs to put the gown on without stressing the joints, tendons, muscles, and nerves of the weak arm.
 3. This may be frustrating and tiring and may cause further damage to the weak arm.
 4. This is unnecessary. The patient should be dressed appropriately.

43. 1. Strong soap can further irritate the skin.
 2. **Loose stool contains digestive enzymes that are irritating to the skin and should be cleaned from the skin as soon as possible after soiling.**
 3. This will not keep stool off the skin.
 4. The patient is mentally impaired and is unaware of needs.

44. 1. **Patients can provide self-care within their abilities. When they have limitations, such as an inability to reach a body area, an activity intolerance, a decreased level of consciousness, or dementia, it is the nurse's responsibility to assist the patient regardless of the type of bath.**
 2. This is impossible if the patient is taking a tub bath or shower.
 3. **Bathing is a private matter and an invasion of personal space. The nurse provides privacy by pulling a curtain, closing a door, and keeping the patient covered as much as possible. These interventions maintain the patient's dignity.**
 4. Providing a bed bath is within the scope of nursing practice, so a practitioner's order is unnecessary. An order is necessary for a tub bath or shower because it requires an activity order and is therefore a dependent function.

5. There is no need for a call bell when a patient is taking a tub bath or a shower because it is unsafe to leave a patient alone.

45. Answer: 2, 3, 4, 6, 1, 5

2. The bath should follow a cephalocaudal progression and based on the principle of from clean to dirty. The face is washed first before soap is place in the bath water.

3. The axilla are less soiled than the hands but are more soiled than the face.

4. The hands are more soiled than the axilla.

6. The water is changed after washing the soiled hands so as not to contaminate other areas of the body.

1. The back is less soiled than the genital area.

5. The genital area is considered the most soiled and should be washed last.

Mobility

KEYWORDS

The following words include English vocabulary, nursing/medical terminology, concepts, principles, or information relevant to content specifically addressed in the chapter or associated with topics presented in it. English dictionaries, nursing textbooks, and medical dictionaries, such as *Taber's Cyclopedic Medical Dictionary*, are resources that can be used to expand your knowledge and understanding of these words and related information.

Alignment
Ambulation
Anterior
Arthroscopy
Atrophy
Axillae
Balance
Base of support
Blanchable erythema
Body mechanics
Bones
Bony prominence
Cane
Cartilage
Contracture
Coordination
Dangle
Deep vein thrombosis
Dermis
Energy
Epidermis
Exercises
- Aerobic
- Anaerobic
- Isometric
- Isotonic

Flaccid
Foot drop
Fracture
Functional alignment
Gait
Gravity
Hemiparesis
Hemiplegia
Hip protector undergarment
Hoyer lift
Hydraulic lift
Ilium
Ischial tuberosities
Joints
Kyphosis
Lateral
Logrolling
Lordosis
Malleolus
Mechanical lift
Misalign
Mobility
Muscles
Occipital
Orthostatic hypotension
Osteoporosis
Paresis
Paraplegia
Pathological fracture
Physical conditioning
Pivot
Popliteal
Positioning devices
- Bed cradle
- Hand roll
- Hand-wrist splint
- Heel and elbow protectors
- Pillow
- Side rail
- Trapeze bar
- Trochanter roll
- Turning and pull sheet

Positions
- Contour
- Dorsal recumbent
- Fowler's (low-, semi-, high-)
- Knee-chest
- Lateral
- Lithotomy
- Orthopneic
- Prone
- Sims'
- Supine
- Trendelenburg

Posture
Pressure relief and reduction devices
- Duoderm
- Mattress overlay

- Air mattress
- Dense foam and gel
- Egg-crate mattress
- Cushions
  - Air
  - Gel
- Heel and elbow protectors
- Sheepskin
- Specialty beds

Pressure ulcer (Stages I, II, III, IV)
Proprioception
Protracted
Quadriplegia
Range-of-motion exercises
- Active
- Active-assistive
- Passive

Range-of-motion movements
- Abduction
- Adduction
- Circumduction
- Eversion
- Extension
- Flexion
  - Dorsal flexion
  - Lateral flexion
  - Plantar flexion
  - Radial flexion
  - Ulnar flexion
- Hyperextension
- Inversion
- Opposition of thumb
- Pronation
- Rotation
  - External
  - Internal
- Supination

Reactive hyperemia
Restraints
- Belt
- Chest
- Elbow
- Four-point
- Mitt
- Poncho
- Vest
- Wrist

Sacral
Scapulae
Sedentary
Shearing force
Skin integrity
Sling
Spasticity
Stability
Strength
Superior
Synovium
Tendons
Torque
Transfer
Transfer belt
Turning and positioning
Venous pooling
Zygomatic arch

QUESTIONS

1. The nurse must transfer a patient from a bed to a chair using a mechanical lift. The nurse should:
1. Ensure that there is a physician's order to move the patient with a mechanical lift
2. Hook the longer straps on the end of the sling closest to the patient's feet
3. Place a sheepskin inside the sling so that it is under the patient
4. Lead with the patient's feet when exiting the bed

2. An emaciated patient is at risk for developing a pressure ulcer. In which position should the nurse avoid placing the patient?
1. Low-Fowler's
2. Side-lying
3. Supine
4. Prone

3. A patient has been experiencing prolonged immobility because of a brain attack resulting in a coma. The nurse should monitor the patient for which local adaptation?
1. Contractures
2. Renal calculi
3. Thrombophlebitis
4. Pathological fracture

4. A patient prefers to remain in the low-Fowler's position the majority of the time. The nurse understands that the greatest potential problem associated with the low-Fowler's position is:
   1. Pressure on the ischial tuberosities of the pelvis
   2. Dorsiflexion contractures of the feet
   3. External rotation of the hips
   4. Adduction of the legs

5. The nurse is making an occupied bed. To prevent plantar flexion, the nurse should:
   1. Tuck in the top linens on just the sides of the bed
   2. Place a toe pleat in the top linens over the feet
   3. Let the top linens hang off the end of the bed
   4. Use trochanter rolls to position the feet

6. The nurse identifies that a patient's pressure ulcer has just partial-thickness skin loss involving the epidermis and dermis. The nurse documents that the patient's pressure ulcer is:
   1. Stage I
   2. Stage II
   3. Stage III
   4. Stage IV

7. Which is the most important nursing action when assisting a patient to move from a bed to a wheelchair?
   1. Applying pressure under the patient's axillae areas when standing up
   2. Lowering the bed to below the height of the patient's wheelchair
   3. Letting the patient help as much as possible when permitted
   4. Keeping the patient's feet within six inches of each other

8. The nurse places a patient in the orthopneic position. This position primarily is used to:
   1. Facilitate respirations
   2. Support hip extension
   3. Prevent pressure ulcers
   4. Promote urinary elimination

9. An immobilized bed-bound patient is placed on a 2-hour turning and positioning program. The nurse explains to the family members that this is done primarily to:
   1. Support comfort
   2. Promote elimination
   3. Maintain skin integrity
   4. Facilitate respiratory function

10. A major reason injuries occur to nurses when moving patients is because nurses:
    1. Use the longer, rather than the shorter, muscles when moving patients
    2. Place their feet wide apart when transferring patients
    3. Pull rather than push when turning patients
    4. Misalign their backs when moving patients

11. The nurse is repositioning a patient on the left side. The nurse should place the patient's:
    1. Right leg resting on top of the left leg
    2. Knees in ninety degrees of flexion
    3. Ankles in plantar flexion
    4. Left shoulder protracted

12. The nurse turns a patient's ankle so that the sole of the foot moves medially toward the midline. This motion is known as:
    1. Inversion
    2. Adduction
    3. Plantar flexion
    4. Internal rotation

13. The nurse is transferring a patient from a bed to a wheelchair. To quickly assess this patient's tolerance to the change in position, the nurse should:
 1. Obtain a blood pressure
 2. Monitor for bradycardia
 3. Determine if the patient feels dizzy
 4. Allow the patient time to adjust to the change in position

14. The nurse is transferring a patient from the bed to a wheelchair using a mechanical lift. Which is a basic nursing intervention associated with this procedure?
 1. Lock the base lever in the open position when moving the mechanical lift
 2. Raise the mechanical lift so that the patient is six inches off the mattress
 3. Keep the wheels of the mechanical lift locked throughout the procedure
 4. Ensure the patient's feet are protected when on the mechanical lift

15. A patient has hemiplegia as a result of a brain attack. Which complication of immobility is of most concern to the nurse?
 1. Dehydration
 2. Incontinence
 3. Contractures
 4. Hypertension

16. Which stage pressure ulcer requires the nurse to measure the extent of undermining?
 1. Stage 0
 2. Stage I
 3. Stage II
 4. Stage III

17. A patient has a cast from the hand to above the elbow because of a fractured ulna and radius. After the cast is removed, the nurse teaches the patient active range-of-motion exercises. The nurse identifies that further teaching is necessary when the patient:
 1. Moves the elbow to the point of resistance
 2. Keeps the elbow flexed after the procedure
 3. Assesses the elbows response after the procedure
 4. Puts the elbow through its full range at least three times

18. Which word is most closely associated with nursing care strategies to maintain functional alignment when patients are bed bound?
 1. Endurance
 2. Strength
 3. Support
 4. Balance

19. The nurse places a patient with a sacral pressure ulcer in the left Sims' position. The nurse should place the patient's right arm:
 1. On a pillow
 2. Behind the back
 3. With the palm up
 4. In internal rotation

20. A patient with impaired mobility is to be discharged within a week from the hospital. Which is the best example of a discharge goal for this patient? The patient will:
 1. Understand range-of-motion exercises
 2. Be taught range-of-motion exercises
 3. Transfer independently to a chair
 4. Be kept clean and dry

21. The nurse concludes that a patient has the potential for impaired mobility. Which assessment reflects a risk factor that precipitated this conclusion?
 1. Exertional fatigue
 2. Sedentary lifestyle
 3. Limited range of motion
 4. Increased respiratory rate

22. The nurse is performing passive range-of-motion exercises for a patient who is in the supine position. Which motion occurs when the nurse bends the patient's ankle so that the toes are pointed toward the ceiling?
1. Supination
2. Adduction
3. Dorsal flexion
4. Plantar extension

23. The nurse is caring for a patient with impaired mobility. Which position contributes most to the formation of a hip flexion contracture?
1. Low Fowler's
2. Orthopneic
3. Supine
4. Sims'

24. A patient is diagnosed with a stage IV pressure ulcer with eschar. Which medical treatment should the nurse anticipate the physician will order for this patient?
1. Heat lamp treatment three times a day
2. Application of a topical antibiotic
3. Cleansing irrigations twice daily
4. Débridement of the wound

25. The nurse knows that raising a patient's arm over the head during range-of-motion exercises is called:
1. Flexion
2. Supination
3. Opposition
4. Hyperextension

26. A patient with a history of thrombophlebitis should not have pressure exerted on the popliteal space. The nurse should avoid placing this patient in which position?
1. Prone
2. Supine
3. Contour
4. Trendelenburg

27. The nurse plans to teach a patient with hemiparesis to use a cane. The nurse should teach the patient to:
1. Move up a step with the weak leg first followed by the strong leg and cane
2. Adjust the cane height twelve inches lower than the waist
3. Hold the cane in the strong hand when walking
4. Look at the feet when walking

28. The nurse is caring for a variety of patients, each experiencing one of the following problems. Which health problem places a patient at the greatest risk for complications associated with immobility?
1. Quadriplegia
2. Incontinence
3. Hemiparesis
4. Confusion

29. Older adults often are afraid of falling. The nurse understands that the most common consequence associated with this concern is:
1. Impaired skin integrity
2. Occurrence of panic attacks
3. Self-imposed social isolation
4. Decreased physical conditioning

30. The nurse is evaluating an ambulating patient's balance. It is most important that the nurse assess the patient's:
1. Posture
2. Strength
3. Energy level
4. Respiratory rate

31. The nurse is planning to help move a patient up in bed. Strain to the nurse can be reduced when the nurse:
1. Moves the patient up against gravity
2. Uses the large muscles of the legs
3. Keeps the knees locked
4. Bends from the waist

32. A patient with an order for bed rest has diaphoresis. What should the nurse use to best limit the negative effects of perspiration on dependent skin surfaces of this patient?
1. Ventilated heel protectors
2. Air-filled rings
3. Air mattress
4. Sheepskin

33. The nurse understands that the primary reason why immobilized people develop contractures is that:
1. Muscles that flex, adduct, and internally rotate are stronger than weaker opposing muscles
2. Muscular contractures occur because of excessive muscle flaccidity
3. Muscle mass and strength decline at a progressive rate weekly
4. Muscle catabolism exceeds muscle anabolism

34. When the nurse turns the palm of a patient's hand downward when performing range-of-motion exercises, it is known as:
1. External rotation
2. Circumduction
3. Lateral flexion
4. Pronation

35. Which nursing action is most effective in relation to the concept *Immobility can lead to occlusion of blood vessels in areas where bony prominences rest on a mattress?*
1. Encouraging the patient to breathe deeply 10 times per hour
2. Performing range-of-motion exercises twice a day
3. Placing a sheepskin pad under the sacrum
4. Repositioning the patient every 2 hours

36. A patient sits for excessive lengths of time in a wheelchair. Which sites should the nurse assess for skin breakdown in this patient?
1. Ischial tuberosities
2. Bilateral scapulae
3. Trochanters
4. Malleoli

37. The nurse plans to use a trochanter roll when repositioning a patient. The nurse should place the trochanter roll:
1. Under the small of the back
2. Behind the knees when supine
3. Alongside the ilium to midthigh
4. In the palm of the hand with the fingers flexed

38. Which is the earliest nursing assessment that indicates permanent damage to tissues because of compression of soft tissue between a bony prominence and a mattress?
1. Nonblanchable erythema
2. Circumoral cyanosis
3. Tissue necrosis
4. Skin abrasion

39. Nurses should monitor for which systemic adaptations in immobilized patients? Check all that apply.

1. _____ Plantar flexion contracture
2. _____ Hypostatic pneumonia
3. _____ Dependent edema
4. _____ Muscle atrophy
5. _____ Pressure ulcer

40. The nurse moves a patient's leg through range of motion demonstrated in the figure. This joint movement is known as:

1. Eversion
2. Circumduction
3. Plantar flexion
4. External rotation

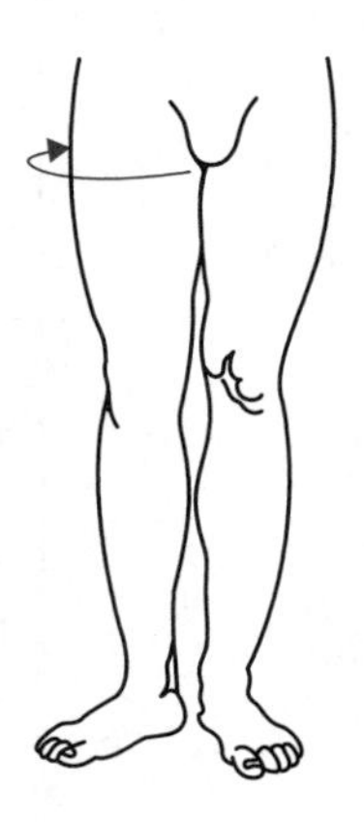

ANSWERS AND RATIONALES

1. 1. Moving patients with a mechanical lift is within the scope of nursing practice and a practitioner's order is unnecessary.
   2. **The longer straps/chains go in the holes for the seat support, which keep the legs and pelvis below the upper body. Appropriate placement of the upper and lower straps/chains creates a bucket seat in which a patient is moved safely.**
   3. This could result in the patient's sliding down and out of the sling during the transfer. Nylon, net, or canvas slings are available.
   4. It does not matter whether the feet or the head exit the bed first as long as functional alignment and safety are maintained.

2. 1. Although in the low-Fowler's position the sacral area is at risk for pressure, the muscles and adipose tissue in the buttocks do provide some protection compared with other vulnerable areas of the body.
   2. **In the side-lying position, the majority of the body weight is borne by the greater trochanter. The bone is close to the surface of the skin, with minimal overlying protective tissue.**
   3. In the supine position the occiput, scapulae, spine, elbows, sacrum, and heels are at risk for pressure; however, the body weight is distributed more evenly than in some other positions.
   4. In the prone position the ears, cheeks, acromion process, anterior superior spinous process, knees, toes, male genitalia, and female breasts are at risk for pressure; however, the body weight is distributed more evenly than in some other positions.

3. 1. **A contracture is a localized response to immobility. When muscle fibers are not able to shorten or lengthen, eventually a permanent shortening of the muscles, and subsequently, of the tendons and ligaments occurs.**
   2. Demineralization of bone is a systemic response to immobility. Without the stress of weight-bearing activity, the bones begin to demineralize and the urine becomes more alkaline. Calcium salts precipitate out as crystals to form calculi.
   3. Thrombophlebitis results from the systemic responses of impaired venous return and hypercoagulability in conjunction with injury to a vessel wall.
   4. Immobility can cause the systemic response of demineralization of bone (disuse osteoporosis) that eventually can result in bone fractures.

4. 1. **In the low-Fowler's position, the majority of the body's weight is borne by portions of the pelvis: bony protuberances of the lower portion of the ischium (ischial tuberosities) and the triangular bone at the dorsal part of the pelvis (sacrum).**
   2. Plantar flexion contractures (foot drop), not dorsiflexion contractures, can occur in the low-Fowler's position.
   3. This is more likely to occur in the supine, rather than the low-Fowler's, position.
   4. Abduction, rather than adduction, of the legs is more likely to occur in the low-Fowler's position.

5. 1. Top sheets tucked in along the sides of the bed still exert pressure on the upper surface of the feet, which may promote plantar flexion. The sides of top sheets, mitered at the foot of the bed, hang feely off the side of the bed.
   2. **Making a vertical or horizontal toe pleat at the foot of the bed over the patient's feet leaves room for the feet to move freely and avoids exerting pressure on the upper surface of the feet, thus minimizing plantar flexion.**
   3. The weight of the top sheets still exerts pressure on the upper surface of the feet, promoting plantar flexion.
   4. Trochanter rolls prevent external hip rotation, not plantar flexion.

6. 1. In a Stage I pressure ulcer the skin is still intact and presents clinically as reactive hyperemia.
   2. **In a Stage II pressure ulcer the partial-thickness skin loss presents clinically as an abrasion, blister, or shallow crater.**
   3. In a Stage III pressure ulcer there is full-thickness skin loss involving the subcutaneous tissue that may extend to the underlying fascia. The ulcer presents clinically as a deep crater with or without undermining.
   4. In a Stage IV pressure ulcer there is full-thickness skin loss with extensive destruction, tissue necrosis, or damage to muscle, bone or supporting structures.

7. 1. This should be avoided because it can injure nerves and blood vessels.

2. The bed should be higher, not lower, than the wheelchair so that gravity can facilitate the transfer.
3. Encouraging the patient to be as self-sufficient as possible ensures that the transfer is conducted at his/her pace, promotes self-esteem, and decreases the physical effort expended by the nurse.
4. This will provide a narrow base of support and is unsafe.

8. 1. Sitting in the high-Fowler's position and leaning forward allows the abdominal organs to drop by gravity, which promotes contraction of the diaphragm. The arms resting on an over-bed table increases thoracic excursion.
2. The hips will be in extreme flexion, not extension.
3. Pressure ulcers can still occur on the ischial tuberosities.
4. Standing by men and sitting on a toilet/commode by women are superior to any bed position for promoting urinary elimination.

9. 1. Although turning the patient to a new position every 2 hours provides variety and increased comfort, these are not the primary reasons for this intervention.
2. Although turning frequently promotes elimination, the upright positions, such as high-Fowler's and sitting, have a greater influence on elimination because of the effect of gravity.
3. Compression of soft tissue greater than 32 mm Hg prevents capillary circulation and compromises tissue oxygenation in the compressed area. Turning the patient relieves the compression of tissue in dependent areas, particularly those tissues overlying bony prominences.
4. Although turning and positioning promotes respiratory functioning, other interventions, such as sitting, deep breathing, coughing, and incentive spirometry, have a greater influence on respiratory status.

10. 1. Nurses should use the longer, stronger muscles of the thighs and buttocks when moving patients to protect their weaker back and arm muscles.
2. Nurses should have a wide base of support when moving patients to provide better stability.
3. Nurses should use a pulling motion to turn patients because the muscles that flex, rather than extend, the arm are stronger and pulling, rather than pushing, creates less friction and therefore less effort.
4. Misaligning the back when moving patients occurs most often when not facing the direction of the move. Twisting (rotation) of the thoracolumbar spine and flexion of the back place the line of gravity outside the base of support, which can cause muscle strain and disabling injuries.

11. 1. The right leg should be supported on a pillow in front of the left leg.
2. This excessive flexion can result in flexion contractures of the hip and knee if left in this position extensively.
3. The ankles should be maintained at 90 degrees.
4. In the left lateral (side-lying) position, the left arm is positioned in front of the body with the shoulder protracted. This reduces the pressure on the joint in the shoulder and the acromial process.

12. 1. Inversion, a gliding movement of the foot, occurs by turning the sole of the foot medially toward the midline of the body.
2. Adduction occurs when an arm or leg moves toward and/or beyond the midline of the body.
3. Plantar flexion occurs when the joint of the ankle is in extension by pointing the toes of the foot downward and away from the anterior portion of the lower leg.
4. Internal rotation of a leg occurs by turning the foot and leg inward so that the toes point toward the other leg.

13. 1. Although a blood pressure reading may indicate the presence of hypotension, the blood pressure should be obtained before and after a transfer to allow a comparison to conclude that the hypotension is orthostatic hypotension.
2. If the patient is experiencing orthostatic hypotension, the heart rate will increase, not decrease.
3. Feeling dizzy is a subjective adaptation to orthostatic hypotension. Obtaining feedback from the patient provides a quick evaluation of the patient's response to the transfer.
4. This is not an assessment. This is a safe intervention for a patient who is experiencing orthostatic hypotension.

14. 1. The width of the base depends on the configuration of the bed, objects in the room, and the ultimate destination. The base usually is locked open when lifting or lowering the patient and locked closed when moving the lift.

2. This is unsafe. The lift should raise the patient high enough to clear the surface of the bed.
3. The wheels must be unlocked to move the lift from under the bed to its ultimate destination.
4. **The legs dangle from the sling and therefore may drag across the linens or hit other objects if not protected.**

15. 1. Dehydration is not an adaptation to immobility.
2. The decreased tone of the urinary bladder and the inability to assume the usual voiding position in bed promotes urinary retention, rather than urinary incontinence.
3. **Contractures result from permanent shortening of muscles, tendons, and ligaments. Contractures are irreversible without surgical intervention.**
4. With immobility, the increased heart rate reduces the diastolic pressure. In addition, there is a decrease in blood pressure related to postural changes from lying to sitting or standing (orthostatic hypotension). This situation is manageable with a priority on maintaining patient safety.

16. 1. There is no Stage 0 in the classification system for staging pressure ulcers.
2. The skin is still intact and there is no undermining in a Stage I pressure ulcer.
3. Tissue damage is superficial and there is no undermining in a Stage II pressure ulcer.
4. **In a Stage III pressure ulcer there is full-thickness skin loss involving damage to subcutaneous tissue that may extend to the fascia and there may or may not be undermining, which is tissue destruction underneath intact skin along wound margins.**

17. 1. This is desirable. Performing range of motion beyond resistance may injure muscles and joints and should be avoided.
2. **This is undesirable because it contributes to a flexion contracture. Functional alignment is preferred because it minimizes stress and strain on muscles and joints.**
3. Response to range of motion must be evaluated and compared with the assessment performed before the procedure.
4. Sequential contraction of muscles tends to be more efficient in facilitating full range of motion.

18. 1. Endurance relates to aerobic exercise that improves the body's capacity to consume oxygen for producing energy at the cellular level.
2. Strength relates to isometric and isotonic exercises, which contract muscles and promote their development.
3. **The line of gravity passes through the center of gravity when the body is correctly aligned; this results in the least amount of stress on the muscles, joints, and soft tissues. Bed-bound patients often need assistive devices such as pillows, sandbags, bed cradles, wedges, rolls, and splints to support and maintain the vertebral column and extremities in functional alignment.**
4. Balance relates to body mechanics and is achieved through a wide base of support and a lowered center of gravity.

19. 1. **In the left Sims' position the patient's right arm and leg are supported on pillows to prevent internal rotation of the shoulder and hip.**
2. The right arm is positioned in front of, not behind, the back.
3. The right hand is positioned in pronation, not supination.
4. The right arm is positioned to maintain the shoulder in functional alignment, not internal, rotation.

20. 1. This goal is not measurable as stated. Understanding is not measurable unless parameters are identified.
2. This is a nursing intervention, not a patient goal.
3. **This is a patient-centered goal and measurable.**
4. This is a nursing intervention, not a patient goal.

21. 1. This is associated with activity intolerance. People who are fatigued are still able to move.
2. This is a contributing factor for activity intolerance. People who are sedentary are still able to move.
3. **Limited range of motion is associated with contracture formation and impaired mobility.**
4. An increased respiratory rate is an adaptation to activity, not impaired mobility.

22. 1. Supination occurs when the hand and forearm rotate so that the palm of the hand is facing upward.
2. Adduction occurs when an arm or leg moves toward and/or beyond the midline of the body.
3. **Dorsal flexion (dorsiflexion) of the joint of the ankle occurs when the toes of the foot point upward and backward toward the anterior portion of the lower leg.**

4. There is no range of motion called plantar extension. Plantar flexion occurs when the joint of the ankle is in extension by pointing the toes of the foot downward and away from the anterior portion of the lower leg.

23. 1. In the low-Fowler's position the hips are slightly flexed.
2. While in the high-Fowler's position the patient is then positioned leaning forward with arms resting on an over-bed table. In this orthopneic position, the hips are extensively flexed creating an angle less than 90 degrees.
3. In the supine position, the hips are extended (180 degrees), not flexed.
4. In the Sims' position, the hip and knee of the upper leg are just slightly flexed.

24. 1. Heat lamp treatments will further dry out the wound and can cause burns.
2. Topical antibiotics are used only when the ulcer is infected, not to treat eschar.
3. Cleansing irrigations are ineffective in removing the thick, fibrin-containing cells of eschar covering the surface of the wound.
4. Thick, leather-like, necrotic devitalized tissue (eschar) must be removed surgically or enzymatically before wound healing can occur.

25. 1. The shoulder, a ball-and-socket joint, flexes by raising the arm from a position by the side of the body forward and upward to a position beside the head.
2. Supination occurs when the hand and forearm rotate so that the palm of the hand is facing upward.
3. Opposition is the touching of the thumb of the hand to each fingertip of the same hand.
4. Hyperextension of the arm occurs by moving an arm from a resting position at the side of the body to a position behind the body.

26. 1. In the prone position, there is pressure in front of, not behind, the knees.
2. In the supine position, the hips and legs are extended, which does not exert pressure on the popliteal spaces.
3. In the contour position, the head of the bed and the knee gatch are slightly elevated. The elevated knee gatch puts pressure on the popliteal spaces.
4. In the Trendelenburg position, the hips and knees are extended, which does not exert pressure on the popliteal spaces.

27. 1. The unaffected leg should be advanced first because the weight of the body is lifted to the next step on the leg with the greatest strength.
2. With the tip of the cane placed 6 inches lateral to the foot, the handle should be at the level of the patient's greater trochanter to ensure that the elbow will be flexed 15 to 30 degrees when using the cane.
3. A cane is a hand-gripped assistive device; therefore, the hand opposite the hemiparesis should hold the cane. Exercises can strengthen the flexor and extensor muscles of the arms and the muscles that dorsiflex the wrist.
4. This will cause flexion of the neck, hips, or waist that will move the center of gravity outside the line of gravity. Proper body alignment is essential for balance, stability, and safe ambulation.

28. 1. Quadriplegia, paralysis of all four extremities, places the patient at greatest risk for pressure ulcers because the patient has no ability to shift the body weight off of bony prominences or change position without total assistance.
2. Patients who are incontinent are not necessarily immobile.
3. Hemiparesis, muscle weakness on one side of the body, does not prevent a person from shifting or changing position to relieve pressure on the skin.
4. Confused patients can move independently when uncomfortable or when encouraged and assisted to move by the nurse.

29. 1. A person who chooses not to ambulate still has the ability to assume many different sitting or lying-down positions.
2. This is not the most common consequence. Anxiety and ultimately panic that is precipitated by a situation can be prevented by avoiding the situation.
3. A person who chooses not to ambulate still can socialize.
4. Most falls occur when ambulating. Fear of falling results in the conscious choice not to place oneself in a position where a fall can occur. Disuse and muscle wasting cause a reduction of muscle strength at the rate of 5 to 10 percent per week so that within 2 months of immobility more than 50 percent of a muscle's strength can be lost. In addition, there is a decreased cardiac reserve. These adaptations result in decreased physical conditioning.

30. 1. Assessing posture will identify whether the patient's center of gravity is in the midline from the middle of the forehead to a midpoint between the feet and, therefore,

balanced within the patient's base of support.
2. Strength has more to do with the exertion of power, not balance.
3. Energy has more to do with endurance, not balance.
4. Assessing the respiratory rate before activity establishes a baseline against which to compare the respiratory rate after activity to determine tolerance for activity, not balance.

31. 1. Muscle strain is reduced when moving patients with gravity, not with the added effort needed to move patients against gravity.
2. To exert an upward lift the gluteal and leg muscles should be used, rather than the sacrospinal muscles of the back. These larger muscles fatigue less quickly, and their use protects the intervertebral disks.
3. The muscles of the legs are used inefficiently when the knees are kept locked. This increases the strain on the other muscles being used.
4. Bending from the waist increases the strain on the sacrospinal muscles and intervertebral disks.

32. 1. This protects only the heels, not the other dependent areas of the body.
2. Air-filled rings usually are made of plastic, which tends to promote sweating. Air rings rarely are used because they are designed for just the sacral area and often they increase, not decrease, pressure.
3. Air mattresses usually are made of plastic, which tends to promote sweating.
4. The soft tuffs of sheepskin allow air to circulate, thereby promoting the evaporation of moisture that can precipitate skin breakdown.

33. 1. The state of balance between muscles that serve to contract in opposite directions is impaired with immobility. The fibers of the stronger muscles contract for longer periods than do those of the weaker, opposing muscles. This results in a change in the loose connective tissue to a more dense connective tissue and to fibrotic changes that limit range of motion.
2. Contractures occur because of muscle spasticity and shortening, not muscle flaccidity.
3. Disuse and muscle wasting cause a reduction in muscle strength at the rate of 5 to 10 percent a week so that within 2 months more than 50 percent of a muscle's strength can be lost. This results in muscle atrophy, not contractures.
4. This is unrelated to contractures. In unused muscles, catabolism exceeds anabolism, and the muscles decrease in size (disuse atrophy).

34. 1. External rotation of the shoulder, a ball-and-socket joint, occurs when the upper arm is held parallel to the floor, the elbow is at a 90-degree angle, and the fingers are pointing toward the floor and the person moves the arm upward so that the fingers point toward the ceiling.
2. Circumduction of the shoulder, a ball-and-socket joint, occurs when an extended arm moves forward, up, back, and down in a full circle.
3. Lateral flexion of the hand occurs with both abduction (radial flexion) and adduction (ulnar flexion). With the hand supinated, radial flexion occurs by bending the wrist laterally toward the thumb and ulnar flexion occurs by bending the wrist laterally toward the fifth finger.
4. Pronation of the hand occurs by rotating the hand and arm so that the palm of the hand is facing down toward the floor.

35. 1. Deep breathing prevents atelectasis and hypostatic pneumonia, not pressure ulcers.
2. Range-of-motion exercises help prevent contractures, not pressure ulcers.
3. Although sheepskin reduces friction and limits pressure, its main purpose is to allow air to circulate under the patient to minimize moisture and maceration of skin.
4. Turning a patient relieves pressure on the capillary beds of the dependent areas of the body, particularly the skin overlying bony prominences, which reestablishes blood flow to the area.

36. 1. When in the sitting position, the hips and knees are flexed at 90 degrees and the body's weight is borne by the pelvis, particularly the ischial tuberosities, which are bony protuberances of the lower portion of the ischium. Using a wheelchair results in prolonged sitting unless interventions are implemented to promote local circulation.
2. Pressure to the scapulae occurs in all back-lying positions, such as the supine and Fowler's positions.
3. Pressure to a trochanter occurs in a side-lying, not the sitting, position.
4. Pressure to the malleolus (medial and lateral) of the ankle occurs in a side-lying, not a sitting, position.

37. 1. This is unsafe. A trochanter roll placed in the small of the back is uncomfortable and produces an excessive lumbar curvature.

2. This is contraindicated because it places unnecessary pressure on the popliteal area.
3. **A trochanter roll is a rolled wedge, pillow, or sandbag placed by the lateral aspect of the leg between the iliac crest and knees to prevent external hip rotation.**
4. The diameter of a trochanter roll is too wide to maintain the hand in functional alignment.

38. 1. **Nonblanchable erythema refers to erythema of intact skin that persists when finger pressure is applied. This is the classic sign of a Stage I pressure ulcer.**
2. Circumoral cyanosis is associated with hypoxia, not pressure ulcers.
3. With necrosis, death of cells has occurred. Necrosis occurs in Stage III and Stage IV pressure ulcers.
4. With an abrasion, the superficial layers of the skin are scraped away. This Stage II, not Stage I, pressure ulcer appears reddened and may exhibit localized serous weeping or bleeding.

39. 1. Plantar flexion contracture (foot drop) is a localized response to prolonged extension of the ankle.
2. Static respiratory secretions provide an excellent media for bacterial growth that can result in hypostatic pneumonia, which is a localized response to immobility.
3. **Decreased calf muscle activity and pressure of the bed on the legs allow blood to accumulate in the distal veins. The resulting increased hydrostatic pressure moves fluid out of the intravascular compartment into the interstitial compartment, causing edema.**
4. **Atrophy is a decrease in the size of a tissue or an organ as a result of inactivity or decreased finction. After 24 to 36 hours of inactivity, muscles begin to lose their contractile strength and begin the process of atrophy.**
5. Prolonged pressure on skin over a bony prominence interferes with capillary blood flow to the skin, which ultimately can result in the localized response of a pressure ulcer.

40. 1. Eversion, a gliding movement of the foot, occurs by turning the sole of the foot away from the midline of the body.
2. Circumduction is a range of motion that is performed with a ball and socket joint. It occurs when an extended extremity moves forward, up, back, and down in a full circle.
3. Plantar flexion occurs when the joint of the ankle is in extension by pointing the toes of the foot downward and away from the anterior portion of the lower leg.
4. **External rotation occurs when the entire leg is rolled outward from the body so that the toes point away from the other leg.**

Nutrition

KEYWORDS

The following words include English vocabulary, nursing/medical terminology, concepts, principles, or information relevant to content specifically addressed in the chapter or associated with topics presented in it. English dictionaries, nursing textbooks, and medical dictionaries such as *Taber's Cyclopedic Medical Dictionary* are resources that can be used to expand your knowledge and understanding of these words and related information.

Alcohol abuse
Amino acids
  Essential
  Nonessential
Anabolism
Anorexia
Anorexia nervosa
Anthropometric measurements
Atherosclerosis
Basal metabolism
Bolus
Cachexia, cachectic
Calorie, kilocalorie
Calorie count
Catabolism
Cholesterol
Cirrhosis of the liver
Creatinine excretion
Dairy foods
Decaffeinated
Dental caries
Diabetes mellitus
Digestion
Dysphagia
Emulsify
Energy
Enteral
Fiber
Fluoride
Food consistency
  Chopped
  Liquid
  Pureed
  Regular
  Soft
Fortified
Gastroesophageal reflux disease (GERD)
Hemoglobin
Hyperglycemia
Hypoglycemia
Ideal body weight
Ingestion
Insoluble fiber
Iron deficiency
Ketones
Ketosis
Lactulose intolerant
Legumes
Lipids
Malnutrition
Mastication
Metabolic
Morbid obesity
Mottling of teeth
My Pyramid
Nausea
Nutrients
  Carbohydrates
  Fats
  Minerals
    Fluoride
    Iodine
    Iron
    Potassium
    Sodium
  Protein
    Complete
    Incomplete
  Water
Obesity
Overweight
Passover
Recommended dietary allowances
Serum albumin
Soluble fiber
Stomatitis
Supplements
Swallowing impairment
Synthesis
Tetany
Therapeutic diets
  Clear liquid
  Full liquid
  2-gm sodium

Low residue
Mechanical soft
Protein restricted
Total cholesterol
Transferrin level
Triglycerides
Tube feedings
Continuous
Enteral
Gastrostomy
Intermittent
Jejunostomy
Nasogastric
Underweight
Vegan
Vitamins
Fat soluble (A, D, E, K)
Water soluble
C (ascorbic acid)
B_1 (thiamine)
B_2 (riboflavin)
B_3 (niacin)
B_6 (pyridoxine)
B_{12} (cobalamin)
Biotin
Folic Acid
Pantothenic acid
Vomiting
Water-soluble fiber

QUESTIONS

1. The practitioner orders a clear liquid diet for a patient. Which food should the nurse teach the patient to avoid when following this diet?
1. Strawberry Jell-O
2. Decaffeinated tea
3. Strong coffee
4. Ice cream

2. The nurse is caring for a patient who is expending energy that is greater than the caloric intake. Which human response most likely will occur?
1. Fever
2. Anorexia
3. Malnutrition
4. Hypertension

3. The nurse teaches a postoperative patient about foods high in protein that will promote wound healing. The nurse identifies that the teaching is successful when from a list of foods the patient selects:
1. Milk
2. Meat
3. Bread
4. Vegetables

4. Which nutrient should the nurse encourage a patient to include in the diet to provide vitamin D?
1. Green leafy vegetables
2. Vegetable oils
3. Fortified milk
4. Organ meats

5. The nurse is reviewing the laboratory findings of a patient to assess the patient's nutritional status. The nurse understands that the laboratory finding that is the best indicator of inadequate protein intake is a:
1. High hemoglobin
2. Low serum albumin
3. Low specific gravity
4. High blood urea nitrogen

6. A patient of Asian heritage is recommended to follow a low-fat diet to lose weight. The nurse understands that a food low in fat that generally is consumed by members of an Asian population is:
   1. Egg rolls
   2. Spareribs
   3. Crispy noodles
   4. Hot and sour soup

7. A patient is scheduled for surgery and the nurse is teaching the patient about the importance of vitamin C in wound healing. Which source of vitamin C should the nurse include in the teaching plan?
   1. Potatoes
   2. Yogurt
   3. Beans
   4. Milk

8. The nurse is teaching a patient about the importance of balancing protein, carbohydrates, and fats in the diet. The nurse identifies that the teaching about carbohydrates is understood when the patient states, "Carbohydrates are best known for providing:
   1. Electrolytes."
   2. Vitamins."
   3. Minerals."
   4. Energy."

9. A patient has been blind in one eye for several years because of the complications associated with diabetes mellitus. The patient is admitted to the hospital with a detached retina and resulting loss of sight in the other eye. What should the nurse do to assist this patient with meals?
   1. Feed the patient
   2. Order finger foods that are permitted on the patient's diet
   3. Encourage eating one food at a time according to the preference of the patient
   4. Explain to the patient where items are located on the plate according to the hours of a clock

10. The nurse understands that the balance of calcium in the body is unrelated to:
    1. Osteoporosis
    2. Vitamin D
    3. Tetany
    4. Iron

11. A patient is admitted to the hospital with a history of liver dysfunction associated with hepatitis. The nurse understands that this patient may have problems with:
    1. Emulsifying fats
    2. Digesting carbohydrates
    3. Manufacturing red blood cells
    4. Reabsorbing water in the intestines

12. The nurse is assessing a patient who is admitted to the hospital with withdrawal from alcohol. The nurse knows that excessive alcohol intake directly contributes to health problems because it:
    1. Lengthens passage time of stool through the intestinal tract
    2. Decreases the absorption of many important nutrients
    3. Accelerates the absorption of medications
    4. Interferes with the absorption of glucose

13. An obese resident of a nursing home who is receiving a 1500-calorie weight reduction diet has not lost weight in the past 2 weeks. The nurse should:
    1. Inform the primary care physician of the patient's lack of progress
    2. Instruct the patient to limit intake to 1000 calories per day
    3. Schedule a multidisciplinary team conference
    4. Keep a log of the oral intake for 3 days

14. A patient with a Latino heritage is to eat a low-fat diet. The patient tells the nurse, "I am going to have a hard time giving up my favorite family recipes." Which food should the nurse recommend that is low in fat and generally is included in the Latino culture?
1. Salsa
2. Pasta
3. Steamed fish
4. Refried beans

15. A patient is diagnosed with a vitamin A deficiency. Which food should the nurse encourage the patient to ingest?
1. Blueberry pie
2. Pumpkin pie
3. Cherry pie
4. Pecan pie

16. A patient is anorexic because of stomatitis related to chemotherapy. When planning care for this patient, the nurse should be most concerned about:
1. Aspiration
2. Dehydration
3. Malnutrition
4. Constipation

17. A patient is diagnosed with osteoporosis. The nurse understands that the vitamin most commonly associated with weak bones is:
1. D
2. K
3. B
4. E

18. The patient has a decreased hemoglobin because of a low intake of dietary iron. The nurse should teach the patient that the food that is the best source of iron is:
1. Eggs
2. Fruit
3. Meat
4. Bread

19. The physician orders a low-residue diet. Which food should the nurse teach the patient to include in the diet?
1. Scrambled eggs
2. Orange juice
3. Green beans
4. Rye bread

20. An older adult is admitted to the hospital for multiple health problems. Assessment reveals that the patient has no teeth and is having difficulty eating. The nurse should encourage the physician to order which diet for this patient?
1. Liquid supplements
2. Mechanical soft
3. Pureed
4. Soft

21. The nurse teaches a patient about the prescribed low-fat diet. The nurse evaluates that the teaching is understood when the patient selects from a list which food low in fat?
1. Eggs
2. Liver
3. Cheese
4. Chicken

22. The nurse is caring for patients with a variety of nutrition-related problems. Which problem eventually may require the patient to have a nasogastric feeding tube inserted?
1. Malabsorption syndrome
2. Difficulty swallowing
3. Nausea and vomiting
4. Stomatitis

23. A patient is to have a test with contrast that contains iodine. To prevent erroneous results, the nurse teaches the patient to avoid which food?
1. Grapefruit
2. Salmon
3. Grains
4. Beans

24. A patient is confused and disoriented. An excellent food for the nurse to select for this patient is chicken:
1. Soup
2. Salad
3. Fingers
4. Casserole

25. The patient has a high-serum cholesterol level. What food should the nurse teach the patient to avoid?
1. Egg yolks
2. Skim milk
3. Turkey burger
4. Sliced bologna

26. An older adult tends to bruise easily and the physician recommends that the patient eat foods high in vitamin K. In addition to teaching the patient about foods sources of vitamin K, the nurse teaches the patient that the nutrient that must be ingested for vitamin K to be absorbed is:
1. Carbohydrates
2. Starches
3. Proteins
4. Fats

27. The school nurse is preparing a health class about vitamins. Which information about vitamins that is based on a scientific principle should the nurse include?
1. Eating a variety of foods prevents the need for supplements
2. Megadoses of vitamins have proven to be most effective in preventing illness
3. Taking a prescribed vitamin supplement is the best way to ensure adequate intake
4. Vitamins from more expensive manufacturers are more pure than those from cheaper companies

28. The nurse understands that which situation results in ketosis in a healthy person?
1. Inadequate intake of carbohydrates
2. Increased intake of protein
3. Excessive intake of starch
4. Decreased intake of fiber

29. The nurse teaches a patient that fat in the diet is unnecessary to absorb:
1. Vitamin C
2. Vitamin A
3. Vitamin E
4. Vitamin D

DAKE

30. An occupational nurse is facilitating a weight reduction group discussion. The nurse understands that the most common contributing factor of obesity is a(n):
1. Sedentary lifestyle
2. Low metabolic rate
3. Hormonal imbalance
4. Excessive caloric intake

31. A patient has multiple fractures from a skiing accident. To best facilitate bone growth the nurse should encourage the patient to eat more foods high in calcium. The nurse identifies that the patient understands the teaching when from a list of foods the patient selects:
   1. Orange juice
   2. Peanut butter
   3. Cottage cheese
   4. Baked flounder

32. When the nurse evaluates the effectiveness of a nutritional program, which is the best short-term indicator of an improved nutritional status?
   1. Weight gain of two pounds daily
   2. Increasing transferrin level
   3. Decreasing serum albumin
   4. Appropriate skin turgor

33. A patient is diagnosed with iron deficiency anemia. The nurse understands that the major cause of iron deficiency is:
   1. Metabolic problems
   2. Inadequate diets
   3. Malabsorption
   4. Hemorrhage

34. When collecting data about a patient, which nursing assessment best reflects a healthy behavior?
   1. Eating foods low in fat
   2. Visiting a physician when ill
   3. Displaying no signs of illness
   4. Wanting to lose twenty pounds

35. The nurse understands that a human response commonly resulting from a fluoride deficiency is:
   1. Stomatitis
   2. Dental caries
   3. Bleeding gums
   4. Mottling of the teeth

36. The nurse identifies that a vegetarian understands the importance of eating kidney beans when the patient says, "Kidney beans are essential because they are a great source of:
   1. Carbohydrates."
   2. Minerals."
   3. Protein."
   4. Fats."

37. The most common independent nursing intervention to help hospitalized older adults maintain body weight is:
   1. Making meal time a social activity
   2. Taking a thorough nutritional history
   3. Providing assistance with the intake of meals
   4. Encouraging dietary supplements between meals

38. It is most significant for the nurse to teach a low-cholesterol diet to an adult female whose total cholesterol level is:
   1. 200 milligrams per deciliter
   2. 190 milligrams per deciliter
   3. 150 milligrams per deciliter
   4. 100 milligrams per deciliter

39. An older adult is admitted to the hospital with a diagnosis of congestive heart failure, malnutrition, and macrocytic anemia. In addition to other medications, the physician orders folic acid 0.8 mg p.o. once daily. A strip of unit dose tablets of 0.4 mg/tablet is sent to the unit from the hospital pharmacy. How many tablets should the nurse administer?
Answer:____________ Tablets.

40. A patient is admitted to the hospital with a diagnosis of alcoholism. The physician orders thiamine hydrochloride (vitamin B_1) 50 mg IM t.i.d. The drug is supplied 100 mg/mL. How much solution should the nurse administer?
Answer:____________ mL.

ANSWERS AND RATIONALES

1. 1. Jell-O is a clear liquid that is a solid when refrigerated and a liquid at room temperature. It is permitted in either form on a clear liquid diet.
   2. Caffeinated or decaffeinated tea is permitted on a clear liquid diet.
   3. Weak or strong and caffeinated or decaffeinated coffee is permitted on a clear liquid diet.
   4. **Milk and milk products are not included on a clear liquid diet. Ice cream contains a high-solute load, including fat and proteins, which stimulates the digestive process.**

2. 1. During the states of malnutrition and starvation, the basal metabolic rate (BMR) decreases because the lean body mass decreases. Fever is associated with an increased, not decreased, BMR.
   2. When energy expended is greater than the caloric intake an individual will experience hunger, not anorexia. Hunger is a dull or acute pain felt around the epigastric area caused by a lack of food. Anorexia is the loss or lack of appetite.
   3. **When energy expenditure exceeds caloric intake, eventually body fat and muscle mass breaks down to supply the fuel needed for metabolism. Malnutrition results when the body's cells have a deficiency or excess of one or more nutrients.**
   4. When a person is malnourished, eventually the serum protein will be low, which may result in a decreased colloid osmotic pressure and then to the movement of fluid from the intravascular compartment into the peritoneal cavity. When the circulating blood volume decreases, the blood pressure decreases, not increases.

3. 1. One cup of milk contains only 8 grams of protein.
   2. **Food from animal sources (meat, poultry, fish, eggs, and cheese) provides complete proteins and, therefore, are the best sources of protein. Three ounces of meat or poultry contain approximately 19 to 25 grams of protein depending on the type of meat or poultry.**
   3. Although a serving of a grain product contains approximately 2 grams of protein, it primarily provides carbohydrates and fiber.
   4. The majority of vegetables provide only 1 to 3 grams of protein.

4. 1. Green leafy vegetables are an excellent source of vitamin K, not D.
   2. Vegetable oils are an excellent source of vitamin E, not D.
   3. **Not many foods contain vitamin D; therefore, it should be supplemented with fortified food, such as milk. One quart of fortified milk contains the Recommended Daily Allowance (RDA) of vitamin D for children.**
   4. Liver is an excellent source of vitamin K, not D.

5. 1. Hemoglobin concentration of the blood correlates closely with the red blood cell count. Elevated hemoglobin suggests hemoconcentration from increased numbers of red blood cells (polycythemia) or dehydration.
   2. **Serum proteins, particularly albumin, reflect a person's skeletal muscle and visceral protein status. An expected serum albumin level ranges between 3.5 and 5.0 g/dL. Mild depletion ranges between 2.8 and 3.4 g/dL. Moderate depletion ranges between 2.1 and 2.7 g/dL. Severe depletion is less than 2.1 g/dL.**
   3. Specific gravity is a urine test that measures the kidney's ability to concentrate urine. A low specific gravity reflects dilute urine that suggests a high urine volume, diabetes insipidus, kidney infections, or severe renal damage with disturbances in concentrating and diluting abilities.
   4. Blood urea nitrogen (BUN) measures the nitrogen fraction of urea, a product of protein metabolism. An elevated BUN suggests renal disease, reduced renal perfusion, urinary tract obstruction, and increased protein metabolism.

6. 1. Egg rolls are a fried food. Frying involves cooking food in a solution consisting of saturated or unsaturated fat, which is composed mostly of fatty acids. Fatty acids combine with glycerol to form triglycerides.
   2. Spareribs are high in saturated fat and cooked with sauces that are high in saturated or unsaturated fat.
   3. Crispy noodles are a fried food that should be avoided. Frying involves cooking food with a saturated or unsaturated fat solution, which is composed mostly of fatty acids. Fatty foods on a low-fat diet should be eaten raw or cooked by broiling, baking, or boiling.

4. **Hot and sour soup contains less fat than the other food choices listed.**

7. 1. **Potatoes are an excellent source of vitamin C (ascorbic acid). One ½-pound potato contains approximately 26 mg of vitamin C.**
   2. Eight ounces of yogurt contains only 1 mg of vitamin C.
   3. Dry beans (legumes) contain no vitamin C. One cup of green beans contains only 12 mg of vitamin C.
   4. One cup of milk contains only 2 mg of vitamin C.

8. 1. An electrolyte is a chemical substance that, in solution, dissociates into electrically charged particles. Electrolytes maintain the chemical balance between cations and anions in the body, which is essential for acid-base balance.
   2. Vitamins are organic compounds that do not provide energy, but are needed for the metabolism of energy.
   3. Minerals are inorganic elements or compounds essential for regulating body functions. The major minerals of the body are calcium, phosphorus, sodium, potassium, magnesium, chloride, and sulfur.
   4. **Carbohydrates, a group of organic compounds, such as saccharides, starch, cellulose, and gum, are the main fuel sources for energy. Athletes competing in endurance events often adhere to a diet that increases carbohydrates to 70% of the diet for the last three days before a race (carbohydrate loading) to maximize muscle glycogen storage.**

9. 1. This does not promote independence and may precipitate feelings of low self-esteem.
   2. This is unnecessary and limits the patient's food choices.
   3. This is unnecessary and may decrease the patient's appetite.
   4. **The clock system, which identifies where certain foods are on a plate in relation to where numbers are located on a clock, allows the patient to be independent when eating. Independence with activities of daily living supports self-esteem.**

10. 1. Osteoporosis is a disease characterized by a decrease in total bone mass and deterioration of bone tissue that leads to bone fragility and the risk of fractures. Adequate calcium is necessary for building and strengthening bones and preventing osteoporosis.
    2. Vitamin D promotes bone mineralization by producing transport proteins that bind calcium and phosphorus. This increases intestinal absorption, stimulates the kidneys to return calcium to the bloodstream, and stimulates bone cells to use calcium and phosphorus to build and maintain bone tissue.
    3. A decrease in calcium in the blood (hypocalcemia) can eventually lead to tetany, which is characterized by muscle spasms, paresthesias, and convulsions.
    4. **Iron is unrelated to calcium balance. Iron is essential for hemoglobin formation.**

11. 1. **Bile is produced and concentrated in the liver and stored in the gallbladder. As fat enters the duodenum, it precipitates the release of cholecystokinin, which stimulates the gallbladder to release bile. Bile, an emulsifier, enlarges the surface area of fat particles so that enzymes can digest the fat.**
    2. The liver is not involved with carbohydrate digestion. Ptyalin (secreted by the parotid glands), amylase (secreted by the pancreas), and sucrase, lactase, and maltase (secreted by the walls of the small intestine) digest carbohydrates.
    3. The liver is not involved with red blood cell production. People who are deficient in iron and protein have difficulty with red blood cell production.
    4. The large intestine, not the liver, is involved with reabsorbing water. The majority of the water in chyme is reabsorbed in the first half of the colon, leaving the remainder (approximately 100 mL) to form and eliminate feces.

12. 1. Alcohol increases intestinal motility so that it decreases, not increases, the length of time it takes intestinal contents to pass through the body.
    2. **Alcohol interferes with vitamin intake, absorption, metabolism, and excretion. It specifically interferes with the absorption of vitamins A, D, K, thiamin, folic acid, pyridoxine, and B_{12}.**
    3. The damaging effects of alcohol decrease, not increase, the efficiency of the process of absorption of medications in the stomach and intestines. However, alcohol can potentiate the action of drugs, such as central nervous system depressants.
    4. Alcohol interferes with the absorption of thiamin, which is essential to oxidize, not absorb, glucose.

13. 1. This is premature. The nurse is abdicating the responsibility to help the patient.

2. A change in diet requires a practitioner's order. Generally, calories should not be restricted below 1200 cal/day for women or 1500 cal/day for men so that there are adequate amounts of essential nutrients.
3. This may eventually be done, but it is premature at this time.
4. **When the expected outcome of an intervention is not attained, the situation must be reassessed to determine the problem and the plan changed appropriately. A record of a dietary intake provides complete objective information about the amounts and types of food consumed. This information provides data about nutrient deficiencies or excesses, eating patterns, behaviors associated with eating, and potential problems and needs.**

14. 1. **Salsa predominantly contains the vegetables: tomatoes, onions, and peppers, all which are low in fat.**
2. Pasta contains predominantly carbohydrates, not fat. In addition, in the Latino culture, rice and beans are preferred over pasta. Pasta is associated with the Italian culture.
3. Although steamed fish is low in fat, foods in the Latino culture are generally stewed or fried. Vegetables, legumes, and meat usually are preferred over fish.
4. Refried beans are a fried food that should be avoided on a low-fat diet. Frying involves cooking food with a saturated or unsaturated fat solution, which is composed mostly of fatty acids. Fatty acids combine with glycerol to form triglycerides.

15. 1. One piece of blueberry pie contains only 14 µgRE (Retinol Equivalents) of vitamin A.
2. **Pumpkin is an excellent source of vitamin A. One piece (1/6 of a 9-inch diameter pie) contains 3750 µgRE (Retinol Equivalents) of vitamin A.**
3. One piece of cherry pie contains only 70 µgRE of vitamin A.
4. One piece of pecan pie contains only 115 µgRE of vitamin A.

16. 1. Although in some patients stomatitis may cause difficulty with swallowing (dysphagia), which may contribute to aspiration, a bland diet soft in consistency will help to minimize dysphagia.
2. Fluids promote a softer stool and activity increases peristalsis. Ingesting adequate amounts of fluid generally is not a problem as long as acidic fluids are avoided because they irritate the lesions of the mucous membranes.
3. **Stomatitis, inflammation of the mucous membranes of the oral cavity, can be painful. Patients with stomatitis frequently avoid eating to limit discomfort, which can lead to inadequate nutritional intake and malnutrition.**
4. Although a loss of appetite may contribute to constipation, an increase in fluid intake and activity can help prevent constipation.

17. 1. **Vitamin D (also regarded as a hormone) promotes bone mineralization by producing transport proteins that bind calcium and phosphorus, which increases intestinal absorption, stimulates the kidneys to return calcium to the bloodstream, and stimulates bone cells to use calcium and phosphorus to build and maintain bone tissue.**
2. Vitamin K promotes blood clotting by increasing the synthesis of prothrombin by the liver; it does not promote strong bones.
3. The B-complex vitamins are related to protein synthesis and cross-linking of collagen fibers, which are essential for integrity of the integumentary system, not to strong bones.
4. Vitamin E prevents the oxidation of unsaturated fatty acids and thereby prevents cell damage; it does not promote strong bones.

18. 1. One egg contains only 1.0 mg of iron.
2. One serving of fruit contains less than 1.0 mg of iron.
3. **Meat, especially liver, is an excellent source of iron. Three ounces of meat contains approximately 1.6 to 5.3 mg of iron depending on the type of meat and whether it is a regular or lean cut.**
4. One slice of bread contains approximately 0.7 to 1.4 mg of iron depending on the type of bread.

19. 1. **All eggs, except fried, are permitted on a low-residue diet. A low-residue diet is easily digested and absorbed and limits bulk in the intestines after digestion.**
2. Orange and grapefruit juice contain pulp, a soluble fiber, which is not permitted on a low-residue diet.
3. Green beans contain polysaccharides that provide structure to plants and result in a residual after digestion that is not permitted on a low-residue diet. One cup of green beans contains 4.19 grams of dietary fiber.
4. Whole-grain breads, breads with seeds or nuts, and bread made with bran consist of insoluble fibers that are not permitted on a low-residue diet.

20. 1. A person with few, or no teeth, should be able to meet all daily nutrient requirements without liquid supplements.
 2. A mechanical soft diet is modified only in texture. It includes moist foods that require minimal chewing and eliminates most raw fruits and vegetables and foods containing seeds, nuts, and dried fruit.
 3. A person with few, or no teeth, can handle a more substantial diet than pureed foods. A pureed diet is a soft diet processed to a semisolid consistency.
 4. A person with few, or no teeth, can handle a more substantial diet than a soft diet. A soft diet is moderately low in fiber and lightly seasoned. A soft diet usually is ordered for patients who are unable to tolerate a regular diet after surgery as a transition between liquids and a regular diet.

21. 1. Eggs should be avoided on a low-fat diet. One egg contains 1.7 grams of saturated fat.
 2. Liver should be avoided on a low-fat diet. Three ounces of liver contain 2.5 grams of saturated fat.
 3. Cheese should be avoided on a low-fat diet. Depending on the cheese, one ounce contains approximately 4.4 to 6.2 grams of saturated fat.
 4. Chicken is permitted on a low-fat diet. Three ounces of chicken contains 0.9 gram of saturated fat. A low-fat food should contain less than 1 gram of saturated fat per serving.

22. 1. This is not an appropriate therapy for a patient with malabsorption syndrome. A gastrostomy tube permits a formula to be instilled into the stomach, which then progresses to the small intestine where absorption takes place. Depending on the etiology, it can cause gastrointestinal irritation, increased intestinal motility, diarrhea, and dehydration.
 2. Difficulty swallowing (dysphagia) that does not respond to dysphagia diets (mechanical soft, soft, blended or pureed liquids) may need the insertion of a gastrostomy tube so that formula feedings can be administered to meet nutritional needs and minimize the risk of aspiration.
 3. Gastric tube feedings are contraindicated in the presence of vomiting because of the potential for aspiration. The cause of the nausea and vomiting should be identified and treated.
 4. This is a drastic measure for stomatitis. Stomatitis, an inflammation of the mouth, usually is a temporary problem that responds to pharmacologic therapy and frequent, appropriate oral hygiene.

23. 1. Grapefruit does not contain iodine. Grapefruit is a source of vitamin C (ascorbic acid) and potassium.
 2. Foods naturally high in iodine include saltwater fish, shellfish, and seaweed because they are derived from seawater.
 3. Although some grains contain iodine because of iodated dough conditioners, they are not a rich source. Grains provide carbohydrates and fiber.
 4. The iodine in plant sources, such as beans, depends on the mineral content of the soil in which they are grown, and are not rich sources of iodine.

24. 1. A confused patient may not know how to manipulate the spoon to eat the soup. This may result in spillage and frustration.
 2. Eating chicken salad requires the use of a utensil that may be beyond the patient's cognitive ability.
 3. This is a single food item that usually is familiar to most people in the United States. A single familiar food is an easier symbol to decode cognitively than food mixed together on a plate or in a casserole. In addition, the fingers, rather than a utensil, can handle a piece of chicken.
 4. Eating a casserole requires the use of a utensil that may be beyond the patient's ability. In addition, food mixed together is more confusing than food that is presented individually.

25. **1. Egg yolks are high in cholesterol and should be avoided by people with high cholesterol. One egg yolk contains 272 mg of cholesterol.**
 2. One cup of skim milk contains only 18 mg of cholesterol.
 3. Three ounces of turkey contain only 45 mg of cholesterol.
 4. Two slices of bologna contain only 31 mg of cholesterol.

26. 1. Carbohydrates are not necessary for the absorption of vitamin K.
 2. Starch is not necessary for the absorption of vitamin K.
 3. Proteins are not necessary for the absorption of vitamin K.
 4. Vitamin K is one of the fat-soluble vitamins (A, D, E, and K) that are absorbed with fat in chylomicrons, which enter the lymphatic system before circulating in the

bloodstream. Vitamin K plays an essential role in the production of the clotting factors II (prothrombin), VII, IX, and X.

27. **1. A balanced diet with choices in moderation from a variety of foods will provide the recommended daily allowances of essential nutrients without the need for supplements.**
    2. Megadoses of vitamins no longer operate as nutritional agents and excesses are detrimental to the body, particularly to the liver and brain.
    3. Vitamins by themselves will not ensure an adequate intake. Their action contributes to chemical reactions (i.e., they act as catalysts), and they must have their substrate material to work on, which are carbohydrates, protein, and fats and their metabolites.
    4. This may or may not be true.

28. **1. When the amount of carbohydrates ingested does not meet the energy requirements of an individual, the body will break down stored fat to meet its energy needs. Ketone bodies are produced during the oxidation of fatty acids.**
    2. An increased intake of protein helps meet energy demands because when the energy from carbohydrates is depleted, the body converts protein and fatty acids to glucose (gluconeogenesis).
    3. Starch is the major source of carbohydrates in the diet and it yields simple sugars on digestion.
    4. Fiber is unrelated to ketosis.

29. **1. Vitamin C (ascorbic acid) is a water-soluble vitamin. The presence of fat or bile salts are unnecessary for its absorption.**
    2. Vitamin A is a fat-soluble vitamin that requires fat and bile salts to be absorbed.
    3. Vitamin E is a fat-soluble vitamin that requires fat and bile salts to be absorbed.
    4. Vitamin D is a fat-soluble vitamin that requires fat and bile salts to be absorbed.

30. 1. This is only one theory associated with the cause of obesity.
    2. This is only one theory associated with the cause of obesity.
    3. This is only one theory associated with the cause of obesity.
    4. This is the basis of all weight gain regardless of the etiology. Excess ingested nutrients are stored in adipose tissue (fat) and muscle, which increases body weight. Obesity is body weight 20% or greater than ideal body weight. Glucose is stored as glycogen in the liver and muscle with surplus amounts being converted to fat. Glycerol and fatty acids are stored as triglycerides in adipose tissue. Excess amino acids are used for glucose formation or are stored as fat.

31. 1. One cup of orange juice contains only 27 mg of calcium.
    2. One tablespoon of peanut butter contains only 5 mg of calcium.
    3. Cottage cheese has the highest amount of calcium of all the options and is an excellent source of calcium, which is essential for bone growth. One cup of cottage cheese contains 155 mg of calcium. The NIH Consensus Conference—Optimal Calcium Intake recommends an average intake of 1000 to 1500 mg of calcium daily for an adult depending on various factors.
    4. Three ounces of baked flounder contains only 13 mg of calcium.

32. 1. A rapid weight gain indicates fluid retention, not nutritional status. One liter of fluid weighs 2.2 pounds.
    2. Serum transferrin is a marker for protein status. Because its half-life is 8 days compared with albumin, which is 20 days, serum transferrin levels will provide earlier objective information concerning a person's increasing or decreasing nutritional status.
    3. A decreasing serum albumin indicates a deteriorating, not improving, nutritional status. A serum albumin level should range between 3.5 and 5.0 g/dL. Mild depletion values range between 2.8 and 3.4 g/dL. Moderate depletion values range between 2.1 and 2.7 g/dL. In severe depletion, values are less than 2.1 g/dL.
    4. Appropriate skin turgor, fullness, and elasticity that allow the skin to spring back to its previous state after being pinched reflect an adequate fluid, not nutritional, balance.

33. 1. Although the inability to form hemoglobin in the absence of other necessary factors, such as vitamin B_{12} (pernicious anemia), can result in iron deficiency, it is not the major cause of iron deficiency.
    2. The most common nutrient deficiency in the United States is iron deficiency caused by an inadequate supply of dietary iron. The major condition indicating iron deficiency is anemia.
    3. Malabsorption of iron is not the major cause of iron deficiency, although a lack of

gastric hydrochloric acid necessary to help liberate iron for absorption and the presence of phosphate or phytate, inhibitors of iron absorption, all can precipitate malabsorption of iron.

4. Although hemorrhage can precipitate iron deficiency, it is not the major etiologic factor.

34. 1. **Eating foods low in fat is a healthy behavior because it is an action that promotes a healthy lifestyle. Implementing health-promotion behaviors is based on the perceived benefits of the actions.**
2. This is a behavior, but it is in response to an illness, not associated with the promotion of health and the prevention of illness.
3. This is one aspect of a person's health status.
4. This reflects cognition, not behavior.

35. 1. Stomatitis, inflammation of the mucous membranes of the mouth, is most often caused by infectious sources (herpes simplex virus, *Candida albicans*, and hemolytic streptococci) or chemotherapy, not fluoride deficiency.
2. **Fluroide strengthens the ability of the tooth structure to withstand the erosive effects of bacterial acids on the teeth. The recommended daily intake of fluoride for adults is 1.5 to 4.0 mg.**
3. Bleeding gums is caused by inflammation of the gums (gingivitis), not fluoride deficiency.
4. This is not specifically caused by fluoride deficiency. Yellow, brown, or black discoloration may indicate problems, such as staining, a partial or total nonviable nerve, or tetracycline administration during the prenatal period or early childhood.

36. 1. Although kidney beans are an excellent source of carbohydrates, a vegetarian diet has many other foods that can be selected to provide this nutrient.
2. Although kidney beans are an excellent source of minerals, especially sodium, potassium, and phosphorus, a vegetarian diet has many other foods that can be selected to provide this nutrient.
3. **Kidney beans are high in protein. One cup of kidney beans contains 15 grams of protein. Complete proteins come from animal sources, such as meat, poultry, and fish, but they are not included on a vegetarian diet. Kidney beans combined with a grain are a substitute for a complete protein.**
4. One cup of kidney beans contains only 1 gram of fat.

37. 1. Although this is desirable, it may be impractical or impossible in an acute-care facility. Patient rooms may be private or semiprivate, which limits exposure to other patients, and patients often are too sick to socialize.
2. Although this can be done, the information will not necessarily improve intake.
3. **Sick older adults often are debilitated, lack energy, and do not feel well. Assistance with meals conserves the patient's energy and demonstrates a caring concern, which may increase the intake of food.**
4. This is a dependent function of the nurse and requires a practitioner's order.

38. 1. **A total cholesterol level of 200 mg/dL in a woman is on the high side of the acceptable range. A total cholesterol level should be ≤ 200 mg/dL. Patients should be taught the foods to avoid that are high in cholesterol to prevent excessive cholesterol levels.**
2. 190 mg/dL is an acceptable level of cholesterol for an adult woman.
3. 150 mg/dL is an acceptable level of cholesterol for an adult woman.
4. 100 mg/dL is an acceptable level of cholesterol for an adult woman.

39. Answer: 2 Tablets. Solve the problem by using ratio and proportion.

$$\frac{\text{Desire}}{\text{Have}} \quad \frac{0.8\text{ mg}}{0.4\text{ mg}} = \frac{x\text{ Tab}}{1\text{ Tab}}$$

$$0.4x = 0.8$$
$$x = 0.8 \div 0.4$$
$$x = 2\text{ Tablets}$$

40. Answer: 0.5 mL. Solve the problem by using ratio and proportion.

$$\frac{\text{Desire}}{\text{Have}} \quad \frac{50\text{ mg}}{100\text{ mg}} = \frac{x\text{ mL}}{1\text{ mL}}$$

$$100x = 50$$
$$x = 50 \div 100$$
$$x = 0.5\text{ mL}$$

Oxygenation

KEYWORDS

The following words include English vocabulary, nursing/medical terminology, concepts, principles, or information relevant to content specifically addressed in the chapter or associated with topics presented in it. English dictionaries, nursing textbooks, and medical dictionaries, such as *Taber's Cyclopedic Medical Dictionary*, are resources that can be used to expand your knowledge and understanding of these words and related information.

Abdominal thrusts
Accessory muscles of respiration
Activity intolerance
Aerosol therapy
Airway clearance
Airway obstruction
Airway resistance
Alveoli
Apical
Arterial blood gases
Artificial airway
Aspiration
Asthma
Atelectasis
Auscultation
Blood coagulability
Breathing, types of
  Abdominal
  Apnea
  Bradypnea
  Deep
  Diaphragmatic
  Pursed-lip
  Tachypnea
  Thoracic
Breath sounds
  Adventitious
    Crackles (rales)
    Gurgles (rhonchi)
    Pleural friction rub
    Stridor
    Wheezes
  Normal
    Bronchial
    Bronchovesicular
    Vesicular
Bronchial spasm
Bronchoscopy
Capillary refill
Cardiac output
Cardiac workload
Cardiopulmonary resuscitation
Cardiovascular
Chest physiotherapy
Chest tube
Chest x-ray
Choking
Chronic bronchitis
Cilia
Circumoral cyanosis
Cough
  Nonproductive
  Productive
Cyanosis
Diffusion
Dyspnea
Dysrhythmias
Electrocardiogram
Endotracheal tube
Excursion
Exertion
Exhale
Expectorate
Expiration
Extubation
Fatigue
Heimlich maneuver
Hemoglobin saturation
Hemoptysis
Hemorrhage
Humidify
Hypercapnia
Hypertension/hypotension
Hyperventilation/hypoventilation
Hypostatic pneumonia
Hypovolemic shock
Hypoxemia
Hypoxia
Incentive spirometer
Inhale
Inspiration
Intrathoracic pressure

Intubation
Iron deficiency anemia
Laryngeal spasm
Liquefy
Metered-dose inhaler (MDI)
Mucous membranes
Mucus
Nares
Nasal prongs
Nebulizer
Oral/nasal pharyngeal airway
Oropharynx
Orthopnea
Orthostatic hypotension
Oxygen delivery systems
  Face mask
  Nasal cannula
  Nonrebreather mask
  Venturi mask
Oxygen gauge
Oxygen liter flow
Oxygen saturation
Oxygen therapy
Pallor
Palpable
Patency
Patent
Percussion
Peripheral pulses
Pneumothorax
Positive pressure ventilation
Postural drainage
Postural hypotension
Pulmonary embolus
Pulmonary function tests
Pulse oximetry
Secretions
Sedentary
Sputum
Sternum
Suctioning
  Nasal
  Oropharyngeal
  Tracheal
Systemic
Tenacious secretions
Thoracentesis
Thoracotomy
Thoracic
Thrombophlebitis
Tidal volume
Tissue perfusion
Tracheostomy
Valsalva's maneuver
Vasoconstriction
Vasodilation
Ventilation
Ventilators
Vibration
Viscous secretions
Vital capacity
Xiphoid process

QUESTIONS

1. The nurse is assessing a patient with a respiratory problem. Which is most reflective of an early adaptation to hypoxia?
1. Apnea
2. Cyanosis
3. Restlessness
4. Dysrhythmias

2. The nurse in the Post-Anesthesia Care Unit is monitoring several patients who received general anesthesia. Which patient adaptation causes the most concern?
1. Pain
2. Stridor
3. Lethargy
4. Diaphoresis

3. When administering oxygen via a wall-outlet system, the nursing action that is unnecessary for a low liter flow as opposed to a high liter flow is:
1. Attaching a flowmeter to the wall outlet
2. Providing oral hygiene whenever necessary
3. Hanging an *Oxygen in Use* sign outside the patient's room
4. Humidifying the oxygen before it is delivered to the patient

4. The nurse is teaching a patient how to use an incentive spirometer. The nurse should assist the patient to assume which position?
   1. Sitting
   2. Side-lying
   3. Orthopneic
   4. Low-Fowler's

5. Which is the most important action by the nurse after a patient has a thoracotomy?
   1. Ensure the patient's intake is at least 3000 mL of fluid per 24 hours
   2. Provide the patient with adequate medication for pain relief
   3. Maintain the integrity of the patient's chest tube
   4. Reposition the patient every 2 hours

6. The nurse is assessing a postoperative patient. Which complication has most likely occurred when the patient experiences purulent sputum, dyspnea, and chest pain?
   1. Hypostatic pneumonia
   2. Hypovolemic shock
   3. Thrombophlebitis
   4. Pneumothorax

7. An obese patient has limited mobility after an open reduction and internal fixation of a fractured hip. The nurse should monitor this patient for the most serious complication of increased blood coagulability precipitated by immobility which is:
   1. Muscle atrophy
   2. Pain in the calf
   3. Hypotension
   4. Bradypnea

8. When assessing a patient, which adaptation indicates the presence of respiratory distress?
   1. Rate of fourteen breaths per minute
   2. Productive cough
   3. Sore throat
   4. Orthopnea

9. When attempting to apply a pulse oximetry probe, the nurse identifies that a patient's hands are edematous. The priority action should be to:
   1. Attach the probe to one of the patient's toes
   2. Connect the probe to one of the patient's earlobes
   3. Wash the patient's hand before attaching the probe to the finger
   4. Encourage the patient to perform active range-of-motion exercises of the hand

10. The practitioner's order reads, "6 L Oxygen Via Face Mask." The patient, who has been extremely confused since being in the unfamiliar environment of the hospital, becomes agitated and repeatedly pulls off the mask. The nurse should:
    1. Tighten the strap around the head
    2. Reapply the mask every time the patient pulls it off
    3. Provide an explanation of why the oxygen is necessary
    4. Request that the order for oxygen be changed to a nasal cannula

11. The nurse teaches a patient how to use an incentive spirometer. The nurse understands that the most appropriate expected outcome associated with the use of an incentive spirometer is:
    1. Coughing will be stimulated
    2. Sputum will be expectorated
    3. Inspiratory volume will be increased
    4. Supplemental oxygen use will be reduced

12. When applying a warm compress, the nurse explains to the patient that the primary reason heat is used instead of cold is that heat:
    1. Minimizes muscle spasms
    2. Prevents hemorrhage
    3. Increases circulation
    4. Reduces discomfort

13. The physician orders chest physiotherapy with percussion and vibration for a newly admitted patient. The nurse should question this order when, during the admission assessment, the patient informs the nurse of a history of:
    1. Emphysema
    2. Osteoporosis
    3. Cystic fibrosis
    4. Chronic bronchitis

14. The nurse teaches a patient about pursed-lip breathing. The nurse identifies that the teaching is effective when the patient says its purpose is to:
    1. Precipitate coughing
    2. Help maintain open airways
    3. Decrease intrathoracic pressure
    4. Facilitate expectoration of mucus

15. What should the nurse do first if a patient is choking on food?
    1. Sweep the patient's mouth with a finger
    2. Hit the middle of the patient's back firmly
    3. Determine if the patient can make any verbal sounds
    4. Apply sharp upward thrusts over the patient's xiphoid process

16. A patient has thick tenacious respiratory secretions. To best help liquefy the patient's respiratory secretions, the nurse should:
    1. Change the patient's position every two hours
    2. Encourage the patient to drink more fluid
    3. Obtain an order for an antitussive agent
    4. Teach effective deep breathing

17. Which action is most effective in meeting the needs of a patient experiencing laryngospasm after extubation?
    1. Ensuring hyperextension of the head
    2. Providing positive pressure ventilation
    3. Instituting cardiopulmonary resuscitation
    4. Administering oxygen by using a face mask

18. A patient's hemoglobin saturation via pulse oximetry indicates inadequate oxygenation. What should the nurse do first?
    1. Administer oxygen at three liters per minute
    2. Encourage deep breathing
    3. Raise the head of the bed
    4. Call the physician

19. The nurse is reviewing the laboratory results of a patient with the preliminary diagnosis of anemia. Which diagnostic test reflects an adaptation to iron deficiency anemia?
    1. Hemoglobin
    2. Platelet count
    3. Serum albumin
    4. Blood urea nitrogen

20. The nurse understands that the physiological factor that places the older adult at the greatest risk during surgery is a decrease in:
    1. Skin elasticity
    2. Bladder emptying
    3. Tolerance for pain
    4. Respiratory excursion

21. A patient is admitted with the diagnosis of peripheral arterial disease. Which is a specific desirable outcome for a patient with this diagnosis?
1. Respirations within the expected range
2. Oriented to the environment
3. Palpable peripheral pulses
4. Prolonged capillary refill

22. The physician orders bed rest for a patient. The nurse understands that bed rest primarily is used to:
1. Conserve energy
2. Maintain strength
3. Reduce peristalsis
4. Enhance protein synthesis

23. The major difference between pursed-lip breathing and diaphragmatic breathing is with diaphragmatic breathing the patient:
1. Inhales through the mouth
2. Exhales through pursed lips
3. Raises both shoulders while breathing deeply
4. Tightens the abdominal muscles while exhaling

24. A meal tray arrives for a patient who is receiving 24% oxygen via a Venturi mask. To meet this patient's needs, the nurse should:
1. Request an order to use a nasal cannula during meals
2. Discontinue the oxygen when the patient is eating meals
3. Obtain an order to change the mask to a nonrebreather mask during meals
4. Arrange for liquid supplements that can be administered via a straw through a valve in the mask

25. Which nursing assessment best indicates a patient's ability to tolerate activity?
1. Results of vital signs before and after activity
2. Presence of adventitious breath sounds
3. Flexibility of muscles and joints
4. Complaints of weakness

26. The nurse is caring for a patient who has a chest tube after thoracic surgery. The nurse should:
1. Clamp the tube when providing for activities of daily living
2. Position the collection device at the same level as the chest
3. Maintain an airtight dressing over the puncture wound
4. Empty chest tube drainage every eight hours

27. The nurse understands that the most serious complication associated with thrombophlebitis caused by immobility is:
1. Postural hypotension
2. Blanchable erythema
3. Dependent edema
4. Acute chest pain

28. An unconscious patient who had oral surgery is admitted to the post-anesthesia care unit. In which position should the nurse place the patient?
1. Prone position
2. Supine position
3. Lateral position
4. Fowler's position

29. A physician orders chest physiotherapy with percussion and vibration for a patient. After the physician leaves, the patient says, "I still don't understand the purpose of this therapy." The nurse's best reply is, "It:
1. Eliminates the need to cough."
2. Limits the production of bronchial mucus."
3. Helps clear the airways of excessive secretions."
4. Promotes the flow of secretions to the base of the lungs."

30. When the head of the bed is elevated to facilitate breathing, the main principle that explains how this action facilitates respiration is based on the science of:
1. Physics
2. Biology
3. Anatomy
4. Chemistry

31. Which adaptation is of most concern when the nurse assesses pulmonary changes associated with immobility?
1. Shallow respirations
2. Increased oxygen saturation
3. Decreased chest wall expansion
4. Respirations that sound gurgling

32. The nurse teaches a patient to make a series of short, forceful exhalations just before actually coughing (huffing). The purpose of this action is to:
1. Conserve the patient's energy
2. Liquefy the respiratory secretions
3. Limit the pain precipitated by coughing
4. Raise the sputum to a level where it can be expectorated

33. Which are the most effective leg exercises the nurse should encourage a patient to perform to prevent circulatory complications during the postoperative period?
1. Flexing the knees
2. Isometric exercises
3. Dorsiflexion exercises
4. Passive range of motion

34. Which outcome best reflects achievement of the goal, "The patient will expectorate lung secretions with no signs of respiratory complications?"
1. Absence of adventitious breath sounds
2. Deep breathing and coughing nonproductively
3. Drinking 3000 mL of fluid in the last 24 hours
4. Expectorating sputum three times between 3 PM and 11 PM

35. What should the nurse do first when caring for an infant, a toddler, or a nonverbal patient who is restless, agitated, and irritable?
1. Administer oxygen
2. Suction the oropharynx
3. Reduce environmental stimuli
4. Determine patency of the airway

36. The nurse is caring for a patient receiving oxygen via a nasal cannula. The nurse should:
1. Reassess the nares, cheeks, and ears for signs of pressure every 2 hours
2. Loop the tubing over the patient's ears and adjust the tubing firmly under the chin
3. Ensure physical hygiene includes applying oil-based lubricant to the patient's nares
4. Alternate the position of the prongs curving upward versus downward every 2 hours

37. To increase both the respiratory and the circulatory functions of a patient in a coma, what is the most important thing the nurse should do?
1. Encourage the patient to cough
2. Massage the patient's bony areas
3. Assist the patient with breathing exercises
4. Change the patient's position every two hours

38. A patient sucking on a hard candy inhales while laughing and develops a total airway obstruction. When the nurse implements abdominal thrusts, the nurse is attempting to:
1. Produce a burp
2. Pump the heart
3. Push air out of the lungs
4. Put pressure on the stomach

39. The nurse is caring for a male patient. Which laboratory results place this patient at risk for an impaired ability to tolerate activity? Check all that apply.
1. _____ Hct of 45%
2. _____ Hgb of 14 g/dL
3. _____ O_2 saturation of 90%
4. _____ RBC of $3.8 \times 10^6/mm^3$
5. _____ WBC of $7.5 \times 10^6/mm^3$

40. The nurse teaches a preoperative patient how to use an incentive spirometer. Place the steps of the use of an incentive spirometer in the order in which they should be performed.
1. Inhale slowly
2. Hold the incentive spirometer level
3. Keep the visual indicator at the inspiratory goal for several seconds
4. Maintain a firm seal with the lips around the mouthpiece during inhalation

Answer: _______________

ANSWERS AND RATIONALES

1. 1. Apnea, a complete absence of respirations, is the cause of, not an adaptation to, hypoxia.
   2. Cyanosis, a bluish discoloration of the skin and mucous membranes caused by reduced oxygen in the blood, is a late sign of hypoxia.
   3. **Hypoxia is insufficient oxygen anywhere in the body. An early sign of hypoxia is restlessness, which is caused by the lack of cerebral perfusion of oxygen.**
   4. A dysrhythmia, a pulse with an irregular rhythm, can occur with hypoxia but it is a late adaptation.

2. 1. Pain is an expected response to the trauma of surgery and usually can be managed effectively.
   2. **Stridor is an obvious audible shrill, harsh sound caused by laryngeal obstruction. The larynx can become edematous because of the trauma of intubation associated with general anesthesia. Obstruction of the larynx is life-threatening because it prevents the exchange of gases between the lungs and atmospheric air.**
   3. Lethargy, which is drowsiness or sluggishness, is an expected response to anesthesia and narcotic medications because these medications depress the central nervous system.
   4. Although diaphoresis is a cause for concern, it is not as immediately life-threatening as an adaptation in another option. Diaphoresis can be related to a warm environment, impaired thermoregulation, the General Adaptation Syndrome, or shock.

3. 1. All oxygen systems should have a flowmeter to control and maintain the flow of oxygen gas.
   2. All oxygen is drying to the oral mucosa. Therefore, oral hygiene should be provided frequently to moisten the mucous membranes.
   3. *Oxygen in use* signs should be displayed prominently on the patient's door and bed to alert others that oxygen is in use and that safety precautions should be implemented.
   4. **A low liter flow system administers a volume of oxygen designed to supplement the inspired room air to provide airflow equal to the person's minute ventilation. A high liter flow system administers a volume of oxygen designed to exceed the volume of air required for the person's minute ventilation. The low liter flow system is less drying than the high liter flow system and humidification is unnecessary. A humidifier is a mechanical device that adds water vapor to air in a particle size that can carry moisture to the small airways.**

4. 1. **An upright sitting position in a bed or chair facilitates maximum thoracic excursion because it permits the diaphragm to contract without pressure being exerted against it by abdominal viscera.**
   2. The side-lying position is not ideal for the use of an incentive spirometer because it limits thoracic expansion. The side-lying position allows the abdominal viscera to exert pressure against the diaphragm during inspiration and the lung on the lower side of the body is compressed by the weight of the body.
   3. The orthopneic position raises intra-abdominal and intrathoracic pressures that can limit thoracic excursion.
   4. The low-Fowler's position does not maximize the effects of gravity. Gravity moves abdominal viscera away from the diaphragm and thus facilitates the contraction of the diaphragm, both of which promote thoracic expansion.

5. 1. This is unnecessary. A fluid intake of approximately 2000 mL of fluid is adequate.
   2. Although this is extremely important, it is not the priority.
   3. **A tension pneumothorax may occur if the integrity of the chest drainage system becomes compromised (e.g., open to atmospheric pressure, clogged drainage tube, or mechanical dysfunction). Maintaining respiratory functioning is the priority.**
   4. Although repositioning is done to promote drainage of secretions from lung segments and aeration of lung tissue, it is not the priority.

6. 1. **Hypoventilation, immobility, and ineffective coughing that lead to stasis of respiratory secretions and the multiplication of microorganisms, cause hypostatic pneumonia. Dyspnea results from decreased lung compliance, chest pain results from coughing and the increased work of breathing, and purulent sputum results from fluid and blood moving from the capillaries into the alveoli.**
   2. Hypovolemic shock is characterized by tachycardia, tachypnea, and hypotension.

3. Thrombophlebitis is characterized by localized pain, swelling, warmth, and erythema.
4. Pneumothorax is characterized by a sudden onset of sharp pain on inspiration, dyspnea, tachycardia, and hypotension.

7. 1. Although muscle atrophy can occur with immobility, it is unrelated to hypercoagulability. Muscle atrophy is the decrease in the size of a muscle resulting from disuse.
   2. **Immobility promotes venous vasodilation, venous stasis and hypercoagulability of the blood, which can precipitate the formation of a clot in a vein of the leg (venous thrombosis) and inflammation of the vein (phlebitis).**
   3. Hypotension, an abnormally low systolic blood pressure (less than 100 mm Hg), is not related to hypercoagulability precipitated by immobility.
   4. Bradypnea, abnormally slow breathing (less than 10 breaths per minute), is unrelated to hypercoagulability caused by immobility.

8. 1. A respiratory rate of 14 in an adult is within the expected range of 12 to 20 breaths per minute.
   2. A productive cough indicates that the person is managing respiratory secretions adequately and keeping the airway patent.
   3. A sore throat indicates posterior oropharyngeal irritation or inflammation. This may or may not progress to respiratory distress.
   4. **Orthopnea, the ability to breathe easily only in an upright (standing or sitting) position, is a classic sign of respiratory distress. The upright position permits maximum thoracic expansion because the abdominal organs do not press against the diaphragm and inspiration is aided by the principle of gravity.**

9. 1. The use of a toe for pulse oximetry can result in inaccurate results because of concurrent problems, such as vasoconstriction, hypothermia, impaired peripheral circulation, and movement of the foot.
   2. **An earlobe is an excellent site to monitor pulse oximetry. It is least affected by decreased blood flow, has greater accuracy at lower saturations, and rarely is edematous. This site is used for intermittent, not continuous, monitoring.**
   3. Soap and water will not resolve the edema. In addition, attaching a pulse oximeter clip sensor to an edematous finger is contraindicated because interstitial fluid interferes with obtaining an accurate oxygen saturation level.
   4. The cause of the edema must be identified first because range-of-motion exercises may be contraindicated.

10. 1. This is unsafe because it can compress the capillaries under the strap, which may interfere with tissue perfusion and result in pressure ulcers.
    2. This may increase the patient's agitation and it is impractical.
    3. This will probably be useless because an agitated patient often does not understand cause and effect.
    4. **Agitated, confused patients generally tolerate a nasal cannula better than a face mask. A nasal cannula (nasal prongs) is less intrusive than a mask; masks are oppressive and may cause a patient to feel claustrophobic.**

11. 1. Although the deep breathing associated with the use of an incentive spirometer may stimulate coughing, this is not the primary reason for its use.
    2. Although sputum may be expectorated after the use of an incentive spirometer, this is not the primary reason for its use.
    3. **An incentive spirometer provides a visual goal for and measurement of inspiration. It encourages the patient to execute and maintain a sustained inspiration. A sustained inspiration opens airways, increases the inspiratory volume, and reduces atelectasis.**
    4. Patients who use an incentive spirometer may or may not be receiving oxygen.

12. 1. Both cold and heat relax muscles and thus minimize muscle spasms.
    2. Heat promotes, not prevents, bleeding because it causes vasodilation. Cold causes vasoconstriction, which limits bleeding.
    3. **Heat raises the skin surface temperature promoting vasodilation, which increases blood flow to the area.**
    4. Cold reduces discomfort by numbing the area, slowing the transmission of pain impulses, and increasing the pain threshold. Heat reduces discomfort by relaxing the muscles.

13. 1. These are appropriate interventions for a patient with emphysema. Emphysema is a chronic pulmonary disease characterized by an abnormal increase in the size of air spaces distal to the terminal bronchioles with destructive changes in their walls.
    2. **This intervention provides for patient safety because percussion and vibration with a patient who has osteoporosis**

may cause fractures. Osteoporosis is an abnormal loss of bone mass and strength.

3. These are appropriate interventions for a patient with cystic fibrosis. Cystic fibrosis causes widespread dysfunction of the exocrine glands. It is characterized by thick, tenacious secretions in the respiratory system that block the bronchioles, creating breathing difficulties.
4. These are appropriate interventions for a patient with chronic bronchitis. Bronchitis is an inflammation of the mucous membranes of the bronchial airways.

14. 1. Deep breathing and huff coughing, not pursed-lip breathing, stimulate effective coughing.
2. **Pursed-lip breathing involves deep inspiration and prolonged expiration against slightly closed lips. The pursed lips create a resistance to the air flowing out of the lungs, which prolongs exhalation and maintains positive airway pressure, thereby maintaining an open airway and preventing airway collapse.**
3. Pursed-lip breathing increases, not decreases, intrathoracic pressure.
4. The huff cough stimulates the natural cough reflex and is effective for clearing the central airways of sputum. Saying the word *huff* with short, forceful exhalations keeps the glottis open, mobilizes sputum, and stimulates a cough.

15. 1. This can force the bolus of food further down the trachea and is contraindicated.
2. This should never be done with an adult because if it is a partial obstruction it interferes with the person's own efforts to clear the airway or can cause the bolus of food to lodge further down the trachea. If it is a total obstruction, slapping the back will be useless and delay the initiation of the abdominal thrust maneuver.
3. **When a person is choking on food, the first intervention is to determine if the person can speak because the next intervention will depend on if it is a partial or total airway obstruction. With a partial airway obstruction, the person will be able to make sounds because some air can pass from the lungs through the vocal cords. In this situation, the person's own efforts (gagging and coughing) should be allowed to clear the airway. With a total airway obstruction, the person will not be able to make a sound because the airway is blocked and the nurse should immediately initiate the abdominal thrust maneuver (Heimlich maneuver).**
4. Thrusts to the xiphoid process may cause a fracture that may result in a pneumothorax.

16. 1. Changing positions will mobilize, not liquefy, respiratory secretions.
2. **A fluid intake of 2500 to 3000 mL is recommended to maintain the moisture of the respiratory mucous membranes. Adequate fluid keeps respiratory secretions thin so that they can be moved by ciliary action or coughed up and spit out (expectorated).**
3. Mucolytics, not antitussives, liquefy respiratory secretions. Antitussives prevent or relieve coughing.
4. Deep breathing will mobilize, not liquefy, respiratory secretions.

17. 1. Although tilting the head backward (hyperextension of the neck) elongates the pharynx, reducing airway resistance, this will do nothing to correct the obstruction at the glottis (opening through the vocal cords). Also, the tongue will block the airway unless there is forward pressure applied on the lower angle of the jaw (jaw thrust maneuver).
2. **Positive pressure will push the vocal cords backward toward the wall of the larynx, opening the glottis (space between the vocal cords), which allows ventilation of the lung.**
3. This is unnecessary. The patient is having a respiratory, not cardiac, problem.
4. This is useless because the glottis is obstructed and the oxygenated air will not enter the lung.

18. 1. When administering oxygen in an emergency, the nurse should not exceed two liters per minute because high oxygen levels can depress respirations in people with chronic obstructive lung diseases. Obtaining and setting up the equipment takes time that can be used for other more appropriate interventions first.
2. Although this might be done eventually, it is not the priority at this time. This may or may not help. Inadequate oxygenation can be caused by a variety of problems other than shallow breathing.
3. **A nurse can implement this immediate, independent action. Nurses are permitted to treat human responses. Raising the head of the bed facilitates the dropping of the abdominal organs by gravity away from the diaphragm, which permits the greatest lung expansion.**

4. This is premature. The patient's needs must be met first.

19. 1. **Iron is necessary for hemoglobin synthesis. Therefore, reduced intake of dietary iron results in iron deficiency anemia. Hemoglobin is the main component of red blood cells and transports oxygen and carbon dioxide through the bloodstream.**
2. Platelets are unrelated to iron deficiency anemia. Platelets (thrombocytes) are nonnucleated, round or oval, flattened, disk-shaped, formed elements in the blood that are necessary for blood clotting.
3. Albumin is unrelated to iron deficiency anemia. Albumin is a protein in the blood that helps to maintain blood volume and blood pressure.
4. Blood urea nitrogen is unrelated to iron deficiency anemia. Blood urea nitrogen (BUN) is a test that measures the nitrogen portion of urea present in the blood. It is an index of glomerular function in the production and excretion of urea.

20. 1. Although healing of an incision may take longer in an older adult, it is not as serious as another age-related change. In the older adult, there is atrophy and thinning of both the epithelial and subcutaneous layers of tissue, collagenous attachments become less effective, sebaceous gland activity decreases, and interstitial fluid decreases. These changes lead to decreased skin elasticity.
2. Although there is a greater risk of postoperative urinary complications in older adults, they are not as serious as problems caused by other age-related changes. In the older adult, bladder muscles weaken, bladder capacity decreases, the micturition reflex is delayed, emptying of the bladder becomes more difficult, and residual volume increases.
3. Although an incision in an older adult may be painful, it is not as serious as other age-related changes. In addition, in the older adult there is an increased threshold for sensations of pain, touch, and temperature because of age-related changes in the nerves and nerve conduction.
4. **Age-related changes in the older adult include calcification of costal cartilage (making the trachea and rib cage more rigid), an increase in the anterior-posterior chest diameter, and weakening of the thoracic inspiratory and expiratory muscles. These changes decrease respiratory excursion, which can result in multiple life-threatening postoperative complications, such as atelectasis and hypostatic pneumonia.**

21. 1. This is unrelated to peripheral arterial disease.
2. Peripheral arterial disease usually involves inadequate circulation in the lower extremities, not the brain.
3. **This is an appropriate expected outcome for a patient with arterial vascular disease, which is a decrease in nutrition and respiration at the peripheral cellular level because of a decrease in capillary blood supply. A physiologic adaptation is diminished or absent arterial pulses.**
4. A prolonged capillary refill indicates a continued problem with peripheral tissue perfusion. After compression, blanched tissue should return to its original color within 2 seconds (blanch test).

22. 1. **Bed rest reduces cardiopulmonary demands, muscle contraction, and other bodily functions. All of this reduces the basal metabolic rate, which conserves energy.**
2. Activity, not bed rest, maintains strength.
3. Although bed rest may limit peristalsis, it is not the most common reason bed rest is ordered.
4. Protein synthesis is enhanced by the intake of amino acids, not bed rest.

23. 1. Inhalation is through the nose for both diaphragmatic and pursed-lip breathing.
2. Exhalation through pursed lips is performed only with pursed-lip breathing.
3. This action is not part of diaphragmatic or pursed-lip breathing. The use of these accessory muscles of respiration is a compensatory mechanism that helps to increase thoracic excursion when inhaling.
4. **With diaphragmatic breathing, the contraction of abdominal muscles at the end of expiration helps to reduce the amount of air left in the lungs at the end of expiration (residual volume).**

24. 1. **This intervention will help meet both the nutritional and oxygen needs of the patient. A nasal cannula delivers oxygen via prongs placed in the patient's nares leaving the mouth unobstructed, which promotes talking and eating.**
2. This is unsafe because it can compromise the patient's respiratory status while the oxygen is disconnected.
3. A Venturi mask and a nonrebreather mask are both masks that cover the mouth, which interferes with eating.
4. Liquid supplements are unnecessary. The patient should eat the diet ordered by the physician.

25. **1. Vital signs reflect cardiopulmonary functioning of the body. Vital signs obtained before and after activity provide data that can be compared to determine the body's response to the energy demands of ambulation.**
2. The presence of unexpected (abnormal) breath sounds (adventitious sounds) indicates the presence of a respiratory problem (narrowed airways, presence of excessive respiratory secretions, or pleural inflammation), not a response to activity.
3. Flexibility relates to mobility, not one's physiologic capacity to endure activities that require energy.
4. Although this may reflect a response to activity, this evaluation is subjective and vague. Measurable, specific outcomes that are objective are the best way to evaluate a patient's physiologic response to activity.

26. 1. This is contraindicated because clamping a chest tube may cause a tension pneumothorax.
2. The chest drainage system should be kept below the level of the insertion site to promote the flow of drainage from the pleural space and prevent the flow of drainage back into the pleural space.
3. An airtight dressing seals the pleural space from the environment. If left open to the environment, atmospheric pressure causes air to enter the pleural space, which results in a tension pneumothorax.
4. This is unnecessary. Chest drainage systems are closed, self-contained systems that have a chamber for drainage. At routine intervals, as per hospital policy, the date, time, and nurse's initials mark the level of drainage on the drainage collection chamber.

27. 1. Postural hypotension is unrelated to phlebitis caused by immobility. Postural hypotension (orthostatic hypotension) is a decrease in blood pressure related to positional or postural changes from the lying down to sitting or standing positions.
2. Blanchable erythema is unrelated to phlebitis caused by immobility. Blanchable erythema (reactive hyperemia) is a reddened area caused by localized vasodilation in response to lack of blood flow to the underlying tissue. The reddened area will turn pale with fingertip pressure.
3. Dependent edema is unrelated to phlebitis caused by immobility. Although fluid will collect in the interstitial compartment (edema) around the phlebitis, it is localized, not dependent, edema. Dependent edema is the collection of fluid in the interstitial tissues below the level of the heart; it occurs bilaterally and usually is caused by cardiopulmonary problems.
4. Immobility promotes venous stasis, which in conjunction with hypercoagulability and injury to vessel walls predisposes patients to thrombophlebitis. These three factors are known as Virchow's triad. A thrombus can break loose from the vein wall and travel through the circulation (embolus) where eventually it obstructs a pulmonary artery or one of its branches causing sudden, acute chest pain, dyspnea, coughing, and frothy sputum.

28. 1. Although the prone position allows for drainage from the mouth, it is contraindicated because lying on the side of the face compresses oral tissues, impedes assessment, complicates oral suctioning, and may compromise the airway.
2. The supine position is unsafe. In an unconscious patient, the gag and swallowing reflexes may be impaired, which increases the risk for aspiration as the tongue falls to the back of the oropharynx occluding the airway.
3. The lateral position facilitates the flow of secretions out of the mouth by gravity, keeps the tongue to the side of the mouth maintaining the airway, and permits effective assessment of the oropharynx and respiratory status.
4. The Fowler's position is unsafe. An unconscious patient is unable to maintain an upright position.

29. 1. Chest physiotherapy promotes, not eliminates, the need for coughing.
2. Chest physiotherapy promotes the expectoration of, not limits the production of, bronchial mucus.
3. The forceful striking of the skin over the lung (percussion, clapping) and fine, vigorous, shaking pressure with the hands on the chest wall during exhalation (vibration) mobilize secretions so that they can be coughed up and expectorated.
4. Chest physiotherapy mobilizes secretions facilitating expectoration, interfering with the flow of secretions to the base of the lungs.

30. **1. Raising the head of the bed drops the abdominal organs away from the diaphragm via the principle of gravity, facilitating breathing. Gravity, the tendency of weight to be pulled toward the center of the earth, is a physics principle.**

2. This is not related to biology. Biology is the study of living organisms.
3. This is not related to anatomy. Anatomy is the study of the form and structure of living organisms.
4. This is not related to chemistry. Chemistry is the study of elements, compounds, and atomic relations of matter.

31. 1. Although this is a concern, it is not as serious as an adaptation in another option.
2. Oxygen saturation may be decreased, not increased, with immobility.
3. Although this is a concern, it is not as serious as an adaptation in another option.
4. **Respirations that sound gurgling (gurgles, rhonchi) indicate air passing through narrowed air passages because of secretions, swelling, or tumors. A partial or total obstruction of the airway can occur, which is life threatening.**

32. 1. Regardless of the type of cough, coughing uses, not conserves, energy. However, after the airway is cleared of sputum, the patient's oxygen demands will be met more effectively.
2. An increased fluid intake, not coughing, liquefies respiratory secretions.
3. This is not the purpose of huff coughing. Coughing usually is not painful unless the thoracic muscles are strained or the patient has had abdominal or pelvic surgery.
4. **The huff cough stimulates the natural cough reflex and is effective for clearing the central airways of sputum. Saying the word *huff* with short, forceful exhalations keeps the glottis open and raises sputum to a level where it can be coughed up and expectorated.**

33. 1. Flexing the knee exerts pressure on the veins in the popliteal space; this reduces venous return, which increases, not decreases, the risk of postoperative circulatory complications.
2. These exercises strengthen muscles; they do not prevent postoperative circulatory complications. Isometric exercises change the muscle tension but do not change the muscle length or move joints.
3. **Alternating dorsiflexion and plantar flexion (calf pumping) alternately contracts and relaxes the calf muscles, including the gastrocnemius muscles. This muscle contraction promotes venous return, preventing the venous stasis that contributes to the development of postoperative thrombophlebitis.**
4. Passive range-of-motion exercises are exercises that are done by another person moving a patient's joints through their complete range of movement. This does not prevent postoperative circulatory complications because the power is supplied by a person other than the patient.

34. 1. **Adventitious breath sounds are unexpected (abnormal) breath sounds that occur when pleural linings are inflamed or when air passes through narrowed airways or through airways filled with fluid. The absence of unexpected (abnormal) sounds is desirable.**
2. To expectorate secretions, coughing must be productive, not nonproductive. A nonproductive cough is dry, which means that no respiratory secretions are raised and spit out (expectorated) because of coughing.
3. Drinking fluid is an intervention that will liquefy respiratory secretions, facilitating their expectoration. However, just drinking fluid will not ensure that the secretions will be expectorated.
4. Although spitting out sputum reflects achievement of the goal in relation to expectorating lung secretions, it does not address the absence of respiratory complications which is the ultimate goal of decreasing stasis of respiratory secretions.

35. 1. This may or may not be necessary. The need for oxygen administration will depend on the results of other interventions that should be done first.
2. This is premature. Mucus or sputum may not be the cause of the problem.
3. This intervention is useless at this time and is not the priority.
4. **Early signs of hypoxia are restlessness, agitation, and irritability due to reduced oxygen to brain cells. A partial or completely obstructed airway prevents the passage of gases into and out of the lungs. The ABCs of emergency care identify airway as the priority.**

36. 1. **This ensures that tissue irritation or capillary compression does not occur from the nasal prongs, tubing, or elastic strap. The elastic strap should be snug enough to keep the nasal prongs from becoming displaced but loose enough not to compress or irritate tissue.**
2. This is the correct placement of the tubing; however, it should be secured gently, not firmly, under the chin.

3. A water-based, not oil-based, lubricant should be applied to the nares.
4. The nasal prongs should always be curving downward to follow the natural curve of the nares. Placing the nasal prongs curving upward does not follow the natural curve of the nasal passage, which can cause tissue injury.

37. 1. A patient in a coma is unable to respond.
2. This helps only skin circulation in the small area being massaged.
3. A patient in a coma is unable to respond.
4. This helps respirations by preventing fluid from collecting in the lung, which can cause infection; it helps circulation since activity increases circulation, and it relieves local pressure.

38. 1. Whatever is causing the obstruction is not caught in the esophagus, which leads to the stomach, but in the respiratory system.
2. Pressing on the heart (compression) is used in cardiopulmonary resuscitation (CPR).
3. When trapped air behind an obstruction is forced out, it pushes out what is causing the obstruction.
4. Whatever is causing the obstruction is not caught in the esophagus, which leads to the stomach, but in the respiratory system.

39. 1. This is within the expected range for hematocrit for men (42%–52%) and women (36%–48%).
2. This is within the expected range for hemoglobin for men (14.0 to 17.4 g/dL) and women (12.0 to 16.0 g/dL).
3. An oxygen saturation of 90% is below the expected level of 95% or greater. Adequate oxygen levels are necessary to meet the metabolic demands of activity that requires muscle contraction.
4. This is below the expected range of 4.71 to 5.14 × 10^6/mm^3 for red blood cells for men. Hemoglobin, which carries oxygen, is a component of red blood cells.
5. This is within the expected range of 4.5 to 11 × 10^6/mm^3 for white blood cells (WBCs). WBCs are not related to a patient's oxygenation status; they are related to protecting the patient from infection.

40. Answer: 2, 4, 1, 3
2. Holding the incentive spirometer level prevents factors, such as friction and gravity from altering the correct function of the device.
4. A firm seal around the mouthpiece is necessary during inhalation, but the mouthpiece should be removed during exhalation.
1. Inspiration should be accomplished through a slow, deep breath. A rapid, forceful inhalation can collapse the airway and is contraindicated.
3. When the visual indicator reaches the preset goal during inhalation, the inhalation should be maintained for 2 to 4 seconds to ensure ventilation of the alveoli.

Urinary Elimination

KEYWORDS

The following words include English vocabulary, nursing/medical terminology, concepts, principles, or information relevant to content specifically addressed in the chapter or associated with topics presented in it. English dictionaries, nursing textbooks, and medical dictionaries, such as *Taber's Cyclopedic Medical Dictionary*, are resources that can be used to expand your knowledge and understanding of these words and related information.

- 24-hour urine collection
- Acidic urine
- Anuria
- Bacteruria
- Bladder cues
- Bladder irritability
- Bladder training
- Blood urea nitrogen
- Catheter port
- Commode chair
- Condom catheter
- Credé maneuver
- Cystoscopy
- Detrusor muscles
- Dysuria
- Enuresis
- Excretion
- Filtration
- Foreskin
- Fracture bedpan
- Frequency
- Glomerular filtration rate
- Graduate
- Hematuria
- Hesitancy
- Incontinence, types
  - Functional
  - Overflow
  - Reflex
  - Stress
  - Total
  - Urge
- Incontinence pad
- Incontinent
- Kegel exercises
- Ketones
- Micturition
- Nocturia
- Oliguria
- Perineal care
- Polyuria
- Prostate
- Pyuria
- Reagent strips
- Renal calculi
- Renal dialysis
- Renal perfusion
- Residual urine
- Retention
- Specific gravity
- Suprapubic distention
- Trigone
- Turbidity
- Urea
- Ureter
- Urethra
- Urgency
- Urinary catheters
  - Condom catheter (Texas)
  - Indwelling (retention, Foley)
  - Straight catheter
  - Suprapubic catheter
- Urinary diuresis
- Urinary diversion
- Urinary drainage bag, leg bag
- Urinary meatus
- Urinary obstruction
- Urinary output
- Urinary tract infection
- Urine clarity
- Urine specimens
  - Clean catch
  - From a catheter port
  - Urinalysis
- Void

QUESTIONS

1. What should the nurse monitor to best assess a patient's renal perfusion?
   1. Blood pressure every 15 minutes
   2. Urinary output every hour
   3. Body weight every day
   4. I&O every 24 hours
2. The nurse collects data about a patient regarding a risk for stress incontinence. Which is a major contributing factor for this condition?
   1. Decreased bladder capacity
   2. Spinal cord dysfunction
   3. Cognitive impairment
   4. Weak pelvic muscles
3. A patient has a urinary retention catheter. Which is most important when the nurse cares for this patient?
   1. Ensuring that the catheter remains connected to the collection bag
   2. Wearing sterile gloves when accessing the specimen port
   3. Cleansing the urinary meatus with Betadine daily
   4. Increasing fluid intake to 3000 mL per day
4. The nurse is assessing a patient for the presence of dysuria. The nurse should ask, "Do you:
   1. Feel that you are able to empty your bladder fully each time you void?"
   2. Have a problem stopping or starting the flow of urine?"
   3. Pass a little urine when you cough or sneeze?"
   4. Experience any pain or burning on urination?"
5. The nurse is assessing a patient's urinary status. Which adaptation indicates urinary retention?
   1. Wet bed and undergarments
   2. Burning and pain on voiding
   3. Sudden, overwhelming need to void
   4. Bladder fullness in the absence of voiding
6. The nurse should be most concerned about which problem when patients have bowel and bladder incontinence?
   1. Lowered level of consciousness
   2. Decreased fluid volume
   3. Impaired skin integrity
   4. Imbalanced nutrition
7. When the nurse documents that the patient has polyuria, the nurse is communicating that the patient is:
   1. Excreting excessive amounts of urine
   2. Experiencing pain on urination
   3. Retaining urine in the bladder
   4. Passing blood in the urine
8. A patient is experiencing bladder irritability. Which fluid should the nurse teach the patient to include in the diet?
   1. Beer
   2. Coffee
   3. Orange juice
   4. Cranberry juice
9. What adaptation identified by the nurse most commonly is associated with excessive production of the hormone ADH?
   1. Diuresis
   2. Oliguria
   3. Retention
   4. Incontinence

10. The nurse needs to obtain a urine specimen from a patient. Which nursing intervention is the greatest help to most people who need to void for a urine test?
   1. Exerting manual pressure on the abdomen
   2. Encouraging a backward rocking motion
   3. Running water in the sink
   4. Providing for privacy

11. The nurse has identified that the patient has overflow incontinence. The nurse understands that a major contributing factor is:
   1. Coughing
   2. Mobility deficits
   3. Prostate enlargement
   4. Urinary tract infection

12. The nurse must measure the intake and output for a patient who has a urinary retention catheter in place. The most appropriate way for the nurse to accurately measure urine output from the urinary retention catheter is via a:
   1. Urinal
   2. Graduate
   3. Large syringe
   4. Urine collection bag

13. The patient's urine is cloudy, amber, and has an unpleasant odor. The nurse makes the inference that the patient has:
   1. Urinary retention
   2. A urinary tract infection
   3. Ketone bodies in the urine
   4. A high urinary calcium level

14. The nurse is caring for a debilitated female patient with nocturia. The nursing intervention that is most helpful in meeting this patient's needs is:
   1. Encouraging the use of bladder training exercises
   2. Providing assistance with toileting every 4 hours
   3. Positioning a bedside commode near the bed
   4. Teaching the avoidance of fluids after 5 PM

15. The nurse must collect a urine specimen for culture and sensitivity via a straight catheter. The nurse should:
   1. Use a sterile specimen container
   2. Collect urine from the catheter port
   3. Inflate the balloon with ten mL of sterile water
   4. Have the patient void before collecting the specimen

16. The nurse is caring for a patient with a condom catheter. Which nursing action is most important?
   1. Providing perineal care every shift
   2. Avoiding kinks in the collection tubing
   3. Ensuring that the Velcro strap is snug, not tight
   4. Retracting the foreskin before the catheter is applied

17. The nurse is caring for a patient on bed rest who has a urinary retention catheter. The nurse should:
   1. Irrigate the tubing to ensure patency
   2. Label the tubing with the date of insertion
   3. Ensure the tubing is positioned over the leg
   4. Hang the collection bag on the side rail of the bed

18. Which should the nurse teach the patient to avoid to prevent urinary diuresis?
   1. Narcotics
   2. Caffeine
   3. Activity
   4. Protein

19. The nurse identifies that the constituent found in urine that indicates an abnormality is:
    1. Electrolytes
    2. Protein
    3. Water
    4. Urea

20. A patient is complaining about burning on urination. Which question should the nurse ask to best obtain information about the patient's dysuria?
    1. "Tell me about the problems you have been having with urination?"
    2. "How would you describe your experience with incontinence?"
    3. "What are your usual bowel habits?"
    4. "What color is your urine?"

21. The nurse is caring for a group of patients with a variety of urinary problems. The patient adaptation identified by the nurse that causes the most concern is:
    1. Anuria
    2. Dysuria
    3. Diuresis
    4. Enuresis

22. Which problem identified by the nurse is most associated with urinary incontinence?
    1. Chronic pain
    2. Reduced fluid intake
    3. Disturbed self-esteem
    4. Insufficient knowledge

23. Which characteristic is common to both reflex incontinence and total incontinence?
    1. Urination following an increase in intra-abdominal pressure
    2. Loss of urine without awareness of bladder fullness
    3. Retention of urine with overflow incontinence
    4. Strong, sudden desire to void

24. Which adaptation can the nurse expect when a postoperative patient experiences stress associated with surgery?
    1. Decreased urinary output
    2. Low specific gravity
    3. Reflex incontinence
    4. Urinary hesitancy

25. What is the best nursing action to facilitate bladder continence for the patient who is cognitively impaired?
    1. Offer toileting reminders every two hours
    2. Provide clothing that is easy to manipulate
    3. Encourage avoidance of fluid between meals
    4. Explain the need to call for the nurse for help with toileting

26. The nurse understands that an assessment that is not common to monitoring both urine and stool is:
    1. Constituents
    2. Urgency
    3. Shape
    4. Color

27. Which adaptation indicates that additional nursing assessments are necessary regarding the urinary status of a patient?
    1. Aromatic odor
    2. Pale yellow urine
    3. Specific gravity of 1.035
    4. Output of 50 mL every hour

28. The patient states, "It burns and stings every time I pass urine." The nurse should make the inference that the patient is most likely experiencing:
1. A rentention of urine
2. Reflex incontinence
3. Stress incontinence
4. An infection

29. A patient tells the nurse, "I have to urinate as soon as I get the urge to go." Which is a contributing factor to urinary urgency?
1. Anesthesia
2. Full bladder
3. Dehydration
4. Urinary tract infection

30. A patient has a history of urinary tract infections. The nurse should encourage the patient to drink 8 ounces of cranberry juice daily because it:
1. Dilutes bacterial growth
2. Promotes an acidic urine
3. Prevents urinary retention
4. Stimulates hypoactive detrusor muscles

31. When planning nursing care, which factor in the patient's history places the patient at the greatest risk for stress incontinence?
1. Lumbar spinal cord injury
2. Urinary obstruction
3. Six vaginal births
4. Confusion

32. What is the most effective nursing intervention to prevent urinary tract infections?
1. Teach female patients to wipe from the back to the front after urinating
2. Instruct patients to use bath powder to absorb perineal perspiration
3. Advise patients to report burning on urination to the physician
4. Encourage patients to drink at least two quarts of fluid daily

33. A patient has urinary incontinence. Which is the best nursing intervention for this patient?
1. Drying the area well after perineal care
2. Dusting the perineal area with cornstarch
3. Providing skin care immediately after soiling
4. Using a deodorant soap when providing skin care

34. When the nurse assesses a patient, which adaptations support the presence of urinary retention? Check all that apply
1. _____ Nocturia
2. _____ Hematuria
3. _____ Bladder contractions
4. _____ Suprapubic distention
5. _____ Frequent small voidings

35. The nurse plans to clamp a patient's urinary drainage system to obtain a urine specimen for a urine culture and sensitivity. Indicate with an X, on the figure to the right, where the nurse should clamp the catheter drainage system.

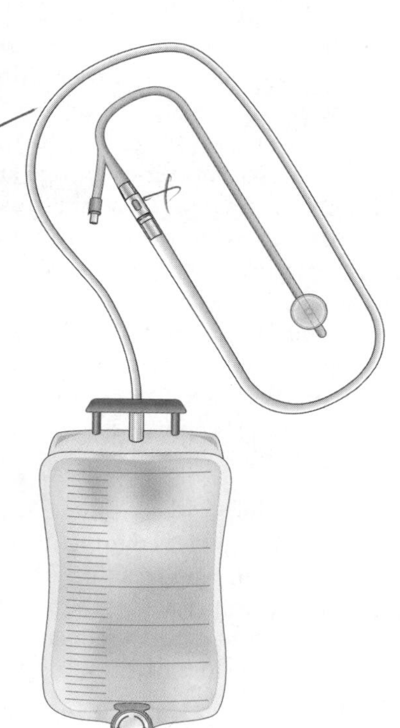

ANSWERS AND RATIONALES

1. 1. Blood pressure measurements do not directly reflect renal perfusion. However, blood pressure measurements reflect cardiac and circulatory functioning and fluid balance, which indirectly provide vague information in relation to renal perfusion.
   2. **Adequate renal perfusion and kidney function are reflected by an hourly urine output of 30 to 50 mL of urine.**
   3. Daily weights reflect fluid balance. One liter of fluid weighs approximately 2.2 pounds.
   4. This is too long a time period to reflect renal perfusion. Intake and output over 24 hours reflects fluid balance.

2. 1. This is related to urge incontinence, not stress incontinence.
   2. This is related to reflex incontinence, not stress incontinence.
   3. This is related to total incontinence, not stress incontinence.
   4. **Stress incontinence is an immediate involuntary loss of urine during an increase in intra-abdominal pressure. It is related to weak or degenerated pelvic muscles and structural supports.**

3. 1. **Maintaining the connection of the catheter to the drainage bag prevents the introduction of microorganisms that can cause infection. A urinary retention catheter is a closed system that should remain closed.**
   2. Clean, not sterile, gloves should be worn. Surgical asepsis (use of a sterile syringe and alcohol swab) is necessary when accessing the specimen port on a urinary retention catheter.
   3. Betadine is irritating to mucous membranes. Soap and water is adequate.
   4. Although increasing fluid intake will increase urinary output, thereby facilitating flushing the bladder, urethera, and urinary meatus of microorganisms, it is not as important as another option.

4. 1. This question might be asked if there is a concern that the person is retaining urine in the bladder after urinating (residual urine).
   2. This question might be asked if there is a concern that the person is experiencing a difficulty initiating urination (hesitancy) or urge incontinence.
   3. This question relates to stress incontinence, which is the immediate involuntary loss of urine during an increase in intra-abdominal pressure.
   4. **This question relates to painful or difficult urination (dysuria). It is most often caused by bladder or urethral inflammation or trauma.**

5. 1. Urine is being passed from, not retained in, the bladder when voiding in bed. Wet bed linens and undergarments indicate urinary incontinence.
   2. Painful or difficult urination is called dysuria, not urinary retention.
   3. A sudden, overwhelming need to void is called urgency, not urinary retention.
   4. **In urinary retention, urine accumulates in and distends the bladder, resulting in bladder fullness, absence of voiding, and suprapubic distention.**

6. 1. Experiencing bowel and bladder incontinence does not alter the level of consciousness. However, a person who has an altered level of consciousness may experience bowel and bladder incontinence because of an inability to recognize elimination cues.
   2. Incontinence is unrelated to deficient fluid volume, which is the state in which an individual is at risk of experiencing vascular, interstitial, or intracellular dehydration.
   3. **With total incontinence, there is a continuous unpredictable loss of urine, and with bowel incontinence, there is an involuntary passage of stool. Urine is acidic and stool contains digestive enzymes, both of which are irritating to the skin unless removed immediately.**
   4. Incontinence is unrelated to imbalanced nutrition, which is the state in which an individual is at risk for an inadequate or excessive intake of, or inability to absorb, or utilize, nutrients for metabolic needs.

7. 1. **Polyuria is an excessive output of urine. This is associated with problems, such as diabetes mellitus, diabetes insipidus, diuresis phase after a burn injury, and reduced antidiuretic hormone.**
   2. This is the definition of dysuria.
   3. This is the definition of urinary retention.
   4. This is the definition of hematuria.

8. 1. Beer contains alcohol, which is irritating to the bladder.

2. Coffee contains caffeine, which is irritating to the bladder.
3. Orange juice, a citrus fruit, is irritating to the bladder.
4. **Cranberries have no constituents that irritate the bladder. In addition, it produces a more acidic environment that is less conducive to the growth of microorganisms and prevents bacteria from adhering to the mucous membranes of the urinary tract, promoting their excretion.**

9. 1. Diuresis occurs when there is inadequate antidiuretic hormone.
2. **Antidiuretic hormone (ADH) increases the reabsorption of water by the kidney tubules, decreasing the amount of urine formed. Oliguria is diminished urinary output relative to intake (less than 400 mL in 24 hours).**
3. With urinary retention, urine is formed, but it accumulates in the bladder and is not excreted.
4. Antidiuretic hormone is unrelated to incontinence.

10. 1. Manual bladder compression (Credé maneuver) is performed when a patient has bladder flaccidity and is not expected to regain voluntary control.
2. This rocking motion is used to promote a bowel movement, not voiding.
3. Although running water in the sink may be helpful, it is not as effective as an intervention in another option.
4. **Few people can void on demand with an audience. Tending to bodily functions is a personal, private activity in the North American culture. Providing privacy supports patient dignity.**

11. 1. Coughing, which raises the intra-abdominal pressure, is related to stress incontinence, not overflow incontinence.
2. Mobility deficits, such as spinal cord injuries, are related to reflex incontinence, not overflow incontinence.
3. **An enlarged prostate compresses the urethra and interferes with the outflow of urine, resulting in urinary retention. With urinary retention, the pressure within the bladder builds until the external urethral sphincter temporarily opens to allow a small volume (25 to 60 mL) of urine to escape (overflow incontinence).**
4. Urinary tract infections are related to urge incontinence, not overflow incontinence.

12. 1. Although urinals have volume markings on the side, usually they occur in 100-mL increments that do not promote accurate measurements.
2. **A graduate is a collection container with volume markings usually at 25 mL increments that promote accurate measurements of urine volume.**
3. This is impractical. A large syringe is used to obtain a sterile specimen from a Foley catheter.
4. A urine collection bag is flexible and balloons outward as urine collects. In addition, the volume markings are at 100-mL increments that do not promote accurate measurements.

13. 1. These adaptations do not reflect urinary retention. Urinary retention is evidenced by suprapubic distention and lack of voiding or small, frequent voidings (overflow incontinence).
2. **The urine appears concentrated (amber) and cloudy because of the presence of bacteria, white blood cells, and red blood cells. The unpleasant odor is caused by pus in the urine (pyuria).**
3. These adaptations do not reflect ketone bodies in the urine. A reagent strip dipped in urine will measure the presence of ketone bodies.
4. These adaptations do not reflect excessive calcium in the urine. Urine calcium levels are measured by assessing a 24-hour urine specimen.

14. 1. Although this should be done, something else must also be done to ensure safe urination at night.
2. This may be too often or not often enough for the patient. A bladder-retraining program should be individualized for the patient.
3. **The use of a commode requires less energy than using a bedpan or walking to the bathroom. Sitting on a commode uses gravity to empty the bladder fully and thus prevent urinary stasis.**
4. Fluids may be decreased during the last two hours before bedtime, but they should not be avoided completely after 5 PM. Some fluid intake is necessary for adequate renal perfusion.

15. 1. **A culture attempts to identify the microorganisms present in the urine, and a sensitivity identifies the antibiotics that are effective against the isolated microorganisms. A sterile specimen container is used to prevent contamination of the specimen by microorganisms outside the body (exogenous).**

2. The urine from a straight catheter (single lumen tube) flows directly into the specimen container. Collecting a urine specimen from a catheter port is necessary when the patient has a urinary retention catheter.
3. A straight catheter has a single lumen for draining urine from the bladder. A straight catheter does not remain in the bladder and therefore does not have a second lumen for water to be inserted into a balloon.
4. This may result in no urine left in the bladder for the straight catheter to collect. A minimum of 3 mL of urine is necessary for a specimen for urine culture and sensitivity.

16. 1. This is unnecessary. Perineal hygiene should be performed at least once a day, after a bowel movement, and whenever the catheter is changed or replaced.
2. Although this is important to promote the flow of urine from the patient to the drainage bag, it is not as important as an action in another option.
3. The anchoring device (e.g., Velcro, elastic, self-adhesive, inflatable ring) must be snug enough to prevent the condom from falling off, but not so tight that it interferes with blood circulation to the penis.
4. This is contraindicated. If left in this position it can constrict the penis resulting in edema and tissue injury.

17. 1. This is contraindicated because it may introduce microorganisms into the bladder that can cause an infection. Irrigation of a urinary retention catheter is not done prophylactically.
2. This information should be documented on the patient's hospital record, not the tubing.
3. This prevents pressure of the leg on the drainage tube that can interrupt the flow of urine out of the bladder.
4. A urine drainage bag should hang on the bed frame. If left on a side rail, the catheter may inadvertently be pulled out when the side rail is moved. In addition, it must be kept below the level of the bladder to promote the flow of urine out of the bladder by gravity and prevent a flow of urine back into the bladder from the catheter.

18. 1. Narcotics are central nervous system depressants that can cause urinary retention, not diuresis.
2. Drinks with caffeine (e.g., coffee, tea, and some carbonated beverages) promote diuresis, which is secretion and excretion of large amounts of urine.
3. Although activity may increase renal perfusion, which may increase urinary output, the increased fluid lost during activity usually is through insensible losses (e.g., perspiration, moisture in exhaled breaths).
4. Avoiding protein does not prevent diuresis. The presence of protein in the urine indicates that the glomeruli have become too permeable, which occurs in kidney disease. Most plasma proteins are too large to move out of the glomeruli and the small proteins that enter the filtrate are reabsorbed by pinocytosis.

19. 1. Electrolytes are usual constituents of urine, and they fluctuate to help maintain fluid and electrolyte and acid-base balance.
2. The presence of protein in the urine indicates that the glomeruli have become too permeable, which occurs with kidney disease. Most plasma proteins are too large to move out of the glomeruli, and the small proteins that enter the filtrate are reabsorbed by pinocytosis.
3. Urine usually is composed of 95% water.
4. Urea is an expected constituent of urine. It is formed by liver cells when excess amino acids are broken down (deaminated) to be used for energy production.

20. 1. This open-ended question encourages the patient to talk about the problem from a personal perspective. Follow-up questions can be more specific.
2. Dysuria is not necessarily related to incontinence.
3. Dysuria is a problem associated with urine, not fecal, elimination.
4. Although an abnormal color of urine may indicate a potential urinary tract infection, which is associated with dysuria, the question is too narrow because it focuses on only one issue.

21. 1. The inability to produce urine (anuria) is a life-threatening situation. If the cause is not corrected, the patient will need dialysis to correct fluid and electrolyte imbalances and rid the body of the waste products of metabolism.
2. Although this is a concern because it may indicate a urinary tract infection, it is not as serious as an adaptation in another option.
3. The secretion and excretion of large amounts of urine (diuresis) is a concern but it is not as serious as an adaptation in another option.
4. Involuntary discharge of urine after an age when bladder control should be established

(enuresis) is a concern, but it is not as serious as an adaptation in another option.

22. 1. Urinary incontinence usually is not related to chronic pain. Chronic pain is the state in which an individual experiences pain that is persistent or intermittent and lasts for longer than 6 months.
2. A deficient fluid intake is unrelated to urinary incontinence. A reduced fluid intake places an individual at risk of experiencing vascular, interstitial, or intracellular dehydration.
3. Disturbed self-esteem is the state in which an individual experiences, or is at risk of experiencing, negative self-evaluation about self or capabilities. Incontinence may be viewed by the patient as regressing to child-like behavior and has a negative impact on feelings about the self.
4. Urinary incontinence may be unpreventable and uncontrollable. Sufficient knowledge may, or may not prevent, or promote, continence. Deficient knowledge is the state in which an individual or group experiences a deficiency in cognitive knowledge, or psychomotor skills, concerning the condition, or treatment plan.

23. 1. This is related to stress incontinence, which is an immediate involuntary loss of urine during an increase in intra-abdominal pressure.
2. Involuntary voiding, and a lack of awareness of bladder distention, are related directly to both reflex incontinence and total incontinence. Reflex incontinence is the predictable, involuntary loss of urine with no sensation of urgency, of the need to void, or bladder fullness. Total incontinence is the continuous unpredictable loss of urine without distention or awareness of bladder fullness.
3. This is related to urinary retention, which is the chronic inability to void followed by involuntary voiding (overflow incontinence).
4. This is related to urge incontinence, which is an involuntary loss of urine associated with a strong, sudden desire to void.

24. **1. During the General Adaptation Syndrome, the posterior pituitary secretes antidiuretic hormone that promotes water reabsorption in the kidney tubules. Also, the anterior pituitary secretes adrenocorticotropic hormone (ACTH) that stimulates the adrenal cortex to secrete aldosterone, which reabsorbs sodium and thus water.**
2. A low specific gravity reflects dilute urine. With the stress response, the urine will be concentrated and the specific gravity will be elevated.
3. The stress response is unrelated to reflex incontinence. Reflex incontinence is a predictable, involuntary loss of urine with no sensation of urgency, the need to void, or bladder fullness.
4. The stress response is unrelated to urinary hesitancy. Hesitancy is the involuntary delay in initiating urination.

25. **1. A cognitively impaired person may not be able to receive, interpret, or respond to cues for voiding. Reminding the person to void every 2 hours empties the bladder, which limits episodes of incontinence.**
2. Although this might be done, it is not the most important intervention. A cognitively impaired person may or may not have problems with handling clothing when voiding.
3. Restriction of fluid intake is an inappropriate way to manage urinary incontinence. The body needs fluids throughout the day to maintain renal perfusion, kidney function, and fluid balance.
4. A cognitively impaired person may not be able to receive, interpret, or respond to cues for voiding, understand cause and effect, or follow directions.

26. 1. Both urine and stool have usual constituents. Urine has organic constituents (e.g., urea, uric acid, creatinine) and inorganic constituents (e.g., ammonia, sodium, chloride, potassium, calcium). Feces have waste residues of digestion (e.g., bile, intestinal secretions, bacteria) and inorganic constituents (e.g., calcium, phosphorus).
2. A person can feel an overwhelming need to void as well as defecate.
3. Only stool can be assessed regarding shape. Stool usually is tubular in shape. Urine is a liquid that assumes the shape of the container in which it is collected.
4. Both urine and stool can be assessed for color. Stool usually is brown and urine usually is yellow, straw-colored, or amber depending on its concentration.

27. 1. This is the usual odor of urine.
2. Urine usually is pale yellow, straw-colored, or amber depending on its concentration.
3. Specific gravity is the measure of the concentration of dissolved solids in the urine. The acceptable range is 1.010 to

1.025. A specific gravity of 1.035 indicates concentrated urine.

4. Adequate renal perfusion and kidney function are reflected by an hourly urine output of 30 to 50 mL of urine.

28. 1. This adaptation is not associated with urinary retention, which is the inability to void eventually followed by involuntary voiding (overflow incontinence).
2. This adaptation is not associated with reflex incontinence, which is the predictable, involuntary loss of urine with no sensation of urgency, the need to void, or bladder fullness.
3. This adaptation is not associated with stress incontinence, which is the immediate involuntary loss of urine during an increase in intra-abdominal pressure.
4. **Burning on urination (dysuria) is associated with mucosal inflammation that occurs with urinary tract infections.**

29. 1. Anesthesia is a central nervous system depressant that tends to cause urinary retention, not urgency.
2. The urinary bladder does not have to be full to precipitate the urge to void. The urge to void can be felt when 150 to 200 mL of urine collects in the urinary bladder.
3. Dehydration causes a decrease in renal perfusion that results in a diminished capacity to form urine (oliguria), not urgency.
4. **Feeling the need to void immediately (urgency) occurs most often when the urinary bladder is irritated. In the adult, the bladder usually holds 600 mL of urine, although the desire to urinate can be sensed when it contains as little as 150 to 200 mL. As the volume increases, the bladder wall stretches, sending sensory messages to the sacral spinal cord, and parasympathetic impulses stimulate the detrusor muscle to contract rhythmically. Bladder contractions precipitate nerve impulses that travel up the spinal cord to the pons and cerebral cortex where the person experiences a conscious need to void.**

30. 1. Cranberry juice does not dilute bacterial growth. The constituents of cranberries, not the volume of fluid, help prevent urinary tract infections (UTIs). Older adults have a greater risk for UTIs because of decreased bladder tone and increased urine residual.
2. **Foods that promote an acid urine (e.g., cranberries, prunes, plums, eggs, meat, and whole grain breads) create an environment that is not conducive to the growth of bacteria in urine. Microorganisms grow more readily in an alkaline urine.**
3. Cranberry juice does not prevent urinary retention.
4. Cranberry juice does not stimulate hypoactive detrusor muscles.

31. 1. A person with a spinal cord injury will experience reflex incontinence, not stress incontinence.
2. A person with a urinary tract obstruction will experience urinary retention, not stress incontinence.
3. **Stress incontinence is an immediate involuntary loss of urine during an increase in intra-abdominal pressure. It is associated with weak pelvic muscles and structural supports resulting from multiple pregnancies, age-related degenerative changes, and overdistention between voiding.**
4. Confused people may experience total, not stress, incontinence because they do not recognize bladder cues.

32. 1. The opposite should be done to prevent microorganisms from the intestines (e.g., *Escherichia coli*) from being drawn from the anus toward the urinary meatus.
2. This should be avoided because it has been implicated as a precipitating cause of gynecological cancer.
3. This will not prevent a urinary tract infection. Burning on urination (dysuria) is an adaptation to acidic urine flowing over inflamed mucous membranes and is a sign of a urinary tract infection.
4. **Drinking a minimum of 2000 mL of fluid a day produces adequately dilute urine, washes out solutes, and flushes microorganisms out of the distal urethra and urinary meatus.**

33. 1. Although this is done, it is not the best intervention of the options offered.
2. This should be avoided. Cornstarch can accumulate in folds of the skin and when damp can become like sandpaper and cause friction upon movement.
3. **As soon as possible after an incontinence episode, the patient should receive thorough perineal care with soap and water and the area dried well. This action removes urea from the skin, which can contribute to skin breakdown.**

4. Plain soap, not deodorant soap, is all that is necessary when providing perineal care after urinary or bowel incontinence.

34. **1. Excessive urination at night is called nocturia. A person with urinary retention will have small, frequent voidings or dribbling (overflow incontinence) rather than a complete discharge of urine from the bladder.**

2. Hematuria is the presence of red blood cells in the urine. It is associated with bladder inflammation, infection, or trauma, not urinary retention.

3. Urinary retention may produce an atonic bladder rather than bladder contractions.

4. The bladder lies in the pelvic cavity behind the symphysis pubis. When it fills with urine (600 mL), it extends above the symphysis pubis, and when greatly distended (2000 to 3000 mL), it can reach to the umbilicus.

5. With urinary retention the bladder fills with urine causing distention. Eventually the external urethral sphincter temporarily opens to allow a small volume of urine to pass out of the bladder (overflow incontinence, retention with overflow).

35. **The tubing from the collection bag that is attached to the catheter inserted into the bladder should be clamped 2–3 inches below the collection port. This location allows urine to collect above the port. The catheter inserted into the bladder should not be clamped to prevent trauma to the catheter lumen or the lumen leading to the inflated balloon.**

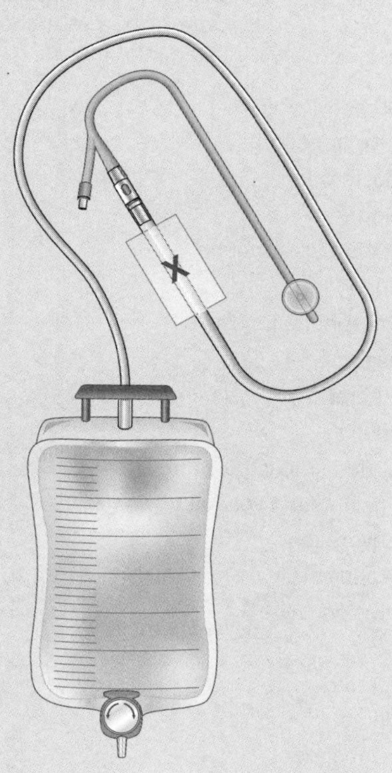

Fluids and Electrolytes

KEYWORDS

The following words include English vocabulary, nursing/medical terminology, concepts, principles, or information relevant to content specifically addressed in the chapter or associated with topics presented in it. English dictionaries, nursing textbooks, and medical dictionaries, such as *Taber's Cyclopedic Medical Dictionary*, are resources that can be used to expand your knowledge and understanding of these words and related information.

Acid
Active transport
Aldosterone
Anion
Antidiuretic hormone
Anuria
Atmospheric pressure
Base
Catheter
Cation
Colloid osmotic pressure
Deficient fluid volume
Dehydration
Diaphoresis
Diffusion
Diluent
Diuretic
Edema
- Dependent
- Peripheral
- Pitting
- Sacral

Electrolytes
- Calcium
- Magnesium
- Phosphorus
- Potassium
- Sodium

Filtration
Fluid compartments
- Extracellular
- Interstitial
- Intracellular
- Intravascular
- Third-compartment spacing

Fluid restriction
Fluid volume deficit
Fluid volume excess
Hydrostatic pressure
Hypercalcemia
Hyperkalemia
Hypermagnesemia
Hyperosmolar
Hypertension
Hypertonic
Hypervolemic
Hypocalcemia
Hypokalemia
Hypomagnesemia
Hypo-osmolar
Hypotension
Hypotonic
Hypovolemic
Icteric
Infiltrate
Infusion port
Insensible fluid loss
Ion
Irrigant
Isotonic
Macrodrip
Microdrip
Milliequivalent
Oncotic pressure
Osmolality
Osmolarity
Osmosis
Osmotic pressure
Primary infusion line
Residual
Secondary infusion line
Sensible fluid loss
Skin turgor
Solute
Specific gravity
Tenting
Thirst
Tonicity
Vaporization

QUESTIONS

1. The physician orders a 2-gram sodium diet for a patient with hypertension. Which food should the nurse teach a patient to avoid?
   1. American cheese
   2. Shredded wheat
   3. Potatoes
   4. Cashews

2. A patient receiving a tube feeding develops diarrhea. The nurse understands that the primary reason tube feedings cause diarrhea is because they are:
   1. Icteric
   2. Isotonic
   3. Hypotonic
   4. Hypertonic

3. When the nurse assesses a patient, which adaptation indicates a potassium deficiency?
   1. Increased blood pressure
   2. Muscle weakness
   3. Chest pain
   4. Dry hair

4. The nurse suspects that an older patient may have a problem with excess fluid volume when the patient's skin appears:
   1. Dry and scaly
   2. Taut and shiny
   3. Red and irritated
   4. Thin and inelastic

5. The nurse determines that inflammation of a vein may have occurred at an intravenous insertion site if when touching the area it:
   1. Feels soft
   2. Seems cool
   3. Produces pallor
   4. Causes discomfort

6. When a patient is under extreme stress there is an increased production of antidiuretic hormone (ADH) and aldosterone. Considering the effect of these hormones in the body, the nurse should expect a decrease in the patient's:
   1. Blood pressure
   2. Urinary output
   3. Body temperature
   4. Insensible fluid loss

7. The nurse checks a meal tray for a patient on a clear liquid diet. The item that is acceptable is:
   1. Ginger ale
   2. Lemon sherbet
   3. Vanilla ice cream
   4. Cream of chicken soup

8. The nurse is caring for a patient who has a reduced fluid intake. The nurse understands that this reduced intake will contribute to:
   1. A decreased urine output
   2. Incontinence of urine
   3. A retention of urine
   4. Frequent urination

9. The nurse is providing dietary teaching for a patient with the diagnosis of osteoporosis. The nurse should teach the patient that the best source of calcium is:
   1. Cheese
   2. Lettuce
   3. Peppers
   4. Oranges

10. The nurse is monitoring a patient who is receiving intravenous fluid. The nurse identifies that the patient is experiencing a fluid overload when assessment reveals:
   1. Chills, fever, and generalized discomfort
   2. Blood in the tubing close to the insertion site
   3. Dyspnea, headache, and increased blood pressure
   4. Pallor, swelling, and discomfort at the insertion site

11. When caring for a patient with hypertension, the nurse should anticipate that the physician will first limit the patient's intake of:
   1. Potassium
   2. Sodium
   3. Protein
   4. Fluids

12. The nurse should notify the physician when a critically ill patient's hourly urine output first falls below:
   1. 20 mL
   2. 30 mL
   3. 60 mL
   4. 120 mL

13. The nurse understands that excess fluid in the interstitial compartment results from increased:
   1. Oncotic pressure
   2. Diffusion pressure
   3. Hydrostatic pressure
   4. Intraventricular pressure

14. When the nurse evaluates a patient's fluid intake and output, the fluid intake should be:
   1. Slightly more than the fluid output
   2. Lower than the urine output
   3. Higher than the fluid output
   4. Equal to the urine output

15. The physician orders hydrochlorothiazide, a diuretic for a patient who is retaining fluid. The nurse should encourage the patient to ingest nutrients rich in:
   1. Magnesium
   2. Potassium
   3. Calcium
   4. Sodium

16. To encourage a confused patient to drink more fluid, the nurse should:
   1. Serve fluid at a tepid temperature
   2. Explain the reason for the desired intake
   3. Offer the patient something to drink every hour
   4. Leave a pitcher of water at the patient's bedside

17. When the nurse cares for an older adult, which assessment best reflects fluid and electrolyte balance?
   1. Intake and output results
   2. Serum laboratory values
   3. Condition of the skin
   4. Presence of tenting

18. A patient has a continuous bladder irrigation. What should the nurse do with the irrigant on the I&O sheet when calculating the fluid balance for this patient?
    1. Add it to the oral intake column
    2. Deduct it from the total urine output
    3. Subtract it from the intravenous flow sheet as output
    4. Document the intake hourly in the urine output column

19. When the nurse identifies patient adaptations that include either oliguria or polyuria, the nurse should be most concerned about a risk for:
    1. Diarrhea
    2. Cachexia
    3. Fluid volume deficit
    4. Impaired skin integrity

20. The patient is receiving a diuretic that contributes to the loss of potassium. The nurse should teach the patient that the best source of potassium is:
    1. Baked potato
    2. Bran flakes
    3. Lean meat
    4. Table salt

21. The physician orders a patient's IV fluids to be discontinued. When discontinuing a patient's intravenous infusion, it is essential that the nurse:
    1. Withdraw the catheter along the same angle of its insertion
    2. Use an alcohol swab to scrub the insertion site
    3. Flush the line with normal saline
    4. Don sterile gloves

22. A patient is admitted to the hospital for a fever of unknown origin. The nursing assessment reveals profuse diaphoresis, dry, sticky mucous membranes, weakness, disorientation, and a decreasing level of consciousness. The nurse infers that the patient has:
    1. Hyperkalemia
    2. Hypercalcemia
    3. Hypernatremia
    4. Hypermagnesemia

23. The physician progresses a patient's diet from clear liquid to full liquid. Which can the nurse include on the full-liquid diet that is not included on the clear-liquid diet?
    1. Cranberry juice
    2. Ginger ale
    3. Jell-O
    4. Milk

24. When a patient exhibits an increasing blood pressure and 2-pound weight gain over two days, the nurse should further assess the patient for:
    1. A decrease in heart rate
    2. An increase in skin turgor
    3. An increase in pulse volume
    4. A decrease in pulse pressure

25. Which is most important when the nurse assesses adult patients for the effects of vomiting?
    1. Electrolyte values
    2. Mouth condition
    3. Bowel function
    4. Body weight

26. When assessing a patient, the nurse understands that an adaptation common to both excess fluid volume and deficient fluid volume is:
    1. Hypotension
    2. Weakness
    3. Agitation
    4. Dyspnea

27. The physician orders an intravenous infusion containing potassium. Before administering this solution to the patient, it is essential that the nurse:
 1. Assess the skin turgor
 2. Obtain the blood pressure
 3. Measure the depth of edema
 4. Determine the presence of urinary output

28. When teaching a patient about a 2-gram sodium diet, which is the best choice for an appetizer?
 1. Pigs in a blanket
 2. Stuffed mushrooms
 3. Cheese and crackers
 4. Fresh vegetable sticks

29. The nurse is monitoring a patient who is receiving fluids intravenously. The nurse identifies that the IV has infiltrated when the insertion site is:
 1. Red
 2. Firm
 3. Inflamed
 4. Edematous

30. The nurse is documenting a patient's intake and output. What should be recorded at approximately ½ its volume?
 1. Ice chips given by mouth
 2. A continuous bladder irrigation
 3. A tube feeding of ½ formula and ½ water
 4. Solution used to maintain patency of a tube

31. When patients are taking supplemental calcium, it is important that the nurse teach them to maintain their fluid intake at a minimum of 2500 mL a day to prevent the:
 1. Formation of kidney stones
 2. Occurrence of muscle cramps
 3. Irritation of the bladder mucosa
 4. Mobilization of calcium from bone

32. A patient receiving a diuretic is encouraged to increase the intake of potassium. The nurse evaluates that the patient understands the teaching when for dinner the patient selects:
 1. Baked salmon fillet
 2. Cooked chicken liver
 3. Cream of chicken soup
 4. Lettuce and tomato salad

33. The nurse is assessing a patient's fluid status. What assessment indicates that the patient has a deficient fluid volume?
 1. Negative balance of intake and output
 2. Decreased body temperature
 3. Increased blood pressure
 4. Shortness of breath

34. When the nurse evaluates the effectiveness of patient teaching, which food selections by a patient indicate understanding regarding an abundant source of calcium? Check all that apply.
 1. _____ Bread
 2. _____ Yogurt
 3. _____ Spinach
 4. _____ Green beans
 5. _____ Peanut butter

35. A patient in the hospital emergency department tells the nurse, "I feel lousy and I've had bad diarrhea for several days. It must have been something I ate. I have nausea and I don't feel like eating or drinking." The physical assessment reveals a weight loss of 4 pounds in 3 days and tenting of the skin. The nurse obtains the vital signs and the practitioner orders laboratory studies. Based on these assessments the nurse identifies that the patient may be experiencing:
 1. Hypokalemia
 2. Hypervolemia
 3. Metabolic acidosis
 4. Respiratory alkalosis

CHART/EXHIBIT

Vital Signs: Oral temperature: 101.2°F
Pulse: 92 bpm, regular, thready
Respirations: 26, deep
Blood pressure: 100/60 mm Hg

Laboratory Values: Urine specific gravity: 1.036
Serum potassium: 5.3 mEq/L
Arterial blood gases:
pH: 7.30
$PaCO_2$: 24 mEq/L
HCO_3: 18 mEq/L

ANSWERS AND RATIONALES

1. 1. **One ounce of American cheese contains 406 mg of sodium and should be avoided on a 2-gram sodium diet.**
   2. Two-thirds of a cup of shredded wheat cereal contains 3 mg of sodium and is permitted on a 2-gram sodium diet.
   3. One ½-pound baked potato contains approximately 16 mg of sodium and is permitted on a 2-gram sodium diet.
   4. One ounce of natural roasted cashews, with no added salt, contains approximately 4 mg of sodium and is permitted on a 2-gram sodium diet.

2. 1. Icteric is unrelated to tube feedings and fluid shifts. Icteric pertains to, or resembles, jaundice.
   2. Isotonic solutions have the same concentration of solutes as the blood. With isotonic solutions there is no net transfer of water across two compartments separated by a semipermeable membrane.
   3. Hypotonic solutions have a lesser concentration of solutes than does the blood. A hypotonic tube feeding will result in fluid being absorbed from the gastrointestinal tract into the intravascular and intracellular compartments.
   4. **Hypertonic solutions have a greater concentration of solutes than does the blood. The high osmolarity of a hypertonic tube feeding exerts an osmotic force that pulls fluid into the stomach and intestine, resulting in intestinal cramping and diarrhea.**

3. 1. Hypertension is associated with hypervolemia, not a potassium deficiency.
   2. **Potassium is an essential component in the sodium-potassium pump, cellular metabolism, and muscle contraction. Patient adaptations associated with a potassium deficiency (hypokalemia) include muscle weakness, fatigue, lethargy, leg cramps, and depressed deep-tendon reflexes.**
   3. Chest pain is associated with a myocardial infarction (heart attack) and pulmonary embolus, not a potassium deficiency
   4. Dry hair is associated with malnutrition and hypothyroidism, not a potassium deficiency.

4. 1. These are signs of aging and dehydration, not excessive fluid volume.
   2. **With excessive fluid volume, the increased hydrostatic pressure moves fluid from the intravascular compartment into the interstitial compartment. As fluid collects in the interstitial compartment (edema), the skin appears taut and shiny.**
   3. These are signs of the local inflammatory response, not of excessive fluid volume.
   4. These are characteristics of skin in the older adult because of a loss of subcutaneous fat and a reduced thickness and vascularity of the dermis, not of excessive fluid volume.

5. 1. The localized edema associated with the inflammatory response causes the affected area to feel firm, not soft.
   2. The localized vasodilation associated with the inflammatory response increases blood flow to the affected area, which causes it to feel warm, not cool.
   3. The localized vasodilation associated with the inflammatory response increases blood flow to the affected area, which causes erythema, not pallor.
   4. **The physiologic response associated with the inflammation of a vein (phlebitis) causes a movement of fluid from the intravascular compartment into the interstitial compartment. Pressure of fluid on nerve endings causes local discomfort.**

6. 1. The blood pressure will increase, not decrease, when the circulating fluid volume increases in response to these hormones.
   2. **Both hormones are involved with water reabsorption, which conserves fluid and results in a decreased urinary output. With decreased kidney perfusion, the juxtaglomerular cells of the kidneys release angiotensin II, which stimulates the release of aldosterone from the adrenal cortex. Aldosterone promotes the excretion of potassium and reabsorption of sodium, which results in the passive reabsorption of water. As the concentration of the blood (osmolality) increases, the anterior pituitary releases antidiuretic hormone (ADH). ADH causes the collecting ducts in the kidneys to become more permeable to water, promoting its reabsorption into the blood.**
   3. ADH and aldosterone do not regulate body temperature.
   4. ADH and aldosterone influence the kidneys to maintain fluid balance. They do not affect

insensible fluid loss through the lungs, skin, or intestinal tract.

7. 1. **Ginger ale is an easily ingested and digested liquid that is permitted on a clear liquid diet. It relieves thirst, prevents dehydration, and minimizes stimulation of the gastrointestinal tract.**
   2. Sherbet contains milk, which is not permitted on a clear liquid diet.
   3. When ice cream melts, it is not a clear liquid and therefore is not permitted on a clear liquid diet. Milk contains protein and lactose, which stimulates the digestive process; this is undesirable when a patient is receiving a clear liquid diet.
   4. Cream of chicken soup contains milk and small particles of chicken, both of which are contraindicated on a clear liquid diet.

8. 1. **When the serum osmolarity increases because of insufficient fluid intake, antidiuretic hormone (ADH) increases the permeability of the collecting tubules in the kidneys, which increases the reabsorption of water and decreases urine output.**
   2. Involuntary urination (incontinence) is not associated with a reduced fluid intake.
   3. The accumulation of urine in the bladder with an inability to empty the bladder (urinary retention) is unrelated to a decreased fluid intake.
   4. Frequent urination occurs with increased, not decreased, fluid intake.

9. 1. **Cheese, a dairy product, is an excellent dietary source of calcium. One ounce of cheese contains approximately 150 mg to 406 mg of calcium depending on the type of cheese.**
   2. Lettuce is not high in calcium. One cup of shredded loose leaf lettuce contains approximately 38 mg of calcium.
   3. Peppers are not high in calcium. One pepper contains approximately 4 mg of calcium.
   4. Oranges are not high in calcium. One orange contains approximately 52 mg of calcium.

10. 1. These are signs of an infection, not excess fluid volume.
    2. This occurs when the IV bag is held lower than the IV insertion site and is an undesirable occurrence.
    3. **IV fluid flows directly into the circulatory system via a vein. Excess intravascular volume (hypervolemia) causes hypertension, pulmonary edema, and headache.**
    4. These are signs of an IV infiltration, not excess fluid volume.

11. 1. Potassium restriction is a therapy associated with kidney disease, not hypertension. If diuretics are used to treat a patient's hypertension, potassium supplementation through diet or medications may be employed.
    2. **In the stepped-care approach to the management of hypertension, sodium intake is restricted in Step I.**
    3. Protein intake may be restricted when a patient has kidney disease, not hypertension.
    4. Fluid restriction is not part of the 4-part stepped-care management of hypertension. Adequate fluids (a minimum of 1500 to 2000 mL) are necessary for fluid balance. Fluids may be restricted as an intervention for kidney disease or pulmonary edema, not hypertension.

12. 1. The physician should be notified long before the hourly urine output reaches 20 mL.
    2. **The circulating blood volume perfuses the kidneys, producing a glomerular filtrate of which varying amounts are either reabsorbed or excreted to maintain fluid balance. When a person's hourly urine output is only 30 mL, it indicates a deficient circulating fluid volume, inadequate renal perfusion, and/or kidney disease. The physician should be notified.**
    3. An hourly urine output of 60 mL is close to the expected range of 1400 mL to 1500 mL per 24 hours or 30 mL to 50 mL per hour.
    4. The physician does not have to be notified about this. An hourly urine output of 120 mL indicates that there is adequate kidney perfusion. The intake and output should be monitored to ensure that volume depletion does not occur over time.

13. 1. Oncotic (colloid osmotic) pressure is the force exerted by colloids (such as proteins) that pull or keep fluid within the intravascular compartment. Oncotic pressure is the major force opposing hydrostatic pressure in the capillaries.
    2. Diffusion is a continual intermingling of molecules with movement of molecules from a solution of higher concentration to a solution of lower concentration.
    3. **Hydrostatic pressure is the pressure exerted by a fluid within a compartment, such as blood within the vessels. Hydrostatic pressure moves fluid from an area of greater pressure to an area of lesser pressure. Hydrostatic pressure within vessels of the body moves fluid out**

of the intravascular compartment into the interstitial compartment. Interstitial fluid is extracellular fluid that surrounds cells.

4. Intraventricular pressure is the pressure that exists in the left and right ventricles of the heart. These pressures do not move fluid from the intravascular compartment to the interstitial compartment.

14. 1. **The volume and composition of body fluids are kept in a delicate balance (total intake is slightly more than total output) by a harmonious interaction of the kidneys and the endocrine, respiratory, cardiovascular, integumentary, and gastrointestinal systems.**

2. If the total intake is lower than the urine output, the patient will develop a deficient fluid volume.
3. If the total intake is higher than the total output, the patient will develop an excess fluid volume.
4. If intake and urine output are equal, the patient will develop a deficient fluid volume because of fluid loss through routes other than the kidneys. In addition to urine output, the body has insensible fluid loss through the skin, in feces, and as water vapor in expired air.

15. 1. Although loop and thiazide diuretics enhance magnesium excretion, which may produce a mild hypomagnesemia, it does not require supplementation.

2. **Most diuretics affect the renal mechanisms for tubular secretion and reabsorption of electrolytes, particularly potassium. Because of potassium's narrow therapeutic window of 3.5 to 5.0 mEq/L and its role in the sodium-potassium pump and muscle contraction, depleted potassium must be supplemented by increasing the dietary intake of foods high in potassium and/or the administration of potassium drug therapy.**
3. Serum calcium levels vary depending on the diuretic. Loop diuretics increase calcium excretion, which may produce hypocalcemia. Thiazide diuretics decrease calcium excretion, which may produce hypercalcemia.
4. Although sodium deficit (hyponatremia) may occur with diuretics, usually it is mild and does not require supplementation.

16. 1. Fluids should be administered at the temperature usually associated with the fluid. For example, cool temperatures for juice, soda, and milk and warm temperatures for tea, coffee, and soup. Hot liquids should be avoided for safety reasons.

2. This probably will be ineffective because a confused person has difficulty understanding cause and effect.
3. **Frequent smaller volumes of fluid (50 to 100 mL/hour) are better tolerated physiologically and psychologically than infrequent larger volumes of fluid.**
4. A confused patient, having difficulty understanding cause and effect, may ignore a pitcher of water.

17. 1. This assesses only fluid balance.

2. **Laboratory studies provide objective measurements of indicators of fluid, electrolyte, and acid-base balance. Common diagnostic tests include serum blood studies such as electrolytes (particularly sodium, potassium, chloride, and calcium), osmolarity, hemoglobin, hematocrit, and arterial blood gases.**
3. This assesses only fluid balance. In addition, the changes in the integumentary system as a person ages complicate assessment of the skin for fluid balance disturbances in the older adult. Skin changes include loss of dermal and subcutaneous mass (thin and wrinkled), decreased secretion from sebaceous and sweat glands (dry skin), and less organized collagen and elastic fibers (wrinkles, decreased elasticity).
4. This assesses only fluid balance. *Tenting* occurs when the skin of a dehydrated person remains in a peak or tent position after the superficial layers of the skin are pinched together. Caution is advised when assessing an older person because some degree of tenting may occur even when hydrated because of the decrease in skin elasticity and tissue fluid associated with aging. The skin over the sternum is the area that should be tested for tenting.

18. 1. The irrigant of a continuous bladder irrigation is instilled into the urinary bladder, not the mouth.

2. **When a continuous bladder irrigation is in use, drainage from the urinary bladder will consist of both urine and the instilled irrigant. To determine the patient's urinary output, the amount of the irrigant instilled must be deducted from the total urinary output.**
3. The IV flow sheet should not contain any information regarding intake and output other than the amount and type of fluid that is instilled into the circulatory system.

4. Intake anywhere in the body should be recorded in the appropriate intake column, not in the urinary output column.

19. 1. Frequent, loose, liquid stools, not oliguria or polyuria, are associated with diarrhea.
2. Oliguria and polyuria are related to fluid balance and kidney functioning, not nutrition. Cachexia is a profound state of malnutrition.
3. **The production of excessive amounts of urine by the kidneys without an increase in fluid intake can precipitate a fluid volume deficit. Oliguria, the production of excessively small amounts of urine by the kidney, is reflected as a negative balance in the intake and output. A negative balance of intake and output is a characteristic of fluid volume deficit.**
4. Oliguria and polyuria are related to fluid balance and kidney functioning, not skin integrity. However, because oliguria may be related to fluid retention and subsequent edema and polyuria may ultimately cause dehydration and dry skin, the patient may eventually be at risk for impaired skin integrity.

20. 1. **This is the best source of potassium of the foods listed. A ½-pound baked potato contains approximately 844 mg of potassium.**
2. Bran flakes do not contain any potassium.
3. Depending on the type of meat, 3 ounces of meat contains only 57 mg to 323 mg of potassium and is not the best choice of the options offered.
4. One teaspoon of salt contains only trace amounts of potassium.

21. 1. **Removing a catheter by withdrawing it along the same path of its insertion minimizes injury to the vein and trauma to the surrounding tissue. This action limits seepage of blood and promotes healing of the puncture wound.**
2. Scrubbing the area with an alcohol wipe is unnecessary. The area should be compressed with a sterile gauze pad. Pressure helps stop the bleeding and prevents the formation of a hematoma. A sterile gauze pad provides for surgical asepsis, which prevents infection.
3. This is unnecessary.
4. Clean, not sterile, gloves should be worn by the nurse to prevent exposure to the patient's body fluids.

22. 1. Although muscle weakness and lethargy are associated with hyperkalemia, the other adaptations are not.
2. Although weakness and lethargy are associated with hypercalcemia, the other adaptations are not.
3. **With profuse diaphoresis, the water loss exceeds the sodium loss resulting in hypernatremia. Excess serum sodium precipitates changes in the musculoskeletal (weakness), neurologic (disorientation and decreased level of consciousness), and integumentary (dry, sticky mucous membranes) systems.**
4. Although muscle weakness, lethargy, and drowsiness are associated with hypermagnesemia, the other adaptations are not.

23. 1. Cranberry juice is a clear liquid.
2. Ginger ale is a clear liquid.
3. Jell-O is a clear liquid that is a solid when refrigerated and a liquid at room temperature. It is permitted in either form on a clear liquid diet.
4. **Milk is not on a clear liquid diet. It contains a high solute load, including fat and proteins, which precipitates the digestive process.**

24. 1. With an excess fluid volume the heart rate will increase, not decrease, in an attempt to maintain adequate cardiac output.
2. In the early stages of an excess fluid volume, a change in skin turgor may not be evident. One liter of fluid is equal to approximately 2.2 pounds.
3. **With an excess fluid volume the amount of circulating blood volume increases, resulting in full, bounding peripheral pulses.**
4. The pulse pressure is the difference between the systolic and diastolic pressures of a blood pressure measurement, and the acceptable range is 30 to 50 mm Hg. With an excess fluid volume, the pulse pressure increases, not decreases.

25. 1. **Vomiting results in a loss of chloride (greatest amount), sodium (next greatest amount), and potassium (least amount, but of greatest importance because it can cause dysrhythmias and cardiac arrest).**
2. Although the mouth is assessed and oral care is provided, it is performed for comfort, not because there is a life-threatening problem.
3. This will be done, but it is not the priority.
4. Although this will be done to assess fluid volume deficit (2.2 pounds equals approximately 1 liter of fluid), it is not as critical as another assessment.

26. 1. A decrease in blood pressure is associated with fluid volume deficit, not excess, because of the decreased circulating blood volume.
    2. **Muscle weakness is a musculoskeletal adaptation to both increased fluid volume and decreased fluid volume because the fluid imbalances alter cellular and body metabolism.**
    3. Agitation and restlessness are neurologic adaptations associated with fluid volume deficit, not excess.
    4. Dyspnea is associated with fluid volume excess, not deficit, because fluid overload causes pulmonary congestion.

27. 1. This is unnecessary for the administration of potassium. This is part of the assessment of a patient's hydration status, particularly when the patient is at risk for dehydration.
    2. Although all the vital signs should be measured when a patient is receiving any fluids or electrolytes, monitoring the heart rate and rhythm are more significant assessments than the blood pressure in relation to the administration of potassium. Both a serum potassium decrease (hypokalemia) and increase (hyperkalemia) cause cardiac dysrhythmias.
    3. This is unnecessary for the administration of potassium. This is part of the assessment when a patient has a fluid volume excess in dependent tissues where the hydrostatic capillary pressure is high.
    4. **Serum potassium has a narrow therapeutic window (3.5 to 5.0 mEq/L). When kidney function is impaired, potassium can accumulate in the body and exceed the therapeutic level of 5.0 mEq/L, which can cause cardiac dysrhythmias and arrest.**

28. 1. One tenth of a pound of frankfurters contains approximately 168 mg of sodium and should be avoided on a 2-gram sodium diet.
    2. Although mushrooms are low in sodium, when stuffed with seasoned bread crumbs (1/3 cup contains approximately 370 mg of sodium) they should be avoided on a 2-gram sodium diet.
    3. One ounce of cheese contains approximately 106 to 400 mg of sodium depending on the cheese. Two crackers contain approximately 44 to 165 mg depending on the product. These foods should be avoided on a 2-gram sodium diet.
    4. **As a food group, fresh vegetables have low-sodium content. The sodium content of vegetables include 1 cup of broccoli, 17 mg; 1 cup of cauliflower, 20 mg; 1 carrot, 25 mg; 1 pepper, 2 mg; 1 radish, 1 mg; 1 cup of mushrooms, 3 mg; and 6 slices of cucumber, 1 mg.**

29. 1. When the insertion site of an IV is reddened, swollen, warm to the touch, and painful, the patient has phlebitis, not an infiltration of an IV.
    2. When IV fluid flows into the tissue surrounding a vein (infiltration), the area will feel soft and spongy, not hard.
    3. When the area at the insertion site of an IV appears inflamed, the patient has phlebitis, not an infiltration of an IV.
    4. **When an IV line moves out of a vein and into subcutaneous tissue, the IV fluid will begin to collect in the interstitial compartment causing swelling (edema).**

30. 1. **Ice chips are particles of frozen water that take up more volume when they are frozen than when they melt. When ice chips change from a solid to a liquid, the resulting fluid is approximately ½ the volume of the ice chips.**
    2. The total amount of the irrigant instilled into the urinary bladder is accounted for as intake. The total volume that was instilled is then deducted from the total urinary output to determine the patient's urinary output.
    3. When a tube feeding solution consists of ½ formula and ½ water, the final combined volume of the formula and water is recorded on the appropriate intake column of the intake and output record.
    4. Whatever volume of solution is instilled into a catheter, the full volume used is recorded when the nurse documents the intervention.

31. 1. **A high fluid intake increases the volume of urine produced. The resulting frequent urination of dilute urine prevents the formation of renal calculi, which may occur because of the increased precipitation of calcium salts associated with calcium supplementation.**
    2. Excessive supplementation of calcium causes hypercalcemia. Muscle tremors and cramps are associated with hypocalcemia, not hypercalcemia.
    3. Neither hypocalcemia nor hypercalcemia irritates the bladder mucosa.
    4. Calcium supplementation and weight bearing, not an increased fluid intake, prevent bone demineralization.

32. 1. Three ounces of baked salmon contains only 305 mg of potassium.
    2. One cooked chicken liver contains only 28 mg of potassium.

3. One cup of cream of chicken soup contains only 273 mg of potassium.
4. **Lettuce and tomatoes are excellent sources of potassium. One 6-inch diameter head of iceberg lettuce contains 852 mg of potassium, and one 2 ¾-inch diameter tomato contains 255 mg of potassium.**

33. 1. **A patient has a negative balance of intake and output when the output exceeds the intake. This is a characteristic of deficient fluid volume.**
 2. An elevated temperature is characteristic of a deficient fluid volume.
 3. A low blood pressure is characteristic of a deficient fluid volume.
 4. Shortness of breath is a characteristic of excess fluid volume, not deficient fluid volume.

34. 1. Grain products are not high in calcium. One slice of bread contains approximately 20 to 49 mg of calcium depending on the type of grain.
 2. **Yogurt is an excellent dietary source of calcium. Eight ounces of yogurt contain 415 mg of calcium.**
 3. **One cup of cooked fresh spinach contains 245 mg of calcium.**
 4. Green beans are not high in calcium. One cup of green beans contains approximately 60 mg of calcium.
 5. Peanut butter is not high in calcium. One tablespoon of peanut butter contains approximately 5 mg of calcium.

35. 3. **Metabolic Acidosis**

CHART/EXHIBIT

Vital Signs:
Oral temperature: 101.2°F
Pulse: 92 bpm, regular, thready
Respirations: 26, deep
Blood pressure: 100/60 mm Hg

Laboratory Values:
Urine specific gravity: 1.036
Serum potassium: 5.3 mEq/L
Arterial blood gases: pH: 7.30
$PaCO_2$: 24 mEq/L
HCO_3: 18 mEq/L

ANSWERS AND RATIONALES:
1. Hyperkalemia, not hypokalemia, is associated with metabolic acidosis. The potassium is more than the acceptable range of 3.5–5.0 mEq/L.
2. The patient has hypovolemia, not hypervolemia, because of dehydration. The pulse is rapid and thready and the urine specific gravity is increased. An abrupt weight loss indicates fluid loss (2.2 pounds is equal to 1 liter of fluid) and the patient is exhibiting decreased intracellular and interstitial fluid as evidenced by tenting of the skin. Also, the blood pressure is on the low extreme of the acceptable range of 90 to 119 mm Hg for systolic and 60 to 79 mm Hg for diastolic.
3. **Intestinal secretions distal to the pyloric sphincter contain large amounts of bicarbonate which is lost through diarrhea. The arterial blood gases indicate uncompensated metabolic acidosis: the pH is less than the acceptable range of 7.35 to 7.45; the HCO_3 is less than the acceptable range of 21 to 28 mEq/L; and the $PaCO_2$ is within the acceptable range of 23 to 30 mEq/L.**
4. With respiratory alkalosis the pH will be >7.45, the $PaCO_2$ will be <35 mm Hg, and the HCO_3 will be within the acceptable range of 21 to 28 mEq/L. Respiratory alkalosis usually is caused by hyperventilation precipitated by conditions such as anxiety, thyrotoxicosis, mechanical ventilation, early sepsis, and high fever.

Gastrointestinal

KEYWORDS

The following words include English vocabulary, nursing/medical terminology, concepts, principles, or information relevant to content specifically addressed in the chapter or associated with topics presented in it. English dictionaries, nursing textbooks, and medical dictionaries, such as *Taber's Cyclopedic Medical Dictionary*, are resources that can be used to expand your knowledge and understanding of these words and related information.

Abdominal
Abdominal distention
Anus
Borborygmi
Bowel flora
Bowel habits
Bowel sounds
Bowel training
Bulk
Cathartic
Colon
Colorectal
Colostomy
Constipation
Defecate
Defecation reflex
Diarrhea
Distention
Diverticulitis
Diverticulosis
Endoscopic
Enema
- Cleansing
- Harris drip (flush)
- Hypertonic
- Hypotonic
- Isotonic
- Large volume
- Oil retention
- Saline
- Soapsuds
- Tap water

Evacuate, evacuation
Fecal
Fecal diversion
Fecal impaction
Feces
Flatus/flatulence
Fracture bedpan
Gastrocolic reflex
Hemoccult test, guaiac
Hemorrhoids
Hypermotility
Hypomotility
Ileostomy
Irrigation
Laxative
Mucosal
Nasogastric tube
Occult blood
Ostomy
Ova and parasites
Paralytic ileus
Perianal
Perineal
Peristalsis
Pinworms
Prolapse
Rectal fullness
Rectal tube
Rectum
Seepage
Sigmoidoscopy
Sitz bath
Spastic colon
Sphincter
Steatorrhea
Stoma
Stool
Straining
Suppository
Tarry stool

QUESTIONS

1. Which word is unique regarding how a soapsuds enema works on the mucosa of the bowel?
   1. Dilating
   2. Irritating
   3. Softening
   4. Lubricating
2. The nurse is caring for an patient with an intestinal stoma. Which intervention is most important?
   1. Cleansing the stoma with cool water
   2. Spraying an air-freshening deodorant in the room
   3. Selecting a bag with an appropriate-size stomal opening
   4. Wearing sterile nonlatex gloves when caring for the stoma
3. The nurse is caring for a group of patients with a variety of gastrointestinal problems. Which factor can influence the occurrence of both diarrhea and constipation?
   1. Increased metabolic rate
   2. High-solute tube feedings
   3. Side effects of medications
   4. Inability to perceive bowel cues
4. The nurse identifies that when compared with other nasogastric tubes used for gastric decompression, a Salem sump tube is uniquely designed to:
   1. Minimize the risk of bowel obstruction
   2. Ensure drainage of the intestines
   3. Prevent gastric mucosal damage
   4. Promote gastric rest
5. A patient is admitted with a diagnosis of upper GI bleeding. The nurse should expect the color of this patient's stool to be:
   1. Red
   2. Pink
   3. Black
   4. Brown
6. When administering a small-volume hypertonic enema to an adult, the nurse should:
   1. Insert the rectal tube 1 to 1.5 inches into the rectum
   2. Position the enema bottle 12 inches above the level of the patient's anus
   3. Direct the rectal tube toward the vertebrae as it is inserted into the rectum
   4. Maintain the compression of the enema container until after withdrawing the tube
7. Before collecting a stool sample for occult blood, the nurse should:
   1. Plan to collect the first specimen of the day
   2. Secure a sterile specimen container
   3. Wash the patient's perianal area
   4. Ask the patient to void
8. Which is a defining characteristic of the nursing diagnosis Bowel Incontinence?
   1. Frequent, soft stools
   2. Involuntary passage of stool
   3. Impaired rectal sphincter control
   4. Greenish-yellow color to the stool
9. The nurse is collecting a bowel elimination history for a newly admitted patient with a medical diagnosis of possible bowel obstruction. Which question takes priority?
   1. "Do you use anything to help you move your bowels?"
   2. "When was the last time you moved your bowels?"
   3. "What color are your usual bowel movements?"
   4. "How often do you have a bowel movement?"

10. When obtaining a patient's health history the patient tells the nurse, "I've got gastroesophageal reflux disease." Which most serious adaptation associated with this disorder should the nurse expect the patient to develop?
    1. Diarrhea
    2. Heartburn
    3. Gastric fullness
    4. Esophageal erosion

11. The nurse determines that a fracture bedpan should be used for the patient who:
    1. Has a spinal cord injury
    2. Is on bed rest
    3. Has dementia
    4. Is obese

12. A patient with the diagnosis of diverticulosis is advised to eat a diet high in fiber. To best increase the bulk in fecal material, the nurse should recommend that the patient eat:
    1. Whole wheat bread
    2. White rice
    3. Pasta
    4. Kale

13. Which statement by a patient with an ileostomy alerts the nurse to the need for further education?
    1. "I don't expect to have much of a problem with fecal odor."
    2. "I will have to take special precautions to protect my skin around the stoma."
    3. "I'm going to irrigate my stoma so I have a bowel movement every morning."
    4. "I should avoid gas-forming foods like beans to limit funny noises from the stoma."

14. The nurse is assessing a patient with a fecal elimination problem. The nurse understands that a major defining characteristic for the nursing diagnosis Diarrhea is:
    1. Spastic colon
    2. Impaired sphincter control
    3. Inability to respond to rectal cues
    4. Loose stools more than three times a day

15. A patient is straining excessively when attempting to have a bowel movement. The nurse discourages the patient from straining on defecation primarily because it may precipitate:
    1. Incontinence
    2. Dysrhythmias
    3. Fecal impaction
    4. Rectal hemorrhoids

16. When teaching a health class about bodily functions, the school nurse includes the fact that mucus in the gastrointestinal tract:
    1. Activates digestive enzymes
    2. Protects the gastric mucosa
    3. Enhances gastric acidity
    4. Emulsifies fats

17. A patient complains of constipation. The nurse should encourage the patient to eat:
    1. Applesauce
    2. Bananas
    3. Cheese
    4. Beans

18. A patient is experiencing constipation. Which independent nursing action facilitates defecation of a hard stool?
    1. Applying a lubricant to the anus
    2. Encouraging a sitz bath after defecation
    3. Instilling warm mineral oil into the rectum
    4. Positioning cold compresses against the anus

19. The nurse is caring for a patient with a nasogastric tube attached to suction. The most important nursing action when caring for the nasogastric tube is:
    1. Using sterile technique when irrigating the tube
    2. Recording the intake and output every 2 hours
    3. Maintaining suction at the prescribed level
    4. Providing oral hygiene every 4 hours

20. The nurse is caring for a patient who is experiencing diarrhea. About which should the nurse be most concerned?
    1. Dehydration
    2. Malnutrition
    3. Excoriated skin
    4. Urinary incontinence

21. A patient's colostomy stoma appears pale. What should the nurse do?
    1. Notify the physician
    2. Listen for bowel sounds
    3. Wash the area with warm water
    4. Gently massage around the stoma

22. A patient with flatulence is concerned about the production of unpleasant odors. The nurse should encourage the patient to avoid:
    1. Alcohol
    2. Raisins
    3. Coffee
    4. Eggs

23. The nurse is caring for a group of patients. The nurse determines that the person at the greatest risk for bowel incontinence is the person who is:
    1. Ninety years old
    2. On a program of sedation for sleep
    3. Disoriented to time, place, and person
    4. Receiving multiple antibiotic medications

24. A patient is admitted with lower gastrointestinal tract bleeding. The nurse expects that the patient will have:
    1. Tarry-colored stool
    2. Green-mucoid stool
    3. Orange-colored stool
    4. Bright-red–tinged stool

25. The nurse determines that the teaching about a guaiac test of stool is understood when the patient states, "This test can detect the presence of:
    1. Bile."
    2. Bacteria."
    3. Hidden blood."
    4. Ova and parasites."

26. The nurse must collect a specimen for the presence of pinworms. Which action is most essential to ensure accuracy of the specimen?
    1. Press the sticky side of nonfrosted cellophane tape across the anus before the patient goes to bed at night
    2. Pass a rectal swab beyond the internal rectal sphincter and rotate gently to collect a specimen
    3. Perform the procedure the first thing in the morning before the first bowel movement
    4. Wash the rectal area gently with soap and water before collecting the specimen

27. The nurse identifies that the patient understands the need to reestablish bowel flora after a week of diarrhea when the patient states, "I'm going to:
    1. Wean myself off of the antibiotics one day after my temperature is normal."
    2. Eat a container of yogurt every day for a few days."
    3. Add rice to my diet one meal each day."
    4. Drink eight glasses of water today."

28. The nurse teaches a patient with a history of constipation that the excessive use of laxatives should be avoided primarily because it:
1. Weakens the natural response to defecation
2. Results in distention of the intestines
3. Causes abdominal discomfort
4. Precipitates incontinence

29. The nurse is assisting a patient with a bedpan. Which nursing action is most important?
1. Position the patient slightly off the back edge of a regular bedpan
2. Fold the top linen out of the way when putting the patient on the bedpan
3. Place the flat part of the rim of the fracture bedpan toward the patient's feet
4. Once on the bedpan raise the head of the bed so that the patient is in the Fowler's position

30. The nurse identifies that a patient has tarry stools. The nurse understands that tarry stools indicate:
1. Upper gastrointestinal bleeding
2. Pancreatic dysfunction
3. Lactulose intolerance
4. Inadequate bile salts

31. The nurse is providing dietary teaching to a patient with diverticulosis. The nurse should encourage the patient to increase the intake of which food?
1. Tofu
2. Oatmeal
3. Corn on the cob
4. Cucumber spears

32. The nurse is teaching a patient with a cardiac condition to avoid the Valsalva's maneuver. The nurse should teach the patient to:
1. Exhale while contracting the abdominal muscles
2. Attempt to have a bowel movement every day
3. Take a cathartic on a regular basis
4. Eat rice several times a week

33. When the nurse uses a cone attached to a colostomy irrigation catheter it works by:
1. Stopping the outflow of enema solution during the procedure
2. Dilating the stoma so that the enema tube can be inserted
3. Facilitating the elimination of drainage from the colon
4. Preventing prolapse of the bowel during peristalsis

34. Which goal is most appropriate for a patient with the nursing diagnosis Perceived Constipation? "The patient will:
1. Defecate every day."
2. Drink eight glasses of water per day."
3. Verbalize the rationale for the use of laxatives."
4. Have a bowel movement without the use of a laxative."

35. A patient consistently is incontinent of feces. The nurse understands that bowel incontinence is unrelated to:
1. Overdistention of the rectum
2. Anal sphincter dysfunction
3. Cognitive impairment
4. Pain on defecation

36. Which action is most important for the nurse to teach patients about the intake of bran to facilitate defecation?
1. Eat three tablespoons of bran each morning
2. Drink at least eight glasses of fluids each day
3. Have a bowel movement right after ingesting the bran
4. Take a cathartic that will supplement the action of bran

37. The nurse must administer a large-volume tap-water enema. Which mechanism associated with this type of enema increases peristalsis?
   1. Bowel distention
   2. Hypertonic action
   3. Irritating the bowel
   4. Absorption of fluid by stool

38. The nurse understands that a tap-water enema usually is given to:
   1. Reduce abdominal gas
   2. Drain the urinary bladder
   3. Empty the bowel of stool
   4. Limit nausea and vomiting

39. Which statements by a patient with diverticulosis alerts the nurse that the patient needs additional health teaching? Check all that apply.
   1. _____ "I am allowed to eat high-fiber cereal."
   2. _____ "I love to eat poppy seed bagels in the morning."
   3. _____ "I sit on the toilet for ten minutes after breakfast every day."
   4. _____ "I am going to drink eight glasses of water a day when I get home."
   5. _____ "I should hold my breath and bear down when having a bowel movement."
   6. _____ "I like to massage my lower abdomen when I'm trying to have a bowel movement."

40. The nurse is caring for a patient with a colostomy, and the patient's stool has a pasty consistency. Place an X over the area of the intestine where the nurse can expect a colostomy to usually produce stool with a pasty consistency.

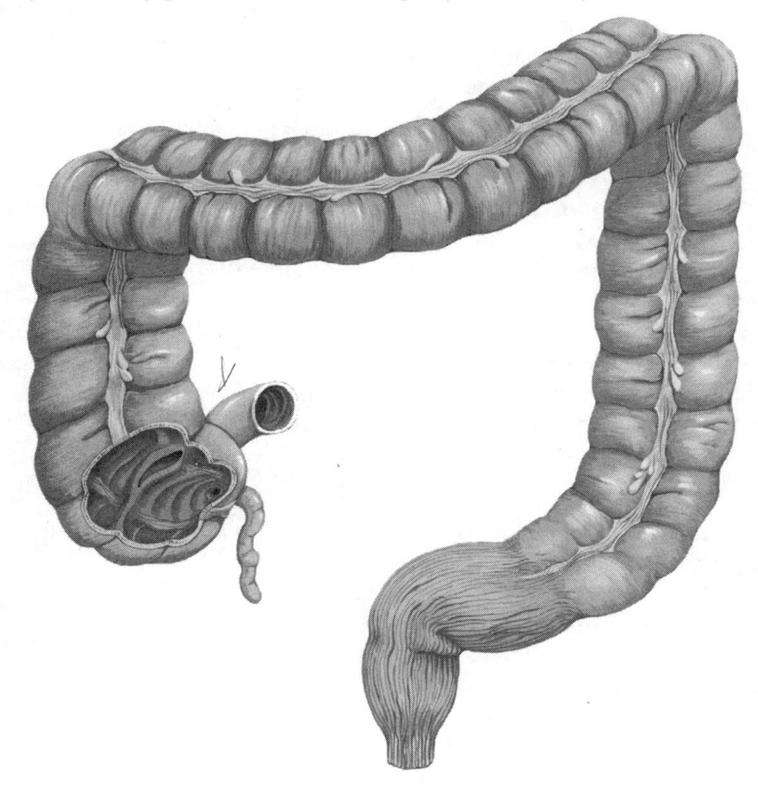

ANSWERS AND RATIONALES

1. 1. High-volume (not soapsuds) enemas, such as tap-water or saline enemas work by distending (dilating) the lumen of the intestine.
   2. **Although a soapsuds enema works by increasing the volume in the colon, its unique attribute is that soap is irritating to the intestinal mucosa. Irritation of the mucosa precipitates peristalsis, which facilitates the evacuation of fecal material.**
   3. An oil-retention enema, a small-volume enema, introduces oil into the rectum and sigmoid colon; this softens the feces and lubricates the rectum and anal canal, facilitating defecation.
   4. An oil-retention, not soapsuds, enema lubricates the rectum and anal canal, facilitating the passage of feces.

2. 1. Although a stoma can be cleaned with water as long as it is not at the extremes of hot or cold, it is not the priority.
   2. Although this might be done, it is not the priority.
   3. **The opening of the appliance must be large enough to encircle the stoma to within 1/8 to 1/6 inch to protect the surrounding tissue from the enzymes present in the intestinal discharge without impinging on the stoma. Pressure against the stoma can damage delicate mucosal tissue or impede circulation to the stoma, both of which can impair the viability of the stoma.**
   4. Clean, not sterile, gloves should be worn when caring for a stoma. Medical, not surgical, asepsis should be practiced. Latex or nonlatex gloves can be worn as long as the patient or nurse does not have a latex allergy.

3. 1. An increased metabolic rate will increase peristalsis and possibly result in diarrhea, not constipation.
   2. A high-solute tube feeding has a greater osmotic pressure than surrounding interstitial tissue; it draws fluid into the gastrointestinal tract, which may result in diarrhea, not constipation.
   3. **Medications, depending on their physiologic action, side effects, and toxic effects, can cause either constipation or diarrhea.**
   4. An inability to perceive bowel cues for defecation results in a lack of response that further weakens the defecation reflex, ultimately causing constipation, not diarrhea.

4. 1. Nasointestinal tubes, attached to suction, remove the fluid that collects behind an intestinal obstruction. They help treat, not prevent, an intestinal obstruction.
   2. All nasogastric tubes attached to suction remove drainage from the stomach, not the intestine. Nasointestinal tubes attached to suction remove fluid from the intestine.
   3. **A Salem sump tube is a double-lumen, rather than a single-lumen, tube. The second lumen (blue pigtail) is open to environmental (atmospheric) air, which is drawn into the stomach to equalize the outside pressure with the pressure inside the stomach. This prevents the catheter tip from attaching to the gastric mucosa when the drainage lumen is attached to suction, limiting mucosal damage.**
   4. All nasogastric tubes attached to suction empty the stomach contents in an effort to promote gastric and intestinal rest. Gastric glands produce up to 4 to 5 liters of fluid a day that stimulate the intestine unless removed.

5. 1. Red-colored stool indicates lower, not upper, gastrointestinal bleeding.
   2. Pink-colored stool, although uncommon, may indicate lower gastrointestinal bleeding mixed with mucus or intestinal fluid.
   3. **Black (tarry) stool indicates upper gastrointestinal bleeding. Enzymes acting on the blood turn it black. In addition, iron supplements, excessive intake of red meat, and dark green vegetables can cause black stools.**
   4. Brown is the expected color of stool. This color is caused by the presence of stercobilin and urobilin, which are derived from a pigment in bile (bilirubin).

6. 1. This will not permit safe administration of the enema solution. The rectal tube must be inserted 3 to 4 inches to ensure that the catheter is beyond both the external and internal sphincters.
   2. A small-volume enema bottle is held directly outside the anus because the solution container is attached to the prelubricated nozzle. The container of a large-volume enema should not exceed a height of 12 inches above the anus.

3. This will injure the intestinal mucosa. The catheter should be directed toward the umbilicus, not the vertebrae.
4. **This prevents suctioning back of the fluid that has just been instilled. Releasing compression on the bottle causes a vacuum at the tip of the nozzle that can injure mucous membranes.**

7. 1. This is unnecessary.
   2. This is unnecessary. Medical, not surgical, asepsis should be followed.
   3. This is unnecessary. However, the nurse may assist the patient to perform perineal hygiene after the stool specimen has been obtained.
   4. **Emptying the urinary bladder before attempting to have a bowel movement prevents accidental contamination of the specimen by urine.**

8. 1. This is not a defining characteristic of any nursing diagnosis, but it is similar to the defining characteristics for the nursing diagnosis Diarrhea, which is loose, liquid stools and/or increased frequency of stools (more than three times a day).
   2. **An involuntary passage of stool is a major defining characteristic of the nursing diagnosis Bowel Incontinence, which is the state in which an individual experiences a change in usual bowel habits characterized by involuntary passage of stool.**
   3. Impaired rectal sphincter control is a related factor, not defining characteristic, for the nursing diagnosis Bowel Incontinence.
   4. This is unrelated to the nursing diagnosis Bowel Incontinence. A green or orange color to the stool indicates intestinal infection.

9. 1. Although this question may be asked, it is not the priority at this time.
   2. **A cardinal sign of a bowel obstruction is the lack of a bowel movement (obstipation).**
   3. Although this will be asked, this information relates more to malabsorption, biliary problems, and gastrointestinal bleeding.
   4. Although this will be asked to obtain baseline information about intestinal elimination, it is not specific to the presenting problem.

10. 1. Diarrhea is not associated with GERD.
    2. Pain occurring behind the sternum (heartburn) and sore throat are the predominant symptom of GERD. Although these adaptations are a concern, they can be treated.
    3. Although feeling full, distended, or bloated can occur with GERD, it is not life threatening and the patient can be taught interventions to limit its occurrence.
    4. **With GERD a backflow of the contents of the stomach into the esophagus occurs. Gastric juices are acidic (pH less than 3.5), which can cause erosion of the mucous membranes of the esophagus necessitating surgery.**

11. 1. **A fracture bedpan has a low back that promotes function of the patient's lower back while on the bedpan.**
    2. A regular bedpan is appropriate for this patient.
    3. A regular bedpan is appropriate for this patient.
    4. A regular bedpan is appropriate for this patient.

12. 1. One slice of whole wheat bread contains only 1.5 grams of dietary fiber.
    2. A serving of a ½ cup of white rice contains only 0.8 gram of dietary fiber.
    3. A serving of 3½ ounces of cooked pasta contains only 1.6 grams of dietary fiber.
    4. **Kale is an excellent source of dietary fiber. A serving of 3½ ounces of kale contains 6.6 grams of dietary fiber.**

13. 1. The odor from drainage is minimal because fewer bacteria are present in the ileum compared to the large intestine. An ileostomy is an opening into the ileum (distal small intestine from the jejunum to the cecum).
    2. Cleansing the skin, skin barriers, and a well-fitted appliance are precautions to protect the skin around an ileostomy stoma. The drainage from an ileostomy contains enzymes that can damage the skin.
    3. **This statement is inaccurate in relation to an ileostomy and indicates that the patient needs more teaching. An ileostomy produces liquid fecal drainage that is constant and cannot be regulated.**
    4. An ileostomy stoma does not have a sphincter that can control the flow of flatus or drainage, resulting in noise.

14. 1. Spastic colon is a pathophysiological related factor, not a defining characteristic, for the nursing diagnosis Diarrhea.
    2. Impaired sphincter control is a related factor for the nursing diagnosis Bowel Incontinence, not Diarrhea.
    3. An inability to recognize, interpret, or respond to rectal cues is a situational-related factor for the nursing diagnosis Bowel Incontinence.
    4. **The major defining characteristics for the nursing diagnosis Diarrhea are increased**

frequency of stools (more than three times a day) and/or loose, liquid stools. Diarrhea is the state in which an individual experiences, or is at risk for experiencing, frequent passage of liquid stool or unformed stool.

15. 1. The loss of the voluntary ability to control the passage of fecal or gaseous discharges through the anus (bowel incontinence) is caused by impaired functioning of the anal sphincter or its nerve supply, not straining on defecation.
    2. Straining on defecation requires the person to hold the breath while bearing down (Valsalva's maneuver). This maneuver increases the intrathoracic and intracranial pressures, which can precipitate dysrhythmias, brain attack (stroke), and respiratory difficulties; all of these can be life threatening.
    3. Fecal impaction is caused by prolonged retention and the accumulation of fecal material in the large intestine, not straining on defecation.
    4. Although straining on defecation can contribute to the formation of hemorrhoids, this is not the primary reason straining on defecation is discouraged. Hemorrhoids, although painful, are not life threatening.

16. 1. The presence of fluid, or food, activates digestive enzymes, not mucus.
    2. Mucus, secreted by mucous membranes and glands, is a viscous, slippery fluid containing mucin, white blood cells, water, inorganic salts, and exfoliated cells. Mucin, a mucopoly saccharide, is a lubricant that protects body surfaces from friction and erosion.
    3. Mucus does not enhance gastric acidity. Gastric acidity enhances digestion.
    4. The low surface tension of bile salts contributes to the emulsification of fats in the intestine.

17. 1. Applesauce thickens, not softens, stool.
    2. Bananas thicken, not soften, stool.
    3. Cheese thickens, not softens, stool.
    4. Beans contain both soluble and insoluble fibers and are second only to bran as the best plant source of fiber. They increase bulk and absorb many times their weight in water to produce a larger, softer stool.

18. **1. A lubricant reduces friction, which facilitates the passage of a hard, dry stool through the anus. Nurses are legally permitted to diagnose and treat human responses. Constipation is a human response, and applying a lubricant to the anus is an independent function of the nurse.**
    2. A sitz bath requires a practitioner's order and is a dependent, not independent, function of the nurse. A sitz bath will not promote the passage of a hard, dry stool, but it may promote hygiene and comfort after the bowel movement.
    3. An oil retention enema softens the feces and lubricates the rectum and anus. However, it requires a practitioner's order and is a dependent, not independent, function of the nurse.
    4. Warm, not cold, compresses may facilitate defecation. Warm compresses may relax the surrounding muscles and the external sphincter, promoting defecation.

19. 1. Medical, not surgical, asepsis is necessary.
    2. It is unnecessary to monitor the intake and output this frequently. The intake and output must be recorded at routine intervals as per hospital policy, usually every 8 and 24 hours.
    3. The level of suctioning is part of the physician's order for nasogastric decompression. Low suction pressure is between 80 and 100 mm Hg and high suction pressure is between 100 and 120 mm Hg. Suctioning must be maintained continuously with a Salem sump to prevent reflux of gastric secretions into the vent lumen, which will obstruct its functioning and result in mucosal damage. A single-lumen tube requires low intermittent suction to prevent the tube from adhering to the stomach mucosa.
    4. Oral hygiene should be provided more frequently than every 4 hours. Because there is no food or fluid to stimulate salivary gland secretion and the tube in the nose may interfere with breathing, precipitating mouth breathing, the mouth becomes dry.

20. **1. Usually digestive juices of approximately 3.5 to 5 liters are secreted and reabsorbed by the body daily. With diarrhea, the transit time through the intestine is decreased, interfering with the reabsorption of water, resulting in frequent, loose watery stools and dehydration.**
    2. Although malnutrition may be related to diarrhea, particularly if it is prolonged, it is neither life-threatening, nor the priority in comparison to another option.
    3. Although the skin may become excoriated in the presence of diarrhea because the enzymes

in fecal material can erode the skin, it is neither life-threatening, nor the priority in comparison to another option.
4. Diarrhea is unrelated to urinary incontinence.

21. 1. **A pale stoma indicates that the circulation to the stoma is compromised and viability of tissue is questionable without immediate intervention. The physician should be notified immediately.**
2. Although this might be done, it is not the priority. Active bowel sounds indicate peristalsis and the presence of flatus in the small intestines, which can occur even if there is an impending problem in the large intestine.
3. This is inappropriate. This will not improve circulation to the stoma and will waste valuable time.
4. This is inappropriate. This will not improve circulation and may injure surrounding tissue.

22. 1. Alcohol may cause gas, but it does not produce an odor.
2. Raisins may cause gas, but they do not produce an odor.
3. Coffee may have a laxative effect, but it does not produce an odor.
4. **Eggs will produce odorous gas and should be avoided. In addition, the patient should be taught to avoid other odor-producing foods, such as asparagus, fish, garlic, green peppers, mustard, onions, radishes, and spicy foods.**

23. 1. Constipation, not bowel incontinence, is more common in the older adult than other age groups. Constipation in the older adult is caused by decreased bowel motility, inadequate hydration, lack of fiber, sedentary lifestyle, abuse of laxatives, and side effects of medications.
2. Sedatives depress the central nervous system, which may precipitate constipation, not bowel incontinence.
3. **When a person is disoriented to time, place, and person, the individual may not have the cognitive ability to perceive and interpret fecal distention and rectal pressure cues to defecate, resulting in bowel incontinence.**
4. Antibiotic medications are known for causing diarrhea, not bowel incontinence.

24. 1. Tarry-colored stool indicates upper gastrointestinal bleeding.
2. Green-mucoid stool indicates the presence of infection.
3. Orange-colored stool indicates the presence of infection.
4. **Bright-red–tinged stool is the cardinal sign of lower gastrointestinal bleeding. When bleeding occurs close to the anus, enzymes have not digested the blood, so the blood has not turned black.**

25. 1. Bile is an expected constituent of fecal material and is not detected with the guaiac test.
2. Bacteria are identified in feces through a stool culture, not the guaiac test.
3. **Testing the feces for occult blood is called the guaiac test or Hemoccult test. This test uses a chemical reagent to detect the presence of the enzyme peroxidase in the hemoglobin molecule. Occult blood is hidden, obscure, and may not be visable to the naked eye.**
4. Ova and parasites are identified through microscopic examination of feces, not the guaiac test.

26. 1. Specimen collection is done immediately after awakening from sleep, not before sleep.
2. This is unnecessary and can injure the anal and rectal mucosa.
3. **This ensures that there will be eggs available for collection at the perianal area. The adult pinworm (*Enterobius vermicularis*) exits the anus at night to lay eggs. The cellophane-tape (Scotch-tape) test is performed first thing in the morning before a bowel movement or bathing so that these eggs are not disrupted or removed before obtaining a specimen for testing.**
4. This will remove any eggs that are present in the perianal area, which will interfere with accurate test results.

27. 1. This will not reestablish bowel flora. Discontinuing antibiotics before the full course of therapy is completed can result in a return of the original infection or precipitate the development of a superinfection.
2. **Yogurt is merely milk that is curdled by the addition of bacteria, specifically *Lactobacillus bulgaricus* and *Streptococcus thermophilus*. Eating yogurt helps to restore bacterial balance of the resident flora of the intestine.**
3. Although rice helps to limit diarrhea, it will not reestablish bowel flora.
4. Although water is essential for all body processes, and to replace fluid lost in the diarrhea, it does not reestablish bowel flora.

28. 1. **Laxatives cause a rapid transit time of intestinal contents. When used excessively,**

the bowel's natural responses to fecal distention and rectal pressure weaken, resulting in chronic constipation.

2. Laxatives increase peristalsis, which helps evacuate the bowel, preventing, not promoting, abdominal distention from flatus or intestinal contents.
3. Although excessive laxative use can cause cramping, it is temporary and does not have long-term implications, as does the problem in another option.
4. The loss of the voluntary ability to control the passage of fecal or gaseous discharges through the anus (bowel incontinence) is caused by impaired functioning of the anal sphincter, or its nerve supply, not excessive laxative use.

29. 1. This is unsafe and uncomfortable. The patient should be positioned so that the buttocks rest on, not slightly off of, the smooth, rounded rim of a regular bedpan.
2. This is unnecessary. The top linen can be draped over the patient in such a way as to promote placement of the bedpan while maintaining the privacy and dignity of the patient.
3. The opposite is true. A fracture bedpan should be placed with the flat, low end under the patient's buttocks.
4. **Raising the patient to a Fowler's position assumes the familiar, usual position for having a bowel movement. The more vertical position utilizes gravity and hip flexion raises intra-abdominal pressure, both of which maximize evacuation of feces.**

30. 1. **When blood from bleeding in the upper gastrointestinal tract is exposed to the digestive process, the fecal material becomes black (tarry). In addition, exogenous iron, red meat ingestion, and dark green vegetables can make the stool look black.**
2. Pancreatic dysfunction results in impaired digestion of fats (by lipase), protein (by trypsin and chymotrypsin), and carbohydrates (by amylase). Pancreatic dysfunction results in pale, foul-smelling, bulky stools, not tarry stools.
3. A reduction or lack of the secretion of lactase from the wall of the small intestine results in the inability of the body to break down lactose to glucose and galactose. Lactose intolerance causes diarrhea, gaseous distention, and intestinal cramping, not tarry stools.
4. Inadequate bile salts result in less bile entering the intestinal tract. The brown color of stool is caused by the presence of stercobilin and urobilin, which are derived from a pigment in bile (bilirubin). With inadequate bile salts the stool will appear clay-colored.

31. 1. Tofu is a soy product that is low in fiber and calories but high in protein and calcium.
2. **One cup of oatmeal contains 2.2 grams of dietary fiber. A high-fiber diet is recommended for people with diverticulosis because it produces a bulky stool that prevents constipation. Constipation results in straining when defecating, which raises the intraintestinal pressure and promotes the development of diverticuli.**
3. Although a ½ cup of corn contains 2.9 grams of dietary fiber, it is contraindicated for people with diverticular disease because it contains a husk.
4. Although cucumbers are high in dietary fiber, they are contraindicated for people with diverticular disease because they contain seeds.

32. 1. **Exhaling requires the glottis to be open, which prevents the Valsalva's maneuver. The Valsalva's maneuver is bearing down while holding the breath by closing the glottis.**
2. This may result in straining, which employs the use of the Valsalva's maneuver. Also, the patient may not need to have a daily bowel movement.
3. Ordering a cathartic is a dependent, not an independent, function of the nurse. Regular use of a cathartic is contrindicated because it leads to dependence.
4. Rice thickens stool, which promotes the development of constipation. Constipation may result in straining on defecation, which employs the Valsalva's maneuver.

33. 1. **The cone advances into the stoma until it effectively fills the opening, which prevents a reflux of solution while the irrigating solution is being instilled. In addition, it helps prevent accidental perforation of the bowel with the rectal catheter.**
2. This is not the purpose of the cone. The catheter is threaded through the center of the cone.
3. The cone is removed before the bowel evacuates its contents.
4. The stoma of a colostomy should never prolapse. If this should occur, the physician should be notified immediately.

34. 1. The need to have a bowel movement every day is unnecessary, unrealistic, and a

myth. Patterns of bowel elimination vary considerably depending on a multitude of factors.
2. This is an intervention, not a goal. Although desirable for everyone, it does not specifically relate to the nursing diagnosis Perceived Constipation.
3. Although knowledge is essential, behavioral outcomes determine if a goal has been achieved.
4. **This is the most appropriate goal for a patient with the nursing diagnosis Perceived Constipation because a defining characteristic of this diagnosis is the excessive use of laxatives to achieve a daily bowel movement.**

35. 1. An overdistention of the rectum may impair the person's ability to control the external sphincter, resulting in bowel incontinence.
2. Anal sphincter dysfunction is related to bowel incontinence. The internal and external anal sphincters and their nerve supply must be intact to maintain bowel control.
3. People who are cognitively impaired do not perceive or respond to the cues to defecate and, as a result, experience bowel incontinence.
4. **When people experience pain when having a bowel movement, they postpone or ignore the urge to defecate; this results in constipation, not bowel incontinence. As fecal material is retained in the intestines, water continues to be reabsorbed resulting in a hard, dry stool.**

36. 1. This is too stimulating for the intestines initially. Bran use should begin with 1 tablespoon and gradually increased as tolerated because it can cause flatus and distention.
2. **Bran is an insoluble fiber that increases bulk in the intestines. Eight glasses of water daily keeps the body well hydrated and the stool soft. Intestinal elimination is dependent on the relationship among fiber, water, and activity.**
3. This is too soon to expect a physiologic response to the bran.
4. This is counterproductive. Cathartic use will weaken the bowel's natural responses to fecal distention and rectal pressure, resulting in chronic constipation.

37. 1. **A large-volume enema dilates the intestine by exerting pressure against the intestinal wall. This pressure stimulates peristalsis, which propels intestinal contents toward the anus.**
2. The constituents of the enema solution, not its volume, exert a hypertonic or hypotonic action. Hypertonic solutions exert a greater osmotic pressure than the surrounding interstitial fluid, which draws fluid from the interstitial compartment into the colon.
3. A large-volume enema exerts pressure within the intestinal lumen; it does not irritate the intestinal mucosa. Castile soap, used with a soapsuds enema, irritates the intestinal mucosa, which precipitates peristalsis and subsequent defecation.
4. Medications, not enemas, influence the relationship between fecal material and water. Emollient/stool-softener laxatives soften and delay the drying of feces, which permit fat and water to penetrate feces. Wetting-agent/stool-softener laxatives lower the surface tension of feces, which helps water to penetrate the feces.

38. 1. A Harris drip (Harris flush) helps eliminate intestinal gas.
2. A urinary catheter (Foley or retention catheter) drains the urinary bladder of urine, not a tap-water enema.
3. **A tap-water enema puts fluid into the large intestine; the pressure of this volume causes the colon to empty of stool.**
4. A tap-water enema will not affect nausea and vomiting; nothing by mouth, or medication, can be used to limit nausea and vomiting.

39. 1. High-fiber foods are encouraged because they prevent constipation. Constipation increases intraluminal intestinal pressure, which promotes intestinal mucosal outpouching.
2. **This patient needs further teaching because people with diverticulosis should avoid foods with husks and seeds. Poppy seeds are tiny seeds that may become lodged in diverticula. Fecal material may combine with these seeds and cause a fecalith that is capable of causing inflammation and perforation of the intestine.**
3. This is an accepted practice. Bowel elimination should follow a familiar routine, and attempting to defecate after breakfast takes advantage of the gastrocolic reflex.
4. This is desirable for effective bowel function. An adequate intake of fluid ensures that after water is reabsorbed through the large intestines for essential body processes there is enough water left in the intestine to create a soft, formed stool.
5. **The Valsalva's maneuver increases intraluminal intestinal pressure, which promotes intestinal mucosal outpouching and should be avoided.**

6. This is an accepted practice. Light stroking of the skin (effleurage) reduces abdominal muscle tension, which may facilitate defecation.

40. An X anywhere along the highlighted area is the correct answer. Stool in the ascending colon is the most liquid, but as it travels through the transverse colon, fluid is reabsorbed and stool becomes pasty in consistency. In the descending colon, stool becomes more dry, solid, and formed.

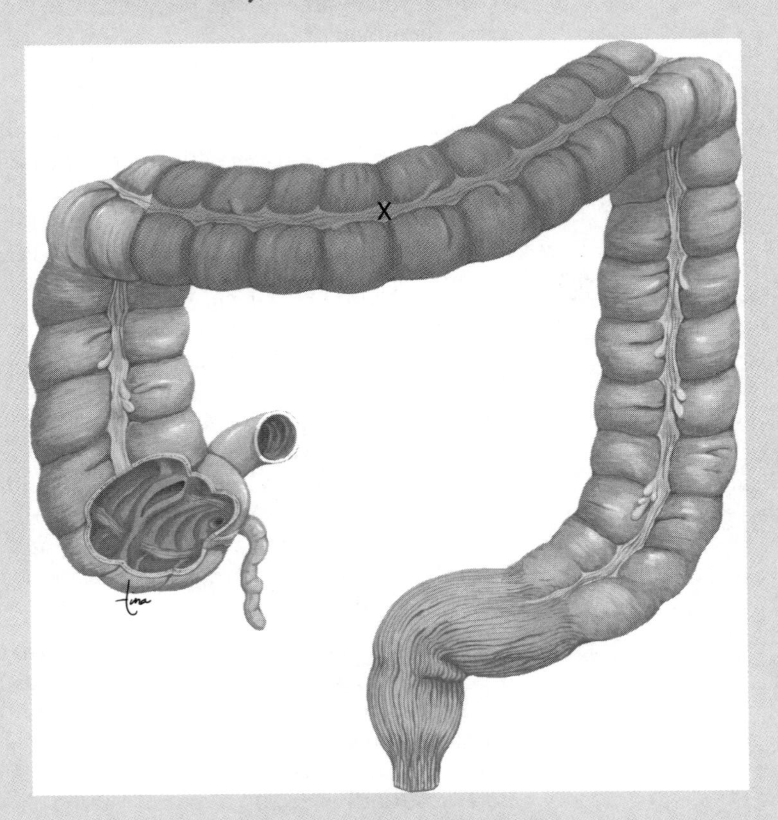

Pain, Comfort, Rest, and Sleep

KEYWORDS

The following words include English vocabulary, nursing/medical terminology, concepts, principles, or information relevant to content specifically addressed in the chapter or associated with topics presented in it. English dictionaries, nursing textbooks, and medical dictionaries, such as *Taber's Cyclopedic Medical Dictionary*, are resources that can be used to expand your knowledge and understanding of these words and related information.

Addiction
Back rub
Bedtime routines
Biofeedback
Breakthrough pain
Circadian rhythm
Cold therapy
Contralateral stimulation
Continuous positive airway pressure (CPAP)
Distraction techniques
Enuresis
Epidural analgesia
Fatigue
Gate control theory
Grimacing
Guarding behaviors
Guided imagery
Heat therapy
Hypnosis
Intensive care unit psychosis, ICU psychosis
Intrathecal analgesia
Massage
Meditation
Nocturia
Nonopioid analgesics
Opioid analgesics
Pain, characteristics
- Aggravating factors
- Duration
- Intensity
- Onset
- Quality
- Relieving factors

Pain scale
Pain threshold
Pain tolerance
Pain, types
- Acute
- Chronic
- Episodic
- Intermittent
- Intractable
- Malignant
- Neuropathic
- Phantom
- Radiating
- Remittent
- Visceral

Patient-controlled analgesia (PCA)
Physical dependence
Placebo
Progressive muscle relaxation
Psychological dependence
Rest
Self-splinting
Sleep
- Non-Rapid Eye Movement sleep (NREM)
- Rapid Eye Movement sleep (REM)

Sleep disorders
- Bruxism
- Hypersomnia
- Insomnia
- Narcolepsy
- Night terrors
- Parasomnia
- Restless legs
- Sleep apnea
- Sleep deprivation
- Somnambulism

Sleepiness
Sleep rituals
Snoring
Sundowning
Transcutaneous electrical nerve stimulation

QUESTIONS

1. The nurse understands that a patient who has difficulty sleeping may have shortened NREM sleep. Therefore, the nurse should assess this patient for:
   1. Decreased pain tolerance
   2. Excessive sleepiness
   3. Confusion
   4. Irritability
2. The nurse understands that the shortest-acting pain relief method is:
   1. Patient-controlled analgesia
   2. Intramuscular sedatives
   3. Intravenous narcotics
   4. Regional anesthesia
3. Which concept associated with sleep must the nurse understand to best plan nursing care?
   1. Bedtime routines are associated with an expectation of sleep
   2. Alcohol intake interferes with one's ability to fall asleep
   3. Sleep needs remain consistent throughout the life span
   4. Total time in bed gradually decreases as one ages
4. A patient has been in the intensive care unit for two weeks. Which nursing diagnosis associated with sleep deprivation is most appropriate for this patient?
   1. Risk for Disturbed Thought Processes
   2. Impaired Gas Exchange
   3. Disuse Syndrome
   4. Powerlessness
5. The nurse understands that the internal stimulus that most commonly interferes with sleep is:
   1. Ringing in the ears
   2. Bladder fullness
   3. Hunger
   4. Thirst
6. The nurse is giving a back rub. The stroke that is most effective in inducing relaxation at the end of the procedure is:
   1. Percussion
   2. Effleurage
   3. Kneading
   4. Circular
7. A patient states, "The pain moves from my chest down my left arm." The nurse identifies that the characteristic of pain associated with this statement is:
   1. Pattern
   2. Duration
   3. Location
   4. Constancy
8. Which best supports the nursing diagnosis Fatigue?
   1. Muscle weakness
   2. Exertional dyspnea
   3. Activity intolerance
   4. Exhaustion unrelieved by rest
9. The nurse understands that with obstructive sleep apnea, the aspect of sleep that most often is affected is its:
   1. Amount
   2. Quality
   3. Depth
   4. Onset

10. A patient is being admitted to the hospital and the nurse is performing a complete assessment. Which is the most therapeutic open-ended question the nurse can ask about the quality of the patient's sleep?
    1. "How would you describe your sleep?"
    2. "Do you consider your sleep to be restless or restful?"
    3. "Is the number of hours you sleep at night good for you?"
    4. "Does your bed partner complain about your sleep behaviors?"

11. The nurse is caring for a patient who is experiencing pain. The nurse understands that a common psychological patient response to pain is:
    1. Experiencing fear related to loss of independence
    2. Developing an increased tolerance to the drug
    3. Asking for pain medication to relieve the pain
    4. Verbalizing the presence of nausea

12. The most appropriate goal for an adult who has disturbed sleep because of nocturi12a is, "The patient will:
    1. Report fewer early morning awakenings because of a wet bed."
    2. Demonstrate a reduction in nighttime bathroom visits."
    3. Resume sleeping immediately after voiding."
    4. Use an incontinence device at night."

13. The nurse understands that a contributing factor to fatigue that is not related to pregnancy is:
    1. Increased basal metabolic rate
    2. Changes in hormonal levels
    3. Decreased cardiac output
    4. Low hemoglobin level

14. Which concept associated with rest and sleep must the nurse understand to plan nursing care?
    1. Metabolic rates increase during rest
    2. Energy requirements increase with age
    3. Sleep requirements increase during stress
    4. Catabolic hormones increase during sleep

15. A patient has a total abdominal hysterectomy and debulking for fourth-stage ovarian cancer. What should the nurse do first when on the second postoperative day this patient complains of abdominal pain at level 5 on a 1-to-10 pain scale?
    1. Reposition the patient
    2. Offer a relaxing back rub
    3. Use distraction techniques
    4. Administer the ordered pain medication

16. A patient is diagnosed with narcolepsy. The nurse's primary intervention should address the patient's:
    1. Inability to provide self-care
    2. Altered thought processes
    3. Excessive fatigue
    4. Risk for injury

17. When caring for patients who have problems sleeping, it is important for the nurse to remember that an adaptation uniquely associated with shortened REM sleep is:
    1. Hyporesponsiveness
    2. Immunosuppression
    3. Irritability
    4. Vertigo

18. A patient is experiencing discomfort associated with gastroesophageal reflux. The nurse should teach the patient to sleep in which position?
   1. Semi-Fowler's
   2. Right lateral
   3. Prone
   4. Sims'

19. A patient complains of pain. When caring for this patient, the most important thing the nurse must recall is that:
   1. The extent of pain is directly related to the amount of tissue damage
   2. Administering opioids for pain will eventually lead to addiction
   3. The person experiencing the pain is the authority about the pain
   4. Behavioral adaptations are congruent with statements about pain

20. A patient is experiencing anxiety. Which aspect of sleep should the nurse expect will be affected as a result of the anxiety?
   1. Onset
   2. Depth
   3. Stage II
   4. Duration

anxiety - Sympathetic - sleep onset

21. A patient requests pain medication. What should the nurse do first when responding to this patient's request for pain medication?
   1. Use distraction to minimize the patient's perception of pain
   2. Place the patient in the most comfortable position possible
   3. Administer pain medication to the patient quickly
   4. Assess the various aspects of the patient's pain

22. With children, which is a major defining characteristic of the nursing diagnosis Disturbed Sleep Pattern?
   1. Hyperactivity
   2. Respiratory disorders
   3. Resisting going to bed
   4. Early morning awakenings

23. A patient has the medical diagnosis of obstructive sleep apnea. A common intervention the nurse can employ is:
   1. Teaching the use of devices that support airway patency
   2. Encouraging sleeping in the supine position
   3. Positioning two pillows under the head
   4. Administering sedatives

24. Which statement by the patient to a nurse indicates a precipitating factor associated with pain?
   1. "I usually feel a little dizzy and think I'm going to vomit when I have pain."
   2. "I usually have pain after I get dressed in the morning."
   3. "My pain usually comes and goes throughout the night."
   4. "My pain feels like a knife cutting right through me."

25. Of the options presented, the most important nursing intervention that supports a patient's ability to sleep in the hospital setting is:
   1. Providing an extra blanket
   2. Limiting unnecessary noise on the unit
   3. Shutting off lights in the patient's room
   4. Pulling curtains around the bed at night

26. A patient has a history of severe chronic pain. One of the most important guidelines associated with providing nursing care to this patient is:
   1. Determining the level of function that can be performed without pain
   2. Focusing on pain management intervention before pain is excessive
   3. Providing interventions that do not precipitate pain
   4. Asking what is an acceptable level of pain

27. The nurse needs to remember that when assessing pain:
    1. The lack of expression of pain does not always equate with the pain being experienced
    2. Pain medication can significantly increase a patient's pain tolerance
    3. The majority of cultures value the concept of suffering in silence
    4. Most people experience approximately the same pain tolerance

28. The nurse understands that the most common cause of sleep deprivation in the hospital setting is:
    1. Fragmented sleep
    2. Early awakening
    3. Restless legs
    4. Sleep apnea

29. The nurse is performing an admitting interview. Which patient statement about pain causes the most concern?
    1. "At home I take something for pain before it gets too bad."
    2. "They say my pain may get worse, and I can't stand it now."
    3. "My pain medication works, but I'm afraid of becoming addicted."
    4. "I try to pretend that it is not part of me, but it takes a lot of effort."

30. A patient has been in the intensive care unit for three days. For which common adaptation indicating ICU psychosis associated with sleep deprivation should the nurse assess the patient?
    1. Hypoxia
    2. Delirium
    3. Lethargy
    4. Dementia

31. The nurse is caring for a patient who is verbalizing feeling fatigued. Which is a major defining characteristic of the nursing diagnosis Fatigue?
    1. Lacking interest in surroundings
    2. Exhaustion that is relieved by rest
    3. Inability to maintain usual routines
    4. Compromised physical conditioning

32. The concept associated with sleep that the nurse must understand to best plan nursing care for the hospitalized patient is:
    1. People require eight hours of uninterrupted sleep to meet energy needs
    2. Frequency of nighttime awakenings decreases with age
    3. Fear can contribute to the need to stay awake
    4. Bed rest decreases the need to sleep

33. The nurse is assessing a patient in pain. The nurse understands that a word that reflects the pattern of pain is:
    1. Episodic
    2. Phantom
    3. Moderate
    4. Tenderness

34. The nurse is obtaining a health history from a newly admitted patient. Which patient statement about alcohol intake is based on a common physiologic response?
    1. "After I go drinking, I have to urinate during the night."
    2. "When I drink, I get hungry in the middle of the night."
    3. "Falling asleep is hard, but once asleep I sleep great."
    4. "If I drink too much, I oversleep in the morning."

35. The nurse is assessing a patient in pain. Which characteristic is more common with acute pain than with chronic pain?
1. Self-focusing
2. Sleep disturbances
3. Guarding behaviors
4. Variations in vital signs

36. Preemptive analgesia is used when a nurse medicates the patient:
1. Before a patient goes to sleep
2. Equal distant times around the clock
3. As soon as a patient complains of pain
4. Before doing a dressing change that has been painful in the past

37. A patient is diagnosed with chronic fatigue syndrome. It is most important that the nurse explore the extent of the patient's:
1. Ability to provide self-care
2. Physical mobility
3. Social isolation
4. Gas exchange

38. When caring for patients in pain, it is important for the nurse to understand that patients:
1. Are able to describe qualities of their pain
2. Who are in pain will request pain medication
3. Need to know that the nurse believes what they say about their pain
4. Will demonstrate vital signs that are congruent with the intensity of pain

39. A patient is experiencing interrupted sleep. For which adaptation associated with shortened NREM sleep should the nurse assess the patient?
1. Anxiety
2. Hyperactivity
3. Delayed healing
4. Aggressive behavior

40. A patient is experiencing lack of sleep because of pain. Which is the most appropriate goal for this patient? The patient will:
1. Be provided with a back massage every evening before bedtime
2. Report feeling rested after awakening in the morning
3. Request less pain medication during the night
4. Experience four hours of uninterrupted sleep

41. The nurse is helping a patient who is experiencing mild pain to get ready for bed. Which nursing action is most effective?
1. Assisting with relaxing imagery
2. Obtaining an order for an opioid
3. Encouraging the patient to take a warm shower
4. Recommending that the patient be more active during the day

42. The nurse understands that people tend to be the sleepiest between:
1. 12 noon and 2 PM
2. 6 AM and 8 AM
3. 2 AM and 4 AM
4. 6 PM and 8 PM

43. Which patient statement indicates that the patient is experiencing bruxism?
1. "I walk around in my sleep almost every night, but I don't remember it."
2. "I annoy the whole family with the loud snoring noises I make at night."
3. "I occasionally urinate in bed when I am sleeping, and it's embarrassing."
4. "I am told by my wife that I make a lot of noise grinding my teeth when I sleep."

44. When assessing patients who have difficulty sleeping, the nurse understands that there are common psychological and physiological adaptations to insomnia. Check all those that are physiological adaptations to insomnia.
   1. _____ Vertigo
   2. _____ Fatigue
   3. _____ Headache
   4. _____ Irritability
   5. _____ Frustration

45. The phyician orders oxycodone (Roxicozone) oral solution 15 mg every 6 hours. The drug is supplied in a 500-mL bottle that indicates 5 mg/5 mL. How much oral solution should the nurse administer?
   Answer: ___________ mL.

ANSWERS AND RATIONALES

1. 1. An increased sensitivity to pain is associated with disturbed Rapid Eye Movement (REM), not Non-Rapid Eye Movement (NREM), sleep.
   2. **During Non-Rapid Eye Movement (NREM) sleep the parasympathetic nervous system dominates and the vital signs and metabolic rate are low; also growth hormone is consistently secreted, which provides for anabolism. Shortened NREM sleep decreases these restorative processes resulting in excessive sleepiness.**
   3. REM, not NREM, sleep is essential for maintaining mental and emotional equilibrium, and when interrupted, results in confusion, irritability, excitability, restlessness, and suspiciousness.
   4. Irritability, excitability, and restlessness are associated with disturbed REM, not NREM, sleep.

2. 1. Patient-controlled analgesia delivers an intermittent dose of an opioid on demand within safe limitations. Pain relief can be maintained for hours to days.
   2. Intramuscular injections of analgesics usually are effective for 3 to 6 hours.
   3. **Intravenous analgesics act within 1 to 2 minutes but drug inactivation (biotransformation) also is fast, so there is a short duration of action.**
   4. With regional anesthesia (e.g., nerve block, Bier block, spinal, epidural), an anesthetic agent is instilled around nerves to block the transmission of nerve impulses, thus reducing pain for many hours.

3. 1. **An expectation of an outcome of behavior usually becomes a self-fulfilling prophecy. Bedtime rituals include activities that promote comfort and relaxation (e.g., music, reading, praying) and hygienic practices that meet basic physiologic needs (e.g., bathing, brushing the teeth, toileting).**
   2. Alcohol hastens the onset of sleep.
   3. The need for sleep varies and depends on factors, such as age, activity level, and health.
   4. The healthy older adult spends more time in bed, spends less time asleep, awakens more often, stays awake longer, and naps more often. REM sleep and Stage IV NREM sleep are reduced, resulting in less restorative sleep. Naps lead to desynchronization of the sleep-wake cycle.

4. 1. **Sleep deprivation and dysfunction of the sleep-wake cycle cause ICU psychosis, resulting in Disturbed Thought Processes evidenced by inaccurate interpretations of internal or external stimuli.**
   2. Impaired Gas Exchange relates to problems that interfere with an exchange of oxygen and carbon dioxide between the alveoli of the lungs and the vascular system.
   3. Disuse Syndrome relates to a deterioration of body systems or alteration in function because of prescribed or unavoidable musculoskeletal inactivity.
   4. Sleep deprivation is not related to the nursing diagnosis of Powerlessness, which is the state in which an individual perceives a lack of personal control over certain events or situations that affects outlook, goals, and lifestyle.

5. 1. Although tinnitus can interfere with sleep, it is not the most common problem.
   2. **Bladder fullness causes pressure in the pelvic area that interrupts sleep. Awakening to void during the night is a common occurrence, particularly in older adult men.**
   3. Although hunger can interfere with sleep, it is not the most common problem. A light evening snack or glass of milk prevents hunger.
   4. Although thirst can interfere with sleep, it is not the most common problem. Thirst is prevented by drinking water as part of the bedtime routine.

6. 1. Percussion involves gentle tapping of the skin. Percussion is stimulating and usually is performed during the middle of a back massage.
   2. **Effleurage involves long, smooth strokes sliding over the skin. When performed slowly with light pressure at the end of a back massage, it has a relaxing, sedative effect.**
   3. Kneading (petrissage) involves squeezing the skin, subcutaneous tissue, and muscle with a lifting motion. Kneading is stimulating and usually is performed during the middle of a back massage.
   4. Circular strokes usually are performed in the area around the buttocks, lower back,

and scapulae. They are stimulating and are performed during the beginning of a back rub.

7. 1. The pattern of pain refers to time of onset, duration, recurrence, and remissions.
   2. Duration refers to how long the pain lasts, which is an aspect of the pattern of pain.
   3. **This is referred pain, which is pain felt in a part of the body that is a distance from the tissues causing the pain. Referred pain is related to location of pain.**
   4. Constancy refers to whether the pain is continuous or if there are periods of relief from pain, both of which relate to the pattern of pain.

8. 1. One of the major defining characteristics of the nursing diagnosis of Activity Intolerance is exertional fatigue three minutes after stopping activity. Although somewhat related, Fatigue and Activity Intolerance are two separate nursing diagnoses.
   2. This is the major defining characteristic of the nursing diagnoses Activity Intolerance and Impaired Gas Exchange
   3. Activity Intolerance is a separate nursing diagnosis that relates to a reduction in one's physiologic capacity to endure activities to the degree desired or required.
   4. **The nursing diagnosis Fatigue is the self-recognized state in which an individual experiences an overwhelming sustained sense of exhaustion and decreased capacity for physical and mental work that is not relieved by rest.**

9. 1. The amount of time spent sleeping usually is not affected.
   2. **Sleep apnea is the periodic cessation of breathing during sleep. Episodes occur during REM sleep (interfering with dreaming) and NREM sleep (interfering with restorative sleep), both of which reduce the quality of sleep.**
   3. Patients still reach the depth of Stage IV NREM sleep.
   4. Sleep apnea does not influence the onset of sleep.

10. 1. **This open-ended question requires patients to explore the topic of sleep as it relates specifically to their own experiences.**
    2. This direct question gathers information about only one aspect of sleep.
    3. This direct question precipitates just a yes or no response.
    4. This direct question precipitates just a yes or no response about only one aspect of sleep.

11. 1. **Psychologic or affective responses to pain relate to feelings and emotional distress. Fear of being dependent on others or loss of self-control are psychologic adaptations to pain.**
    2. Tolerance to a drug is not an adaptation to pain. Tolerance to a drug can be physiologic and/or psychologic.
    3. Requesting pain medication is a behavioral response to pain.
    4. Nausea is a physiologic response to pain.

12. 1. This relates to enuresis, which is recurrent involuntary urination that occurs during sleeping.
    2. **This is an appropriate goal for nocturia, which is voluntary urination during the night.**
    3. This relates to insomnia, which is difficulty initiating or maintaining sleep.
    4. This is an intervention, not a goal.

13. 1. During pregnancy, the basal metabolic rate rises gradually to an increase of 25%. Pregnancy mimics a mild hyperthyroid state to provide the energy required to maintain the pregnancy and promote the development of the fetus.
    2. There are major hormonal changes associated with pregnancy. Triiodothyronine (T_3), thyroxine (T_4), cortisol, insulin, parathyroid hormone (PTH), estrogen, progesterone, human chorionic gonadotropin (hCG), relaxin, and human placental lactogen (HPL) increase during pregnancy. Oxytocin is secreted late in pregnancy and prolactin is secreted after birth in response to breastfeeding. Follicle-stimulating hormone (FSH) and luteinizing hormone (LH) cease during pregnancy.
    3. **Cardiac output, the amount of blood pumped from the heart in 1 minute, increases by 30 to 50 percent early in the first trimester.**
    4. Anemia (low hemoglobin level) associated with pregnancy is called hemodilution of pregnancy. Most of the increased blood volume is plasma, causing an imbalance between the ratio of RBCs to plasma that results in a decreased hematocrit.

14. 1. Metabolic rates decrease by 5% to 25% during rest.
    2. Energy requirements decrease with age as metabolic processes slow and older adults become more sedentary.
    3. **Stress precipitates the sympathetic nervous system increasing cortisone,**

norepinephrine, and epinephrine, which increase the metabolic rate. Physical and psychic energy expended is restored through rest and sleep.

4. Catabolic hormones (cortisol and epinephrine) increase with activity, not during sleep. Catabolism is the breaking down of muscle and lean body mass to produce glucose to meet energy needs (gluconeogenesis).

15. 1. Repositioning is effective for mild, not severe, pain.
2. A back massage is ineffective for acute, severe pain; however, it may relax the patient and increase the effectiveness of analgesic medication.
3. Guided imagery is more effective for mild pain, not acute, severe pain.
4. **Major abdominal surgery involves extensive manipulation of internal organs and a large abdominal incision that require adequate pharmacologic intervention to provide relief from pain.**

16. 1. Although the overwhelming daytime sleepiness associated with narcolepsy may interfere with the ability to perform some self-care activities, this is not the major problem related to narcolepsy.
2. Narcolepsy does not involve disturbed thought processes, which is the state in which an individual experiences a disruption in mental activities, such as conscious thought, reality orientation, problem solving, and judgment.
3. Although a person with narcolepsy may verbalize a lack of energy, this is not the primary concern associated with narcolepsy.
4. **Narcolepsy is excessive sleepiness in the daytime that can cause a person to fall asleep uncontrollably at inappropriate times (sleep attack) and result in physical harm to self or others.**

17. 1. Hyporesponsiveness, withdrawal, apathy, flat facial expression, and excessive sleepiness are physiologic responses associated with a lack of NREM sleep.
2. A depressed immune response is a physiologic adaptation to a lack of NREM sleep.
3. **REM sleep is essential for maintaining mental and emotional equilibrium and when interrupted results in irritability, excitability, restlessness, confusion, and suspiciousness.**
4. Shortened NREM sleep can result in vertigo, which is a physiologic response to sleep deprivation.

18. 1. **Gastric secretions increase during REM sleep. The semi-Fowler's position limits gastroesophageal reflux because gravity allows the abdominal organs to drop, which reduces pressure on the stomach and results in less stomach contents flowing upward into the esophagus.**
2. This is a horizontal position that increases the pressure of the abdominal organs against the stomach and increases gastric reflux.
3. This is a horizontal position that increases the pressure of the abdominal organs against the stomach and increases gastric reflux.
4. This is a horizontal position halfway between lateral and prone. Direct pressure exerted on the stomach, particularly in the left Sims' position, promotes gastric reflux.

19. 1. This may or may not be true.
2. This is not a true statement. The judicious use of opioids does not necessarily result in addiction. In addition, there are many nonopioid drugs, such as nonsteroidal anti-inflammatory drugs, antidepressants, and anticonvulsants, all of which relieve pain.
3. **Pain is a personal experience. Margo McCaffery, a pain researcher, has indicated that pain is whatever the person in pain says it is and exists whenever the person in pain says it exists.**
4. This may or may not be true. There may be behavioral signs of pain, such as guarding, grimaces, and clenching the teeth, at the same time that there are no verbal statements indicating the presence of pain. In some cultures, it is unacceptable to complain about pain, or tolerance of pain signifies strength and courage.

20. 1. **Anxiety increases norepinephrine blood levels through stimulation of the sympathetic nervous system, which results in prolonged sleep onset.**
2. Patients with anxiety still reach the depth of Stage IV NREM sleep.
3. Stage IV, not Stage II, of NREM sleep is affected.
4. The duration of sleep is affected indirectly, not directly, because of the prolonged onset of sleep.

21. 1. This is premature without information about the intensity of the pain. Distraction is not effective for severe pain.
2. There is not enough information to indicate that this intervention may be effective. In addition, the position the patient considers

most comfortable may be contraindicated based on physician orders or safety issues.
3. This is a hasty, impulsive response that may or may not be necessary.
4. **All the factors that affect the pain experience should be assessed, including location, intensity, quality, duration, pattern, aggravating and alleviating factors, and physical, behavioral, and attitudinal adaptations. Assessment must precede intervention.**

22. 1. Agitation is a minor defining characteristic for the nursing diagnosis of Disturbed Sleep Pattern in an adult, not a child.
2. Respiratory disorders, such as obstructive sleep apnea, are related factors, not defining characteristics, for the nursing diagnosis of Disturbed Sleep Pattern.
3. **Children may be reluctant to retire at night because of fear, enuresis, or inconsistent adherence to routines by parents.**
4. Early morning awakenings occur with older adults or people who have consumed alcohol.

23. 1. **A continuous positive airway pressure (CPAP) mask worn over the nose when sleeping keeps the upper airway patent through continuous positive airway pressure.**
2. This increases the episodes of sleep apnea because the structures of the mouth and oropharynx (i.e., tonsils, adenoids, mucous membranes, uvula, soft palate, and tongue) drop by gravity and ultimately obstruct the airway.
3. This flexes the neck, which narrows the upper airway and thus contributes to episodes of sleep apnea. Pillows under the upper shoulders and head or small blocks under the head of the bed may assist in keeping the upper airway open.
4. Sedatives do not limit episodes of sleep apnea.

24. 1. These are physiologic adaptations, not precipitating factors, associated with the pain experience.
2. **Anything that induces or aggravates pain is considered a precipitating factor of pain. For example, precipitating factors may be physical (exertion associated with ADLs, Valsalva's maneuver), environmental (extremes in temperature, noise), or emotional (anxiety, fear).**
3. This statement reflects the pattern (onset, duration, and intervals) of the pain experience.
4. This statement reflects the quality of the pain. Descriptive adjectives, such as knife-like, burning, or cramping explain how the pain feels.

25. 1. Although meeting the basic physiologic need to feel warm is appropriate, a hospital's environment generally is warm, so a top sheet and spread are adequate.
2. **Noise is a serious deterrent to sleep in a hospital. The nurse should limit environmental noise (i.e., distributing fluids, providing treatments, rolling drug and linen carts) and staff communication noise.**
3. This is unsafe. Dim the lights or put a night light on to provide enough illumination for safe ambulation to the bathroom.
4. Although this provides privacy, it does not limit the environmental factors that usually interfere with sleeping in a hospital.

26. 1. Although the nurse and patient attempt to do this, there may be unavoidable activities that may precipitate pain.
2. **Administration of analgesics around the clock (ATC administration) at regularly scheduled intervals or by long-acting controlled release transdermal patches maintains therapeutic blood levels of analgesics, which limit pain at levels of comfort acceptable to patients.**
3. Although the nurse will attempt to do this, there may be significant interventions that must be performed that may precipitate pain.
4. Although the nurse will ask this question to determine the patient's level of pain tolerance, it is not the priority.

27. 1. **An obvious response to pain is not always apparent because psychosociocultural factors may dictate behavior. Fear of the treatment for pain, lack of validation, acceptance of pain as punishment for previous behavior, and the need to be strong, courageous, or uncomplaining are factors that influence behavioral responses to pain.**
2. The opposite may be true. As a person experiences relief from pain, the person may be unwilling to endure previously acceptable levels of pain.
3. This is not a true statement. Although a generalization, many groups such as Jewish, Italian, Greek, and Chinese are able to express their pain.
4. Pain tolerance varies widely among people and is influenced by experiential, psychologic, and sociocultural factors.

28. 1. **Sleep deprivation occurs with frequent interruptions of sleep because the sleeper returns to Stage I rather than to the stage that was interrupted. There is a greater loss of Stage III and IV NREM sleep, which is essential for restorative sleep.**
2. Although early awakenings often do occur in hospital settings, it is not the most common cause of sleep deprivation in the hospital.
3. Restless legs syndrome, an intrinsic sleep disorder, is not the most common cause of sleep deprivation in the hospital.
4. Only 1 to 4 percent of the population have sleep apnea.

29. 1. This is desirable because it keeps pain under control before it becomes excessive.
2. **The level of pain tolerance is exceeded. The present pain must be relieved and the patient assured that future pain also will be controlled.**
3. The concern of addiction is not the priority among these statements. The nurse can respond to this common concern through education and judicious medication administration.
4. This is not the statement of greatest concern. Nonpharmacologic measures to relieve pain, such as imagery and self-hypnosis, use the mind-body (psyche-soma) connection to reduce pain. The nurse should encourage the use of these measures and validate the energy expended.

30. 1. Hypoxia is associated with obstructive sleep apnea because episodes of upper airway obstruction occur 50 to 600 times a night.
2. **Melatonin, the "hormone of darkness," regulates the circadian phases of sleep. Environmental triggers called synchronizers adjust the sleep-wake cycle to a 24-hour solar day. With ICU psychosis, bright lights and increased sensory input cause disorientation to day and night and interrupt sleep. Interrupted sleep results in lability of mood, irritability, excitability, suspiciousness, confusion, and delirium.**
3. Lethargy and fatigue are earlier signs of sleep deprivation than an adaptation in another option.
4. Sleep deprivation may cause impaired memory, confusion, illusions, and visual or auditory hallucinations, not dementia.

31. 1. This is a minor, not a major, defining characteristic of the nursing diagnosis Fatigue.
2. Exhaustion relieved by rest relates to the nursing diagnosis Activity Intolerance. The nursing diagnosis Fatigue is related to a sustained sense of exhaustion that is unrelieved by rest.
3. **An inability to maintain usual routines along with verbalization of distress and an unremitting and overwhelming lack of energy are the major defining characteristics of the nursing diagnosis Fatigue.**
4. Compromised physical conditioning caused by factors that compromise oxygen transport relates to the nursing diagnosis Activity Intolerance.

32. 1. Although uninterrupted sleep is advantageous for restorative sleep, the number of hours required depends on the individual.
2. In older adults, the length of Stage IV sleep is markedly decreased; they awaken more frequently, and it takes them longer to go back to sleep.
3. **Fear of loss of control, the unknown, and potential death results in the struggle to stay awake, which interferes with the ability to relax sufficiently to fall asleep.**
4. Bed rest does not decrease the need to sleep. The body still needs Stage IV restorative sleep. Often the physiologic problems requiring the bed rest increase the need for sleep.

33. 1. **The word episode refers to an incident, occurrence, or time period; therefore, episodic refers to patterns of pain and is concerned with time of onset, duration, recurrence, and remissions.**
2. Phantom pain is related to location of pain. Phantom pain is a painful sensation perceived in a body part that is missing.
3. The description of pain as being moderate is related to intensity of pain.
4. Tenderness is a sensory word that describes pain and is related to the quality of pain.

34. 1. **Alcoholic beverages are fluids that have a mild diuretic effect. Frequent nighttime awakenings to empty a full bladder is called nocturia.**
2. Excessive drinking usually causes nausea and vomiting rather than hunger.
3. Alcohol hastens, not delays, the onset of sleep.
4. Alcohol disrupts sleep and causes early morning awakenings.

35. 1. Self-focusing is associated with chronic, not acute, pain because its unrelenting, prolonged nature interferes with pursuing a normal life.

As a result, there may be changes in family dynamics, sexual functioning, financial status, and self-esteem that result in introspection and depression.
2. Pain is an internal stimulus that can interrupt sleep. Because chronic pain is unrelenting and prolonged, over time, interrupted sleep results in sleep deprivation.
3. Guarding behaviors occur in both acute and chronic pain. However, because of the unrelenting prolonged nature of chronic pain, behavioral adaptations, such as guarding, stooped posture, and altered gait may become permanent adaptations.
4. **Acute pain stimulates the sympathetic nervous system, which responds by increasing pulse, respirations, and blood pressure. Chronic pain stimulates the parasympathetic nervous system, which results in lowered pulse and blood pressure.**

36. 1. Hour of sleep (h.s., hora somni) medications usually are sedatives that promote rest and sleep.
2. Medications administered *around the clock at regularly scheduled intervals* (ATC) usually maintain therapeutic drug levels regardless of other factors influencing the patient.
3. Medication administered when necessary at the patient's request will have a physician's order that states *p.r.n.* (**p**ro **r**e **n**ata).
4. **The word preemptive means preventive, anticipatory, and defensive. Therefore, preemptive analgesia is administered before activity or interventions that may precipitate pain in an attempt to limit the anticipated pain.**

37. 1. **Chronic fatigue syndrome is a condition characterized by the onset of disabling fatigue after an initial viral-like illness. The fatigue is so overwhelming and consuming it interferes with the activities of daily living.**
2. Chronic fatigue syndrome does not impair mobility. Impaired physical mobility is the state in which an individual experiences limitation of physical movement, but is not immobile.
3. The fatigue of chronic fatigue syndrome may be unrelated to social isolation, which is a state in which an individual experiences or perceives a desire for increased involvement with others, but is unable to make that contact.
4. Although fatigue is related to impaired gas exchange, the fatigue caused by hypoxia is unrelated to chronic fatigue syndrome, which is a very different condition.

38. 1. Patients, particularly children and those who are cognitively impaired, often have problems describing the quality of pain because of difficulty interpreting painful stimuli or having never experienced the sensation before.
2. Psychosociocultural factors influence patients' lack of request for medication when experiencing pain. Patients may not request medication because they fear the possibility of addiction, consider the pain as punishment for previous behavior, or need to be strong, courageous, or uncomplaining.
3. **Pain is a personal experience, and the nurse must validate its presence and severity as perceived by the patient. This conveys acceptance and respect and promotes the development of trust.**
4. Acute pain increases vital signs because of sympathetic nervous system stimulation, but chronic pain will not.

39. 1. Rapid Eye Movement (REM) sleep is essential for maintaining mental and emotional equilibrium, and when interrupted, results in anxiety, irritability, excitability, restlessness, confusion, and suspiciousness.
2. Interrupted REM, not NREM, sleep is associated with hyperactivity, excitability, and restlessness.
3. **During Non-Rapid Eye Movement (NREM) sleep, growth hormone is consistently secreted, which provides for protein synthesis, anabolism, and tissue repair.**
4. Interrupted REM, not NREM, sleep is associated with excitability, emotional lability, and suspiciousness. Interrupted NREM sleep is associated with apathy, withdrawal, and hyporesponsiveness.

40. 1. This is a planned nursing intervention, not a goal.
2. **Sleep is a sensory experience that restores cerebral and physical functioning. Evaluations related to sleep are based on patient reports because effectiveness of sleep is subjective.**
3. This is a goal that relates to relieving pain.
4. Four hours of sleep is not enough for most adults. Most adults require 6 to 8 hours of sleep.

41. 1. **Imagery, the internal experience of memories, dreams, fantasies, or visions, uses positive images to distract, which**

reduces stress, limits mild pain, and promotes relaxation and sleep.

2. The use of opioids should be a last resort. Nursing interventions or nonopioid medications usually are effective in limiting mild pain.
3. Bathing preferences are highly individual, and the patient may not prefer a shower. In addition, a shower is stimulating and may be contraindicated.
4. Although daytime activity does promote sleep at night, patients with pain may be reluctant to be active.

42. 1. At this time of day, most people are engaged in stimulating activities and generally are not sleepy.
2. By this time of the sleep cycle, most people have had sufficient sleep and are beginning to awaken.
3. **Research has demonstrated that most people experience sleep-vulnerable periods between 2 AM and 6 AM and between 2 PM and 5 PM.**
4. At this time of day, most people are engaged in stimulating activities, such as preparing and eating dinner.

43. 1. Somnambulism, sleepwalking, is a parasomnia that occurs during Stages III and IV NREM sleep.
2. Snoring relates to obstructive sleep apnea, which is a periodic cessation of airflow during inspiration that results in arousal from sleep.
3. Nocturnal enuresis, bedwetting, is a parasomnia that occurs when moving from Stages III to IV of NREM sleep.
4. **Bruxism, clenching and grinding of the teeth, is a parasomnia that occurs during Stage II NREM sleep. Usually, it does not interfere with sleep for the affected individual but rather the sleeper's partner.**

44. 1. **Shortened NREM sleep can result in vertigo, which is a physiologic response to sleep deprivation.**
2. **Interrupted REM and NREM sleep can result in fatigue, which is a physiologic response to sleep deprivation.**
3. **Shortened NREM sleep can result in headache, which is a physiologic response to sleep deprivation.**
4. Irritability is a psychological response to sleep deprivation. As the difficulty of initiating or maintaining sleep continues, the person becomes progressively more upset about the lack of the amount and quality of sleep, further precipitating insomnia.
5. Frustration is a psychological response to sleep deprivation.

45. Answer: 15 mL. Solve the question by using ratio and proportion.

$$\frac{\text{Desired}}{\text{Have}} \quad \frac{15\text{ mg}}{5\text{ mg}} \times \frac{x\text{ mL}}{5\text{ mL}}$$

$$5x = 75$$

$$x = \frac{75}{5}$$

$$x = 15\text{ mL}$$

Perioperative Nursing

KEYWORDS

The following words include English vocabulary, nursing/medical terminology, concepts, principles, or information relevant to content specifically addressed in the chapter or associated with topics presented in it. English dictionaries, nursing textbooks, and medical dictionaries, such as *Taber's Cyclopedic Medical Dictionary*, are resources that can be used to expand your knowledge and understanding of these words and related information.

- Abdominal binder
- Anesthesia, types
  - Epidural
  - General
  - Local
  - Nerve block
  - Regional
  - Spinal
- Anesthesiologist
- Anesthetist
- Antiembolism stockings
  - Elastic
  - Sequential compression devices
- Bowel preparation
- Certified Registered Nurse Anesthetist
- Circulating nurse
- Collagen production
- Conscious sedation
- Débridement
- Deep breathing and coughing
- Drains, types
  - Penrose
  - Portable wound drainage systems
    - Hemovac
    - Jackson-Pratt
- Dressings, types
  - Alginates (exudate absorbers)
    - Debrisan
    - Sorbsan
  - Dry sterile dressing
  - Hydrocolloids
    - DuoDerm
    - Tegasorb
  - Impregnated
    - Adaptic
    - Xeroform
  - Transparent
    - Bioclusive
    - Op-Site
    - Tegaderm
  - Wet-to-moist
- Granulation
- Hypostatic pneumonia
- Incision
- Informed consent
- Laparoscopic
- Latex allergy
- Leg exercises
- Nasogastric decompression
- Negative pressure
- NPO status
- Pain management
- Patient-controlled analgesia (PCA)
- Perioperative
  - Intraoperative
  - Postoperative
  - Preoperative
- Postoperative complications
  - Aspiration
  - Deep vein thrombosis
  - Dehiscence
  - Evisceration
  - Malignant hyperthermia
  - Pneumonia
  - Postoperative ileus
  - Pulmonary embolus, emoboli
  - Wound infection
- Positioning
- Post-Anesthesia Care Unit
- Preoperative checklist
- Preoperative medication
- Radiation safety
- Residual limb
- Skin preparation
- Skin staple
- Surgical asepsis
- Surgery, purposes of
  - Ablative
  - Constructive
  - Diagnostic
  - Palliative
  - Reconstructive
  - Transplant
- Surgery types

- Ambulatory surgery
- Elective surgery
- Urgent surgery
- Emergency surgery
- Minor surgery
- Major surgery
- Suture
- Turning and positioning
- Wound
- Wound drainage
  - Purulent
  - Sanguineous
  - Serosanguineous
  - Serous

QUESTIONS

1. The nurse understands that the difference between a Jackson-Pratt and a Hemovac is:
   1. The size of the collection container
   2. How the pressure within the collection container is reestablished
   3. The type of pressure that promotes drainage to the collection container
   4. Where the collection container should be placed in relation to the insertion site
2. The nurse is caring for several patients who received general anesthesia. The nurse identifies that the patient who is at the greatest risk is the patient with:
   1. Gastroesophageal reflux disease
   2. Reduced reflexes
   3. Hypothyroidism
   4. Emphysema
3. The nurse is caring for a patient who had abdominal surgery. Which type of incisional drainage should the nurse expect four hours after surgery?
   1. Serous wound drainage
   2. Purulent wound drainage
   3. Sanguineous wound drainage
   4. Serosanguineous wound drainage
4. A surgical patient is transferred from the Post-Anesthesia Care Unit to a medical–surgical unit. When reviewing the physician's orders, the nurse is on alert for which vitamin that commonly is ordered for postoperative patients?
   1. Vitamin A
   2. Vitamin B
   3. Vitamin C
   4. Vitamin K – help blood clotting.
5. A patient spikes a temperature during the first postoperative day. The nurse understands that usually this indicates a potential problem involving the:
   1. Intestines
   2. Bladder
   3. Wound
   4. Lungs
6. The nurse is assessing a patient's status while in the Post-Anesthesia Care Unit. Which patient adaptation is of most concern?
   1. Pain
   2. Incontinence
   3. Mental confusion
   4. Limited airway clearance
7. The nurse is to apply a transparent wound barrier over a patient's incision. Which nursing action is appropriate?
   1. Clean the skin with normal saline before applying the dressing
   2. Stretch the transparent wound barrier snugly over the entire wound
   3. Cover the transparent wound barrier with a gauze dressing and secure with paper tape
   4. Ensure the reinforcing tape extends several inches beyond the edges of the transparent wound barrier

8. The nurse in the operating room positions a patient for surgery. Which is most important?
   1. Allowing for skeletal deformities
   2. Preventing pressure on bony prominences
   3. Providing for adequate thoracic expansion
   4. Avoiding stretching of neuromuscular tissue

9. Perioperative nursing care begins when the:
   1. Patient is transferred to the operating room
   2. Decision for surgery is made
   3. Consent form is signed
   4. Patient is anesthetized

10. One hour after the reduction of a compound fracture of the ulna and radius and application of a cast, the nurse notices a centimeter circle of drainage on the patient's cast. What should the nurse do first?
    1. Inform the surgeon immediately
    2. Reinforce the cast with a gauze dressing
    3. Nothing, but continue to monitor the area for expansion
    4. Circle the spot with a pen and date, time, and initial the area

11. There are discharge criteria for patients in the Post-Anesthesia Care Unit regardless of the type of anesthesia used and additional criteria for specific types of anesthesia. The criterion specific for the patient who has received spinal anesthesia is:
    1. Oxygen saturation reaches the presurgical baseline
    2. Motor and sensory function returns
    3. Nausea and vomiting are minimal
    4. Headache is considered tolerable

12. A patient is admitted to the Post-Anesthesia Care Unit (PACU). Which nursing action is most important during the patient's stay in the PACU?
    1. Monitoring urinary output
    2. Assessing level of consciousness
    3. Ensuring patency of drainage tubes
    4. Suctioning mucus from respiratory passages

13. A postoperative patient is transferred back to the surgical unit with an abdominal dressing and a Penrose drain. Which is the most important nursing action associated with caring for a patient with a Penrose drain?
    1. Removing the excess external portion until drainage stops
    2. Changing the soiled dressing carefully
    3. Maintaining the negative pressure
    4. Pinning the drain to the dressing

14. A patient who received spinal anesthesia is admitted to the Post-Anesthesia Care Unit. In which position should the nurse place the patient?
    1. Prone
    2. Supine
    3. Right lateral
    4. Trendelenburg

15. What nutrient containing vitamin C should the nurse encouraged a postoperative patient to eat to facilitate wound healing?
    1. Liver
    2. Cheese
    3. Broccoli
    4. Legumes

16. A patient has a tonsillectomy. Which is most appropriate for the nurse to encourage this patient to have during the first 24 hours after surgery?
    1. Warm pudding
    2. Milk shakes
    3. Soft toast
    4. Ice pops

17. A patient has abdominal surgery. To best assess this patient's gastrointestinal status postoperatively, the nurse should:
    1. Identify the time of the first bowel movement
    2. Monitor the tolerance of a clear liquid diet
    3. Palpate for abdominal distention
    4. Auscultate for bowel sounds

18. Four days after abdominal surgery, while being transferred from a bed to a chair, a patient says to a nurse, "My incision feels funny all of a sudden." What should the nurse do first?
    1. Take the vital signs
    2. Apply an abdominal binder immediately
    3. Place the patient in the low-Fowler's position
    4. Encourage slow deep breathing by the patient

19. The nurse understands that the greatest risk for postoperative nausea and vomiting after receiving general anesthesia is caused by:
    1. Obesity
    2. Inactivity
    3. Hypervolemia
    4. Unconsciousness

20. On the second postoperative day after an above-the-knee amputation the patient's elastic dressing accidentally comes off. What should the nurse do first?
    1. Wrap the residual limb with an elastic compression bandage
    2. Apply a saline dressing to the residual limb
    3. Place two pillows under the limb
    4. Notify the physician

21. The nurse is caring for a postoperative patient. The action most effective in preventing postoperative urinary tract infections is:
    1. Eating foods with roughage
    2. Taking sitz baths twice a day
    3. Drinking an adequate amount of fluid
    4. Increasing the intake of citrus fruit juices

22. A patient received conscious sedation during a colonoscopy. The nurse can expect this patient to be:
    1. Unresponsive and pain-free
    2. At risk for malignant hyperthermia
    3. Sleepy but able to follow verbal commands
    4. Positioned in the supine position to prevent headache

23. A patient has a portable wound drainage system after resection of a tumor in the neck. The nurse must ensure that the portable wound drainage system is emptied:
    1. After it is full
    2. Every 2 hours
    3. Every 4 hours
    4. When it is half full

24. Which patient having emergency surgery should the nurse anticipate to be at the greatest risk for postoperative mortality?
    1. Chronic alcoholic
    2. Older adult
    3. Epileptic
    4. Infant

25. The nurse is caring for a patient who had an abdominal hysterectomy. Which intervention best prevents postoperative thrombophlebitis?
1. Elevation of the legs on 2 pillows
2. Utilization of compression stockings at night
3. Deep breathing and coughing exercises daily
4. Leg exercises 10 times per hour when awake

26. The nurse understands that vitamin C is often ordered by the physician for a postoperative patient to:
1. Improve digestion
2. Support collagen production
3. Encourage growth of red blood cells
4. Minimize formation of deep vein thrombosis

27. A patient has abdominal surgery for removal of the gallbladder. Which should the nurse be most concerned about if exhibited by the patient?
1. Constipation
2. Urinary retention
3. Shallow breathing
4. Inability to provide self-care

28. A patient arrives in the Post-Anesthesia Care Unit. Which is the most important information that the nurse needs to know?
1. Type and extent of the surgery
2. Anxiety level before the surgery
3. Type of intravenous fluids administered
4. Special requests that were verbalized by the patient

29. The nurse understands that a central venous catheter inserted into a peripheral vein is preferable to a central venous catheter inserted into a subclavian vein because a peripheral catheter will not:
1. Cause a pneumothroax
2. Be in the superior vena cava
3. Prevent the development of an infection
4. Allow large volumes of fluid to be administered

30. The nurse understands that evidence of a postoperative wound infection usually is not apparent before the:
1. Fifth day
2. Third day
3. Ninth day
4. Seventh day

31. The nurse is assessing a patient who had spinal anesthesia. Which common patient adaptation can the nurse expect?
1. Headache
2. Neuropathy
3. Lower back discomfort
4. Increased blood pressure

32. A hospitalized patient who has been receiving medications via a variety of routes for several days is scheduled for surgery at 10:00 AM. On the day of surgery the nurse should plan to:
1. Use an alternative route for the oral medications
2. Withhold all the previously ordered medications
3. Withhold the oral medications and administer the other drugs
4. Obtain directions from the physician regarding the medications

33. The nurse understands that the most common diet ordered after surgery is:
    1. Clear liquids
    2. Full liquids
    3. Low fiber
    4. Regular

34. Which adaptations identified by the nurse best support the decision to discharge the patient from the Post-Anesthesia Care Unit?
    1. SaO_2 of 95%, vital signs stable for 30 minutes, active gag reflex
    2. Afebrile, presence of adventitious breath sounds, ability to cough
    3. Tolerable pain, ability to move the extremities, dry, intact dressing
    4. Urinary output of 30 mL per hour, awake, turning from side to side

35. The nurse understands that the most important aspect associated with general anesthesia is:
    1. Ensuring the loss of pain sensation
    2. Providing for adequate ventilation
    3. Observing for reflex activity
    4. Monitoring the heart rate

36. A patient has a right abdominal incision. When giving instructions on how to get out of bed, the nurse should teach the patient to:
    1. Exit from the left side of the bed
    2. Ask the nurse to apply an abdominal binder
    3. Hold a pillow against the abdomen with both hands
    4. Use the right elbow to assist in lifting the body to a sitting position

37. A postoperative patient experiences tachycardia, sudden chest pain, and a low blood pressure. Which complication associated with the postoperative period should the nurse conclude that the patient most likely experienced?
    1. Pulmonary embolus
    2. Hemorrhage
    3. Heart attack
    4. Pneumonia

38. The nurse is assessing a postoperative patient. Which patient adaptation identified by the nurse indicates altered renal perfusion?
    1. Oliguria
    2. Cachexia
    3. Yellow sclera
    4. Suprapubic distention

39. When evaluating the effectiveness of nursing interventions for meeting the nutrient needs of patients during the first two days after abdominal surgery, which outcome is most important?
    1. Nausea and vomiting has not occurred
    2. Fluid and electrolytes are balanced
    3. Wound healing is progressing
    4. Oral intake is reestablished

40. After assessing a postoperative patient for a patent airway, which is the next most important assessment made by the nurse?
    1. Condition of drains
    2. Level of consciousness
    3. Stability of the vital signs
    4. Location of surgical dressing

41. The nurse is aware that the nutrients that are the best for supporting collagen production are:
    1. Whole grain breads
    2. Yellow vegetables
    3. Citrus fruits
    4. Red meats

42. When caring for a patient recovering from abdominal surgery, an important action by the nurse that facilitates ventilation is:
1. Preventing abdominal distention
2. Positioning in the side-lying position
3. Monitoring respiratory status every hour
4. Providing passive range-of-motion exercises

43. When preparing a patient who is to undergo perineal surgery, the nurse should place the patient in the:
1. Sims' position
2. Supine position
3. Lithotomy position
4. Trendelenburg position

44. Which nursing actions are most important when applying antiembolism stockings? Check all that apply.
1. _____ Eliminating the wrinkles in the stockings
2. _____ Ensuring the toe window is properly positioned
3. _____ Applying the stockings after the patient is out of bed
4. _____ Flexing the knee as the stocking is pulled over the knee
5. _____ Removing the stocking once a day for at least thirty minutes

45. The nurse is caring for a patient in the ambulatory surgery unit who just had a laparoscopic cholecystectomy. The patient complains of pain that is commonly associated with the migration of CO_2 used to inflate the abdominal cavity to improve visualization during surgery. Shade in the location of this referred pain on the illustration.

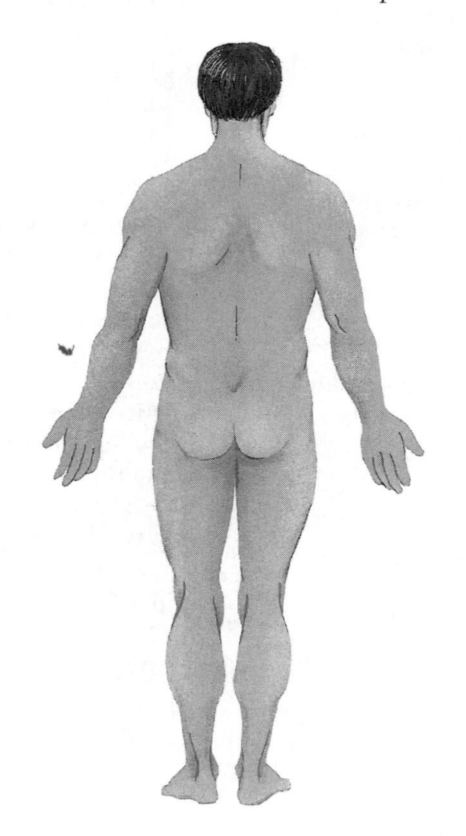

ANSWERS AND RATIONALES

1. 1. **A Hemovac is designed to accommodate 100, 400, or 800 mL of drainage depending on the system used, while a Jackson-Pratt accommodates volumes under 100 mL of drainage.**
   2. Both create a vacuum by closing the drainage port while compressing the device.
   3. Both work by gentle negative pressure that draws fluid from the tissues to the collection chamber.
   4. Both collection chambers should be placed below the site of insertion to allow gravity to work in conjunction with the negative pressure within the self-contained systems.

2. 1. This is not a problem with general anesthesia because of interventions such as NPO status before surgery, use of a cuffed endotracheal tube, and positioning.
   2. Although this is significant to know when monitoring a patient throughout the surgical experience, it does not place a patient at the greatest risk.
   3. Although a decreased metabolism is taken into consideration when monitoring reflexes during the induction, maintenance, and reversal phases of anesthesia, hypothyroidism does not place a patient at the greatest risk.
   4. **Respiratory problems complicate the administration of inhalation anesthesia. Emphysema is characterized by destruction of alveoli, loss of elastic recoil, and narrowing of bronchioles, which result in alveolar hyperinflation and increased airflow resistance.**

3. 1. Serous exudate is a clear, watery fluid consisting mainly of serum. It is the exudate expected before final wound healing.
   2. Purulent exudate is a thick drainage known as pus, which consists of leukocytes, liquefied dead-tissue debris, and bacteria. This is unexpected and indicates the presence of a wound infection. Wound infections become apparent 2 to 11 days postoperatively.
   3. Sanguineous (hemorrhagic) exudate consists of large amounts of red blood cells and is associated with open wounds or hemorrhage.
   4. **Serosanguineous exudate, a combination of serous and sanguineous drainage, consists of plasma and red blood cells and is pale red and watery. This is the initial drainage expected after surgery.**

4. 1. Although vitamin A is associated with epithelial tissue, usually it is not ordered individually, but rather as part of a multivitamin.
   2. Although the B complex vitamins are related to protein synthesis and cross-linking of collagen fibers, they usually are not ordered individually, but rather as part of a multivitamin.
   3. **Vitamin C (ascorbic acid) is essential for collagen formation, the single most important protein of connective tissue. The recommended daily dose is 60 mg; however, a postoperative patient may need up to 1000 mg of vitamin C for tissue repair, necessitating supplementation.**
   4. Although vitamin K promotes blood clotting by increasing the synthesis of prothrombin by the liver, usually it is not ordered individually unless the patient has liver disease or a bleeding tendency.

5. 1. The absence of intestinal motility (paralytic ileus), not infection, is the intestinal adaptation that can occur during the first 24 to 36 hours after surgery. Abdominal distention and absent bowel sounds, not a fever, indicate this problem.
   2. Postoperative bladder infection usually is related to urinary catheterization. A bladder infection will not be apparent during the first 24 hours after catheterization because microorganisms take at least 72 hours to multiply sufficiently to present symptoms.
   3. Microorganisms introduced into the incision at the time of surgery take at least 72 hours to multiply sufficiently to present symptoms.
   4. **When postoperative pneumonia (an inflammation of the lung with consolidation and exudation) occurs, patient symptoms are evident usually any time within 36 hours after surgery.**

6. 1. Although this is important for patient comfort, it is not life threatening.
   2. Patients may become incontinent while, or after, receiving anesthesia; however, it is not life threatening. In addition, this does not occur often because of preoperative bowel preparation and the temporary insertion of a urinary catheter.
   3. Although this can occur as a short-term response to anesthesia, it is not life threatening.

4. **Anesthesia causes a loss of the pharyngeal, laryngeal, and gag reflexes; these losses interfere with the protective mechanisms of coughing and swallowing. Because the patient is unable to clear the airway, oral secretions in the oropharynx and trachea may compromise a patent airway. In addition, occlusion of the airway may occur because of decreased muscle control of the tongue and jaw.**

7. 1. **This removes exudate and ensures adhesion of the dressing. Transparent adhesive films are nonabsorbent semipermeable (which allows oxygen exchange) dressings that are impermeable to water and bacteria.**
   2. This restricts mobility and may exert undue pressure on the surface of the wound. The dressing should be laid gently over the wound and the edges pressed against the skin to ensure adherence.
   3. This defeats one of the purposes of a transparent dressing: wound visualization.
   4. A transparent dressing is self-contained, and reinforcing tape usually is not necessary.

8. 1. Although this always is taken into consideration when positioning a patient during the intraoperative period, it is not the priority.
   2. It is impossible to prevent all pressure on bony prominences during the intraoperative period. Specific positions are necessary to allow exposure and access to the operative area. Positioning devices and padding are used to minimize trauma.
   3. **Facilitating respirations always is the priority because permanent brain damage can result from cerebral hypoxia in as little as 4 to 6 minutes.**
   4. Although stretching of neuromuscular tissue is avoided during the intraoperative period, it is not the priority.

9. 1. The nurse is negligent if nursing care begins at this point in the surgical experience. This is the intraoperative phase of the perioperative experience.
   2. **The surgical experience begins as soon as the decision for surgery is made. Perioperative nursing responsibilities begin immediately and continue throughout the preoperative, intraoperative, and postoperative phases.**
   3. Significant nursing care must be provided before this point in time. The operative consent form is signed during the preoperative phase of the perioperative experience.
   4. The nurse is negligent if nursing care begins only at this point in the surgical experience. This is the intraoperative phase of the perioperative experience.

10. 1. This is premature, because some drainage occurs with a compound fracture.
    2. This is undesirable, because it impedes the ability to assess the site in the future.
    3. This is undesirable, because the determination of expansion will be a subjective assessment without objective parameters.
    4. **This determines objectively the time and extent of the bleeding and the person who performed the assessment. The extent of progression of the bleeding can be established objectively using the original circle as a standard.**

11. 1. The respiratory status of all postoperative patients should be stable and adequate regardless of the type of anesthesia used.
    2. **The ability to move and feel sensations in all four extremities is especially important after receiving spinal anesthesia (subarachnoid block) because it indicates that nerve damage has not occurred because of the lumbar puncture necessary for the introduction of the anesthetic agent into the subarachnoid space.**
    3. Nausea and vomiting are associated with general, not spinal anesthesia.
    4. This is unrealistic. Although a headache may be associated with spinal anesthesia (subarachnoid block), it may manifest after discharge from the Post-Anesthesia Care Unit and persist for several days until the cerebrospinal fluid pressure returns to an acceptable level.

12. 1. Although this is done to ensure that the minimal hourly urine output is 30 mL, it is not the priority.
    2. Although this is part of the routine assessment of a patient recovering from anesthesia, particularly conscious sedation and general anesthesia, it is not the priority.
    3. Although tubes and equipment are always monitored and maintained, the patient is the priority.
    4. **Maintaining a patent airway is always the priority to prevent respiratory distress and hypoxia.**

13. 1. A Penrose drain, a small pliable, flat tube extends beyond the insertion site by approximately 2 inches. This prevents it from being lost inside the wound and allows its placement between gauze dressings to

absorb drainage. As a drain is shortened, it is withdrawn approximately 1 inch and cut to maintain the same 2-inch length outside the body. Although this is done, it is not the priority action associated with a Penrose drain.

2. **This is necessary to prevent inadvertent removal of the Penrose drain because it is placed between several layers of gauze to absorb drainage.**
3. A Penrose drain functions by gravity, not negative pressure.
4. This is not done to avoid inadvertently removing the drain during a dressing change.

14. 1. The prone position limits respiratory excursion, increases the work of breathing, and does not exert pressure on the needle insertion site, which is necessary at this time.
2. **Patients who have received spinal anesthesia (subarachnoid block) are placed in the supine position to limit leakage of cerebrospinal fluid from the needle insertion site. Bed rest in the supine position, pressure against the infusion site, and hydration limit a headache associated with spinal anesthesia.**
3. The right lateral position does not exert pressure on the insertion site, which is necessary to minimize leakage of spinal fluid from the puncture site. A lateral position is used while the lumbar puncture is performed.
4. The Trendelenburg position increases the pressure within the cranial vault, which will increase, not decrease, a headache.

15. 1. Although liver (1 portion 6½ × 2⅜ × ⅜ inches) contains approximately 23 mg of vitamin C, it is noted for being a source of niacin (nicotinic acid) and vitamin D.
2. Cheese does not contain vitamin C; it is noted for containing calcium.
3. **One medium-size spear of broccoli contains 113 mg (cooked) or 141 mg (raw) of vitamin C, which is essential for the formation of collagen. Collagen is a protein substance that adds tensile strength to a healing wound.**
4. Legumes do not contain vitamin C, they are noted for containing protein and phosphorus.

16. 1. Warm liquids and food are contraindicated during the first several days after a tonsillectomy because they cause vasodilation, which may increase bleeding from the vascular mucous membranes of the oropharynx.
2. Milk and milk products are avoided during recovery from oral surgery because some health professionals believe milk increases the consistency of phlegm.
3. Toast is a mechanical irritant to the operative site that may disrupt the healing process and precipitate bleeding.
4. **An ice pop is a frozen clear liquid that promotes vasoconstriction and limits bleeding from the operative site. However, flavors that have a red color are contraindicated because they complicate assessing for bleeding.**

17. 1. A bowel movement will occur long after the first signs of intestinal motility are evident.
2. Administration of fluids before intestinal motility has returned is unsafe and contraindicated. A clear liquid diet is not administered until there are definitive signs of intestinal motility.
3. Although this is done, it is not the best assessment for paralytic ileus. Abdominal distention can be caused by problems other than paralytic ileus, such as hemorrhage, peritonitis, and urinary retention.
4. **Bowel sounds are high-pitched gurgling sounds that vary in frequency, intensity, and pitch; they are caused by the propulsion of intestinal contents through the lower alimentary tract. These sounds are the first indication that intestinal motility is returning.**

18. 1. This should be done eventually, but it is not the priority.
2. An abdominal binder may be used in high-risk patients to prevent, not treat, dehiscence and evisceration.
3. **The low-Fowler's position, a back-lying position, permits inspection of the operative site and promotes retention of abdominal viscera by gravity if dehiscence has occurred. Also, slight flexion of the hips reduces tension on the abdominal musculature.**
4. This is contraindicated because deep breathing increases intra-abdominal pressure, which could cause evisceration.

19. 1. **Obese people have excess adipose tissue that exerts pressure on the abdominal cavity, which raises intra-abdominal pressure. Increased intra-abdominal pressure exerts pressure on the gastrointestinal tract, increasing the risk of nausea and vomiting.**
2. Although inactivity delays recovery of intestinal motility after surgery, a diligent activity and ambulation schedule should

prevent paralytic ileus and its related nausea and vomiting.

3. Intestinal hypomotility, not hypervolemia, is related to postoperative nausea and vomiting. Hypervolemia is an increase in intravascular blood volume.
4. Unconsciousness is not directly related to postoperative nausea and vomiting.

20. 1. **Gentle compression is desirable because it prevents bleeding and promotes molding and shrinkage of the residual limb.**
2. A saline dressing is unsafe because soaking promotes the breakdown of connective tissue fibers (maceration), which impedes wound healing by primary intention.
3. Elevating the limb is unsafe because it promotes hip flexion contractures.
4. This should be done eventually, but caring for the patient is the immediate priority.

21. 1. Dietary roughage prevents constipation, not urinary tract infections.
2. A sitz bath can promote the development of a urinary tract infection if medical aseptic techniques are not followed.
3. **Adequate (approximately 2000 to 3000 mL/day) fluid intake daily promotes a dilute urine and more frequent emptying of the bladder, both of which limit the development of a urinary tract infection. The stasis of concentrated urine promotes microbial growth.**
4. The ingestion of citrus juice causes an alkaline urine, which provides a favorable environment for the multiplication of microorganisms and the development of a urinary tract infection.

22. 1. This occurs with general anesthesia, not conscious sedation.
2. Life-threatening malignant hyperthermia is a rare, autosomal dominant–inherited syndrome that is precipitated by anesthetic inhalation agents and neuromuscular blocking medications used to induce general anesthesia, not conscious sedation.
3. **Conscious sedation involves the use of intravenous opioids and sedatives to decrease the level of consciousness to a degree where the person can still maintain an airway and respond to verbal commands.**
4. Patients who have received spinal anesthesia (subarachnoid block), not conscious sedation, are placed in the supine position to limit leakage of cerebrospinal fluid from the needle insertion site. Bed rest in the supine position, hydration, and pressure against the infusion site, limit headache associated with spinal anesthesia.

23. 1. This is undesirable because of the reduced effectiveness of the system's negative pressure. The power of the suction decreases as the collection chamber fills.
2. Depending on the amount of drainage, this may be unnecessary, or not often enough, to maintain adequate suction. Opening the device increases the risk of infection and should be done only when necessary.
3. Opening the device increases the risk of infection and should be done only when necessary.
4. **The force of the vacuum within the system reduces as the collection chamber fills. Therefore, the collection chamber should be emptied when it is half-full to ensure the effectiveness of suction.**

24. 1. **Chronic alcoholism disrupts the structure and function of the liver. A decrease in the synthesis of bile salts prevents the absorption of vitamin K, which is essential for the production of clotting factors II, VII, IX, and X. Therefore, these patients are at risk for hemorrhage. In addition, malnutrition results in decreased protein synthesis, anemia, and vitamin deficiencies, all of which interfere with fluid and electrolyte balance and wound healing. Lastly, the patient will have to be medically managed to minimize the adaptations to alcohol withdrawal.**
2. Although older adults have a greater surgical risk than younger adults because of the physiologic changes associated with aging (such as prolonged healing and decreased cardiac functioning, homeostatic capacity, and respiratory excursion), they are not at the greatest risk for postoperative mortality as an age group in another option.
3. Although patients with epilepsy have their own unique problems that must be considered, they are not at the greatest risk for postoperative mortality as a group in another option.
4. Although infants have a greater surgical risk than children and young to middle-aged adults because they have a lower total blood volume, larger percentage of body fluid, and difficulty maintaining body temperature as a result of an immature shivering reflex, they are not at the greatest risk for postoperative mortality as a group in another option.

25. 1. This is undesirable because pressure on the popliteal space constricts the vessels, which impedes venous return, promotes venous stasis, and injures tissues. Vessel injury, venous stasis, hypercoagulability, and dehydration all contribute to thrombophlebitis.
2. Although helpful, this will promote venous return for a limited amount of time (approximately 8 hours). The patient will be at risk for the remaining time in the day (approximately 16 hours).
3. This helps to prevent atelectasis and pneumonia, not thrombophlebitis; these should be performed hourly when awake.
4. Leg exercises are an active intervention by the patient that contracts the muscles of the legs. This rhythmically compresses the veins, which promotes venous return and prevents venous stasis.

26. 1. Vitamin C does not improve digestion.
2. Vitamin C (ascorbic acid) promotes collagen production, an essential component of the proliferative phase of wound healing. In addition, vitamin C enhances capillary formation, decreases capillary fragility, increases the tensile strength of the wound, and provides a defense against infection because of its role in the immune response.
3. Vitamin B_{12} (cobalamin), folic acid, and iron promote red blood cell production, not vitamin C.
4. Vitamin C promotes the strength of capillaries, not large veins. Ambulation, leg exercises, and hydration prevent deep vein thrombosis.

27. 1. Although constipation as a result of anesthesia is a concern, it is not life threatening.
2. Although urinary retention as a result of anesthesia is a concern, it is not life threatening.
3. After abdominal surgery, patients frequently have shallow respirations because when the diaphragm contracts with a deep breath, it increases intra-abdominal pressure, which causes pain at the operative site. Shallow breathing may result in atelectasis and/or hypostatic pneumonia.
4. Although a person may experience impaired motor function during recovery from surgery, it is not life threatening.

28. **1. This is significant information because there are unique stressors and expected adaptations to various types of surgery that may direct the plan of care for the patient.**
2. The patient's level of anxiety may be communicated; however, in the immediate postoperative period the physiologic needs of the patient are the priority.
3. Although the type and amount of IV fluids are important and will be communicated, this is only one aspect of the patient's care.
4. Although reasonable requests are honored, the status of the patient or the environment may prohibit them.

29. **1. A pneumothorax is not a concern with a peripherally inserted central venous catheter. Pneumothorax is a complication of a central venous catheter inserted into a subclavian vein because of the close proximity of its insertion site to the apex of the lung.**
2. Both entry sites place the catheter in the superior vena cava.
3. Both entry sites carry a risk of infection because the first line of defense, the skin, has been pierced.
4. Both entry sites allow for the administration of large volumes of fluid because the distal ends of their catheters are both in the superior vena cava.

30. 1. A wound infection is less likely to occur at this time because the proliferative or reconstructive phase of wound healing begins approximately 4 days after tissue damage. By the fifth postoperative day, the wound has filled with highly vascular fibroblastic connective tissue that protects the body from microorganisms.
2. Microorganisms introduced into a surgical site take 72 hours to multiply and present local adaptations of pain, swelling, erythema, warmth, and purulent discharge and systemic adaptations of fever and tachycardia.
3. A wound infection is less likely to occur at this time because by the second postoperative week there is progressive collagen accumulation and the formation of the basic structure of the scar, which protect the body from microorganisms.
4. A wound infection is less likely to occur at this time because by the seventh postoperative day the surface epithelium has the usual thickness and the subepithelial layers are bridged, which protect the body from microorganisms.

31. **1. Leakage of cerebrospinal fluid from the needle insertion site reduces cerebrospinal fluid pressure, which causes a headache.**

2. Neuropathy, due to inflammation or degeneration of the peripheral nerves, is not a response to spinal anesthesia.
3. Although the needle insertion site may feel uncomfortable in some people, it is not a common adaptation after spinal anesthesia.
4. Anesthetic agents cause a decrease, not increase, in blood pressure.

32. 1. This action is beyond the scope of the legal practice of nursing.
2. Withholding medications without a significant reason is unsafe. These medications may be essential to maintain the patient's physical or emotional status.
3. It is unsafe to withhold medications without an important reason. The withheld medications may be essential to maintain the patient's physical or emotional equilibrium.
4. This intervention meets the patient's needs and adheres to the laws that govern the practice of nursing. A change in the route of medication delivery requires an order from a practitioner because medication administration is a dependent function of the nurse.

33. 1. The molecules in clear liquids are less complex and easier to ingest, tolerate, and digest than those in a full-liquid diet or food.
2. This is not the most common diet ordered postoperatively, although a full-liquid diet frequently precedes solid food.
3. A low-fiber diet is ordered for specific problems, such as intestinal inflammation or infection. When able to be tolerated postoperatively, dietary fiber promotes intestinal motility and prevents constipation.
4. This is not the most common diet ordered postoperatively, although most initial postoperative diets eventually progress to a regular diet.

34. 1. These adaptations are essential for discharge from the Post-Anesthesia Care Unit because they reflect the body's vital functions, such as airway, breathing, and circulation.
2. The lack of a fever is not a criterion for discharge from the Post-Anesthesia Care Unit because a low-grade fever is an expected response to the stress of surgery. The other listed adaptations are desirable for discharge.
3. A dry dressing may be unrealistic. Some drainage from a surgical incision is expected in the immediate postoperative period. The other listed adaptations are desirable.
4. A postoperative patient may not be able to turn from side to side, but the patient should be able to move all extremities. The other listed adaptations are desirable for discharge.

35. 1. Although this is essential to proceed with the surgery, it is not as high a priority as another option.
2. During stage III surgical anesthesia the patient experiences a loss of the pharyngeal, laryngeal, and gag reflexes, as well as spontaneous respirations (apnea). Maintaining a patent airway and ventilation are the priorities.
3. Although the reflexes are assessed as the patient progresses through the induction, maintenance, and reversal stages of anesthesia, it is not as high a priority as another option.
4. Although the heart rate is monitored throughout the surgical experience, it is not as great a priority as another option.

36. 1. When exiting from the left side of the bed, the left lateral side of the abdomen will be compressed against the bed by body weight. The left, not right, side of the abdomen will absorb the majority of the muscular strain exerted by the transfer.
2. Although this might be done for patients at high risk for dehiscence, abdominal binders are not used routinely because they increase intra-abdominal pressure; this exerts a force against the diaphragm that impedes maximum respiratory excursion.
3. This is unsafe. At least one upper extremity should be used to help raise the body to a sitting position and promote balance during the transfer out of bed.
4. This places an unnecessary strain on the abdominal muscles in the area of the incision.

37. 1. These are the classic signs of a pulmonary embolus. Chest pain results from local tissue hypoxia, tachycardia from systemic hypoxia, and hypotension from decreased cardiac output. A pulmonary embolus is caused by a thrombus lodging in a vessel in the pulmonary circulation, occluding blood supply to the capillary side of the alveolar-capillary membrane.
2. Although tachycardia and hypotension occur with hemorrhage, chest pain does not.
3. Although tachycardia and chest pain occur with a myocardial infarction (heart attack), the blood pressure probably will increase, not decrease. If cardiogenic shock occurs, the blood pressure decreases eventually.

4. Pneumonia, inflammation of the lung with consolidation and exudation, is associated with tachycardia and chest discomfort. However, it does not have a sudden onset and the blood pressure will increase, not decrease.

38. **1. Oliguria is diminished urine secretion in relation to fluid intake, which is indicated by a negative balance in the intake and output record or hourly urine outputs of less then 30 mL. Oliguria is caused by decreased renal perfusion or kidney disease.**
2. Cachexia is not an adaptation related to altered renal perfusion. Cachexia is malnutrition and emaciation associated with serious diseases such as cancer.
3. Yellow sclera indicates jaundice. Jaundice is the accumulation of bile pigments in tissue, which is associated with liver or biliary problems, not altered renal perfusion.
4. Suprapubic distention indicates urinary retention, which is an inability of the bladder to empty, not a problem with renal perfusion. If it occurs, usually it becomes evident 6 to 8 hours after surgery.

39. 1. This is an unrealistic expectation considering all the stressors that can contribute to these problems. Essential nutrient needs can be met despite the presence of nausea and vomiting.
2. Fluid is the most basic nutrient of the body and it contains compounds such as electrolytes. Electrolytes help maintain fluid balance, contribute to acid-base balance, and facilitate enzyme and neuromuscular reactions. The narrow safe limits of the volumes and composition of fluid compartments are essential for the life-sustaining processes of nutrition, metabolism, and excretion.
3. Wound healing takes time, and it is difficult to evaluate during the inflammatory phase, which lasts approximately 1 to 4 days.
4. Oral intake should not be reestablished until intestinal motility returns, which may take several days.

40. 1. Although the condition of drains ultimately will be assessed, the physiologic status of the patient is the priority.
2. Although the patient's level of consciousness eventually will be assessed, it is not the priority at this time.
3. Assessment in acute situations always follows the ABCs: Airway, Breathing, Circulation. Respirations and pulse reflect the cardiopulmonary status of the patient.
4. Both the location and status of the dressing should be assessed, but not until more critical assessments are completed.

41. 1. Whole grains contain trace amounts or none of the vitamin necessary for collagen production. Whole grains are noted primarily for containing vitamin E and potassium.
2. Yellow vegetables are noted for being a major source of vitamin A, which is not the vitamin most responsible for collagen production.
3. Citrus fruits are the best sources of vitamin C. Vitamin C promotes collagen production, which is essential in the proliferative and maturation phases of wound healing.
4. Red meat contains trace amounts or none of the vitamin necessary for collagen formation with the exception of liver (1 portion equals 6½ × 2⅜ × ⅜ inches), which contains 23 mg of vitamin C.

42. **1. Abdominal distention raises the pressure within the abdominal cavity, which exerts pressure against the diaphragm, impeding its contraction and limiting thoracic excursion.**
2. When in a side-lying position, aeration of the dependent side of the lung is limited because of pooling of secretions and the weight of the body compressing the dependent part of the body.
3. This is not an active intervention to facilitate respirations, but it is an important assessment to evaluate the patient's response to surgery and interventions used to facilitate respirations.
4. Passive range-of-motion exercises do not facilitate respirations; they help prevent contractures.

43. 1. The Sims' position is not used during the intraoperative period for perineal surgery.
2. The supine position is the most common position for abdominal, not perineal, surgery.
3. The lithotomy position, back-lying with the hips and knees flexed and the legs supported in stirrups, provides optimal visualization of and access to the area related to perineal surgery.
4. A patient's legs are adducted when in the Trendelenburg position, which does not permit visualization of or access to the perineal area.

44. **1. Wrinkles create ridges causing unnecessary pressure that can lead to tissue injury.**

2. **The toe window should be positioned over the toes or sole of the feet depending on the manufacturer. This ensures that the stocking is aligned correctly and the distal portion of the foot can be accessed to perform the blanch test to assess peripheral circulation.**
3. The stockings should be applied before, not after, the patient gets out of bed. Standing permits the development of dependent edema because of the force of gravity. Putting them on while still in bed helps prevent dependent edema. If stockings are applied after getting out of bed, they will compress edematous tissues and cause injury.
4. Flexion impedes, while extension promotes, application of an antiembolism stocking. Most antiembolism stockings are knee high rather than thigh high.
5. This is inadequate. Antiembolism stockings should be removed every 8 hours for 30 minutes. This permits inspection and physical hygiene.

45. **The CO_2 that is used to insufflate the abdominal cavity during a laparoscopic cholecystectomy that is not released, or absorbed by the body, can be trapped in the subdiaphragmatic recesses. This can irritate the diaphragm causing referred pain to the right shoulder and scapular area. In addition to irritation of the diaphragm, CO_2 can irritate the phrenic nerve causing dyspnea. Positioning the patient in the left Sims' position will help move the gas away from the diaphragm. Discharge orders may include an order for a heating pad for 20 minutes every few hours and an analgesic. The nurse should encourage the patient to periodically walk and breathe deeply once the patient has fully recovered from anesthesia.**

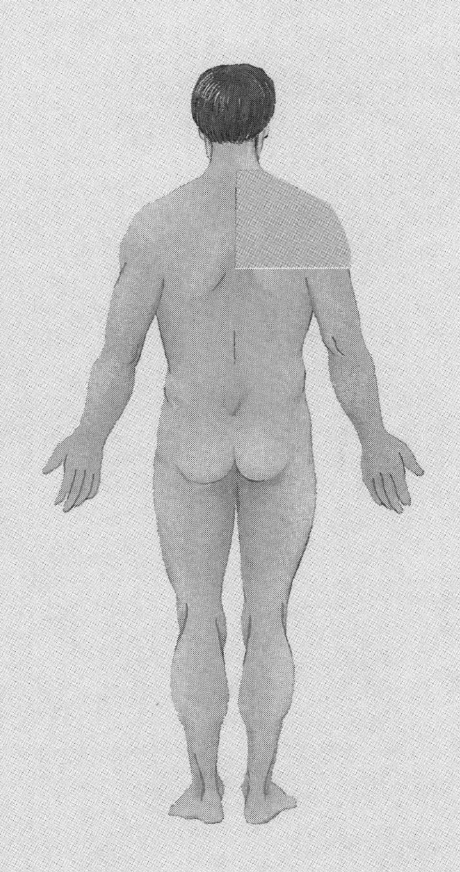

Alternate Item Formats

NCLEX Examinations include multiple-choice questions and alternate item format questions. A typical multiple-choice question presents a statement or situation and then requires the test taker to identify the correct answer from among four presented options. Alternate item formats use the benefits of computer technology to assess knowledge via methods other than the four-option, multiple-choice item. Alternate item formats include questions that require test takers to identify multiple answers, identify priorities, perform a mathematical calculation, or respond to a question in relation to a graphic image, picture, table or chart/exhibit. These alternate item formats are able to measure entry-level nursing competence in ways that are different from the typical multiple-choice format. It is believed that some nursing content is more readily and authentically evaluated using alternate item formats. This chapter includes 40 questions that use formats other than the multiple-choice questions.

ALTERNATE ITEM FORMATS

Multiple-Response Items

A multiple-response item presents a statement or situation that asks a question that will have more than one answer among the presented options. The test taker is required to identify all the options that are correct.

1. A patient who had a total abdominal hysterectomy 2 days ago is ambulating and complains of dyspnea and stabbing chest pain on inspiration. A nursing assessment reveals a pulse of 110 and respirations of 35. While many of the following actions may be implemented, which three take priority?
   1. ____ Administer oxygen
   2. ____ Assess breath sounds
   3. ____ Take vital signs every 30 minutes
   4. ____ Return the patient to bed by wheelchair
   5. ____ Place the patient in the high-Fowler's position

2. A patient comes to the emergency department with a lacerated thumb. The nurse identifies the common signs and symptoms of the Local Adaptation Syndrome (LAS). Indicate all that apply.
   1. ____ Pain
   2. ____ Heat
   3. ____ Erythema
   4. ____ Increased heart rate
   5. ____ Decreased blood pressure
   6. ____ Elevated blood glucose level

3. The nurse is assisting a postoperative patient to ambulate. Which postoperative complications will ambulation help prevent? Select all that apply.
   1. ____ Hypovolemia
   2. ____ Constipation
   3. ____ Dehiscence
   4. ____ Atelectasis
   5. ____ Infection

4. A patient is learning self-care in relation to a 2-gram sodium diet. The nurse knows that further teaching is necessary when the patient selects which foods high in sodium? Check all that apply.
1. ____ Apple juice
2. ____ Corned beef
3. ____ Canned soup
4. ____ Broccoli spears

5. The nurse is monitoring a patient's IV infusion. Which data are necessary to determine that the IV is "on time." Check all that apply.
1. ____ The drip rate per minute
2. ____ The time the bag was hung
3. ____ The solution indicated on the IV bag
4. ____ The volume of solution in the IV bag
5. ____ The milliliters per hour ordered by the physician

6. A patient who was in an automobile collision is brought to the emergency department by ambulance. The patient is exhibiting signs and symptoms of multiple trauma. The nurse identifies the common adaptations to hemorrhage. Indicate all that are relevant.
1. ____ Bradypnea
2. ____ Tachycardia
3. ____ Flushed skin
4. ____ Bounding pulse
5. ____ Delayed capillary refill

7. The nurse is caring for several postoperative patients and understands that common nursing interventions involve the principle of gravity. Check each therapeutic intervention that involves the principle of gravity.
1. ____ Foley catheter
2. ____ Penrose drain
3. ____ Hemovac drain
4. ____ Tap-water enema
5. ____ Gastric decompression

8. The nurse is supervising a nursing team consisting of two nurses and two nursing asssistants. Which tasks can the nurse delegate to the nursing assistants? Check all that apply.
1. ____ Helping a patient who is constipated choose foods from a diet menu
2. ____ Teaching a patient how to walk with a walker
3. ____ Applying Duoderm to unbroken skin
4. ____ Weighing a patient using a bed scale
5. ____ Emptying a Foley collection bag

9. Which actions reflect principles of surgical asepsis? Check all that apply.
1. _____ Washing hands
2. _____ Keeping a sterile field dry
3. _____ Holding sterile objects above the waist
4. _____ Wearing personal protective equipment
5. _____ Considering the outer half inch of the sterile field as contaminated

10. The nurse receives the following information about patients at the change-of-shift report. Although all the patients should be assessed, indicate which two patients should be assessed before the others.
1. ____ A patient who just was informed of having cancer
2. ____ A patient who was complaining of feeling nauseated
3. ____ A patient who is receiving a titrated medication via an infusion pump
4. ____ A patient who received an analgesic by mouth for pain immediately before report
5. ____ A patient whose vital signs include an irregular a pulse and labored respirations

Hot-Spot Items

A hot-spot item asks a question in relation to an illustration. The test taker must identify a location on the illustration that answers the question.

1. A patient with a physician's order for bed rest consistently lies in the right lateral position. Which bony prominence should the nurse assess because it has the greatest risk for the development of a pressure ulcer? Mark an X over the area.

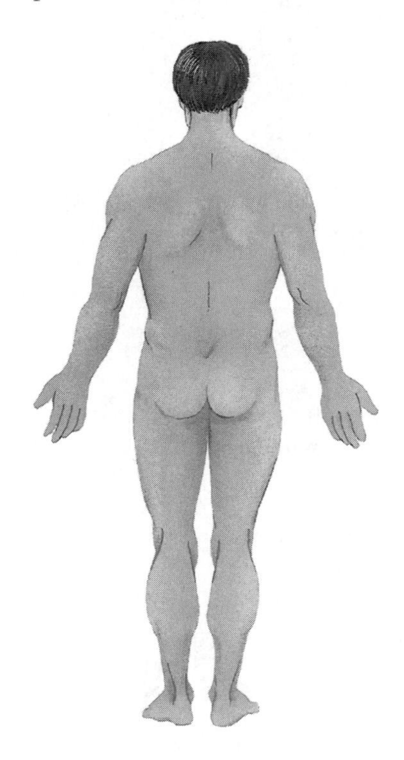

2. The nurse is caring for a patient who had the creation of a colostomy. Place an X over the large intestine that produces the most liquid stool, thereby placing the patient at greatest risk for skin breakdown.

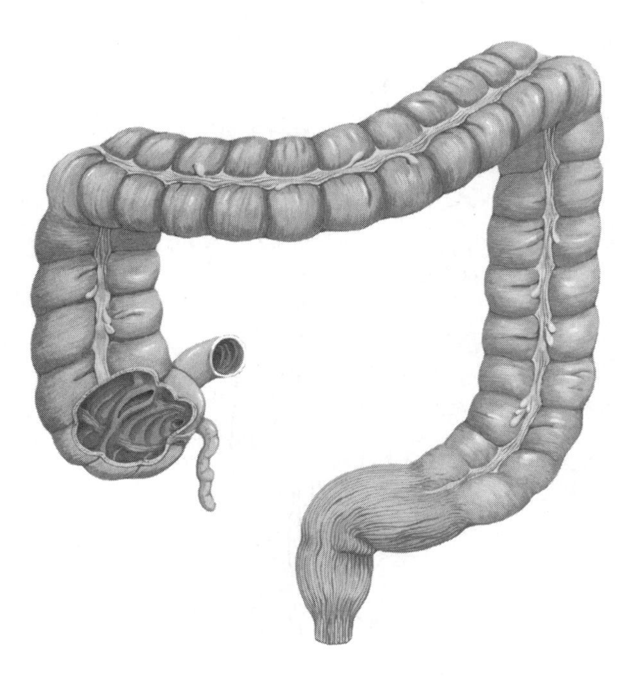

3. The nurse is to administer an intermittent tube feeding via a nasogastric tube. Mark an X where the nurse should place a stethoscope when assessing for placement of the nasogastric tube.

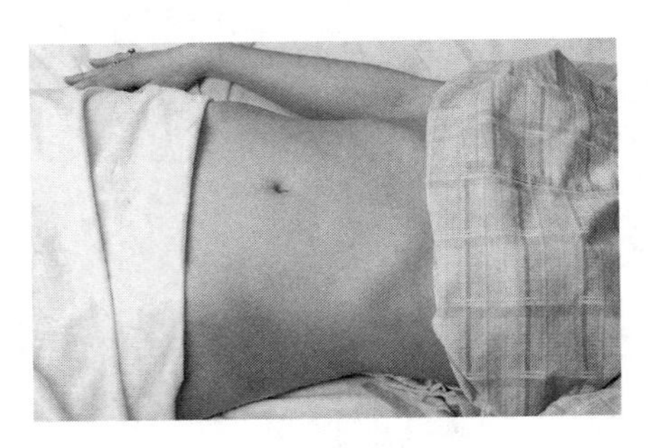

4. The physician orders heparin 5000 units sub-Q twice a day. Place an X over the site that is most commonly used by the nurse to administer this medication.

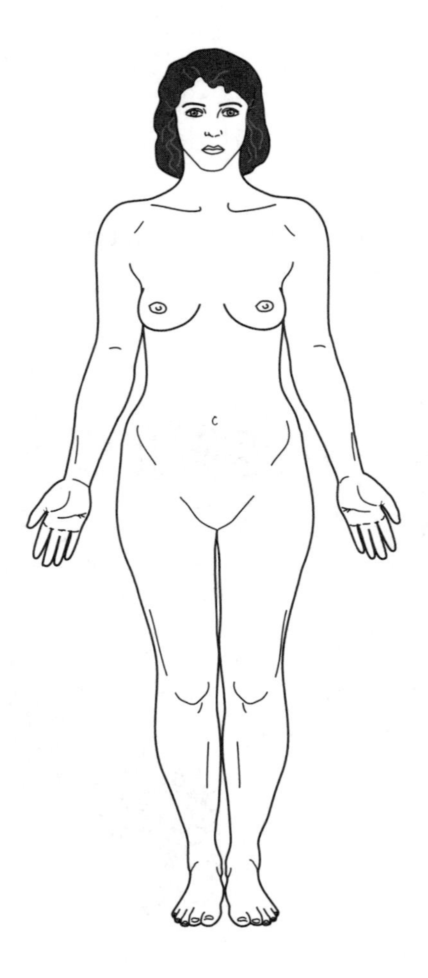

5. Two nurses are performing CPR on a postoperative patient. One nurse performs sternal compressions and the other delivers breaths and monitors the patient. Place an X over the preferred site to obtain this patient's pulse.

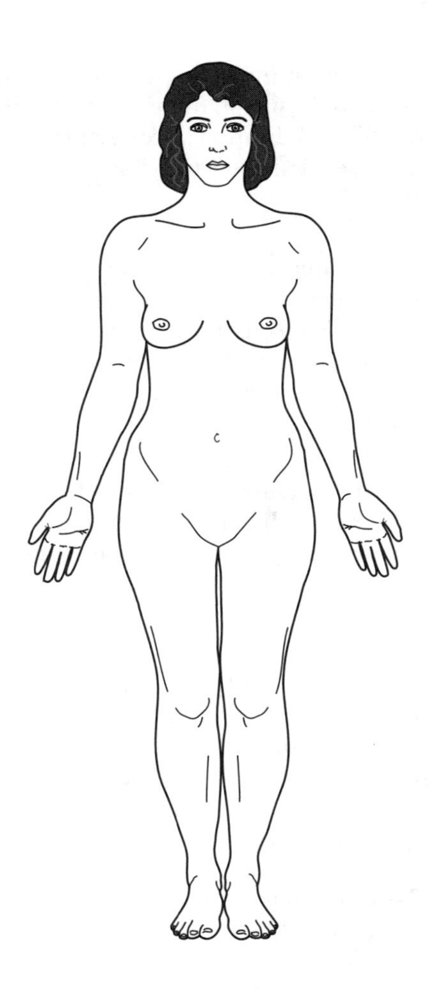

Fill-In-the-Blank Items

A fill-in-the-blank item asks a question that requires the test taker to perform a calculation. Fill-in-the-blank items are associated with pharmacological and parenteral therapies.

1. The primary care practitioner orders an antidysrhythmic medication of 2g IV per 1000 mL D_5W at 4 mg per minute. At what rate should the nurse set the infusion pump?
   Answer: _______mL/hr.
2. The primary care provider orders an antibiotic of 400,000 units IVPB every 6 hours. The medication vial contains 1,000,000 units with the following directions. Add 4.6 mL of diluent to yield a concentrated solution of 200,000 units per mL. How much solution of the antibiotic should the nurse administer?
   Answer:_________mL.
3. The physician orders digoxin (Lanoxin) 0.25 mg po once daily. Available are tablets that contain 0.125 mg. How many tablets should the nurse administer?
   Answer:________Tablets.
4. The physician orders diphenhydramine (Benadryl) elixir 25 mg po twice a day for 3 days. The bottle of Benadryl states that there are 12.5 mg per mL. When preparing the first dose, how much solution should the nurse administer?
   Answer:________mL.

5. The physician orders human recombinant erythropoietin (Epogen) 100 units/kg/dose sub-Q t.i.d. for a patient who weighs 110 pounds. The medication states that there are 2000 units/mL. How much solution should the nurse administer?
Answer: __________mL.

6. The physician orders ondansetron hydrochloride (Zofran) 6 mg to be administered via oral suspension to a 12-year-old child 30 minutes before chemotherapy and then every 8 hours for 2 more doses. The medication states that there are 4 mg/5 mL. How much oral solution should the nurse administer per dose?
Answer: __________mL.

7. A patient initially received ramipril (Altace) 1.25 mg daily. The dose was increased to 2.5 mg once a day for several days, and finally the physician orders the dose to be increased to 5 mg every day. The patient says to the nurse, "I still have a lot of 1.25 mg tablets left. Can I use these up with the new dose the doctor ordered?" How many 1.25 mg tablets should the nurse instruct the patient to take?
Answer: __________Tablets.

8. The physician orders warfarin sodium (Coumadin) 10 mg p.o. once a day on the even days of the month and 15 mg on the odd days of the month. The 10 mg tablets supplied are scored. How many tablets should the nurse administer on the 5th day of the month?
Answer: __________Tablets.

9. The physician orders an IV infusion of 1000 mL of D5W with 20 mEq of potassium chloride to be administered at 125 mL/hour. The infusion set has a drop factor of 15/mL. At how many drops per minute should the nurse set the IV infusion?
Answer: __________drops/minute.

10. A patient has an order for Regular insulin coverage a.c. The order states:

Blood glucose		
	71–150:	no insulin
	151–200:	3 units
	201–250:	5 units
	251–300:	7 units
	301–350:	9 units
	351–400:	11 units and call MD

The patient's blood glucose at 11:30 AM is 230. How many units of Regular insulin should the nurse administer?
Answer: __________Units.

Items Using a Chart, Table, or Graphic Image

An item using a chart, table, or graphic image requires you to refer to the illustration presented to arrive at the correct answer. It tests your ability to identify, calculate, analyze, or interpret data from a chart, table, or graphic image to arrive at the correct answer.

1. The nurse is reviewing the patient's temperatures over the course of hospitalization. What was the patient's temperature on June 7th at 4 PM?
   1. 97.8°F
   2. 99.2°F
   3. 101.2°F
   4. 102.6°F

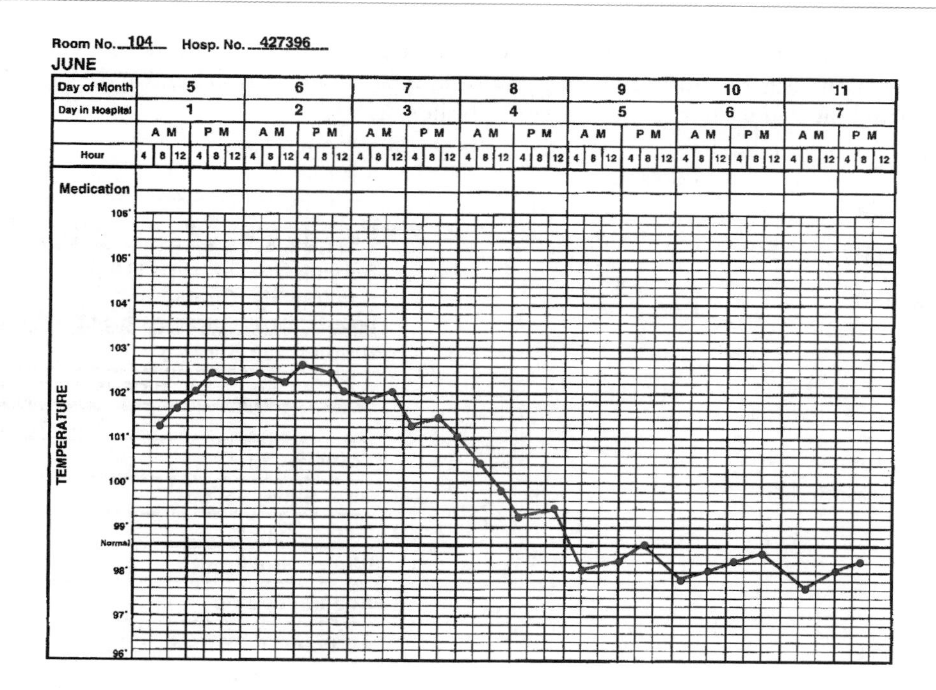

2. The nurse is caring for a patient who has Intake and Output ordered by the physician. Referring to the Intake and Ouput flow sheet, what was the patient's total output for the hours between 7 AM and 3 PM?

1. 355
2. 720
3. 1300
4. 1405

DAILY INTAKE AND OUTPUT RECORD

DATE JUNE 5

INTAKE								OUTPUT			
I.V. FLUIDS							ORAL	URINE	EMESIS	N.G. TUBE	HEMOVAC
Time	Bottle	Amount	Solution	Medication and Dosage	* ABS.	∓ LIB					
8	1	1000	NS	20 mEq KCl				650			
8:30							360				
10:00							120				
11:30							240	150			
12:00									160		
1:40									90		60
2:15								250			
3:00					525	475					45
7-3 TOTAL		8-HR TOTAL			525	475	720	1050	250		105
3-11 TOTAL		8-HR TOTAL									
11-7 TOTAL		8-HR TOTAL									
24 HOUR TOTAL											

INTAKE GRAND TOTAL ______ OUTPUT GRAND TOTAL ______

* ABS. = amount absorbed ∓ LIB = Left in bag

3. The nurse is teaching a patient how to read a food label. Based on the label provided, the patient asks the nurse how many calories are contained in the entire package. Calculate how many calories are contained in the package.

 1. 90
 2. 120
 3. 360
 4. 480

Nutrition Facts

Serving Size 1/2 cup (114g)
Servings Per Container 4

Amount Per Serving

Calories 90	Calories from Fat 30
	% Daily Value *
Total Fat 3g	**5%**
Saturated Fat 0g	**0%**
Trans Fat 0g	**0%**
Cholesterol 0mg	**0%**
Sodium 300mg	**13%**
Total Carbohydrate 13g	**4%**
Dietary Fiber 3g	**12%**
Sugars 3g	
Protein 3g	

Vitamin A	80%	•	Vitamin C	60%
Calcium	4%	•	Iron	4%

* Percent Daily Values are based on a 2,000 calorie diet. Your daily values may be higher or lower depending on your calorie needs:

	Calories	2,000	2,500
Total Fat	Less than	65g	80g
Sat Fat	Less than	20g	25g
Cholesterol	Less than	300mg	300mg
Sodium	Less than	2,400mg	2,400mg
Total Carbohydrate		300g	375g
Dietary Fiber		25g	30g

Calories per gram:
Fat 9 • Carbohydrate 4 • Protein 4

4. A patient is admitted to the Emergency Department for treatment after stepping on a rusty nail at a job site. The physician orders Tetanus Immune Globulin 250 units IM stat. Which illustration indicates the angle at which this injection should be administered by the nurse?

 1. A
 2. B
 3. C
 4. D

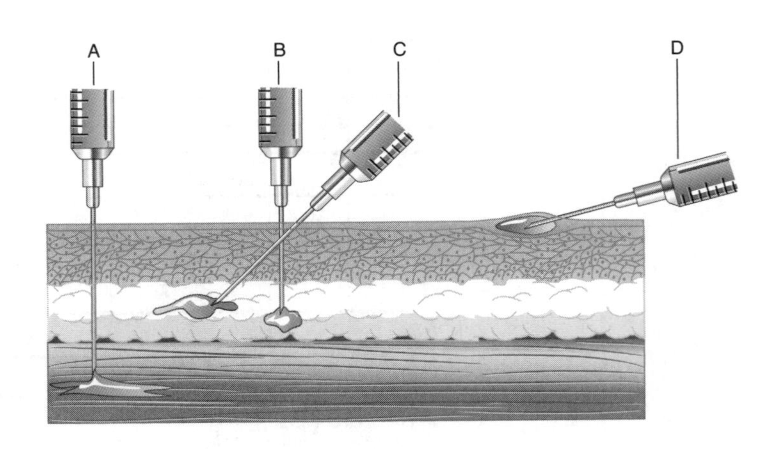

5. A patient is admitted to the hospital with the diagnosis of a brain attack resulting in left-sided hemiplegia. On the first day of admission, the nurse begins passive range-of-motion exercise on the patient's left upper and lower extremities. Which movement is indicated in the illustration?
   1. Inversion
   2. Adduction
   3. Supination
   4. Opposition

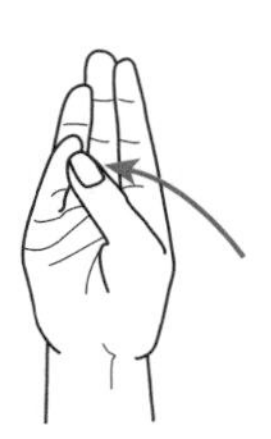

Drop and Drag/Ordered Response Items

A Drop and Drag/Ordered Response item presents a situation followed by a list of statements. You are asked to place the statements in order of priority.

1. At the beginning of a 7 AM to 7 PM shift a nurse receives a report, which is completed by 7:20 AM. Place in order of priority the tasks that should be performed by the nurse.
   1. Give a prn pain medication to a patient in pain
   2. Change a patient's dressing that must be done 2 times a day
   3. Administer the ordered 8:00 AM medications to the patients on the unit
   4. Obtain the vital signs of a patient who is complaining of shortness of breath

   Answer: ______________

2. When assessing a patient's abdomen, the nurse should follow a logical sequence. Place these assessments in the order in which they should be performed.
   1. Percuss the suprapubic area to determine bladder distention
   2. Auscultate the four quadrants of the abdomen for bowel sounds
   3. Observe the abdomen for contour and visible signs of peristalsis
   4. Palpate the abdomen to determine the presence of tenderness and fluid

   Answer: ______________

3. The professional nurse must always be prepared for, and ready to respond to, a fire that may occur on a hospital unit. Place the following activities in the order that they should be implemented by the nurse.
   1. Know the location and use of alarms and extinguishers
   2. Rescue patients in danger when a fire is identified
   3. Pull the fire alarm to notify others about the fire
   4. Close doors and windows on the unit
   5. Be alert for the signs of a fire

4. The nurse plans to reposition an unconscious patient from the supine position to the right side-lying position. Initially, the nurse explains the care to the patient, closes the door for privacy, and performs handwashing before touching the patient. Place the following nursing actions in the order they should be performed.
   1. Move the right shoulder and arm forward and downward
   2. Place the patient's arms across the chest and the left foot over the right foot
   3. Place pillows behind the patient's back and under the head, left arm and left leg
   4. Roll the patient toward the right side using one hand behind the patient's shoulder and the other behind the patient's hip

   Answer: ______________

5. The physician orders a soapsuds enema for an adult patient. The nurse explains the procedure to the patient and arranges for the bathroom to be available. The nurse then performs handwashing, collects the equipment, and begins to prepare the enema equipment. Arrange these interventions in the order they should be performed.
   1. Lubricate the catheter tip with water-soluble jelly
   2. Fill the container with 1000 mL of 110°F water
   3. Flush the tubing with water
   4. Add soap to the container
   5. Clamp the tubing

   Answer: _______________

Exhibit Items

An exhibit item asks a question that requires you to analyze and interpret data that is organized in sections commonly found in a patient's medical record and arrive at a conclusion as to which is the correct answer.

1. An older adult with multiple health problems is admitted to the hospital after passing out in the supermarket. An electrocardiogram reveals the presence of a dysrhythmia and the patient is scheduled for a cardiac catheterization. Twelve hours after admission the nurse on the evening shift reads the collected information about the patient and performs a physical assessment. The nurse concludes that the patient is exhibiting which human response?
   1. Systemic infection
   2. Anaphylactic shock
   3. Fluid volume excess
   4. Orthostatic hypotension

Health History: *Health Problems:*
Hypothyroidism
Atherosclerosis
Osteoarthritis
Heart failure
Daily Medications:
acetaminophen
digoxin (Lanoxin)
furosemide (Lasix)
levothyroxine sodium (Synthroid)

Vital Signs on Admission: Oral Temp: 100.2°F
Pulse: 94/min, irregular
Respirations: 24/min
Blood Pressure: 150/92

Physical Assessment: *Subjective:*
Headache
Loss of appetite
Extreme fatigue
Short of breath
Objective:
1+ pitting edema of ankles
Crackles in base of lungs
VS: P 100, R 26, BP 170/96

2. A 75-year-old man, who had been having transient ischemic attacks (TIAs), is admitted to the hospital after experiencing a brain attack (cerebrovascular accident, CVA). The patient is semicomatose and has right hemiplegia. The nurse reviews the chart and performs a physical assessment. The nurse identifies that this patient is at risk for developing:
   1. Diarrhea
   2. Hemorrhage
   3. Pressure ulcers
   4. Diabetes mellitus

Physical Assessment: Height: 5 feet 9 inches tall
Weight: 106 pounds
Right hemiplegia
Muscle flaccidity
Urinary and fecal incontinence
Responsive only to painful stimuli

Health History: *Health Problems:*
Atherosclerosis
Iron deficiency anemia
Benign prostatic hyperplasia

Laboratory Tests: RBC: 3.5 mil/μl
WBC: 9,000 mil/μl
Hb: 10.0 g/dL
Ferritin: 14 ng/mL
Glucose (FBG): 85 mg/dL

3. The nurse in the Post-Anesthesia Care Unit is monitoring a patient who had a hysterectomy, salpingo-oophorectomy, and debulking for cancer of the ovary. At 11:00 AM the patient complains of difficulty breathing. The nurse performs a focused physical assessment and reviews the patient's hospital record. The nurse concludes that the patient is experiencing what complication?
   1. Pulmonary embolus
   2. Myocardial infarction
   3. Postoperative hemorrhage
   4. Subcutaneous emphysema

Vital Signs: 10 AM–P 72, R 16, BP 120/72
10:15 AM–P 74, R 18, BP 122/70
10:30 AM– P 70, R 20, BP 118/74
10:45 AM–P 74, R 18, BP 120/68

Physical Assessment: Dyspnea
Pale skin
Coughing
Diaphoresis
Right-sided chest pain
Abdomen flat and nontender
Abdominal dressing dry and intact
Decreased breath sounds on right side
VS: P 92; R 28; shallow, labored; BP 160/92
ECG: Normal sinus rhythm

4. The nurse on a surgical unit is caring for a patient who had abdominal surgery at 8:00 AM, 12 hours ago. The patient has an abdominal dressing, 2 portable wound drainage systems at the surgical site, an IV of 1000 mL of sodium chloride 0.95% with 20 mEq of KCl at 125 mL/hr, a PCA pump with an analgesic, and a urinary retention catheter in place. When the patient complains of abdominal discomfort, the nurse collects data and concludes that the patient may be experiencing:
   1. Pain
   2. Hemorrhage
   3. Urinary retention
   4. Excess fluid volume

Vital Signs: 4:00 PM–P 76, R 18, BP 116/72
6:00 PM–P 80, R 20, BP 120/76

I&O: 8:00 AM–8 PM: Intake: IVF–1500 mL
Output: Urine–1050 mL
Wound drainage systems–210 mL

Physical Assessment at 8 PM: Dressing dry and intact
No suprapubic distention
Pain of 8 on a scale of 1 to 10
IVF intact and infusing at 125 mL/hr
Retention catheter draining clear amber urine
Vital Signs: P 86, R 24, BP 136/80

5. A 76-year-old man, diagnosed with dehydration, is admitted to the hospital for rehydration therapy. The nurse collects a health history, obtains the vital signs, and performs a physical assessment. The nurse determines that the patient is at the highest risk for:
   1. Infection
   2. Aspiration
   3. Malnutrition
   4. Constipation

Health History: 76 yrs old
5 feet 10 inches tall
Weighs 175 pounds
Parkinson's disease for 5 years
Benign prostatic hyperplasia for 10 years
Flu and pneumonia vaccines within last 6 mo
carbidopa-levodopa (Sinemet) daily

Vital Signs: Oral temperature: 99.6°F
Pulse: 88, regular rhythm
Respirations: 22, shallow
Blood pressure: 109/68

Physical Assessment: Lethargic
Dysphagia
Dysarthria
Abdomen is soft
Diminished gag reflex
Upper and lower dentures
Skin dry, exhibiting "tenting"
Urinated 500 mL of clear yellow urine
Borborygmi auscultated in all 4 quadrants

ANSWERS AND RATIONALES

Multiple-Response Items

1. 1. **The patient most likely experienced a pulmonary embolus. Administering oxygen is essential to facilitate gas exchange.**
   2. While important, this is not one of the three actions that take priority.
   3. Vital signs should be taken more frequently than every 30 minutes in this situation.
   4. **Using a wheelchair limits muscle activity. Activity can contribute to more emboli and increase the demand on the heart and lungs.**
   5. **The high-Fowler's position facilitates thoracic expansion and ventilation, which are necessary for this patient.**

2. 1. **Pain is caused by irritation of nerve tissue by chemical substances and the pressure of fluid congestion in the area of local trauma.**
   2. **Heat is caused by an increased blood flow in response to the release of histamine at the site of local trauma.**
   3. **Erythema is caused by an increased blood flow in response to the release of histamine and an increased capillary permeability in response to kinins at the site of local trauma or infection.**
   4. This is unrelated to the Local Adaptation Syndrome (LAS). An increased heart rate is associated with activation of the sympathetic nervous system seen in the General Adaptation Syndrome (GAS).
   5. This is unrelated to the LAS. An increased, not decreased, blood pressure is associated with activation of the sympathetic nervous system seen in the GAS.
   6. This is unrelated to the LAS. An elevated blood glucose level occurs in response to the secretion of glucocorticoids in the GAS.

3. 1. Ambulation will not prevent blood loss that results in hypovolemia.
   2. **Ambulation promotes intestinal peristalsis that results in a bowel movement.**
   3. Supporting the incisional site during coughing and deep breathing helps to prevent dehiscence.
   4. **Ambulation promotes deep breathing that helps the alveoli expand.**
   5. The use of sterile technique and handwashing will help prevent infection.

4. 1. Apple juice contains approximately 7 mg of sodium per cup and is permitted on a 2-gm sodium diet.
   2. **Corned beef contains approximately 800 mg of sodium per 3 ounces and should not be included in a 2-gm sodium diet.**
   3. **Most canned soups contain between 800 and 1000 mg of sodium per cup and are contraindicated on a 2-gm sodium diet.**
   4. One broccoli spear contains approximately 20 mg of sodium and is permitted on a 2-gm sodium diet.

5. 1. This is not necessary to know when determining whether an IV is "on time."
   2. **This is one of three pieces of data that the nurse needs to know to determine whether an IV is "on time." The nurse needs to identify how many minutes/hours the IV has been running and then multiply this number by the milliliters of solution ordered by the physician per minute/hour. This volume is then deducted from the original volume in the IV bag. The actual volume that is in the bag should be compared with the volume that should be in the bag. If the volumes match, the IV is "on time," if there is more fluid than should be in the bag, then the IV is "behind schedule," if there is less fluid than should be in the bag, then the IV is "ahead of schedule."**
   3. This is necessary to know to ensure that it is identical to the solution ordered by the physician, not to determine whether an IV is "on time."
   4. **Same as #2.**
   5. **Same as #2.**

6. 1. Tachypnea, not bradypnea, occurs in response to sympathetic nervous system stimulation as the body attempts to deliver more oxygen to body tissues.
   2. **This occurs in response to sympathetic nervous system stimulation as the body attempts to deliver more oxygen to body tissues.**
   3. The skin becomes pale and cold, not flushed, in response to hemorrhage as peripheral vasoconstriction occurs in an attempt to shunt blood to vital organs of the body.
   4. This is reflective of fluid overload (hypervolemia), not hypovolemia associated with hemorrhage.

5. **This occurs in response to peripheral vasoconstriction in an attempt to shunt blood to vital organs.**

7. 1. **Gravity is the force that pulls mass toward the center of the earth. Urine flows by gravity out of the bladder through a tube (indwelling catheter, Foley catheter) into a collection bag.**
   2. **A Penrose drain is a flexible collapsible tube with a potential diameter of approximately 1 inch that drains fluid from inside a surgical site to a dressing via gravity.**
   3. A Hemovac, is a closed wound drainage system, that uses negative pressure, not gravity, to drain secretions from an incisional site.
   4. **Enema fluid flows from a container through a rectal tube into the large intestine via gravity. The force of the flow is regulated by raising or lowering the height of the enema bag in relation to the rectum. Raising the bag increases the force; lowering the bag decreases the force.**
   5. A nasogastric tube removes fluid from the stomach via negative pressure, not gravity.

8. 1. This is outside the scope of practice of a nursing assistant. It requires knowledge about foods, fiber, and teaching principles.
   2. Patient teaching is an independent role of the nurse, not a nursing assistant. This task requires an understanding of anatomy and principles of physics and teaching.
   3. Duoderm is a type of dressing. Applying dressings is a dependent function of the nurse and requires a physician's order or facility protocol. Assessment of the area and correct application of Duoderm is within the scope of nursing practice.
   4. **This is within the scope of practice of the nursing assistant. Nursing assistants can collect vital statistics such as patient's weight, temperature, pulse, respiration, and intake and output.**
   5. **This is within the scope of practice of the nursing assistant. Nursing assistants have been taught to implement medical aseptic principles and standard precautions.**

9. 1. This is a principle of medical, not surgical, asepsis.
   2. **Moisture contaminates a sterile field by facilitating the movement of microorganisms from the unsterile surface below the field to the sterile field by capillary action.**
   3. **Sterile items, including sterile gloved hands, should be held above the waist; when held below the waist, they are considered contaminated.**
   4. This protects the caregiver and is a principle of medical, not surgical, asepsis.
   5. A one-inch, not half-inch, border is considered contaminated.

10. 1. **This information may have precipitated a crisis for this patient. Psychosocial needs of patients are as important as physiologic needs.**
    2. This is not a life-threatening adaptation. Other patient situations are a greater priority.
    3. Although this patient should be monitored, infusion pumps deliver fluid volumes safely. Other patient situations are a greater priority.
    4. An analgesic by mouth takes approximately 20 to 30 minutes to be effective. This patient's response to the medication can be evaluated after other patients' needs are met.
    5. **These vital signs are outside the expected range; therefore, this patient should be assessed first because these adaptations may indicate a life-threatening situation.**

Hot-Spot Items

1. **This site is at risk because it is dependent when lying in a right lateral position; the majority of body mass overlies this area and it bears a greater part of the body's weight.**

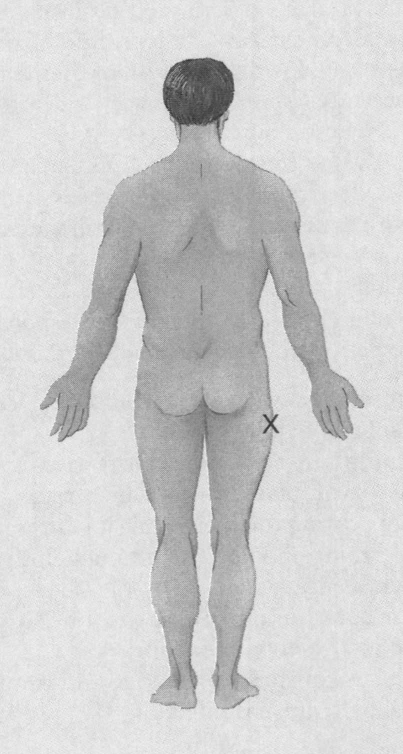

2. **An X anywhere along the highlighted area is the correct answer. This site is the ascending colon, which contains the most liquid stool because it is at the beginning of the large intestine. As stool moves through the large intestine, fluid is reabsorbed and stool becomes more dry and formed.**

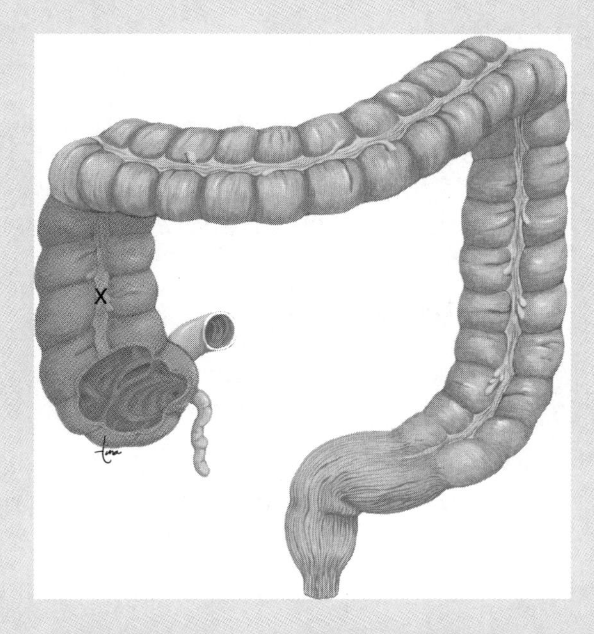

3. **Auscultating over the left upper quadrant slightly to the left of the midsternal line will detect whooshing, gurgling, or bubbling sounds in the stomach, as air is instilled through a nasogastric tube.**

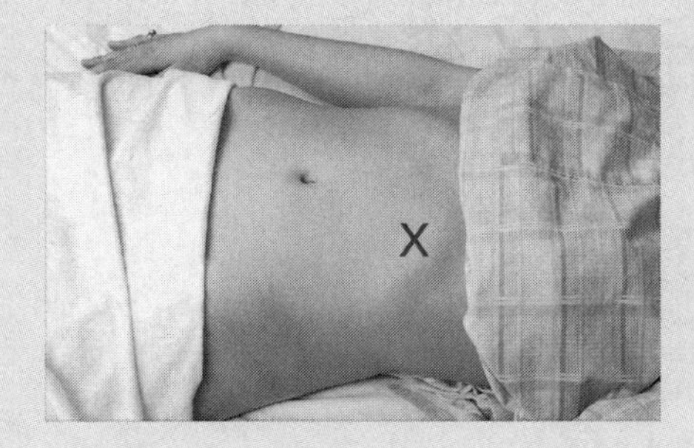

4. **The abdomen even with or below the level of the umbilicus is the preferred site for a Sub-Q injection of 5000 units of heparin. The nurse must avoid the area 2 inches around the umbilicus. The abdomen generally provides a layer of fat located below the dermis and above the muscle for the heparin to be administered deep into the subcutaneous tissue. Also, it allows for faster absorption than subcutaneous sites on the thighs and buttocks. A large area of subcutaneous tissue which is generally found over the abdomen is preferred because if heparin is accidentally administered intramuscularly, it may cause a hematoma and pain.**

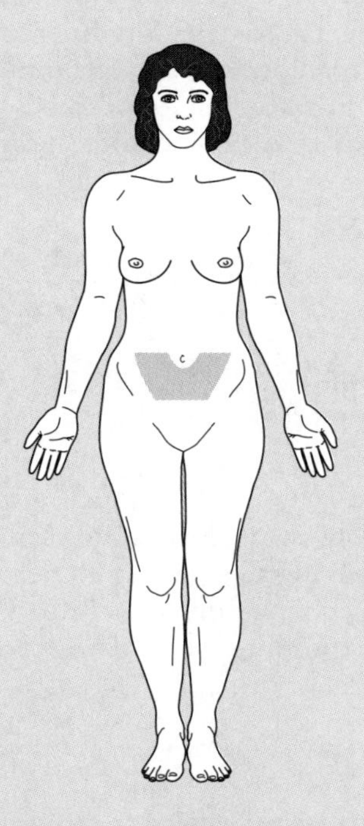

5. **The nurse performing sternal contractions is next to the patient's chest and abdomen. The nurse delivering breaths and monitoring the patient is next to the patient's head. The preferred site to assess the pulse is the carotid artery (either the right or left carotid artery) because the nurse monitoring the patient is next to the patient's head and the carotid arteries are in close proximity to the heart.**

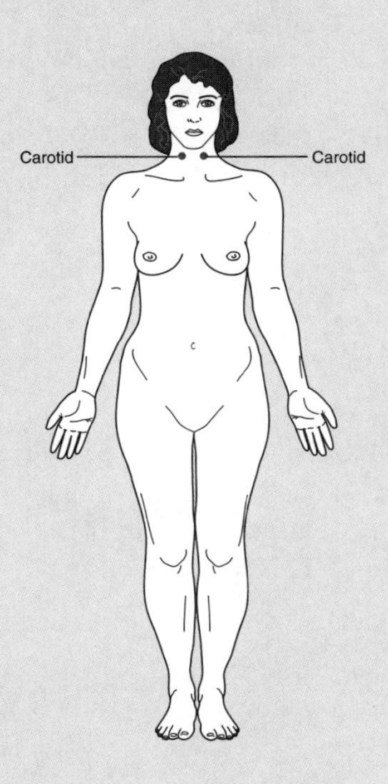

Fill-In-the-Blank Items

1. Answer: 2 mL.

   The nurse has to calculate how many milliliters to administer per minute to deliver 4 mg per minute. Solve for *x* using ratio and proportion after converting 2 grams to its equivalent of 2000 milligrams.

   $$\frac{\text{Desired}}{\text{Have}} \quad \frac{4\ \text{mg}}{2000\ \text{mg}} = \frac{x\ \text{mL}}{1000\ \text{mL}}$$

   $2000x = 4000$
   $x = 4000 \div 2000$
   $x = 2$ mL

   The hourly volume to be infused is calculated by multiplying the milliliters per minute (2) by the number of minutes (60). Therefore, the infusion pump should be set at 120 mL per hour.

2. Answer: 2 mL.
   Solve for x using ratio and proportion.

   $$\frac{\text{Desired}}{\text{Have}} \quad \frac{400{,}000\ \text{mg}}{200{,}000\ \text{mg}} = \frac{x\ \text{mL}}{1\ \text{mL}}$$

   $200{,}000x = 400{,}000$
   $x = 400{,}000 \div 200{,}000$
   $x = 2$ mL of the antibiotic solution

3. Answer: 2 Tablets.
   Solve for x by using ratio and proportion.

   $$\frac{\text{Desired}}{\text{Have}} \quad \frac{0.25\ \text{mg}}{0.125\ \text{mg}} = \frac{x\ \text{Tab}}{1\ \text{Tab}}$$

   $0.125x = 0.25$
   $x = 0.25 \div 0.125$
   $x = 2$ Tablets

4. Answer: 10 mL.
   Solve for x using ratio and proportion.

   $$\frac{\text{Desired}}{\text{Have}} \quad \frac{25\ \text{mg}}{12.5\ \text{mg}} = \frac{x\ \text{mL}}{5\ \text{mL}}$$

   $12.5x = 125$
   $x = 125 \div 12.5$
   $x = 10$ mL

5. Answer: 2.5 mL.
   Use ratio and proportion to convert 110 pounds to kilograms.

   $$\frac{\text{Desire}}{\text{Have}} \quad \frac{110\ \text{pounds}}{2.2\ \text{pounds}} = \frac{x\ \text{kg}}{1\ \text{kg}}$$

   $2.2x = 110$
   $x = 110 \div 2.2$
   $x = 50$ (50 kg is equal to 110 pounds)

   Now calculate the milliliters required using ratio and proportion.

   $$\frac{\text{Desire}}{\text{Have}} \quad \frac{50\ \text{mg}}{1\ \text{kg}} = \frac{x\ \text{units}}{100\ \text{units}}$$

   $1x = 5000$ units

   Now convert the 5000 units to milliliters using ratio and proportion.

   $$\frac{\text{Desire}}{\text{Have}} \quad \frac{5000\ \text{units}}{2000\ \text{units}} = \frac{x\ \text{mL}}{1\ \text{mL}}$$

   $2000x = 5000$
   $x = 5000 \div 2000$
   $x = 2.5$ mL

6. Answer: 7.5 mL.
   Solve the problem by using ratio and proportion.

   $$\frac{\text{Desire}}{\text{Have}} \quad \frac{6\ \text{mg}}{4\ \text{mg}} = \frac{x\ \text{mL}}{5\ \text{mL}}$$

   $4x = 30$ mL
   $x = 30 \div 4$
   $x = 7.5$ mL

7. Answer: 4 Tablets.
   Solve the problem by using ratio and proportion.

   $$\frac{\text{Desire}}{\text{Have}} \quad \frac{5\ \text{mg}}{1.25\ \text{mg}} = \frac{x\ \text{Tab}}{1\ \text{Tab}}$$

   $1.25x = 5$
   $x = 5 \div 1.25$
   $x = 4$ Tablets

8. Answer: 1.5 Tablets.
   Solve the problem by using ratio and proportion.

$$\frac{\text{Desire}}{\text{Have}} \quad \frac{15 \text{ mg}}{10 \text{ mg}} = \frac{x \text{ Tab}}{1 \text{ Tab}}$$

$10x = 15$

$x = 15 \div 10$

$x = 1.5$ Tablets

9. **Answer: 31 drops/minute.**
   Solve the problem by using the following formula.

$$\frac{\text{Total volume to be infused} \times \text{drop factor}}{\text{Total time in minutes}}$$

$$\frac{125 \text{ mL} \times 15 \text{ drops per mL}}{1 \text{ hour} \times 60 \text{ minutes}}$$

$$\frac{1875 \text{ mL}}{60} = 31.25$$

   Since 0.25 is less than half a drop, round the answer down to 31 drops per minute

10. **Answer: 5 Units of Regular insulin.** According to the physician's orders, when the patient's blood glucose level is between 201 and 250 the nurse should administer 5 Units of Regular insulin.

Items Using a Chart, Table, or Graphic Image

1. 1. This temperature occurred on the 6th day of hospitalization (June 10th) at 4 AM.
   2. This temperature occurred on the 4th day of hospitalization (June 8th) at 4 PM.
   3. Find the box in the top left that indicates "Day of Month." Read toward the right across the row until you see the box with the 7 (indicating the 7th day of the month also called the 3rd day in hospital, as indicated in the box below it). Look two rows down below the box with the 7 until you see the box with PM. Now look below the PM box for the box with the 4. Guide your eye down the column until you find a dot on a line. From the dot on the line, guide your eye left across the row until you reach the numbers running along the left end of the graph. The nearest dark line below the row with the dot that indicates a full degree of temperature is 101. The dot in the 4 PM column is one light-colored line above the 101 line indicating 2 tenths of a degree of temperature. Therefore, the dot in the 4 PM column indicates a temperature of 101.2°F.
   4. This temperature occurred on the 2nd day of hospitalization (June 6th) at 4 PM.

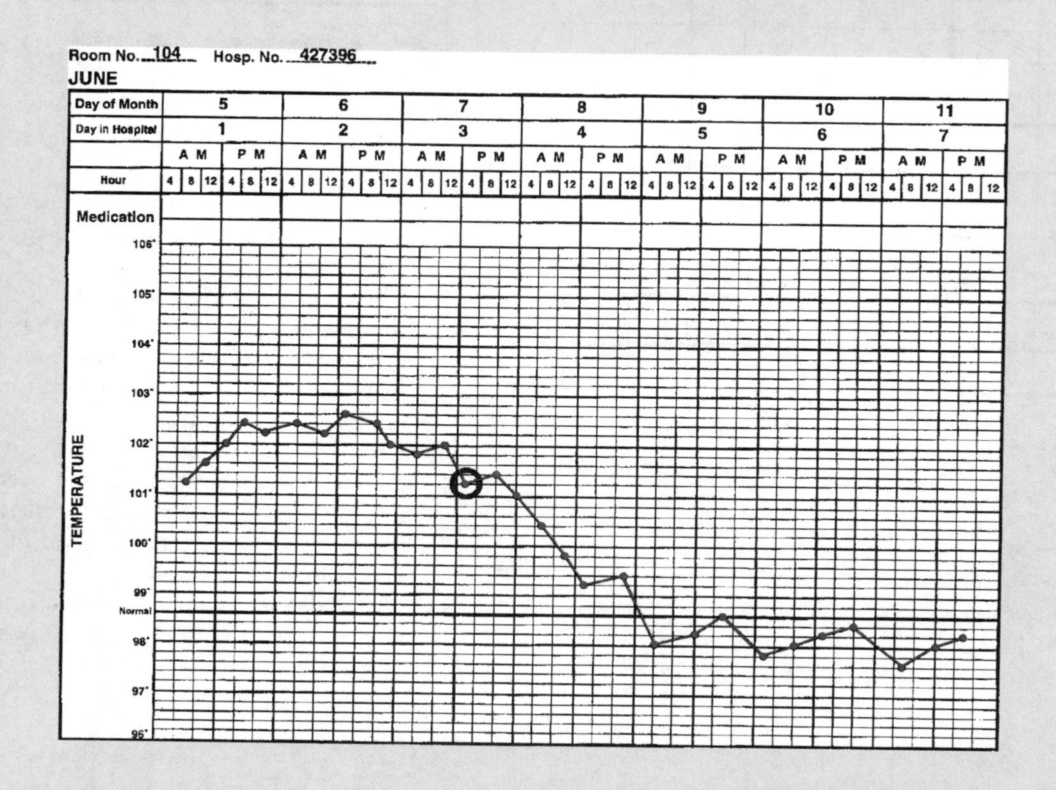

2. 1. This is an incorrect calculation.
   2. This is an incorrect calculation.
   3. This is an incorrect calculation.
   4. **The total ouput between the hours of 7 AM and 3 PM is 1405 mL. The nurse must first calculate the urine, emesis and hemovac totals and insert the amounts in the "7 to 3 Total" row under the appropriate column. Then the nurse must add the totals of the three columns to arrive at the overall total output for the hours between 7 AM and 3 PM.**

DAILY INTAKE AND OUTPUT RECORD

DATE JUNE 5

INTAKE								OUTPUT			
I.V. FLUIDS							ORAL	URINE	EMESIS	N.G. TUBE	HEMOVAC
Time	Bottle	Amount	Solution	Medication and Dosage	* ABS.	‡ LIB					
8	1	1000	NS	20 mEq KCl				650			
8:30							360				
10:00							120				
11:30							240	150			
12:00									160		
1:40									90		60
2:15								250			
3:00					525	475					45
7-3 TOTAL		8-HR TOTAL			525	475	720	1050	250		105
3-11 TOTAL		8-HR TOTAL									
11-7 TOTAL		8-HR TOTAL									
24 HOUR TOTAL											

INTAKE GRAND TOTAL ______ OUTPUT GRAND TOTAL ______

* ABS. = amount absorbed ‡ LIB = Left in bag

3. 1. This is an incorrect calculation.
   2. This is an incorrect calculation.
   3. **The label indicates that the package contains 4 servings and each serving has 90 calories. Multiply 90 calories by 4 servings to arrive at 360 calories.**
   4. This is an incorrect calculation.

Nutrition Facts

Serving Size 1/2 cup (114g)
Servings Per Container 4

Amount Per Serving

Calories 90 Calories from Fat 30

	% Daily Value *
Total Fat 3g	5%
Saturated Fat 0g	0%
Trans Fat 0g	0%
Cholesterol 0mg	0%
Sodium 300mg	13%
Total Carbohydrate 13g	4%
Dietary Fiber 3g	12%
Sugars 3g	
Protein 3g	

Vitamin A 80% • Vitamin C 60%
Calcium 4% • Iron 4%

* Percent Daily Values are based on a 2,000 calorie diet. Your daily values may be higher or lower depending on your calorie needs:

	Calories	2,000	2,500
Total Fat	Less than	65g	80g
Sat Fat	Less than	20g	25g
Cholesterol	Less than	300mg	300mg
Sodium	Less than	2,400mg	2,400mg
Total Carbohydrate		300g	375g
Dietary Fiber		25g	30g

Calories per gram:
Fat 9 • Carbohydrate 4 • Protein 4

4. 1. **Intramuscular injections generally use a 1.5-inch–length needle that is administered at 90 degrees into the muscle tissue and is standard for an IM injection.**
   2. This indicates a medication being administered with a 5/8th-length needle inserted at 90 degrees into the subcutaneous tissue and is considered standard for a subcutaneous injection.
   3. This indicates a medication being administered with 5/8th-length needle inserted at 45 degrees into the subcutaneous tissue and is considered standard for a subcutaneous injection.
   4. This indicates an intradermal injection whereby solution is injected just beneath the skin surface.

5. 1. Inversion is when the foot is turned inward medially.
   2. Adduction is when a body part (e.g., leg, arm) is moved toward the midline.
   3. Supination is when the forearm and hand are turned facing upward.
   4. **Opposition is when the thumb is moved so that it touches the tip of each finger.**

Drop and Drag/Ordered Response Items

1. **Answer: 4, 1, 3, 2**
   4. **The basics of assessment should follow the ABCs–Airway, Breathing, Circulation. Shortness of breath reflects a potential respiratory or cardiac problem and a further assessment is the priority.**
   1. **Relieving pain is a basic physiologic and safety/security need. Relief from pain is not as high a priority as maintaining a patient's respiratory status, but is more important than routine tasks.**
   3. **Administering medications is a dependent function of the nurse. It is accepted practice that medications ordered for 8:00 AM can be dispensed up to 1 hour before or 1 hour after the ordered time.**
   2. **A task ordered twice a day gives the nurse a range in the time frame in which it must be performed. Among the tasks presented, this task can be performed last because the others have greater priority.**

2. **Answer: 3, 2, 4, 1**
   3. **Inspection uses purposeful observation in a systematic manner. It does not require touching the patient; therefore, it will not precipitate a change that will influence future assessments.**
   2. **Auscultation involves listening to sounds produced within the body. It requires the gentle placement of a warmed stethoscope progressively over all four quadrants of the abdomen; it will minimally influence future assessments.**
   4. **Palpation is the use of touch to assess temperature, turgor, texture, dampness, vibration, shape, and presence of fluid. Areas of tenderness are palpated last in the palpation process. Light palpation may cause changes that influence future assessments, but it is less invasive than percussion.**
   1. **Percussion is striking a part of the body with short, sharp blows of the fingers. The sound obtained helps to determine the size, position and density of the underlying body parts. It should be performed last in the assessment process because it is the most disruptive.**

3. **Answer: 1, 5, 2, 3, 4**
   1. **Knowing where fire alarms/extinguishers are located saves time in the event of an actual fire.**
   5. **When identifying a fire in an early stage, it may be extinguished quickly before it becomes a danger to patients.**
   2. **Once the presence of a fire is identified, patients in danger must be rescued before activating the fire alarm.**
   3. **The fire alarm should be activated once patients in the immediate vicinity of the fire are rescued from danger.**
   4. **Once patients in danger are rescued, the fire alarm activated, the nurse should close all doors and windows on the unit to contain the fire.**

4. **Answer: 2, 4, 1, 3**
   2. **Crossing the arms facilitates turning and protects the patient's arms. Crossing the left leg over the right leg uses the patient's weight to facilitate movement.**
   4. **Turning the patient with the hands spread apart and at strategic points of the patient's anatomy permits the body to turn along its vertical axis minimizing strain on the patient's vertebral column.**
   1. **This minimizes pressure on the ball and socket joint and rotator cuff of the shoulder.**
   3. **Pillows under the head and extremities keep them in functional alignment. A pillow behind the back, maintains the patient on the side and keeps the vertebral column in functional alignment.**

5. **Answer: 5, 2, 3, 4. 1**
   5. **Clamping the tubing allows the water to collect in the container.**
   2. **Soapsuds enema for an adult should be 500 to 1000 mL of water at 105°F to 110°F. The volume is sufficient to distend the intestinal lumen, and the temperature is slightly more than body temperature to provide for comfort.**
   3. **This expels air from the tubing, preventing air from entering the intestine.**
   4. **Soap is added after the container is full to prevent the formation of bubbles and after the tubing is flushed to ensure that the soap is diluted in the total volume of**

solution (3 to 5 mL of soap per 1000 mL of water).

1. The catheter is lubricated to limit trauma as the catheter is inserted into the patient's anus and rectum.

Exhibit Item

1. **Answer: 3, Fluid volume excess**

Health History:

Health Problems:
Hypothyroidism
Atherosclerosis
Osteoarthritis
Heart failure

Daily Medications:
acetaminophen
digoxin (Lanoxin)
furosemide (Lasix)
levothyroxine sodium (Synthroid)

Vital Signs on Admission:
Oral Temp: 100.2°F
Pulse: 94/min, irregular
Respirations: 24/min
Blood Pressure: 150/92

Physical Assessment:

Subjective:
Headache
Loss of appetite
Extreme fatigue
Short of breath

Objective:
1+ pitting edema of ankles
Crackles in base of lungs
VS: P 100, R 26, BP 170/96

ANSWER AND RATIONALES:

1. Systemic infection is caused by invasion of a microorganism. Human responses include increased T, P, R, and BP; chills; diaphoresis; malaise; **and** change in mental status.
2. Anaphylactic shock is caused by exposure to an allergen. Human responses include anxiety, tachypnea, throat tightness, stridor, diaphoresis, flushing, **and** urticaria.
3. **Fluid volume excess in this situation is caused by the inefficient pumping action of the heart. A decreased cardiac output results in decreased renal perfusion which stimulates a renin/angiotensin response; this precipitates vasoconstriction and the increased release of aldosterone which causes sodium and fluid retention resulting in a fluid volume excess (FVE). The patient has a history of heart failure and has been receiving digoxin, which slows and strengthens the heart rate and acts as a mild diuretic, and furosemide, which is a loop diuretic. Objective Data: The vital signs have increased, particularly the BP which indicates an increase of fluid in the intravascular compartment and the pulse and respirations, which indicate an attempt to increase the amount of oxygen being delivered to body cells. Pitting edema results because of the movement of excess fluid from the intravascular to the interstitial compartment. Crackles in the lungs indicate pulmonary edema associated with fluid moving from the capillaries in the lung into the alveoli. Subjective Data: These symptoms all support a FVE as the body responds to the excess accumulated fluid.**
4. Orthostatic hypotension is caused by inefficient vasomotor responses in the circulatory system. Patient adaptations include: lightheadedness, vertigo, weakness, and diaphoresis when transferring from a lying down to sitting or sitting to standing position.

2. **Answer: 3, Pressure ulcers**

Physical Assessment:
Height: 5 feet 9 inches tall
Weight: 106 pounds
Right hemiplegia
Muscle flaccidity
Urinary and fecal incontinence
Responsive only to painful stimuli

Health History:

Health Problems:
Atherosclerosis
Iron deficiency anemia
Benign prostatic hyperplasia

Laboratory Tests:
RBC: 3.5 mil/μl
WBC: 9,000 mil/μl
Hb: 10.0 g/dL
Ferritin: 14 ng/mL
Glucose (FBG): 85 mg/dL

ANSWER AND RATIONALES:

1. The patient is unable to control the passage of stool (fecal incontinence) and does not have diarrhea. Diarrhea is the passage of 3 or more liquid or unformed stools a day.
2. No data indicate the presence of hemorrhage. The CVA may be related to the development of a thrombus or embolus associated with the history of atherosclerosis and TIAs.
3. **The patient is anemic. Older males should have: RBC of 3.7 to 6.0 µl; Hb of 11.0 to 17.0 g/dL; and serum ferritin of 18 to 270 ng/mL. The patient is underweight and has less subcutaneous fat because of aging. Urine and feces are irritating to the skin because of their acidity and enzyme content, respectively. The presence of inadequate nutrition, the inability to move the right side of the body, the potential presence of urine and feces on the skin, and the characteristics of skin in the aged all create a risk for pressure ulcers.**
4. The patient's blood glucose is within the acceptable range for an older adult (70 to 120 mg/dL).

3. Answer: 1, Pulmonary embolus

Vital Signs:

10 AM–P 72, R 16, BP 120/72
10:15 AM–P 74, R 18, BP 122/70
10:30 AM–P 70, R 20, BP 118/74
10:45 AM–P 74, R 18, BP 120/68

Physical Assessment:

Dyspnea
Pale skin
Coughing
Diaphoresis
Right-sided chest pain
Abdomen flat and nontender
Abdominal dressing dry and intact
Decreased breath sounds on right side
VS: P 92; R 28; shallow, labored; BP 160/92
ECG: Normal sinus rhythm

ANSWER AND RATIONALES:

1. **When an embolus obstructs an artery in the lung it interrupts gas exchange at the cellular level. This precipitates unilateral chest pain, coughing, and respirations that become rapid, shallow, and labored (dyspnea). Decreased breath sounds occur over the affected alveoli as a result of the lack of gas exchange. All the vital signs increase, and pallor and diaphoresis occur as a result of the release of epinephrine.**
2. The patient is not experiencing a myocardial infarction. The ECG is not displaying a problem, and the chest pain usually is on the left thorax, under the sternum, and/or radiating to the jaw or left arm.
3. The patient is not experiencing hemorrhage. The dressing is dry and intact, and the abdomen is flat and nontender. Also, the blood pressure increased rather than decreased. If the patient were hemorrhaging, the blood pressure would decrease as a result of hypovolemia.
4. The patient is not experiencing subcutaneous emphysema. Subcutaneous emphysema is the presence of air in the subcutaneous tissue; this may occur with an open pneumothorax or around the side of a thoracotomy tube.

4. Answer: 1, Pain

Vital Signs:

4:00 PM–P 76, R 18, BP 116/72
6:00 PM–P 80, R 20, BP 120/76

I&O: 8:00 AM–8 PM

Intake: IVF–1500 mL
Output: Urine–1050 mL
Wound drainage systems–210 mL

Physical Assessment at 8 PM:

Dressing dry and intact
No suprapubic distention
Pain of 8 on a scale of 1 to 10, IVF intact and infusing at 125 mL/hr
Retention catheter draining clear amber urine
Vital Signs: P 86, R 24, BP 136/80

ANSWER AND RATIONALES:

1. **The patient is in pain as evidenced by a rating of 8 on a pain scale of 1 to 10. The increase in the pulse,**

respirations, and blood pressure reflects the response to the stress-related catecholamines.

2. The patient is not hemorrhaging. If the patient were hemorrhaging, the blood pressure should have decreased not increased, the portable wound drainage systems would contain more than 210 mL output, and the dressing may have evidence of blood.
3. The patient is not experiencing urinary retention. The urinary retention catheter is draining clear amber urine, the suprapubic area is not distended, and the I&O is approximately equal, taking into consideration the fluid lost during surgery.
4. If the patient were experiencing excess fluid volume, the blood pressure would be much higher and the fluid intake would exceed the output on the I&O record.

5. **Answer: 2, Aspiration**

Health History:
76 yrs old
5 feet 10 inches tall
Weighs 175 pounds
Parkinson's disease for 5 years
Benign prostatic hyperplasia for 10 years
Flu and pneumonia vaccines in last 6 mo
carbidopa-levodopa (Sinemet) daily

Vital Signs:
Oral temperature: 99.6°F
Pulse: 88, regular rhythm
Respirations: 22, shallow
Blood pressure: 109/68

Physical Assessment:
Lethargic
Dysphagia
Dysarthria
Abdomen is soft
Diminished gag reflex
Upper and lower dentures
Skin dry, exhibiting "tenting"
Urinated 500 mL of clear yellow urine
Borborygmi auscultated in all 4 quadrants

ANSWER AND RATIONALES:

1. Although older adults have a diminished immune system, the patient is not at high risk for an infection because of medical aseptic practices in the hospital and the fact that the patient has received appropriate immunizations.
2. **The patient is exhibiting imperfect articulation of speech (dysarthria), difficulty swallowing (dysphagia), a diminished gag reflex, and lethargy. These adaptations place the patient at high risk for aspiration. Airway is the priority as per the ABCs (Airway, Breathing, Circulation) of patient assessment.**
3. The patient's weight is appropriate for his height. With a mechanical soft diet and supervision during meals, the patient should ingest adequate nutrients to prevent malnutrition.
4. Although constipation may occur in the patient because of lethargy and decreased peristalsis associated with aging, this is not the priority. The patient has borborygmi in all 4 quadrants of the abdomen indicating the presence of intestinal peristalsis. Also, if constipation occurs, it can be diminished with stool softeners.

COMPREHENSIVE FINAL BOOK EXAM

QUESTIONS

1. A patient has a diagnosis of osteoporosis. The nurse should encourage this patient to eat:
   1. Rice
   2. Celery
   3. Sardines
   4. Tomatoes

2. Which early adaptation indicates to the nurse that the patient is experiencing hypoxia?
   1. Increased heart rate
   2. Difficulty breathing
   3. Bradypnea
   4. Pallor

3. A patient has a history of chronic pain because of arthritis, but dislikes taking large doses of analgesics. The nurse understands a concept unique to unrelieved chronic pain is that it:
   1. Generally is better tolerated as the duration of exposure increases
   2. Minimally interferes with activities of daily living
   3. Usually is related to current pathology
   4. Rarely affects the immune response

4. The nurse is assessing several patients who had surgery the previous day. Which sudden patient adaptation should the nurse identify as a life-threatening event?
   1. Slightly elevated temperature
   2. Wound dehiscence
   3. Edema of the legs
   4. Chest pain

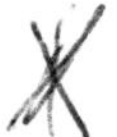

5. The nursing diagnosis of Perceived Constipation is made when the patient states that a bowel movement is expected every day and:
   1. Inspection of the abdomen reveals distention
   2. Hard, dry stools are defecated daily
   3. Laxatives are used excessively
   4. Straining is required

6. The nurse must administer a sedative to a patient before surgery. What should the nurse do first?
   1. Verify that the preoperative checklist is completed
   2. Check that the surgical consent is signed
   3. Ensure an intravenous line is in place
   4. Assess the vital signs

7. The physician orders 500 mg of an antibiotic to be administered IVPB every 6 hours for a patient with a systemic infection. The vial dispensed by the hospital pharmacist contains 1 gram of the prescribed antibiotic in powder form. The instructions on the vial state: Instill 9.6 mL to yield 10 mL. How many milliliters of the antibiotic should the nurse add to the IVPB bag?
   Answer: ____________ mL.

8. Which mechanism is designed to facilitate tracking a patient's progress as a cost containment strategy in managed care?
   1. Primary nursing
   2. Critical pathways
   3. Functional method
   4. Quality management

9. The nurse is assisting a patient who has cognitive deficits with a bed bath. It is most important for the nurse to:
   1. Check the patient every five minutes
   2. Encourage attention to each task of bathing
   3. Arrange the basin within the center of the patient's visual field
   4. Explain in detail everything that will be done during the bath before beginning

10. When interviewing the wife of a patient, which statement about her husband supports the presence of sleep apnea?
   1. "He falls asleep sometimes when he drives, so now I do all the driving."
   2. "He kicks and thrashes so much that the bed linen is upside down by morning."
   3. "He has nightmares that are so scary that he wakes me up because he is afraid."
   4. "He snores and gasps all night long, wakes me up, and then I can't get back to sleep."

11. The physician orders a clear liquid diet for a patient who had abdominal surgery three days ago. The nurse understands that a clear liquid diet is ordered for a patient who had abdominal surgery primarily because it:
   1. Relieves abdominal distention
   2. Stimulates digestive enzymes
   3. Prevents postoperative ileus
   4. Is easily digested

12. The nurse is caring for a patient with prolonged diarrhea. The nurse should assess the patient for signs and symptoms of the common problem of:
   1. Skin breakdown
   2. Deficient self-care
   3. Sexual dysfunction
   4. Disturbed body image

13. The nurse causes harm to a hospitalized patient because of improper use of medical equipment. This is most specifically called:
   1. Battery
   2. Assault
   3. Negligence
   4. Malpractice

14. A patient with a history of diabetes mellitus is experiencing blurred vision, generalized weakness, and fatigue. After receiving a report from the nurse on the previous shift and obtaining additional information from the medical record, the nurse comes to the conclusion that the patient is experiencing which emergency?
   1. Brain attack
   2. Kidney failure
   3. Hypertensive episode
   4. Hyperglycemic event

CHART/EXHIBIT

Laboratory Results: BUN: 18 mg/dL
Creatinine: 1.2 mg/dL
Hemoglobin A_{1c} : 8.0%
Serum glucose: 350 mg/dL

I&O Record (last 24 hours): Intake: 2400 mL
Output: 4200 mL

Nursing Progress Note: 10 AM–patient complains of being thirsty and "urinating a lot," and has lost 20 pounds over the last two months; has poor skin turgor and dry mucous membranes.

15. A group of nurses on a unit are personally and professionally mature and motivated. Which leadership style should the nurse manager employ when working with this group?
1. Directive
2. Autocratic
3. Democratic
4. Laissez-faire

16. The nurse transfers a patient from a bed to a wheelchair. After placing the patient in the wheelchair, the next most important nursing action is to:
1. Ensure the patient's popliteal areas are not touching the seat edge
2. Attach the patient's transfer belt to clips on the wheelchair
3. Support the patient's back with a pillow
4. Put the patient's feet flat on the floor

17. The statement that supports why a nurse must be aware of the patient's perception of health is that the nurse can:
1. Identify the patient's needs based on Maslow's Hierarchy of Basic Human Needs
2. Provide more meaningful assistance to help the patient regain a state of health
3. Help the patient prevent the occurrence of human responses to disease
4. Choose a place for the patient along the Health-Illness Continuum

18. An older adult asks the nurse, "Now that I am getting older I want to make sure I get enough vitamin A to keep my eyes healthy. What food can I eat?" The nurse should respond, "An excellent source of vitamin A is:
1. Grapefruits."
2. Tangerines."
3. Apricots."
4. Bananas."

19. The most important concept that nurses must understand to make accurate assessments is that nonverbal behavior:
1. Is controlled by the conscious mind
2. Carries less weight than what the patient says
3. Does not have the same meaning for everyone
4. Is generally a poor reflection of what the patient is feeling

20. To identify the left dorsogluteal site for an intramuscular injection, the nurse should:
1. Locate the lower edge of the acromion and the midpoint of the lateral aspect of the arm
2. Identify the line from the posterior superior iliac spine to the greater trochanter
3. Place the heel of the left hand on the greater trochanter
4. Palpate the anterior lateral aspect of the thigh

21. Which level need in Maslow's Hierarchy of Needs is supported when the nurse places the patient's get-well cards where the patient can see them?
1. Love and belonging
2. Safety and security
3. Self-esteem
4. Physiologic

22. The nurse must obtain a urine specimen from a patient with a urinary retention catheter (Foley). What should the nurse do first?
1. Cleanse the exit tube at the bottom of the drainage bag with an alcohol swab
2. Clamp the tubing immediately distal to the collection port
3. Position the patient in a semi-Fowler's position
4. Don a pair of clean gloves

23. Which nursing action is most appropriate in relation to the concept, "Bacteria and enzymes in stool are irritating to the skin?"
1. Wearing a pair of sterile gloves when collecting a patient's stool for culture and sensitivity
2. Applying a moisture barrier to the perianal area of incontinent patients
3. Encouraging a patient to drink eight ounces of cranberry juice daily
4. Toileting a confused patient before each meal

24. The nurse decides to give a partial bath instead of a complete bath. When the nurse made this decision, the nurse was working:
1. Dependently
2. Independently
3. Collaboratively
4. Interdependently

25. The physician orders a 2-gram sodium diet for a patient. The nurse should teach this patient to avoid:
1. Kool-Aid
2. Club soda
3. Lemonade
4. Diet root beer

26. After a patient recovers from general anesthesia, the nurse should monitor for the most serious complication of intubation, which is:
1. Stomatitis
2. Atelectasis
3. Sore throat
4. Laryngeal spasm

27. A patient in pain tells the nurse, "It feels like something is on fire." Which characteristic of pain is associated with this statement?
1. Location
2. Intensity
3. Quality
4. Pattern

28. The nurse places a patient who had abdominal surgery in the semi-Fowler's position. This is done primarily to:
1. Support ventilation
2. Facilitate the passing of flatus
3. Encourage urinary elimination
4. Promote drainage in the portable wound drainage system

29. The nurse is teaching a group of nursing assistants about the administration of enemas. The nurse should teach that the enema solution that works by irritating the intestinal mucosa is:
1. Oil
2. Soap
3. Tap water
4. Normal saline

30. The nurse is administering oral medications to several patients. It is important that the nurse understands that oral medications are absorbed more quickly when they are given:
1. With water
2. In the morning
3. On an empty stomach
4. When the patient is resting

31. The nurse in the Post-Anesthesia Care Unit must meet the needs of patients in pain. The nurse identifies that the age group that is most sensitive to pain is:
1. Infants
2. Adolescents
3. Older adults
4. Pregnant women

32. When caring for a patient who is practicing Orthodox Judaism, the nurse must remember that:
1. Coffee and tea are restricted during Passover
2. Dairy products and eggs are forbidden after sundown on Fridays
3. Dairy foods should not be ingested at the same meal as meats and meat products
4. Shellfish is permitted but must be prepared according to biblical religious rituals

33. A newly admitted patient is exhibiting anxiety associated with being hospitalized. To help reduce the anxiety, it is most important that the nurse:
1. Teach relaxation techniques
2. Validate the anxious feelings
3. Minimize environmental stimuli
4. Explain procedures to the patient

34. The physician orders a vaginal suppository. When administering this medication, the nurse should:
1. Irrigate the vagina with normal saline before inserting the suppository
2. Place the patient in the left-lateral position for the procedure
3. Advance the suppository along the posterior vaginal wall
4. Insert the suppository while wearing sterile gloves

35. The home health-care nurse is helping a patient negotiate the health-care system within the community. Which word best reflects this role of the nurse?
1. Leader
2. Resource
3. Surrogate
4. Counselor

36. The nurse evaluates that teaching about the care of dry skin is effective when the older adult says, "I should:
1. Bathe daily with a moisturizing soap."
2. Wear clothes made of woolen fabrics."
3. Increase the amount of water that I drink."
4. Use baby powder rather than lotion on my skin."

37. The nurse understands that the word that best describes the concept of adaptive capacity is:
1. Treatment
2. Flexible
3. Threat
4. Illness

38. The action taken by the nurse that can limit edema and bleeding through vasoconstriction at the site of pain, thereby reducing pain, is:
1. Applying a cold compress
2. Exerting direct pressure
3. Performing effleurage
4. Providing massage

39. Which adaptation identified by the nurse is the priority for a patient in the Post-Anesthesia Care Unit?
   1. Pain
   2. Nausea
   3. Reduced level of consciousness
   4. Excessive loss of fluid through indwelling drains

40. When the vent of a double-lumen gastric sump tube becomes obstructed, the nurse should first:
   1. Instill 10 mL of air into the vent lumen
   2. Place the patient in the high-Fowler's position
   3. Position the vent below the level of the stomach
   4. Withdraw 30 mL of gastric contents from the drainage lumen

41. The nurse is required to complete an incident report when a:
   1. Nurse left work early without reporting to the supervisor
   2. Patient did not receive a medication ordered by the physician
   3. Visitor ambulated a patient who should have been on bed rest
   4. Patient refused to go to physical therapy as ordered by the physician

42. A patient who has a transdermal analgesic patch for cancer experiences breakthrough pain with activity. The nurse should:
   1. Administer an ordered shorter-acting opiate
   2. Encourage the avoidance of moving around
   3. Obtain an order for an antianxiety medication
   4. Suggest to the physician that the long-acting opiate be increased

43. The nurse must perform a procedure and is unsure of the exact steps of the procedure. What should the nurse do first?
   1. Call the staff education department for educational assistance
   2. Refer to a fundamentals of nursing skills textbook
   3. Check the nursing policy and procedure manual
   4. Refuse to do the nursing procedure

44. The nurse is caring for a patient with a pressure ulcer. The nurse identifies the pressure ulcer as which type of stressor?
   1. Microbiological
   2. Developmental
   3. Physiological
   4. Physical

45. The nurse assesses a patient and concludes that the patient is cachectic. The nurse understands that this patient is at the highest risk for which skin integrity problem?
   1. Altered tissue perfusion
   2. Perineal excoriation
   3. Reduced sensation
   4. Pressure ulcers

46. The patient appears agitated and states, "I'm not sure that I want to go through with this surgery." Which response by the nurse uses the technique of paraphrasing?
   1. "Are you saying that you want to postpone the surgery?"
   2. "You are undecided about having this surgery?"
   3. "You seem upset about this surgery."
   4. "Tell me more about your concerns."

47. The nurse is planning to apply a transdermal patch to a patient. The nurse should:
   1. Use the same area each time to limit skin irritation and excoriation
   2. Rub the area to promote comfort and vasodilation before applying the patch
   3. Shave the area to facilitate adherence of the patch and medication absorption
   4. Remove the old patch 1 hour after applying the new patch to ensure a therapeutic blood level of the drug

48. The nurse in charge is delegating assignments to other members of the nursing team. Which actions should be implemented only by a Registered Nurse? Check all that apply.
1. ______Taking the pulse of a patient with a dysrhythmia
2. ______Teaching a patient how to change a colostomy bag
3. ______Applying a condom catheter on a patient who is incontinent
4. ______Changing the linen on an occupied bed for a comatose patient
5. ______Transferring a patient from a bed to a chair with a mechanical lift

49. The nurse routinely administers digoxin 0.125 mg p.o. to a patient every morning. Before administering the digoxin, which patient adaptation should alert the nurse to withhold the drug?
1. Diplopia
2. Tachypnea
3. Hypertension
4. Hyperthermia

50. A patient receiving an intermittent tube feeding develops diarrhea. The nurse understands that the primary cause of diarrhea in a patient receiving a tube feeding is:
1. A high osmolarity of the feeding
2. An inadequate volume of the feeding
3. Failure to test for a residual before the feeding
4. Lying in the high-Fowler's position during the feeding

51. While in a restaurant, a pregnant woman is exhibiting a total airway obstruction because of a bolus of food. The nurse should modify the abdominal thrust (Heimlich) maneuver by performing the thrusts:
1. While the person is in the supine, rather than standing, position
2. With the fist of the pinkie finger, rather than the thumb, against the person's body
3. Against the middle of the sternum, rather than between the umbilicus and xiphoid process
4. After the person becomes unconscious and discontinuing the thrusts after six tries, if unsuccessful

52. Of the factors presented, the nurse identifies that the one that most commonly interferes with the sleep of people who are hospitalized is:
1. Napping during the day
2. Disrupted bedtime rituals
3. Medication administration
4. Difficulty finding a comfortable position

53. The nurse should teach a person who is a vegan that a food combination that is a substitute for a complete protein is:
1. Yogurt and fruit
2. Bread and cheese
3. Legumes and rice
4. Peanut butter and jelly

54. When the nurse cares for an older adult, the nurse understands that drug toxicity is a concern primarily because of a decrease in:
1. Serum calcium
2. Glomerular filtration
3. Red blood cell count
4. Frequency of voiding

55. The nurse instills medicated drops into the ear of an adult. The nurse should:
1. Pull the pinna of the ear backward and downward
2. Insert the drops into the center of the auditory canal
3. Press the tragus of the ear several times after insertion
4. Roll the patient from the side-lying to the supine position

56. The nurse identifies that an adult patient on a psychiatric unit is exhibiting antisocial behavior. According to Erikson, the negative resolution of which stage of development is most commonly associated with antisocial behavior?
    1. Preschool age
    2. Adolescence
    3. School age
    4. Infancy

57. The nurse must obtain a blood pressure from an average-sized adult male. Which nursing technique will result in an accurate blood pressure measurement?
    1. Wrapping the lower edge of the cuff over the antecubital space
    2. Positioning the sphygmomanometer above the level of the heart
    3. Pumping the cuff about 60 mm Hg above the point where the brachial pulse is lost
    4. Releasing the valve on the cuff so that the pressure decreases at the rate of 2 to 3 mm Hg per second

58. The nurse is providing oral care to an unconscious patient. It is best for the nurse to use:
    1. Gauze-wrapped tongue blades with a saline solution
    2. A small amount of nonfoaming toothpaste
    3. Half-strength mouthwash and saline
    4. Packaged glycerin swabs

59. A patient is admitted to the hospital with a medical diagnosis of diverticulitis. What is the best question the nurse should ask when obtaining an admission history from this patient?
    1. "Have you ever had any previous episodes of diverticulitis?"
    2. "What led up to your coming to the hospital today?"
    3. "How long have you had diverticulitis?"
    4. "What did you eat yesterday?"

60. The physician orders peak and trough levels for a patient receiving an antibiotic. What time should the nurse obtain a blood sample to determine a trough level when the antibiotic was administered at 12:00 noon?
    1. 11:00 AM
    2. 11:30 AM
    3. 12:30 PM
    4. 1:00 PM

61. The nurse is planning care for a patient in the spiritual realm. Which age group generally is more involved with expanding and refining spiritual beliefs?
    1. Adolescents
    2. Older adults
    3. Young adults
    4. Middle-aged adults

62. Which nursing action is specifically related to the principle, *the greater the base of support, the more stable the body*?
    1. Using a walker when ambulating
    2. Locking the wheels of a wheelchair
    3. Holding objects close to the body when walking
    4. Keeping the back straight when lifting an object

63. The most effective nursing intervention to promote sleep that is appropriate for patients in any age group is:
    1. Providing a back rub
    2. Playing relaxing music
    3. Offering a glass of warm milk
    4. Following a routine at bedtime

64. When a patient arrives on the unit from the Emergency Department, the nurse reviews the physician's history and physical and the integrated progress notes. The notes indicate that assessment revealed borborygmi. When admitting the patient to the unit, the nurse performs a nursing assesment. Indicate on the figure of the body where the nurse should place the stethoscope to assess for the presence of borborygmi?

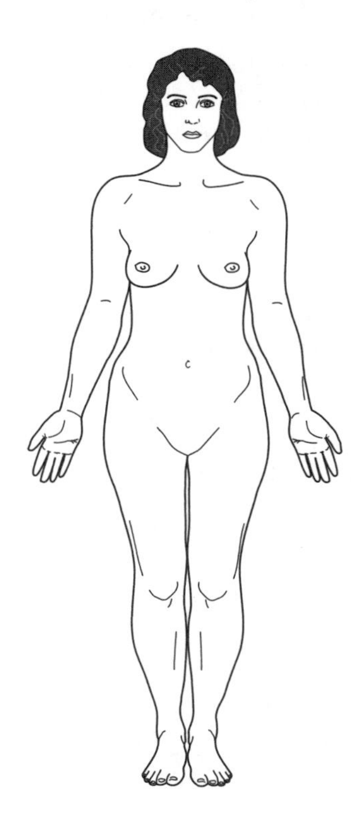

65. Which is the most important nursing intervention to help prevent falls from physical hazards in a hospital?
   1. Using an over-bed table
   2. Ensuring adequate lighting
   3. Storing belongings in a safe place
   4. Positioning the telephone within easy reach

66. Nurses understand that a potential problem associated with the supine position is:
   1. Flexion of the knees
   2. Pressure on the heels
   3. Pressure on the trochanters
   4. Internal rotation of the hips

67. A patient is using the call bell numerous times an hour and requesting assistance with activities that the patient is capable of achieving independently. To best help this patient the nurse should:
   1. Set limits verbally
   2. Alternate care with another nurse
   3. Point out the behavior to the patient
   4. Attempt to see the situation from the patient's perspective

68. The nurse going off duty is making rounds with the nurse coming on duty and provides a report on each patient in the district. Which data given by the nurse is most meaningful?
   1. The patient was given ondansetron eight mg and now has no complaints of nausea
   2. The patient's family members just visited and the patient appears happy
   3. The patient seems less anxious than earlier in the day
   4. The patient's blood pressure is now stable

69. The nurse is bathing a patient. Which nursing action best supports a principle associated with asepsis?
 1. Wearing sterile gloves when washing the perineum
 2. Having the patient void before beginning the bed bath
 3. Replacing the top covers with a clean flannel bath blanket
 4. Washing from the inner canthus to the outer canthus of the eye

70. Health teaching regarding fires in the home should include information about what to do if grease in a frying pan catches on fire. Health educators should teach people to call 911 and then attempt to contain the fire by:
 1. Pouring water in the pan
 2. Putting the lid on the pan
 3. Closing the door to the kitchen
 4. Using a Class A fire extinguisher

71. A patient who self-administers an aerosol medication by a metered-dose inhaler complains of "the nasty taste of the medication." The nurse should encourage the patient to:
 1. Suck on a hard candy after the procedure
 2. Shake the cartridge longer before using it
 3. Perform oral hygiene before inhalation of medication
 4. Attach an aerosol chamber to the metered-dose cartridge

72. The most important purpose of the orientation phase of the assessment interview is to:
 1. Collect data
 2. Build rapport
 3. Identify problems
 4. Establish priorities

73. A patient has a temperature of 102°F and complains of feeling cold. Which additional adaptation should the nurse expect during this onset stage of fever?
 1. Shivering
 2. Diaphoresis
 3. Dehydration
 4. Flushed skin

74. The nurse identifies that the patient who should benefit the most from soaking the feet as part of a bath is the patient who:
 1. Has a preference for taking showers
 2. Is ambulating with paper slippers
 3. Has peripheral vascular disease
 4. Is on bed rest

75. The nurse is assessing the skin of an older adult. Which adaptation is of the greatest concern?
 1. Flat, brown-colored spots on the skin
 2. Thin, translucent skin
 3. Tenting of the skin
 4. Dry, flaky skin

76. The nurse observes a patient using an incentive spirometer. The nurse evaluates that further teaching is necessary when the patient:
 1. Inhales slowly and deeply using the spirometer
 2. Tilts the incentive spirometer while breathing in
 3. Raises the inspiratory goal on the spirometer once a day
 4. Takes several regular breaths and then uses the spirometer again

77. The nurse is providing a back massage for a patient before bedtime. The nurse should:
 1. Use continuous light gliding strokes with fingertips when finishing
 2. Concentrate deep circular motions over the scapulae and sacrum
 3. Knead firmly and quickly over the shoulders and the entire back
 4. Massage gently over the bony prominences of the vertebrae

78. The nurse on a postpartum unit is teaching a class for new mothers about umbilical cord care. The nurse identifies that one mother does not become involved with the discussion and is withdrawn. After the class, the best intervention by the nurse is to:
1. Give the patient written material about cord care
2. Invite the patient to the next class about cord care
3. Bring an audiovisual cassette into the patient's room
4. Provide informal individual instruction for the patient

79. The nurse is assisting a patient with dysphagia to eat. The nurse should encourage the patient to:
1. Tilt the head backward when swallowing
2. Drink fluids when eating bites of solid food
3. Reduce environmental stimuli to a minimum
4. Keep food in the front of the mouth when chewing

80. A patient consistently eats only 25% of every meal. What should the nurse do to encourage the dietary intake of this patient?
1. Persuade the patient to drink between-meal supplements twice daily
2. Encourage the patient to engage in light exercise before meals
3. Teach the patient to avoid fluids and foods that cause flatus
4. Help the patient to select preferred foods

81. The nurse wants to influence a patient's beliefs so that new behaviors can be incorporated into the patient's lifestyle. Within which learning domain does the nurse need to direct teaching?
1. Affective
2. Cognitive
3. Physiologic
4. Psychomotor

82. The nurse is teaching a family member how to perform range-of-motion exercises of the hand. Which motion occurs when the angle is reduced between the palm of the hand and forearm?
1. Hyperextension
2. Opposition
3. Abduction
4. Flexion

83. A patient with terminal cancer says to the nurse, "I've been fairly religious, but sometimes I wonder if the things I did were acceptable to God." The nurse's best response is:
1. "Not knowing what the future brings can be a frightening thought."
2. "God will appreciate that you went to religious services."
3. "If you were good, you have nothing to fear."
4. "In life, all we have to do is try to be good."

84. The nurse is administering a lozenge to a patient's buccal area of the mouth. What should the nurse do?
1. Ensure the medication is dissolved under the tongue
2. Instruct the patient to take occasional sips of water
3. Administer the lozenge one hour before meals
4. Alternate the cheeks from one dose to another

85. Which question by the nurse best assesses a patient's pain tolerance?
1. "At what point on a scale of 1 to 10 do you feel that you must have pain medication?"
2. "What activities help distract you so that you don't feel the need for medication?"
3. "How intense on a scale of 1 to 10 is the pain that you feel right now?"
4. "Do you take pain medication frequently?"

86. The nurse advises an obese patient to lose weight. The patient asks the nurse, "What should I do to help myself lose weight?" Considering the best behavior modification strategy for controlling food intake, the nurse should respond:
1. "Ask family members not to bring tempting food into the house."
2. "Post piggy pictures on the refrigerator."
3. "Avoid snacks between meals."
4. "Maintain a daily food diary."

87. The nurse understands that the most important concept related to the stages of growth and development is that:
1. Individuals experience growth and development at their own pace
2. Each task must be achieved before moving on to the next task
3. Family members provide safe and supportive environments
4. Once a task is achieved regression is minimal

88. The physician orders the insertion of an indwelling urinary catheter (retention, Foley). As part of the patient's preoperative orders. Place these steps of the procedure in the order in which they should be performed by the nurse.
1. ______ Don sterile gloves
2. ______ Open catheterization package
3. ______ Inflate and deflate catheter balloon
4. ______ Place a fenestrated drape over the patient's perineal area
5. ______ Maintain spread of labia while swiping directly over the urinary meatus
6. ______ Maintain spread of labia while swiping each labium with a separate cotton ball

89. The physician orders a vest restraint for a patient in a wheelchair. To prevent the most serious complication associated with the use of a vest restraint, the nurse should:
1. Remove the vest every 2 hours for range of motion
2. Ensure the V opening is positioned in the front
3. Check the circulation every 30 minutes
4. Inspect the skin every 2 hours

90. A patient is admitted to the Emergency Department after sustaining a crushing injury at work. Which characteristic of blood pressure should alert the nurse to impending shock?
1. Rising diastolic
2. Decreasing systolic
3. Korotkoff's sounds
4. Widening pulse pressure

91. The physician orders antiembolism hose for a patient. Which is the most important action the nurse should teach the patient?
1. Monitor the heels and toes for blanchable erythema every eight hours
2. Put them on after the legs have been dependent for several minutes
3. Apply body lotion before putting them on
4. Remove and reapply them once a day

92. The nurse understands that the main effect of Diagnostic Related Groups (DRGs) on the health-care system is:
1. Increased quality of medical care
2. Increased reliability of research statistics
3. Decreased acuity of hospitalized patients
4. Decreased length of an average hospital stay

93. The physician orders 1 gram of an antibiotic to be administered via the intramuscular route b.i.d. Which nursing action reflects the planning step of the nursing process?
1. Identifying body landmarks before giving the injection
2. Sending a copy of the written order to the hospital pharmacy
3. Determining that the medication should be given at 8:00 AM and 8:00 PM
4. Verifying the patient's allergies in the chart and on the patient's allergy band

94. A male patient is told by his physician that he has metastatic lung cancer and he is seriously ill. After the physician leaves the room, the patient has a severe episode of coughing and shortness of breath and says, "This is just a cold, I'll be fine once I get over it." The nurse's best response is:
1. "The doctor talked to you about having a serious illness."
2. "The doctor had some bad news for you today."
3. "Tell me more about your illness."
4. "This is not a cold, it's lung cancer."

95. The nurse is giving a patient a bed bath. To increase circulation, the nurse should:
1. Wash the extremities with firm strokes toward the heart
2. Soak the feet in warm water for at least 20 minutes
3. Expose just the areas that are being washed
4. Ensure that the water is 120°F to 125°F

96. The nurse is predicting the success of a teaching program regarding the learning of a skill. Which factor is most relevant?
1. Cognitive ability of the learner
2. Amount of reinforcement
3. Extent of family support
4. Interest of the learner

97. The nurse is assisting a female patient with care of the hair. It is most important that the nurse:
1. Ensure that the patient's hair is left dry, not wet
2. Ask the patient what should be done with her hair
3. Comb the patient's hair from the proximal to distal end of the hair shaft
4. Avoid tangles in the patient's hair by using rubbing alcohol as a conditioner

98. A patient who is secretly smoking in bed falls asleep and the cigarette ignites the patient's gown. When the nurse discovers the fire, the nurse should first:
1. Close the door
2. Activate the fire alarm
3. Roll the patient from side to side
4. Smother the flames with a blanket

99. The nurse discovers that a patient is taking natural herbal remedies. It is most important that the nurse:
1. Learn about the supplements
2. Think of the supplements as drugs
3. Communicate the supplement use to the physician
4. Include the details about supplement use in the health history

100. A patient sustained a brain injury resulting in neurological deficits after falling off a ladder at work. Which setting is most appropriate for assisting this patient to learn how to live with neurological limitations?
1. Hospice program
2. Acute care setting
3. Extended-care facility
4. Assisted-living residence

COMPREHENSIVE FINAL BOOK EXAM ANSWERS AND RATIONALES

1. 1. Rice, regardless of the type, is not high in calcium. One cup of rice contains approximately 5 to 33 mg of calcium.
   2. Celery is not high in calcium. One stalk of celery contains approximately 15 mg of calcium.
   3. **Sardines are an excellent source of dietary calcium. Three ounces of sardines contains approximately 371 mg of calcium.**
   4. Tomatoes are not high in calcium. One tomato (2¾ inches in diameter) contains approximately 9 mg of calcium.

2. 1. **Hypoxia is insufficient oxygen anywhere in the body. To compensate for this lack of oxygen, the heart increases its rate to improve cardiac output, thereby increasing oxygen to all body cells.**
   2. Difficulty breathing (dyspnea) is a late, not early, sign of hypoxia.
   3. An increase in respirations (tachypnea), not a decrease in respirations (bradypnea), occurs as the body attempts to deliver more oxygen to body cells.
   4. Skin color changes are not early adaptations to hypoxia. Pallor is caused by peripheral vasoconstriction that shunts blood away from the skin to the vital organs and occurs with the stress response.

3. 1. **Persistent chronic pain becomes an unchanging part of life. As the duration of exposure increases, the individual may learn cognitive and behavioral strategies to cope with the pain.**
   2. Chronic pain can markedly impair activities of daily living.
   3. Chronic pain may, or may not, have an identifiable cause.
   4. Acute pain and chronic pain both decrease the efficiency of the immune system.

4. 1. A slight elevation of body temperature is expected after surgery because of the body's response to the stress of surgery.
   2. Dehiscence, separation of the wound margins, is more likely to occur between the fifth and eighth postoperative days, and it is not life threatening.
   3. Dependent edema indicates problems, such as a fluid and electrolyte imbalance, impaired kidney function, or decreased cardiac output. All are serious, but generally manageable.
   4. **An acute onset of chest pain within 24 hours of surgery may indicate myocardial infarction in response to the stress of surgery. Also, it can be caused by a pulmonary embolus, although this is more likely to occur between the seventh and tenth postoperative days. Both of these complications are life threatening.**

5. 1. Abdominal distention is a defining characteristic for the nursing diagnosis Constipation, not Perceived Constipation.
   2. The passage of hard, dry stools is a defining characteristic for the nursing diagnosis Constipation, not Perceived Constipation.
   3. **The defining characteristics for the nursing diagnosis Perceived Constipation are the expectation of a daily bowel movement with the resulting overuse of laxatives, enemas, and/or suppositories and the expected passage of stool at the same time every day.**
   4. Straining at stool is a defining characteristic for the nursing diagnosis Constipation, not Perceived Constipation.

6. 1. Although this is done, it is not the priority.
   2. **The consent for surgery must be signed before preoperative medications are administered because they depress the central nervous system impairing problem solving and decision making.**
   3. This is unnecessary. This can be done at any time during the preoperative phase or at the beginning of the intraoperative phase of surgery.
   4. Although this is done, it is not the priority.

7. **Answer: 5 mL. Use ratio and proportion to first convert 500 milligrams to its equivilant in grams as well as to solve the problem.**

$$\frac{\text{Desire}}{\text{Have}} \quad \frac{500\text{ mg}}{1000\text{ mg}} = \frac{x\text{ gram}}{1\text{ gram}}$$

$$1000x = 500$$
$$x = 500 \div 1000$$
$$x = 0.5 \text{ grams (is equal to 500 mg)}$$

$$\frac{\text{Desire}}{\text{Have}} \quad \frac{0.5\text{ gram}}{1\text{ gram}} = \frac{x\text{ mL}}{10\text{ mL}}$$

$$x = 0.5 \times 10$$
$$x = 5\text{ mL}$$

8. 1. Primary nursing is not a cost containment strategy in managed care, but rather a nursing-care delivery system that ensures a comprehensive and consistent approach to identifying and meeting patients' needs. Primary nursing occurs when one nurse is assigned the 24-hour responsibility for the planning and delivery of nursing care to a specific patient for the duration of the patient's hospitalization.
 2. **Critical pathways are a case management system that identify specific protocols and timetables for care and treatment by various disciplines designed to achieve expected patient outcomes within a specific time frame. The purpose is to discharge patients sooner, thereby reducing the cost of health care.**
 3. Functional method refers to a model of nursing-care delivery that assigns a specific task for a group of patients to one person. Although it is efficient, it is impersonal and contributes to fragmentation of care because it is task oriented rather than patient centered.
 4. Quality management (also known as continuous quality improvement, total quality management, or persistent quality improvement), refers to a program designed to improve, not just ensure, the quality of care delivered to patients. Also, it includes an educational component to support growth and provide for corrective action.

9. 1. Patients with dementia do not have the cognitive ability to perform a procedure independently.
 2. **When progressing through each aspect of the bath, give simple, direct statements to limit the amount of incoming stimuli at one time. This will promote comprehension and self-care.**
 3. The patient has a problem with cognition, not vision.
 4. This intervention may precipitate anxiety. The patient does not have the cognitive ability or attention span to understand a detailed explanation before a procedure.

10. 1. This describes narcolepsy, which is a sudden overwhelming sleepiness (hypersomnia) in the daytime.
 2. This describes Restless Legs Syndrome, a feeling of creeping or itching sensation occurring in the lower extremities causing an irrestible urge to move and kick the legs.
 3. This describes nightmares, which are vivid frightening dreams that occur during REM sleep and awaken the sleeper.
 4. **Episodes of sleep apnea begin with loud snoring followed by silence, during which the person struggles to breathe against a blocked airway. Decreasing oxygen levels cause the person to awaken abruptly with a loud snort.**

11. 1. A clear liquid diet is contraindicated in the presence of abdominal distention because gas has accumulated in the intestines because of a lack of intestinal motility.
 2. This is not the purpose of a clear liquid diet. A full-liquid diet or food will more likely stimulate gastric enzymes.
 3. A clear liquid diet is administered after a postoperative ileus resolves, not to prevent its occurrence.
 4. **The molecules in clear liquids are less complex and easier to ingest, tolerate, and digest than those in a full-liquid diet or food.**

12. 1. **Diarrhea is related directly to a risk for damage to epidermal and dermal tissue. The gastric and intestinal enzymes present in feces are acids capable of eroding the skin.**
 2. Diarrhea is unrelated to the ability to provide self-care. The inability to care for self is the state in which the individual experiences an impaired motor or cognitive function, causing a decreased ability to perform self-care activities.
 3. Diarrhea is not related directly to a sexual dysfunction, which is the state in which an individual experiences or is at risk of experiencing a change in sexual function that is viewed as unrewarding or inadequate.
 4. Diarrhea is not related directly to a body image disturbance, which is the state in which an individual experiences, or is at risk of experiencing, a disruption in the way one perceives one's body image.

13. 1. This is not an example of battery. Battery is the purposeful, angry, or negligent touching of a patient without consent.
 2. This is not an example of assault. Assault is an attempt, or threat, to touch another person unjustly.
 3. This is not an example of negligence. Negligence occurs when the nurse's actions do not meet appropriate standards of care and result in injury to another.
 4. **Malpractice is misconduct, an act of commission or omission, performed in professional practice that results in harm to another.**

14. 4, Hyperglycemia event

Laboratory Results: BUN: 18 mg/dL
Creatinine: 1.2 mg/dL
Hemoglobin A_{1c}: 8.0%
Serum glucose: 350 mg/dL

I&O Record (last 24/hr): Intake: 2400 mL
Output: 4200 mL

Nursing Progress Note: 10 AM–patient complains of being thirsty and "urinating a lot," and has lost 20 pounds over the last two months; has poor skin turgor and dry mucous membranes.

ANSWER AND RATIONALES

1. Generalized weakness and fatigue are not indicative of a brain attack because with a brain attack paresis or paralysis generally is unilateral and focal in nature.
2. Kidney failure can be ruled out because the 4200 mL of urinary output indicates that the kidneys are functioning. Also, with kidney failure, generally there is a weight gain, not loss. The BUN and creatinine levels are within the normal range and indicate that the kidneys are not in failure.
3. There are no data to support the conclusion that this event is a hypertensive episode. With the degree of polyuria, poor skin turgor, and dry mucous membranes, hypotension due to dehydration, not hypertension, is expected.
4. **The serum glucose of 350 mg/dL is excessive and indicates a hyperglycemic event; the acceptable range is 80 to 120 mg/dL. A Hemoglobin A_{1c} greater than 6% to 7% indicates inadequate glucose control over the last 90 to 120 days.**

15. 1. Directive is not one of the four classic leadership styles.
2. The autocratic leadership style is probably the least effective style to use with a professionally mature and motivated staff. Autocratic leaders give orders and directions and make decisions for the group. There is little freedom and a large degree of control by the leader, which frustrates motivated and professionally mature staff members.
3. The democratic leadership style is the second best style to use when the staff is motivated and professionally mature. The democratic style offers fewer opportunities for autonomy for staff members who are mature and motivated than a leadership style in another option.
4. **The laissez-faire leadership style is appropriate for a group of individuals who have an internal locus of control and desire autonomy and independence. Individuals who are professionally mature and motivated more often have an internal locus of control.**

16. 1. **Pressure on the popliteal areas can cause damage to nerves and interferes with circulation and must be avoided.**
2. Transfer belts should be removed once the patient is transferred.
3. This moves the patient too close to the front of the seat and is unsafe.
4. The patient's feet should be positioned flat on the footrests of the wheelchair, not the floor, to protect the feet if the wheelchair is moved.

17. 1. A patient's perceptions are only one part of the data that must be collected before the nurse can establish the priority of the patient's needs. Maslow's Hierarchy of Basic Human Needs helps the nurse to determine the patient's needs in order of priority based on the collected data.
2. **Health perception reflects a person's knowledge, behavior, and attitudes regarding illness, disease prevention, health promotion, and what constitutes a healthy lifestyle. An assessment of these factors captures the uniqueness of each individual and is essential data that must be considered before needs are identified and a plan formulated.**
3. A healthy lifestyle can promote health and prevent some illness or even minimize complications; however, understanding a person's perceptions of health may not prevent human responses to disease.
4. Only a patient, not a nurse, can choose a patient's place along the health-illness continuum. How people perceive themselves is subjective and is influenced by their own attitudes, values, and beliefs.

18. 1. A serving of ½ grapefruit contains only 162 μgRE of vitamin A.
2. One medium-sized tangerine contains only 108 μgRE of vitamin A.
3. **Apricots are an excellent source of vitamin A. Three medium-sized apricots**

contain 867 μgRE (Retinol Equivalents) of vitamin A.

4. One medium-sized banana contains only 69 μgRE of vitamin A.

19. 1. Nonverbal behavior is controlled more by the unconscious than by the conscious mind.
2. Nonverbal behavior carries more, not less, weight than verbal interactions because nonverbal behavior is influenced by the unconscious.
3. **Transculturally, nonverbal communication varies widely. For example, gestures, facial expressions, eye contact, and touch may reflect opposite messages among cultures and among individuals within a culture.**
4. The opposite is true. Nonverbal behaviors often directly reflect feelings.

20. 1. These anatomic landmarks help to identify the deltoid muscle.
2. **These anatomic landmarks help to identify the dorsogluteal site. This site contains the well-developed gluteus muscles, particularly the gluteus maximus, in the buttocks.**
3. This is the initial placement of the hand when identifying landmarks for the ventrogluteal site.
4. This is associated with the vastus lateralis site. It is between one handbreadth above the knee and one handbreadth below the greater trochanter on the anterior lateral aspect of the thigh.

21. 1. **Taping a patient's get-well cards to the wall where the patient can see them supports the patient's need to feel loved and appreciated and meets love and belonging needs according to Maslow's Hierarchy of Needs.**
2. This does not support a patient's safety and security needs. Safety and security needs are related to being and feeling protected in the physiologic and interpersonal realms.
3. This does not support a patient's self-esteem needs. Self-esteem needs are met from within. They are how the patient feels about oneself.
4. This does not support a patient's physiologic needs. Physiologic needs are related to having adequate air, food, water, rest, shelter, and the ability to eliminate and regulate body temperature.

22. 1. This is unnecessary. When obtaining a specimen from a retention catheter, the aspiration port of the catheter (not the exit tube) is wiped with a disinfectant before inserting the syringe. Urine specimens from a retention catheter should come from the port, not the bag, because this urine is the most recently excreted.
2. This should not be done until a step mentioned in another option is performed first. The drainage tubing should be clamped approximately 1 to 2 inches below the aspiration port for 15 to 20 minutes to allow urine to accumulate.
3. This is unnecessary to obtain a urine specimen because only 10 to 30 mL are needed. This position is used to move urine toward the trigone (the triangular area at the base of the bladder where the ureters and urethra enter the bladder) where it is accessible to the catheter, which promotes the flow of urine through the urinary catheter to the drainage bag.
4. **Wearing personal protective equipment, such as clean gloves, is a medical asepsis practice that protects the nurse from the patient's body fluids.**

23. 1. Clean gloves are adequate.
2. **A skin barrier, such as zinc oxide, protects the skin from the digestive enzymes in feces.**
3. Cranberry juice makes urine more alkaline; it does not influence bacteria and enzymes in stool.
4. Patients should attempt to have a bowel movement after a meal to take advantage of the gastrocolic reflex.

24. 1. The nurse does not need a practitioner's order to provide nursing care that is within the realm of nursing practice.
2. **Providing hygiene, an activity of daily living, is within the scope of nursing practice.**
3. The nurse does not need to collaborate with other health-care professionals to provide nursing care.
4. The nurse does not need a practitioner's order, with or without a restriction, to implement nursing care that is within the realm of nursing practice.

25. 1. Kool-Aid contains no sodium and is permitted on a 2-gram sodium diet.
2. Club soda contains no sodium and is permitted on a 2-gram sodium diet.
3. Twelve fluid ounces of lemonade contains approximately 12 mg of sodium and is permitted on a 2-gram sodium diet.
4. **Twelve fluid ounces of diet root beer contains approximately 170 mg of sodium and should be avoided on a 2-gram sodium diet.**

26. 1. Although stomatitis—inflammation of the mouth—can occur from irritation caused by the tube used for delivering general anesthesia to a patient during surgery, it is uncommon and not life threatening.
2. Although atelectasis is serious, it is not as serious as an adaptation in another option. Anesthesia delivered by intubation can interfere with the action of surfactant, resulting in the collapse of alveoli (atelectasis).
3. Although the tube used for intubation commonly does irritate the posterior oropharynx, resulting in a sore throat, it is not as serious as an adaptation in another option.
4. This is a potentially life-threatening complication because it prevents the exchange of gases between the lungs and atmospheric air. Laryngeal spasm can result from irritation caused by the presence of the intubation tube in the glottis (space between the vocal cords) during surgery.

27. 1. The reference is too general to be related to the location of pain, which is the actual site the pain is felt.
2. Intensity refers to the strength or amount of pain experienced, which often is rated from mild to excruciating.
3. Quality refers to the description of the pain sensation.
4. The pattern of pain refers to time of onset, duration, recurrence, and remissions.

28. 1. In the semi-Fowler's position, the abdominal organs drop by gravity, which permits maximum thoracic excursion. In addition, slight flexion of the hips reduces abdominal muscle tension, which limits pressure on the suture line and facilitates diaphragmatic (abdominal) breathing.
2. Resting in bed in any position promotes flatus retention. Ambulation promotes intestinal motility, which promotes the passage of flatus.
3. Inactivity results in decreased detrusor muscle tone, incomplete bladder emptying, and urinary stasis. The high-Fowler's position and ambulation use gravity to promote urinary elimination.
4. This position does not facilitate drainage via a portable wound drainage system. Negative pressure creates the vacuum that draws fluid into a portable wound drainage system.

29. 1. Oil lubricates, not irritates, the intestinal mucosa.
2. Soap irritates the intestinal mucosa and thus stimulates the circular and longitudinal muscles of the intestinal wall, which respond with wave-like movements (peristalsis) that propel intestinal contents toward the anus.
3. Tap water is a hypotonic solution that exerts a lower osmotic pressure than the surrounding interstitial fluid, causing water to move from the colon into interstitial spaces. In addition, the volume of the fluid distends the lumen of the intestine. These processes stimulate peristalsis and defecation.
4. Normal saline, a solution having the same osmotic pressure of surrounding interstitial fluid (isotonic), works by drawing fluid from interstitial spaces into the colon. This fluid, in addition to the original volume of saline instilled, exerts pressure against the intestinal mucosa, which stimulates peristalsis and defecation.

30. 1. Water will not increase the absorption of medications administered orally. Water will facilitate the swallowing of and the movement of the medication down the esophagus to the stomach.
2. The time of day does not influence the rate of absorption of medications administered orally.
3. Food can delay the dissolution and absorption of many drugs; therefore, most oral medications should be administered on an empty stomach. Oral medications should be administered with food only when indicated by the manufacturer's directions.
4. Physical rest does not influence the rate of absorption of medications administered orally.

31. 1. Infants react to pain in an intense way including physical resistance and lack of cooperation. Separation of an infant from the usual comforting contact with parents contributes to separation anxiety, which in turn lowers pain tolerance, which intensifies the pain experience. Infants express pain by irritability, rolling of the head, flexing the extremities, overacting to common stimuli, an inability to be comforted by holding and rocking, and physical responses indicating stimulation of the sympathetic nervous system.
2. Adolescents are less sensitive to pain than an age group in another option. Adolescents generally want to behave in an adult manner and, therefore, demonstrate a controlled behavioral response to pain.
3. Older adults have a decreased capacity to sense pain and pressure. Older adults often fail to notice situations that will cause acute pain in younger people.

4. Pregnant women generally are not more sensitive to pain than when not pregnant.

32. 1. Leavened bread and cake, not coffee and tea, are forbidden during Passover.
2. There are no restrictions on dairy products and eggs after sundown on Fridays.
3. Dairy products and meat/poultry are never served at the same meal or on the same set of dishes. Dairy products are not permitted within 1 to 6 hours after eating meat/poultry. Meat/poultry cannot be eaten for 30 minutes after consuming dairy products. Historically, this was practiced so that one food did not contaminate the other.
4. All crustaceans, shellfish, and fish-like mammals, such as crab, shrimp, and lobster, scallops, oysters, and clams are forbidden.

33. 1. Relaxation techniques are effective ways to reduce the autonomic nervous system response to a threat. However, they do not reduce the stressor contributing to this response.
2. Validating a patient's feelings will help the patient feel accepted, understood, and credible. However, it is not as helpful as another option.
3. Minimizing environmental stimuli may support rest and sleep, which is an essential aspect of stress management in any setting. However, it is not as helpful as another option.
4. Anxiety is a response to an unknown threat to the self or self-esteem. Therefore, explaining what, how, why, when, and where of every procedure to the patient will reduce anxiety by minimizing the unknown.

34. 1. Perineal care, not a vaginal irrigation, should be performed before inserting a vaginal suppository.
2. The patient should be placed in the supine position with the knees flexed (dorsal recumbent) to facilitate insertion of a vaginal suppository. The left-lateral position is used for an enema.
3. This facilitates the placement of the vaginal suppository just outside the cervical os so that when it melts it will eventually disperse through the entire vaginal canal.
4. Medical, not surgical, asepsis is required for the insertion of a vaginal suppository.

35. 1. Although the leadership role is an important role and can be demonstrated on many different levels in the nursing profession, a word in another option has a stronger relationship with the role of the nurse when helping a patient negotiate the health-care system.
2. The health-care delivery system in the United States is complex and can be confusing at a time when patients have the least energy to explore and negotiate intervention options. When functioning as a resource person, the nurse identifies resources, provides information, and makes referrals.
3. The surrogate role is not a professional role of the nurse. A surrogate role is assigned to a nurse when a patient believes that the nurse reminds them of another person and projects that role and the feelings he/she has for the other person onto the nurse.
4. The role of counselor is only one area of nursing practice and a word in another option has a stronger relationship with the role of the nurse when helping a patient negotiate the health-care system. Counseling is related only to helping a patient recognize and cope with emotional stressors, improve relationships, and promote personal growth.

36. 1. Bathing daily, even using a moisturizing soap, is drying to the skin. Two to three times a week is adequate for an older adult who is continent.
2. Woolen fabrics are coarse and irritate the skin, and therefore should be avoided.
3. The percentage of body water dramatically decreases with age, and older adults have altered thirst mechanisms that place them at risk for inadequate fluid intake and dehydration. In addition, the skin of older adults is dryer because of a decreased ability to sweat and a decreased production of sebum.
4. Lotion is preferable to baby powder because lotion lubricates the skin. Also, baby powder should be avoided because when aerosolized, it is a respiratory irritant.

37. 1. Treatment refers to actions designed to help the patient achieve homeostasis, not adaptive capacity.
2. A major component of adaptive capacity is the ability to be flexible in all realms of human dimension, as a person seeks to regain homeostasis or balance. Adaptive capacity refers to the quality and quantity of resources one can draw on to regain balance after one is threatened.
3. The threat that a person perceives is the stressor, not the adaptation.

4. Illness refers to a maladaptive response to a stressor, not to adaptive capacity.

38. **1. Cold lowers the temperature of skin and underlying tissue, which causes vasoconstriction, reducing blood flow to the area. This controls bleeding and slows the passage of fluid from the intravascular to the interstitial compartment, which limits edema.**

2. Direct pressure may limit bleeding but will not affect edema or pain. Acupressure closes the gate mechanism to pain or stimulates areas near pain fibers leading to the brain, thereby blocking the perception of pain.
3. Effleurage—long, smooth strokes sliding over the skin—reduces pain by using the Gate Control Theory of Pain. Peripheral stimuli transmitted via large-diameter nerves close the gate to painful stimuli that use small-diameter nerves, thereby blocking the perception of pain.
4. Massage is cutaneous stimulation that uses the Gate Control Theory of Pain, not vasoconstriction, to limit pain.

39. 1. Although the physical trauma of surgery causes pain and it must be relieved, it is not the priority.

2. Although anesthesia can cause nausea, it is not the priority problem in the Post-Anesthesia Care Unit.
3. **With an altered level of consciousness, the pharyngeal, laryngeal, and gag reflexes may be impaired. The inability to cough or swallow can result in aspiration of oral secretions.**
4. Excessive fluid loss precipitates a deficient fluid volume, but the nurse generally has time to safely meet this need.

40. **1. The only way to reestablish patency of the air vent lumen of a double-lumen nasogastric tube is to instill air into the lumen. The injected air will push the secretions blocking the lumen back into the stomach where the fluid can be removed by the drainage lumen. Keeping the end of the air vent lumen higher than the stomach, prevents reflux of gastric contents into the air vent lumen.**

2. This will not reestablish patency of the air vent lumen. The patient is placed in this position as the tube is being inserted to facilitate its passage into the stomach.
3. This will draw more fluid from the stomach into the air vent lumen by the principle of gravity.
4. This will not reestablish patency of the air vent lumen. This is done to ensure that the catheter is in the correct anatomic location.

41. 1. This action does not require an incident report. The nurse manager should discuss this behavior with the nurse and may document it in the nurse's personnel file.

2. **Not receiving an ordered medication may have the potential to cause harm. Therefore, an incident or adverse occurrence report should be completed to document the incident to add to the data so that similar situations can be prevented in the future.**
3. An incident report does not have to be completed in this instance. The incident should be documented in the patient's medical record.
4. An incident report is unnecessary in this situation. Patients have the right to refuse care; however, the patient's refusal of care and the reasons for the refusal should be documented in the patient's medical record.

42. **1. Intermittent episodes of pain that occur despite continued use of an analgesic (breakthrough pain) can be managed by administering an immediate-release analgesic to reduce pain (rescue dosing). This reduces pain during an unanticipated pain episode without unnecessarily raising the dosage of the long-acting analgesic.**

2. This will not promote absorption via the transdermal patch; it could result in the destructive effects of immobility and may interfere with the quality of life.
3. This is ineffective in this situation. The patient has intractable (malignant) pain that requires an opiate at this time.
4. This is not the priority. Although this may eventually be necessary, the patient's pain must be relieved immediately.

43. 1. This should not be the first thing to do when unsure of the steps in a nursing procedure.

2. Fundamental nursing textbooks are not the best source for a step-by-step review of a nursing skill. Generally, fundamental nursing textbooks do not address every nursing skill in a step-by-step approach, nor do they include intermediate or advanced skills.
3. **This is the first resource the nurse should use when unsure of the steps in a nursing procedure. A review of the procedure in the Procedure Manual may refresh the memory or support the confidence of the nurse so that it is safe to proceed.**

4. This is premature. Another action should be implemented first.

44. 1. A pressure ulcer is not a microbiologic stressor. If an ulcer becomes infected, the organism causing the infection is a microbiologic stressor.
2. A pressure ulcer is not a developmental stressor. Developmental stressors are physiologic changes or transitional life events that occur during the expected stages of growth and development.
3. **Pressure is a physical stressor that stimulates adaptations that cause an ulcer. Once an ulcer is present, the ulcer becomes a secondary stressor and is considered physiologic in nature.**
4. A pressure ulcer is not a physical stressor. The pressure that caused the ulcer is a physical stressor.

45. 1. This is associated with cardiovascular problems.
2. This is associated with bowel and/or urinary incontinence.
3. This is associated with the older adult and people with peripheral neuropathy or neurologic diseases.
4. **Cachexia involves weight loss, muscle atrophy, and decreased subcutaneous tissue, which results in a reduction in the padding between skin and bones, thus increasing the risk of pressure ulcer development.**

46. 1. This is an inference based on inadequate data.
2. **This is an example of paraphrasing, which restates the content of the patient's message in similar words.**
3. This is an example of reflective technique, which focuses on feelings.
4. This is an example of an open-ended statement, which invites the patient to elaborate on the stated concern.

47. 1. Using the same site consistently causes, not limits, skin irritation and excoriation. The sites for a transdermal patch should be rotated.
2. Both irritation of the skin and vasodilation can result from rubbing the skin, which can alter absorption of the medication.
3. **A hairless site will ensure that there is effective contact with the skin.**
4. The old patch should be removed at the same time that the new patch is applied.

48. 1. **A task of this complexity requires the knowledge and judgment of a registered nurse. If the caregiver is unable to assess the patient's condition adequately, this task has great potential for harm. In addition, it requires problem solving that may call for innovation in the form of an individually designed plan of care to address the presence of a dysrhythmia.**
2. **Patient teaching is a complex task. It requires knowledge of principles, such as identifying readiness to learn, progressing from simple to complex information, using motivational theory, and evaluating outcomes. Also, it requires knowledge of principles related to colostomy care such as: the bag opening must be at least ⅛th-inch larger than the stoma, a pale stoma may indicate ischemia, and what to include in an assessment of the characteristics of intestinal output.**
3. Applying a condom catheter is not a complex task. It requires simple problem-solving skills, involves a predictable outcome, and employs a simple level of interaction with the patient. Although this task has the potential to cause harm if the critical elements of the skill are not implemented, it is within the scope of practice of an unlicensed nursing assistant. It does not require the more advanced competencies of a registered nurse.
4. Making an occupied bed is not a complex task. It requires simple problem-solving skills, involves a predictable outcome, and employs a simple level of interaction with the patient. Although this task has the potential to cause harm if the critical elements of the skill are not implemented, it is within the scope of practice of an unlicensed nursing assistant. It does not require the more advanced competencies of a registered nurse.
5. Transferring a patient is not a complex task. It requires simple problem-solving skills, involves a predictable outcome, and employs a simple level of interaction with the patient. Although this task has the potential to cause harm if the critical elements of the skill are not implemented, it is within the scope of practice of an unlicensed nursing assistant. It does not require the more advanced competencies of a registered nurse.

49. 1. **Digoxin (Lanoxin) can cause sensory changes, such as diplopia (double vision), halos, colored vision, blind spots, and flashing lights. If any of these signs of toxicity occur, the medication should be held and a serum digoxin level assessed to determine if the drug is exceeding its therapeutic range of 0.5 to 2 ng/mL.**

2. Tachypnea, an abnormally rapid rate of breathing (usually more than 20 breaths per minute), is not a symptom of digitalis toxicity.
3. Dysrhythmias, not hypertension, are cardiovascular signs of digitalis toxicity.
4. Digoxin does not influence temperature regulation in the body; it is given whether or not the patient has a fever.

50. **1. A tube feeding formula usually is hypertonic, which exerts an osmotic force that pulls fluid into the stomach and intestine, resulting in intestinal cramping and diarrhea.**
2. This may result in fluid volume deficit and malnutrition, not diarrhea.
3. This may result in vomiting, not diarrhea. If there is still fluid remaining from the previous feeding, failure to test for a residual before administering a tube feeding can result in adding more fluid than the stomach can tolerate.
4. Placing a patient in the high-Fowler's position during the administration of a tube feeding is done to prevent aspiration of the formula and will not cause diarrhea.

51. 1. This is unnecessary. This is done when the patient is unconscious.
2. When attempting to clear an airway of an obstruction, the thumb side of the hand should always be against the patient's body regardless of the modification in the maneuver.
3. This is the appropriate modification of the abdominal thrust (Heimlich) maneuver for a pregnant woman. This provides thoracic compression while preventing pressure against the uterus that can result in trauma to the woman or the fetus.
4. Waiting until the person becomes unconscious wastes valuable time and is unsafe. Discontinuing the maneuver before the obstruction is cleared will result in death.

52. 1. The lights, noise, and activity in the hospital environment can interfere with napping during the day. However, naps when they do occur usually are short and rarely reach Stage IV restorative sleep.
2. Hospitalized patients can follow their usual bedtime rituals.
3. Most medications are administered by 10 PM to 11 PM and should not interfere with sleep.
4. Patients frequently find hospital beds unfamiliar and uncomfortable. In addition, therapeutic regimens restrict movement or require patients to assume sleeping positions other than their preference. Studies support the fact that finding a comfortable position is the most common factor that interferes with sleep as reported by hospitalized patients.

53. 1. Yogurt, a dairy product, is not included in a vegetarian diet. Pure vegetarians (vegans) eat only plants. Lacto-vegetarians eat vegetables and milk products, lacto-ovovegetarians eat vegetables, milk products, and eggs (some may occasionally eat fish or poultry).
2. Cheese, a dairy product, is not included in a vegetarian diet. Pure vegetarians (vegans) eat only plants.
3. Grains and legumes lack different amino acids. When these foods are combined, they substitute for a complete protein. Complete proteins supply all eight essential amino acids. Essential amino acids are those that cannot be manufactured by the human body and must be obtained from food sources.
4. Peanut butter combined with a grain, not jelly, is a substitute for a complete protein.

54. 1. Calcium is essential for functioning, but it is unrelated to the risk for drug toxicity in the older adult. Calcium is essential for cell membrane structure, wound healing, synaptic transmission in nervous tissue, membrane excitability, muscle contraction, tooth and bone structure, blood clotting, and glycolysis.
2. The glomerular filtration rate is reduced by as much as 46% at 90 years of age. In addition, decreased cardiac output can reduce the amount of blood flow to the kidneys by as much as 50%. When the glomerular filtration rate declines, the time necessary for half of a drug to be excreted increases by as much as 40%, which places the older adult at risk for drug toxicity.
3. Red blood cells are responsible for delivering oxygen to cells, and are unrelated to the risk for drug toxicity in the older adult.
4. Frequency of voiding is unrelated to the risk for drug toxicity in the older adult.

55. 1. This is done to straighten the ear canal of an infant or a young child, not an adult.
2. This can injure the eardrum. Drops should be directed along the wall of the ear canal.
3. Pressing gently on the tragus facilitates the flow of medication toward the eardrum.
4. This can result in medication flowing out of the ear. The side-lying position with the involved ear on the uppermost side should

be maintained for 2 to 3 minutes after the medication is instilled.

56. 1. Preschoolers (3 to 5 years—Initiative versus Guilt) learn to separate from parents and develop a sense of initiative. Negative resolution will result in guilt, rigidity, and a hesitancy to explore new skills or challenge abilities.
2. **Adolescents (12 to 20 years—Identity versus Role Confusion) strive to develop a personal identity and autonomy. This is a turbulent time as the adolescent internalizes the dramatic physical changes and the psychological stressors of new social conflicts. It is common for adolescents to experience mood swings, make decisions without having all the facts, challenge authority, and assert the self. However, these behaviors are left behind when the developmental tasks of adolescence are positively resolved. Negative resolution results in assertive, rebellious, and antisocial behavior.**
3. School-aged children (6 to 12 years—Industry verses Inferiority) learn to compete, compromise, and cooperate, develop relationships with peers, and win recognition through productivity. Negative resolution results in feelings of inadequacy, low self-esteem, and a reluctance to explore the environment.
4. Infants (birth to 18 months—Trust versus Mistrust) learn to depend on others to meet their needs, thereby developing trust and a beginning sense of self. Negative resolution of this task results in mistrust, dependency, lack of self-confidence, and shallow relationships in later stages of development.

57. 1. This will cover the brachial artery and may interfere with the accurate assessment of blood pressure. The lower edge of the cuff should be approximately 1 inch (2.5 cm) above the antecubital space.
2. This will result in a false low blood pressure reading.
3. The sphygmomanometer should be pumped up 30 mm Hg, not 60 mm Hg, above the palpatory blood pressure reading. This ensures an accurate systolic reading without exerting undue pressure on the tissues of the arm.
4. **Releasing the valve slowly ensures that all 5 Korotkoff's sounds are heard accurately. Deflating the cuff too rapidly, can result in a false low systolic reading and deflating the cuff too slowly can result in a false high diastolic reading.**

58. 1. **Unconscious patients often bite down when something is placed in the mouth. Therefore, a padded tongue blade should be placed between the upper and lower teeth to help keep the mouth open during oral care. Other padded tongue blades, wetted with a small amount of saline, should be used to clean the oral cavity.**
2. Toothpaste should be avoided because it requires flushing the mouth with adequate amounts of water to prevent leaving an irritating residue on the mucous membranes. An unconscious patient usually has a diminished gag reflex and is at risk for aspiration.
3. Although this is used, it is not the best intervention because mouthwash contains ingredients that can be irritating to the mucous membranes.
4. Glycerin swabs are not effective in cleaning the oral cavity.

59. 1. Although this historical information eventually may be obtained, it is not the immediate priority.
2. **This invites the patient to expand on and develop a topic of importance that relates to the current problem.**
3. Although this historical information eventually may be obtained, it is not the immediate priority.
4. This question is too focused.

60. 1. Eleven AM is too soon. The drug will not be at its lowest concentration in the blood.
2. **Thiry minutes before, and up to, the next scheduled dose is the most appropriate time for a trough blood level to be obtained. The serum level of the drug will be at its lowest.**
3. Peak, not trough, levels are obtained thirty minutes after completion of drug administration.
4. The blood level of the drug rises once the drug is administered. A value taken at this time will no longer reflect the lowest serum level, which is the purpose of identifying a trough level.

61. 1. During adolescence, the individual is beginning to question life-guiding values such as spirituality. However, it is not uncommon for the adolescent to turn away from religious practices as part of dealing with role confusion and exploration of self-identity. Faith becomes centered around the peer group and away from the parents. This stage is called

Synthetic-Conventional Faith by James Fowler.
2. Although older adults often refine spiritual beliefs in response to life events, beliefs generally are expanded upon at an earlier stage of development. Some unique adults are able to achieve Universalizing Faith identified by James Fowler, which is a worldview stressing living out the vision of justice, love, and compassion.
3. Young adults are just beginning to think about spirituality more introspectively at this age. Young adults generally enter a reflective period of time as discovery of values in relation to social goals are explored within their own frame of reference rather from the peer group frame of reference as during adolescence. This stage is called Individuative-Reflective Faith by James Fowler.
4. **Middle-aged adults tend to engage in refining and expanding spiritual beliefs through questioning. Middle-aged adults are reported to have greater faith, more reliance on personal spiritual strength, and be less inflexible in spiritual beliefs. Middle-aged adults integrate other viewpoints about faith which introduces tension while working toward resolution of spiritual beliefs. This stage is called Conjunctive Faith by James Fowler.**

62. 1. **Walkers surround a person on three sides and provide 4 points of contact with the floor. This wide base provides the best support available for assisted ambulation.**
2. This follows the principle: *An object with wheels that are locked will remain stationary.*
3. This follows the principle: *The closer an object is held to the center of gravity, the greater the stability and the easier the object is to move.*
4. This follows the principle: *Balance is maintained and muscle strain is limited as long as the line of gravity passes through the base of support.*

63. 1. Back massage is the therapeutic manipulation of muscles and tissues that relaxes tense muscles, relieves muscle spasms, and induces rest or sleep. However, it may be contraindicated, and some people do not like a back rub or consider it an invasion of their personal space.
2. Music can be relaxing or stimulating depending on the music and the individual.
3. Although milk contains the amino acid L-tryptophan that promotes sleep, many people do not like milk or avoid fluids before bedtime to limit nocturia.
4. **Following routines provides consistency and comfort in an unfamiliar environment. Bedtime rituals meet basic physiologic needs and usually include physically and emotionally relaxing behaviors.**

64. An X in any part of the shaded area across the abdomen is a correct answer. The nurse should auscultate all four quadrants of the abdomen to determine the presence of borborygmi. Borborygmi are audible high-pitched, loud, gurgling sounds that occur frequently. Borborygmi are hyperactive bowel sounds that indicate increased intestinal motility usually related to diarrhea, early bowel obstruction, or the use of laxatives.

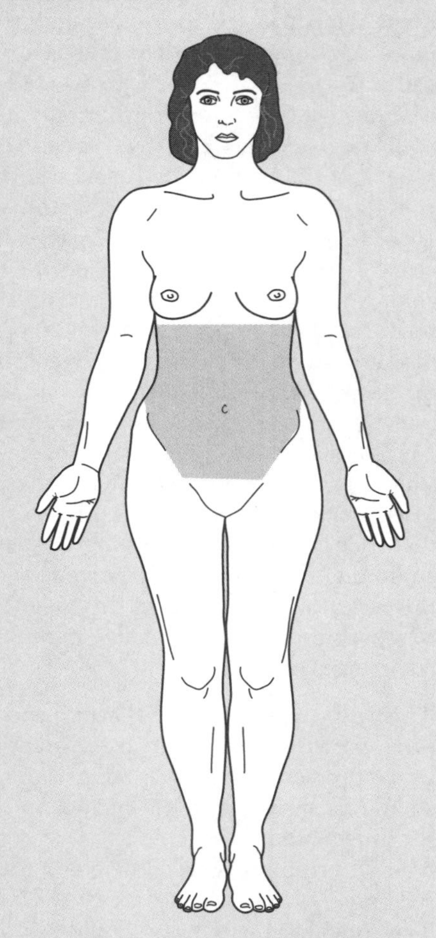

65. 1. This is unsafe. An over-bed table has wheels and therefore cannot provide a firm base of support. Over-bed tables are physical hazards that often contribute to falls if used inappropriately.
2. **This provides for the safety of patients, staff, and visitors within a hospital. Inadequate lighting causes shadows, a dark environment, and the potential for misinterpreting stimuli (illusions), and is**

a major cause of accidents in the hospital setting.

3. Although this should be done, this is not a physical hazard.
4. Although this should be done, and reaching for a phone can result in a loss of balance and a fall, it is not the most important intervention to prevent injury in a hospital.

66. 1. The knees are extended, not flexed, when in the supine position.

2. The supine position is a back-lying position that results in pressure on the heels (calcaneus), which have minimal tissue between the bone and skin, making them vulnerable to the development of pressure ulcers.

3. There is no pressure on either greater trochanter when in the supine position. Pressure on a greater trochanter occurs when the patient is in a lateral (side-lying) position.
4. External, not internal, rotation of the hips tends to occur when a patient is in the supine position.

67. 1. Setting limits will make the patient more anxious and demanding. Demanding behavior generally is an attempt to gain control over events in an effort to protect the Ego.

2. Alternating care with another nurse can be confusing to the patient and increase anxiety. Maintaining continuity in the nurse assignment will support the development of a trusting relationship, enable the nurse to explore the patient's feelings, as well as plan and implement interventions that encourage choices, all of which support feeling in control.
3. Pointing out demanding behavior is too confrontational at this time. Demanding behavior generally is a defense mechanism that reduces anxiety generated by powerlessness. To confront the behavior and take away the patient's coping mechanism will cause the patient to become more anxious.

4. This is an example of empathy, which is understanding a patient's emotional point of view. An empathic response communicates that the nurse is listening and cares.

68. 1. This information includes a nursing intervention and an evaluation of the outcome, which is the most specific and complete of all the options.

2. No data are given to support the assumption that the patient is happy.
3. The words "less anxious" are relative and do not clearly evaluate the patient's status.
4. Every patient has his or her own baseline. Indicating that a blood pressure is stable is unclear.

69. 1. Clean, not sterile, gloves are required during this procedure to protect the nurse because the nurse may be exposed to body fluids.

2. This action is related to a patient's comfort and elimination needs, rather than asepsis.
3. A bath blanket promotes privacy and prevents heat loss during a bath and is unrelated to asepsis. If not soiled, a patient's bath blanket can be reused.

4. The eye should always be washed from the inner to the outer canthus to prevent secretions from entering the lacrimal ducts, which may result in an infection.

70. 1. Water is ineffective against a grease fire. It will scatter the flames and the fire will spread.

2. The lid of the frying pan deprives the fire of oxygen. Without oxygen to support combustion, the fire will go out.

3. Although this will help to contain the fire to the kitchen, there is a more appropriate intervention to contain the fire to the frying pan.
4. This is inappropriate. A class A fire extinguisher is designed for fires consisting of paper, wood, upholstery, rags, and ordinary rubbish.

71. 1. This will not prevent the problem from occurring in the first place.

2. This will ensure that the medication is dispersed throughout solution in the cartridge. It will not change the taste of the medication.
3. Oral hygiene should be performed after the procedure.

4. The aerosolized medication enters the aerosol chamber where the larger droplets fall to the bottom of the chamber. The smaller droplets are inhaled deep into the lungs rather than falling on the patient's tongue.

72. 1. A beginning rapport must be established before information can be collected.

2. The orientation phase (also called the introductory or prehelping phase) of a therapeutic relationship sets the tone for the rest of the relationship. A rapport develops when the patient recognizes that the nurse is willing and able to help and can be trusted.

3. Problems are identified, explored, and dealt with during the working, not orientation, phase of a therapeutic relationship.

4. Prioritiy needs are identified and interventions planned and implemented during the working, not orientation, phase of a therapeutic relationship.

73. 1. **Feeling cold, chills, and shivering are adaptations associated with the onset (chill, initiation) stage of a fever. During this stage, the body responds to pyrogens by conserving heat to raise body temperature and reset the body's thermostat.**
2. Profuse diaphoresis (sweating) occurs during the defervescence (flush) stage of a fever. During this stage, the fever abates and body temperature returns to the expected range.
3. Dehydration can occur during both the febrile (course, plateau) and defervescence (flush) stages of a fever.
4. The patient will have warm, flushed skin during the defervescence (flush) stage of a fever. During this stage, the fever abates and body temperature returns to the expected range.

74. 1. The feet can be washed thoroughly when taking a shower.
2. Extra care with the feet is unnecessary because paper slippers provide a barrier between the feet and the floor.
3. **The warm water used to soak the feet promotes vasodilation, which improves circulation to the most distal portions of the feet. Soaking the feet loosens dirt and limits scrubbing, which prevent trauma to the skin. Soaking the feet should be done for just several minutes because prolonged soaking removes natural skin oils, which dries the skin and makes it prone to cracking.**
4. When on bed rest, the feet do not get soiled with dirt. Bed rest does not necessitate soaking the feet during the bed bath.

75. 1. This is an expected integumentary change in the older adult. Brown spots (lentigo senilis) on the skin are caused by a clustering of melanocytes, pigment-producing cells.
2. A loss of subcutaneous fat and a reduced thickness and vascularity of the dermis that occur with aging result in thin, translucent skin in the older adult.
3. **Tenting occurs when the skin of a dehydrated person remains in a peak or tent position after the skin is pinched together. This is a sign of a fluid volume deficit. Care must be taken when assessing an older person because some degree of tenting may occur, even when hydrated, because of the decrease in skin elasticity and decrease in tissue fluid associated with aging; however, in the hydrated patient tenting will slowly resolve.**
4. A decrease in tissue fluid and sebaceous gland activity associated with aging commonly result in dry, flaky skin.

76. 1. This is the correct way to inhale when using an incentive spirometer; it helps to keep the airways open.
2. **The patient is using the incentive spirometer incorrectly and needs further teaching. An incentive spirometer must be held in an upright position. A tilted flow-oriented device requires less effort to reach the desired inspiratory volume. A tilted volume-oriented device will not function correctly.**
3. This is an acceptable practice. Inspiratory goals should be progressively increased daily or more frequently depending on the patient's ability to continually maximize the inspiratory volume, which promotes alveoli ventilation.
4. This is a desirable practice because it prevents hyperventilation and respiratory alkalosis.

77. 1. **Effleurage involves long, smooth strokes sliding over the skin that have a relaxing, sedative effect. When performed slowly with light pressure at the end of a back massage, it is called "feathering off."**
2. Firm, not deep, circular motions are used with back massage.
3. Kneading (petrissage) is not performed over the vertebrae because it is stimulating and traumatic for the vertebral column and spinal cord.
4. Massage over the vertebrae is contraindicated because it is traumatic to the verterbral column and spinal cord. Massage should be performed on either side of the vertebrae.

78. 1. This assumes that the patient can read at the reading level of the presented material. Also, it does not provide an opportunity for the nurse to communicate with the patient.
2. If the patient was not participating in the present formal class, it is unlikely that the patient will participate in the next class.
3. Although an audiovisual cassette is an excellent strategy to provide instruction, it does not provide the nurse an opportunity to individualize one-on-one instruction.
4. **The nurse identified that the patient was quiet and withdrawn in the group class. Individual instruction provides the nurse**

the opportunity to explore the patient's concerns and address the patient's individual needs in privacy.

79. 1. This increases the risk of aspiration because it straightens the trachea and anatomically makes it easier for food and fluid to enter the trachea rather than the esophagus.
 2. Food and fluid should be consumed separately in the presence of dysphagia. Fluid is more difficult to control with dysphagia and it may flush the solid food toward the trachea where it can cause choking or a partial or total airway obstruction.
 3. A patient with dysphagia should concentrate on the acts of chewing and swallowing. Environmental stimuli can be distracting and can result in inadequate chewing or premature swallowing, which in turn can result in choking and aspiration.
 4. This will increase the risk for aspiration. Food should be placed in the posterior, not anterior, part of the mouth toward the side. The molars in the back of the mouth are designed for chewing. Placing food to the side keeps it close to the molars for chewing and out of direct line with the trachea. Placing food in the posterior of the mouth limits the need for the tongue to manipulate the bolus of food toward the back of the mouth in preparation for swallowing (deglutition).

80. 1. This may further decrease the consumption of food at mealtimes. Supplements are given in addition to, not to replace, the nutrients that are consumed with meals.
 2. Research indicates that exercise decreases appetite and increases the need for calories. Exercise releases beta-endorphin, which results in a state of relaxation and satisfaction with less food.
 3. This intervention is premature. It assumes that the inadequate intake is related to discomfort associated with flatus.
 4. A person's cultural, religious, educational, economic, and experiential background influences eating behaviors and food preferences. When familiar, preferred foods are available and personally selected, patients may feel that the care is individualized and that they are in more control, resulting in eating a greater percentage of the meal.

81. **1. This is an example of learning in the *affective domain*. In the *affective domain*, learning is concerned with feelings, emotions, values, beliefs, and attitudes.**
 2. This is not an example of learning in the *cognitive domain*. In the *cognitive domain*, learning is concerned with intellectual understanding and includes thinking on many levels, with progressively increasing complexity.
 3. There is no learning domain known as physiologic.
 4. This is not an example of learning in the *psychomotor domain*. Learning in the *psychomotor domain* includes using motor and physical abilities to master a skill. It requires the learner to practice to improve coordination and dexterity manipulating the equipment associated with the skill.

82. 1. Hyperextension of the condyloid joint of the wrist is accomplished by bending the fingers and hand backward as far as possible.
 2. Opposition of the thumb, which is a saddle joint, occurs when the thumb touches the top of each finger on the same hand.
 3. Abduction of the fingers (metacarpophalangeal joints—condyloid) occurs when the fingers of each hand spread apart.
 4. Flexion of the wrist, a condyloid joint, occurs when the fingers of the hand move toward the inner aspect of the forearm.

83. **1. This recognizes the patient's feelings.**
 2. This denies the patient's feelings and gives false reassurance.
 3. This denies the patient's feelings and gives false reassurance.
 4. This denies the patient's feelings.

84. 1. This is done with a medication administered via the sublingual, not buccal, route.
 2. Fluid will interfere with the action and absorption of the medication.
 3. It should be administered after, or between, meals. Food will interfere with the action and absorption of the medication.
 4. Alternating cheeks will limit irritation to the mucous membranes in the buccal area.

85. **1. Pain tolerance is the maximum amount and duration of pain that a person is willing to tolerate. It is influenced by psychosociocultural factors and usually increases with age.**
 2. This question focuses on an alleviating factor, distraction, rather than on the concept of pain tolerance.
 3. This question is determining the patient's perception of the intensity of pain, not pain tolerance.

4. This question focuses on an alleviating factor, medication, rather than on the concept of pain tolerance.

86. 1. This imposes on family members. A person must learn to cope with temptation because exposure to desirable foods occurs inside and outside the home.
2. This is degrading and should be avoided. Pictures that reflect a positive outcome are more desirable.
3. The rigidity and limitation of avoiding between-meal snacks may cause periods of hypoglycemia, overeating, and noncompliance. Between-meal snacks should be calculated into the weight-reduction program to meet both physical and emotional needs.
4. Behavior modification strategies are most successful when the person has an internal locus of control and is actively involved in self-care. Research demonstrates that self-monitoring of food intake is the single most helpful strategy in weight reduction.

87. 1. Although there is a predictable sequence to growth and development, there are individual differences in the rate and pace in which developmental milestones are achieved. Therefore, achievement of milestones is measured in ranges of time to allow for individual differences.
2. Task achievement refers to Erikson's Theory of Personality Development, which is only one aspect of growth and development. Erikson believed that each stage of personality development is characterized by the need to achieve a specific developmental task, and that achievement of each task is affected by the social environment and influence of significant others. The success or failure to achieve a task at one stage will influence task achievement in subsequent stages.
3. Unfortunately, not all families provide safe and supportive environments for the growing child. In addition, the family is only one of many factors that influence the stages of growth and development.
4. This is untrue. Regression is possible at any stage when one attempts to cope with a threat to the Ego.

88. Answer: 2, 1, 4, 3, 6, 5
2. The outside of the catheterization package is contaminated and should be opened with hands that have been washed with soap and water.
1. The inside of the catheterization package is sterile. Sterile gloves are on the top of the supplies included because all subsequent equipment in the package must remain sterile.
4. The nurse's sterile gloved hands then place the fenestrated drape over the patient's perineal area to continue with the establishment of a sterile field.
3. The integrity of the balloon (inability to inflate or deflate, presence of leaks) is established before insertion to prevent trauma to the patient.
6. Cleansing the labia moves from areas that are less likely to be contaminated than the urinary meatus as well as reduces the spread of microorganisms toward the urinary meatus.
5. Cleansing the urinary meatus last reduces the possibility of introducing microorganisms into the urinary meatus and bladder.

89. 1. Although a jacket restraint is removed every 2 hours to permit range-of-motion exercises, contractures are not life threatening and therefore are not the most serious complication associated with a vest restraint.
2. The V opening of a jacket restraint should be in the front of the patient to prevent pressure against the neck, particularly the trachea. The rounded side of the restraint goes across the patient's back.
3. This is too often and unnecessary.
4. Although a jacket restraint is removed every 2 hours to permit inspection of the skin, excoriation and skin compression are not the most serious complications associated with a vest restraint.

90. 1. The diastolic blood pressure decreases, not increases, during shock.
2. The initial stage of shock begins when baroreceptors in the aortic arch and the carotid sinus detect a drop in the mean arterial pressure. The systolic pressure is the pressure in the arteries during ventricular contraction.
3. Korotkoff's sounds are the 5 distinct sounds that are heard when auscultating a blood pressure (I—faint, clear tapping; II—swishing sound; III—intense, clear tapping; IV—muffled, blowing sounds; V—absence of sounds).
4. During shock, there will be a narrowing, not widening, of pulse pressure. Pulse pressure is the difference between the systolic and diastolic pressures.

91. 1. **Elastic stockings provide external pressure on the patient's legs to prevent pooling of blood in the veins while not interfering with arterial circulation. Inspecting the skin 3 times a day is adequate.**
2. This is unsafe because pressure injures fluid-filled tissue. They should be applied before, not after, the legs are dependent.
3. When applying elastic stockings, lotion increases friction that can injure tissue.
4. This is unsafe. Elastic stockings should be removed for 30 minutes 3 times a day; some practitioners' orders require elastic stockings to be worn only when the patient is out of bed.

92. 1. The DRGs were not designed to increase the quality of health care.
2. DRGs are unrelated to increasing or decreasing reliability of research statistics. Reliability is the degree of consistency with which a research study measures a hypothesis and depends on how well the measurement tool and the research methods are designed.
3. DRGs have increased, not decreased, the acuity of the hospitalized population. Patients, who in the past, were treated in the hospital are now treated in the home, ambulatory care settings, or in less acute care settings, such as rehabilitation or extended-care centers.
4. **The DRGs, pretreatment diagnoses reimbursement categories, were designed to decrease the average length of a hospital stay, which in turn reduces costs.**

93. 1. Identifying body landmarks before giving an injection is part of the procedure for administering an injection and, therefore, is an example of the implementation step of the nursing process.
2. Obtaining the medication is part of the procedure associated with giving medication and, therefore, this is an example of the implementation step of the nursing process.
3. **Determining when medications should be administered requires planning and, therefore, is part of the planning step of the nursing process.**
4. Collecting data from a patient involves assessment and, therefore, verifying a patient's allergies is an example of the assessment step of the nursing process.

94. 1. This is a challenging statement and is inappropriate. It may take away the patient's coping mechanism, is demeaning, and may cut off communication; the patient is using denial to cope with the diagnosis.
2. This response may take away the patient's coping mechanism, is demeaning, and may cut off communication; the patient is using denial to cope with the diagnosis.
3. **This provides an opportunity to discuss the illness; eventually a developing awareness will occur, and the patient will move on to other coping mechanisms.**
4. This response may take away the patient's coping mechanism, is demeaning, and may cut off communication; the patient is using denial to cope with the diagnosis.

95. 1. **The pressure of firm strokes on the skin moving from distal to proximal areas increases venous return. When venous return increases, cardiac output increases.**
2. Prolonged soaking removes the protective oils on the skin; the result is dry, cracked skin that is prone to further injury.
3. This prevents chilling, not increases circulation.
4. This is too hot for bath water because it may cause tissue injury. Bath water should be 110°F to 115°F.

96. 1. Although a teaching program must be designed within the patient's developmental and cognitive abilities, it is not the most relevant factor when predicting success of the options presented.
2. Although this is important, it is not the most relevant factor when predicting success of the options presented.
3. Although family support is important, it is not the most relevant factor when predicting success of the options presented. Not all patients have a family support system.
4. **The motivation of the learner to acquire new attitudes, information, or skills is the most important component for successful learning; motivation exists when the learner recognizes the future benefits of learning.**

97. 1. After shampooing a patient's hair, it may be dried or just toweled dry until it is free of excess moisture.
2. **The appearance of one's hair is an extension of self-image. Therefore, the patient's personal preferences should be considered before grooming the hair.**
3. Combing or brushing should begin from the ends of the hair, then from the middle to the ends, and finally from the scalp to the ends. This technique limits discomfort and prevents broken ends and damaged hair shafts.

4. The application of alcohol, will help prevent matting and tangles. A small amount of a lubricant, not alcohol, applied to the hair will facilitate the combing out of tangles once they have occurred.

98. 1. This will impede the evacuation of the room if it becomes necessary.
2. This is premature at this time, but it may become necessary eventually.
3. This is unsafe. Rolling the patient from side to side fans the flames, which will increase the intensity of the fire.
4. Smothering the flames with a blanket deprives the fire of oxygen. Without oxygen to support combustion, the fire will go out. Rescuing the patient is the first step of fire safety.

99. 1. It is essential for the nurse to be an informed provider of care, but it is not the priority of care for this patient.
2. Although this should be done, it is not the priority of care for this patient.
3. The practitioner should be notified immediately because the herb may interact with prescribed medications or therapies.
4. Although this should be done, it is not the priority. Medications or therapies may interact with the herb before the physician reads the information in the health history.

100. 1. Hospice care is inappropriate for this patient because the patient is not dying. Hospice programs provide supportive care to dying patients and their family members to promote dying with dignity.
2. This generally is not the best setting to provide extensive rehabilitation services. The acute care setting provides services that medically and emotionally support the patient during the critical and acute phases right after the traumatic event and until the patient is stable and out of danger.
3. An extended-care facility is an inpatient setting where people live while receiving subacute medical, nursing, and rehabilitative care. Extended-care facilities that should meet the needs of this individual include intermediate-care facilities, nursing homes that provide subacute care/skilled nursing care, or rehabilitation centers.
4. Once stabilized and out of danger, the individual in this scenario needs intensive rehabilitation services that generally cannot be provided in an assisted-living residence. An assisted-living residence (e.g., apartment, villa, or condominium) provides limited assistance with activities of daily living, meal preparation, laundry services, transportation, and opportunities for socialization. Residents are relatively independent.

Bibliography

Alfaro-LeFevre, R: *Critical Thinking and Clinical Judgment: A Practical Approach*, ed 3. Philadelphia, W.B. Saunders Company, 2004.

Brookfield, DD: *Developing Critical Thinkers*. SanFrancisco, Jossey-Bass, 1991.

Chaffee, J: *Thinking Critically*, ed 8. Boston, Houghton Mifflin, 2006.

Deglin, JH, and Vallerand, AH: *Davis's Drug Guide for Nurses*, ed 10. Philadelphia, F.A. Davis Company, 2006.

Erikson, EH: *Childhood and Society*. New York, Norton, 1993.

Hopkins, T: *LabNotes: Guide to Lab & Diagnostic Tests*. Philadelphia, F.A. Davis Company, 2005.

Johnson, F, and Johnson, L: The Hazards of Immobility. *American Journal of Nursing*, March 1990: 43–48.

Kübler-Ross, E: *On Death and Dying*. New York, Macmillan, 1969.

Maslow, AH: *Motivation and Personality*, ed 2. New York, Harper & Row, 1970.

Myers, E, and Hopkins, T: *MedSurg Notes: Nurse's Clinical Pocket Guide*, ed 2. Philadelphia, F.A. Davis Company, 2007.

Myers, E: *RN Notes: Nurse's Clinical Pocket Guide*. F.A. Davis Company, 2006.

Nugent, P, and Vitale, V: *Test Success: Test-Taking Techniques for Beginning Nursing Students*, ed 5. Philadelphia, F.A. Davis Company, 2008.

Stanley, M, Blair, KA, and Beare, PG: *Gerontological Nursing: Promoting Successful Aging with Older Adults*, ed 3. Philadelphia, F.A. Davis Company, 2005.

Van Leeuwen, AM, Kranpitz, TR, and Smith, L: *Davis's Comprehensive Handbook of Laboratory and Diagnostic Tests with Nursing Implications*, ed 2. Philadelphia, F.A. Davis Company, 2006.

Venes, D (ed): *Taber's Cyclopedic Medical Dictionary*, ed 20. Philadelphia, F.A. Davis Company, 2005.

Vitale, B: *NCLEX-RN Notes: Core Review & Exam Prep*. Philadelphia, F.A. Davis Company, 2007.

Wilkinson, JM, and Van Leuven, K: *Fundamentals of Nursing: Thinking and Doing*. Philadelphia, F.A. Davis Company, 2007.

Glossary of English Words Commonly Encountered on Nursing Examinations

Abnormality — defect, irregularity, anomaly, oddity

Absence — nonappearance, lack, nonattendance

Abundant — plentiful, rich, profuse

Accelerate — go faster, speed up, increase, hasten

Accumulate — build up, collect, gather

Accurate — precise, correct, exact

Achievement — accomplishment, success, reaching, attainment

Acknowledge — admit, recognize, accept, reply

Activate — start, turn on, stimulate

Adequate — sufficient, ample, plenty, enough

Angle — slant, approach, direction, point of view

Application — use, treatment, request, claim

Approximately — about, around, in the region of, more or less, roughly speaking

Arrange — position, place, organize, display

Associated — linked, related

Attention — notice, concentration, awareness, thought

Authority — power, right, influence, clout, expert

Avoid — keep away from, evade, let alone

Balanced — stable, neutral, steady, fair, impartial

Barrier — barricade, blockage, obstruction, obstacle

Best — most excellent, most important, greatest

Capable — able, competent, accomplished

Capacity — ability, capability, aptitude, role, power, size

Central — middle, mid, innermost, vital

Challenge — confront, dare, dispute, test, defy, face up to

Characteristic — trait, feature, attribute, quality, typical

Circular — round, spherical, globular

Collect — gather, assemble, amass, accumulate, bring together

Commitment — promise, vow, dedication, obligation, pledge, assurance

Commonly — usually, normally, frequently, generally, universally

Compare — contrast, evaluate, match up to, weigh or judge against

Compartment — section, part, cubicle, booth, stall

Complex — difficult, multifaceted, compound, multipart, intricate

Complexity — difficulty, intricacy, complication

Component — part, element, factor, section, constituent

Comprehensive — complete, inclusive, broad, thorough

Conceal — hide, cover up, obscure, mask, suppress, secrete

Conceptualize — to form an idea

Concern — worry, anxiety, fear, alarm, distress, unease, trepidation

Concisely — briefly, in a few words, succinctly

Conclude — make a judgment based on reason, finish

Confidence — self-assurance, certainty, poise, self-reliance

Congruent — matching, fitting, going together well

Consequence — result, effect, outcome, end result

Constituents — elements, component, parts that make up a whole

Contain — hold, enclose, surround, include, control, limit

Continual — repeated, constant, persistent, recurrent, frequent

Continuous — constant, incessant, nonstop, unremitting, permanent

Contribute — be a factor, add, give

Convene — assemble, call together, summon, organize, arrange

Convenience — expediency, handiness, ease

Coordinate — organize, direct, manage, bring together

Create — make, invent, establish, generate, produce, fashion, build, construct

Creative — imaginative, original, inspired, inventive, resourceful, productive, innovative

Critical — serious, grave, significant, dangerous, life-threatening

Cue — signal, reminder, prompt, sign, indication
Curiosity — inquisitiveness, interest, nosiness, snooping
Damage — injure, harm, hurt, break, wound
Deduct — subtract, take away, remove, withhold
Deficient — lacking, wanting, underprovided, scarce, faulty
Defining — important, crucial, major, essential, significant, central
Defuse — resolve, calm, soothe, neutralize, rescue, mollify
Delay — hold up, wait, hinder, postpone, slow down, hesitate, linger
Demand — insist, claim, require, command, stipulate, ask
Describe — explain, tell, express, illustrate, depict, portray
Design — plan, invent, intend, aim, propose, devise
Desirable — wanted, pleasing, enviable, popular, sought after, attractive, advantageous
Detail — feature, aspect, element, factor, facet
Deteriorate — worsen, decline, weaken
Determine — decide, conclude, resolve, agree on
Dexterity — skillfulness, handiness, agility, deftness
Dignity — self-respect, self-esteem, decorum, formality, poise
Dimension — aspect, measurement
Diminish — reduce, lessen, weaken, detract, moderate
Discharge — release, dismiss, set free
Discontinue — stop, cease, halt, suspend, terminate, withdraw
Disorder — complaint, problem, confusion, chaos
Display — show, exhibit, demonstrate, present, put on view
Dispose — to get rid of, arrange, order, set out
Dissatisfaction — displeasure, discontent, unhappiness, disappointment
Distinguish — to separate and classify, recognize
Distract — divert, sidetrack, entertain
Distress — suffering, trouble, anguish, misery, agony, concern, sorrow
Distribute — deliver, spread out, hand out, issue, dispense
Disturbed — troubled, unstable, concerned, worried, distressed, anxious, uneasy
Diversional — serving to distract
Don — put on, dress oneself in
Dramatic — spectacular
Drape — cover, wrap, dress, swathe
Dysfunction — abnormal, impaired
Edge — perimeter, boundary, periphery, brink, border, rim
Effective — successful, useful, helpful, valuable
Efficient — not wasteful, effective, competent, resourceful, capable
Elasticity — stretch, spring, suppleness, flexibility
Eliminate — get rid of, eradicate, abolish, remove, purge
Embarrass — make uncomfortable, make self-conscious, humiliate, mortify
Emerge — appear, come, materialize, become known
Emphasize — call attention to, accentuate, stress, highlight
Ensure — make certain, guarantee
Environment — setting, surroundings, location, atmosphere, milieu, situation
Episode — event, incident, occurrence, experience
Essential — necessary, fundamental, vital, important, crucial, critical, indispensable
Etiology — assigned cause, origin
Exaggerate — overstate, inflate
Excel — to stand out, shine, surpass, outclass
Excessive — extreme, too much, unwarranted
Exhibit — show signs of, reveal, display
Expand — get bigger, enlarge, spread out, increase, swell, inflate
Expect — wait for, anticipate, imagine
Expectation — hope, anticipation, belief, prospect, probability
Experience — knowledge, skill, occurrence, know-how
Expose — lay open, leave unprotected, allow to be seen, reveal, disclose, exhibit
External — outside, exterior, outer
Facilitate — make easy, make possible, help, assist
Factor — part, feature, reason, cause, think, issue
Focus — center, focal point, hub
Fragment — piece, portion, section, part, splinter, chip
Function — purpose, role, job, task
Furnish — supply, provide, give, deliver, equip
Further — additional, more, extra, added, supplementary
Generalize — to take a broad view, simplify, to make inferences from particulars
Generate — make, produce, create
Gentle — mild, calm, tender
Girth — circumference, bulk, weight
Highest — uppermost, maximum, peak, main
Hinder — hold back, delay, hamper, obstruct, impede
Humane — caring, kind, gentle, compassionate, benevolent, civilized
Ignore — pay no attention to, disregard, overlook, discount
Imbalance — unevenness, inequality, disparity
Immediate — insistent, urgent, direct
Impair — damage, harm, weaken
Implantation — to put in
Impotent — powerless, weak, incapable, ineffective, unable

Inadvertent — unintentional, chance, unplanned, accidental

Include — comprise, take in, contain

Indicate — point out, sign of, designate, specify, show

Ineffective — unproductive, unsuccessful, useless, vain, futile

Inevitable — predictable, to be expected, unavoidable, foreseeable

Influence — power, pressure, sway, manipulate, affect, effect

Initiate — start, begin, open, commence, instigate

Insert — put in, add, supplement, introduce

Inspect — look over, check, examine

Inspire — motivate, energize, encourage, enthuse

Institutionalize — to place in a facility for treatment

Integrate — put together, mix, add, combine, assimilate

Integrity — honesty

Interfere — get in the way, hinder, obstruct, impede, hamper

Interpret — explain the meaning of, to make understandable

Intervention — action, activity

Intolerance — bigotry, prejudice, narrowmindedness

Involuntary — instinctive, reflex, unintentional, automatic, uncontrolled

Irreversible — permanent, irrevocable, irreparable, unalterable

Irritability — sensitivity to stimuli, fretful, quick excitability

Justify — explain in accordance with reason

Likely — probably, possible, expected

Logical — using reason

Longevity — long life

Lowest — inferior in rank

Maintain — continue, uphold, preserve, sustain, retain

Majority — the greater part of

Mention — talk about, refer to, state, cite, declare, point out

Minimal — least, smallest, nominal, negligible, token

Minimize — reduce, diminish, lessen, curtail, decrease to smallest possible

Mobilize — activate, organize, assemble, gather together, rally

Modify — change, adapt, adjust, revise, alter

Moist — slightly wet, damp

Multiple — many, numerous, several, various

Natural — normal, ordinary, unaffected

Negative — no, harmful, downbeat, pessimistic

Negotiate — bargain, talk, discuss, consult, cooperate, settle

Notice — become aware of, see, observe, discern, detect

Notify — inform, tell, alert, advise, warn, report

Nurture — care for, raise, rear, foster

Obsess — preoccupy, consume

Occupy — live in, inhabit, reside in, engage in

Occurrence — event, incident, happening

Odorous — scented, stinking, aromatic

Offensive — unpleasant, distasteful, nasty, disgusting

Opportunity — chance, prospect, break

Organize — put in order, arrange, sort out, categorize, classify

Origin — source, starting point, cause, beginning, derivation

Pace — speed

Parameter — limit, factor, limitation, issue

Participant — member, contributor, partaker, applicant

Perspective — viewpoint, view, perception

Position — place, location, point, spot, situation

Practice — do, carry out, perform, apply, follow

Precipitate — to cause to happen, to bring on, hasten, abrupt, sudden

Predetermine — fix or set beforehand

Predictable — expected, knowable

Preference — favorite, liking, first choice

Prepare — get ready, plan, make, train, arrange, organize

Prescribe — set down, stipulate, order, recommend, impose

Previous — earlier, prior, before, preceding

Primarily — first, above all, mainly, mostly, largely, principally, predominantly

Primary — first, main, basic, chief, most important, key, prime, major, crucial

Priority — main concern, giving first attention to, order of importance

Production — making, creation, construction, assembly

Profuse — a lot of, plentiful, copious, abundant, generous, prolific, bountiful

Prolong — extend, delay, put off, lengthen, draw out

Promote — encourage, support, endorse, sponsor

Proportion — ratio, amount, quantity, part of, percentage, section of

Provide — give, offer, supply, make available

Rationalize — explain, reason

Realistic — practical, sensible, reasonable

Receive — get, accept, take delivery of, obtain

Recognize — acknowledge, appreciate, identify, aware of

Recovery — healing, mending, improvement, recuperation, renewal

Reduce — decrease, lessen, ease, moderate, diminish

Reestablish — reinstate, restore, return, bring back

Regard — consider, look upon, relate to, respect

Regular — usual, normal, ordinary, standard, expected, conventional

Relative — comparative, family member
Relevance — importance of
Reluctant — unwilling, hesitant, disinclined, indisposed, adverse
Remove — take away, get rid of, eliminate, eradicate
Reposition — move, relocate, change position
Require — need, want, necessitate
Resist — oppose, defend against, keep from, refuse to go along with, defy
Resolution — decree, solution, decision, ruling, promise
Resolve — make up your mind, solve, determine, decide
Response — reply, answer, reaction, retort
Restore — reinstate, reestablish, bring back, return to, refurbish
Restrict — limit, confine, curb, control, contain, hold back, hamper
Retract — take back, draw in, withdraw, apologize
Reveal — make known, disclose, divulge, expose, tell, make public
Review — appraisal, reconsider, evaluation, assessment, examination, analysis
Ritual — custom, ceremony, formal procedure
Rotate — turn, go around, spin, swivel
Routine — usual, habit, custom, practice
Satisfaction — approval, fulfillment, pleasure, happiness
Satisfy — please, convince, fulfill, make happy, gratify
Secure — safe, protected, fixed firmly, sheltered, confident, obtain
Sequential — chronological, in order of occurrence
Significant — important, major, considerable, noteworthy, momentous
Slight — small, slim, minor, unimportant, insignificant, insult, snub
Source — basis, foundation, starting place, cause
Specific — exact, particular, detail, explicit, definite
Stable — steady, even, constant
Statistics — figures, data, information
Subtract — take away, deduct
Success — achievement, victory, accomplishment
Surround — enclose, encircle, contain
Suspect — think, believe, suppose, guess, deduce, infer, distrust, doubtful
Sustain — maintain, carry on, prolong, continue, nourish, suffer
Synonymous — same as, identical, equal, tantamount
Thorough — careful, detailed, methodical, systematic, meticulous, comprehensive, exhaustive
Tilt — tip, slant, slope, lean, angle, incline
Translucent — see-through, transparent, clear
Unique — one and only, sole, exclusive, distinctive
Universal — general, widespread, common, worldwide
Unoccupied — vacant, not busy, empty
Unrelated — unconnected, unlinked, distinct, dissimilar, irrelevant
Unresolved — unsettled, uncertain, unsolved, unclear, in doubt
Utilize — make use of, employ
Various — numerous, variety, range of, mixture of, assortment of
Verbalize — express, voice, speak, articulate
Verify — confirm, make sure, prove, attest to, validate, substantiate, corroborate, authenticate
Vigorous — forceful, strong, brisk, energetic
Volume — quantity, amount, size
Withdraw — remove, pull out, take out, extract

Index

Note: Page numbers followed by an "f" indicate a figure, page numbers followed by a "b" indicate a box, and page numbers followed by a "t" indicate a table.

A

Affective domain, 12, 143
Affective learning, 139, 140, 142
Alternate item format
  answers and rationales, 353–362
  chart, table, or graphic image, 346–349, 357–359
  drop and drag/ordered response item, 349–350, 359–360
  exhibit item, 350–352, 360–362
  fill-in-the-blank item, 345–346, 356–357
  hot-spot item, 343–345, 354–355
  multiple-response item, 341–342, 353–354
  on NCLEX examination, 341
  questions about, 341–352
Ambiguous, 11
Analysis, 21
Analysis level, 142
Analysis question
  cognitive requirements for, 21
  emphasis of, 12
  RACE Model for answering, 21–24
Application, 18
Application question
  cognitive requirements for, 18
  emphasis of, 12
  RACE Model for answering, 18–21
Assessment, physical
  answers and rationales, 165–171
  keywords for, 158–159
  questions about, 160–164

B

Barrier
  creativity, 11
  effective reflection, 8
  inquisitiveness, 10
  positive mental attitude, 5–6

C

Characterizing level, 141
Chart, items using, 346–349, 357–359
Clinical postconference, 7
Cognitive competency, 2, 3–4, 3f
Cognitive domain, 12, 140, 142, 143
Cognitive learning, 139, 140, 143
Comfort. *See* Pain, comfort, rest, and sleep
Communication
  answers and rationales, 114–119
  keywords for, 108
  questions about, 108–113
Community-based nursing
  answers and rationales, 84–92
  keywords for, 79
  questions about, 79–83
Competency, 3–4, 3f
Comprehension level, 140, 141
Comprehension question
  cognitive requirements for, 15–16
  emphasis of, 12
  RACE Model for answering, 16–18
Comprehensive final book exam
  answers and rationales, 376–392
  questions about, 363–375
Computer-assisted instruction (CAI), 144
Confidence, definition of, 5
Continuing education, 141
Courage, 8
Creativity
  overcoming barriers to, 11
  thinking outside the box, 10–11
Critical thinking
  being positive, 5
  definition of, 2
  hysterical perspective of, 1
  maximizing ability for, 5
  RACE Model, 12–13
    acronym for answering questions, 13
    for analysis questions, 21–24
    for application questions, 18–21
    for comprehension questions, 15–18
    for knowledge questions, 13–15
    for multiple choice questions, 12–13
Curiosity, definition of, 10

D

Decision-Making Process, 2
Demonstration, 139, 144
Diagnostic reasoning, 2
Discipline, definition of, 5
Distractor, 12
Drop and drag/ordered-response items, 349–350, 359–360
Drug. *See* Medication administration; Pharmacology

E

Egocentric thinking, 11
Electrolytes, fluids and
  answers and rationales, 292–297
  keywords for, 286
  questions about, 287–291
Elimination, urinary
  answers and rationales, 280–285
  keywords for, 275
  questions about, 276–279
Evaluation, purpose of, 11

Evaluation level, 141
Exam, comprehensive final book
  answers and rationales, 376–392
  questions about, 363–375
Exhibit items, 350–352, 360–362

F

Fill-in-the-blank item, 345–346, 356–357
Final book exam, comprehensive
  answers and rationales, 376–392
  questions about, 363–375
Fluids and electrolytes
  answers and rationales, 292–297
  keywords for, 286
  questions about, 287–291
Formal reasoning process, types of, 2
Freudian slip, definition of, 1

G

Gastrointestinal system
  answers and rationales, 304–310
  keywords for, 298
  questions about, 299–303
Goal-directed thinking, 4
Graphic image, items using, 346–349, 357–359

H

Health care delivery
  answers and rationales, 70–78
  keywords for, 64–65
  questions about, 65–69
Helix of Critical Thinking
  cognitive versus personal competencies, 3–4, 3f
  concept of, 2–3
  interactive nature of, 4, 4f, 5f
Hot-spot item, 343–345, 354–355
Humility, 8
Hygiene
  answers and rationales, 228–234
  keywords for, 221–222
  questions about, 222–227
Hysterical, definition of, 1

I

Independence of thought, 11
Infection control
  answers and rationales, 177–182
  keywords for, 172–173
  questions about, 173–176
Information
  application of, 18
  memorizing for test, 13–14
  methods of manipulating and processing, 2
Inquiry
  definition of, 8
  examples of, 8–9
Inquisitiveness, overcoming barrier to, 10
Intellectual standards, 2
Investigation, inquiry as, 8
Item
  chart, table, or graphic image, 346–349, 357–359
  definition of, 12
  drop and drag/ordered response, 349–350, 359–360
  exhibit, 350–352, 360–363
  fill-in-the-blank, 345–346, 356–357
  hot-spot, 343–345, 354–355
  multiple-response, 341–342, 353–354

J

Journal, definition of, 6

K

Knowledge level, 143
Knowledge question
  cognitive requirements for, 13
  emphasis of, 12
  RACE Model for answering, 14–15

L

Leadership, management and
  answers and rationales, 57–63
  keywords for, 52
  questions about, 53–56
Learning
  activities for, 140
  cognitive versus affective, 139–140
  domains in nursing, 12
  teaching and
    answers and rationales, 139–146
    keywords for, 133
    questions about, 134–138
Legal issues
  answers and rationales, 46–51
  keywords for, 40–41
  questions about, 41–45
Life span, nursing care across
  answers and rationales, 99–107
  keywords for, 93–94
  questions about, 94–98

M

Management and leadership
  answers and rationales, 57–63
  keywords for, 52
  questions about, 53–56
Mechanism level, 144
Medication administration
  answers and rationales, 201–206
  keywords for, 194–195
  questions about, 195–200
  See also Pharmacology
Mental picture, 6
Mobility
  answers and rationales, 242–247
  keywords for, 235–236
  questions about, 236–241
Motivation, 10, 139
Multiple-response item, 341–342, 353–354

N

NCLEX-RN, 141, 341
Nursing
  community-based
    answers and rationales, 84–92
    keywords for, 79
    questions about, 79–83

continuing education for, 141
critical thinking and, 1
domains of learning, 12
perioperative
answers and rationales, 332–339
keywords for, 325–326
questions about, 325–326
psychosocial
answers and rationales, 99–107
keywords for, 93–94
questions about, 94–98
Nursing care, components of
answers and rationales, 152–157
keywords for, 147–148
questions about, 148–151
Nursing process, 2
answers and rationales, 152–157
Helix of Critical Thinking, 4, 4f
keywords for, 147–148
positive mental attitude, 5
questions about, 148–151
reflective thinking, 6
retrospective reflection, 6–8
Nutrition
answers and rationales, 255–260
keywords for, 248–249
questions about, 249–254

O

Open-minded, 11
Option, 12
Ordered-response items, 349–350, 359–360
Outcome, successful versus unsuccessful, 11
Oxygenation
answers and rationales, 268–274
keywords for, 261–262
questions about, 262–267

P

Pain, comfort, rest, and sleep
answers and rationales, 318–324
keywords for, 311
questions about, 312–317
Perioperative nursing
answers and rationales, 332–339
keywords for, 325–326
questions about, 326–331
Perseverance, definition of, 10
Personal competency, 2, 3–4, 3f
Pharmacology
answers and rationales, 214–220
keywords for, 207–208
questions about, 208–213
See also Medication administration
Physical assessment
answers and rationales, 165–171
keywords for, 158–159
questions about, 160–164
Positive mental attitude, 5
Positive thinking, 5
Problem-Solving Process, 2, 4, 5f
Psychological support
answers and rationales, 126–132
keywords for, 120–121
questions about, 121–125
Psychomotor domain, 12, 140, 143, 144
Psychosocial nursing care
answers and rationales, 99–107
keywords for, 93–94
questions about, 94–98

Q

Question
chart, table, or graphic image, 346–349, 357–359
cognitive levels of, 12
drop and drag/ordered response item, 349–350, 359–360
exhibit item, 350–352, 360–362
fill-in-the-blank item, 345–346, 356–357
hot-spot item, 343–345, 354–355
inquiries as, 8
multiple choice, components of, 12
multiple-response item, 341–342, 353–354
on NCLEX examination, 341
Questionnaire, 142–143

R

RACE Model
acronym for answering questions, 13
for analysis questions, 21–24
for application questions, 18–21
for comprehension questions, 15–18
for knowledge questions, 13–15
for multiple choice questions, 12–13
Rationale, 9
Reasoning process, types of, 2
Reflection
overcoming barriers to, 8
process of, 6
Reflective learning, 141
Rest. *See* Pain, comfort, rest, and sleep
Retrospective reflection
examples of, 7
process of, 6
purpose of, 6–7
Risk-taking, 11
Role-playing, 140, 143

S

Safety
answers and rationales, 188–193
keywords for, 183
questions about, 183–187
Scientific method, 2
Self-assessment, 6
Sleep. *See* Pain, comfort, rest, and sleep
Stem, 12
Survey, 142–143

T

Table, items using, 346–349, 357–359
Teaching and learning
answers and rationales, 139–146
keywords for, 133
questions about, 134–138
Test taking
critical thinking and, 12
inquiry techniques for, 9

Theory-based nursing
answers and rationales, 31–39
keywords for, 31
questions about, 25–30
Thinking
egocentric, 11
goal-directed, 4
outside the box, 10–11
See also Critical thinking
Thought, independence of, 11

U

Urinary elimination
answers and rationales, 280–285
keywords for, 275
questions about, 276–279

V

Valuing, 140
Valuing level, 143